M/B	Market to book ratio
MCC	Marginal cost of capital
NPV	Net present value
P	Price of a share of stock
	P_0 = price of the stock today
P/E	Price/earnings ratio
Pmt	An annuity
PV	Present value
r	(1) Rate of return
	(2) The IRR on a new project
	(3) Correlation coefficient
R_F	Rate of return on a risk-free security
ROA	Return on assets
ROE	Return on equity
ROI	Return on investment
S	(1) Sales
	(2) Stock, total market value
Σ	Summation sign (capital sigma)
σ	Standard deviation (lower case sigma)
t	(1) Tax rate
	(2) Time, when used as a subscript
	(for example, D_t = the dividend in Year t)
TIE	Times interest earned
V	Value
YTM	Yield to maturity

Introduction to Financial Management

Second Edition

Introduction to Financial Management

Second Edition

B.J. Campsey
San Jose State University

Eugene F. Brigham
University of Florida

The Dryden Press
Chicago   Fort Worth   San Francisco   Philadelphia   Montreal   Toronto   London   Sydney   Tokyo

Acquisitions Editor: Ann Heath
Developmental Editor: Judy Sarwark
Project Editor: Cate Rzasa
Design Director: Alan Wendt
Production Manager: Barb Bahnsen
Permissions Editor: Doris Milligan
Director of Editing, Design, and Production: Jane Perkins
Director of IE Production: Johann F. Struth

Text and Cover Designer: C. J. Petlick
Copy Editor: Judith Lary
Indexer: Sheila Ary
Compositor: The Clarinda Company
Text Type: 10/12 ITC Garamond Light

Library of Congress Cataloging-in-Publication Data

Campsey, B. J.
  Introduction to financial management.

  Includes index.
  1. Corporations — Finance.   I. Brigham, Eugene F.,
  1930–   II. Title.
  HG4026.C23   1989   658.1'5   87–31419
  ISBN 0-03-012353-4
  ISBN 0-03-028313-2 (Dryden Press International Edition)

Printed in the United States of America
890-016-98765432

Address orders:
The Dryden Press
Orlando, FL 32887

Address editorial correspondence:
The Dryden Press
908 N. Elm Street
Hinsdale, IL 60521

The Dryden Press
Holt, Rinehart and Winston
Saunders College Publishing

The Dryden Press Series in Finance

Preface

The practice of financial management has changed greatly in recent years. Computers, especially personal computers, are being used increasingly and effectively to analyze financial decisions. This usage has made it more important than ever for financial problems to be set up in a form suitable for quantitative analysis. At the same time the financial environment has become less predictable and more volatile than before. In the late 1970s and early 1980s, strong inflationary pressures pushed interest rates to unprecedented highs, and the resulting volatile cost of capital led to profound changes in corporate financial policies and practices. By the mid-1980s, however, inflationary pressures had been reduced, causing the stock market, a barometer of the country's economic health, to rise to its highest level ever by 1987. Yet uncertainties about the huge federal deficit and the foreign trade imbalance have made financial decision making exceedingly difficult.

In such an uncertain environment, many have turned to academicians for answers. Indeed, academic researchers have made a number of important theoretical advances. Business practitioners gain insights from the use of financial theory and in turn provide feedback from their "real world" perspective. This practitioners' input has led to modifications and improvements in financial theory.

Although theory is an important factor in developing financial practice, this book focuses on the practitioner, particularly one who will own or manage a small- to medium-size business. The book is designed for the general business student, not just for the finance major. It is our opinion that many so-called introductory texts are designed specifically for finance (and accounting) majors. These are excellent textbooks, but in their efforts to include theory (some of which seems to contain little practical usefulness) or detailed models of financial concepts, the nonfinance major is often lost or "turned off" to the study of finance. This is unfortunate, because financial planning affects and in turn is affected by marketing, production, and other business decisions. Thus all business students must have a thorough knowledge of finance. It is our hope that this book will provide that knowledge in a manner that is interesting and enjoyable to all business students, regardless of major.

INTENDED MARKET AND USE

As indicated by its title, *Introduction to Financial Management,* second edition, is intended for use in an introductory course in financial management. The main parts of the text can be covered in a one-term course, but when supplemented with cases and some outside readings, the text can also be used over two terms.

If the book is to be used in a one-term course, the instructor will probably want to cover only selected chapters, leaving the others for students to examine on their own or to use as references in conjunction with work in other courses. In our own courses, we seldom are able to complete an entire book. The material we tend to omit is contained in Chapters 22 through 24. Our students cover these topics in subsequent finance courses. Other instructors have indicated that they often save material in Chapters 16, 20, and 21 for an advanced course. Where a money and banking course is required, instructors may wish to omit parts of Chapters 3, 4, and 5; in schools that do not require such a course, instructors may wish to expand the material covered in these chapters. Still other instructors may wish to use the material in Chapters 13, 17, and 18 earlier in the course than the chapter sequence indicates. Thus many other course structures are possible, and we trust that it will be quite easy to cover chapters in a sequence different from the one in the book. The Glossary and Appendix F (which summarizes the equations contained in the text) make alternative sequences easy to follow.

SPECIAL FEATURES OF THIS TEXT

1. *Streamlined Quantitative Material*
A conscious effort has been made to streamline as much of the quantitative material as possible without lowering the quality of the text. Thus, where possible, very detailed mathematical formulas or concepts have been simplified or deleted. For example, our chapter on risk assumes no previous statistical knowledge. Further, the chapters on the diverse areas of international finance, mergers, and changes in credit policy have received a practical orientation.

2. *Decisions in Finance*
Each chapter begins with an actual financial decision faced by a firm. The actual resolution to the decision is given at the end of the chapter. For example, Chapter 1 begins with the story of Bendix Corporation's bid for Martin Marietta — one of the messiest corporate takeover attempts ever. We hope these sections challenge students to consider how knowledge of the material contained in the chapter would help the financial decision maker.

3. *Industry Practice*
In most chapters we present a real-world industry practice section that highlights or expands on key issues. For example, the industry practice section in Chapter 3 explains how the SEC is working to prevent illegal

insider trading. These illustrations also help to enliven the material in the chapter.

4. *Focus on Small Business*
Several chapters contain small business sections, written by Professor Christopher Barry of Texas Christian University. For example, the small business section in Chapter 8 explains how franchising is implemented to develop a good idea when resources are limited. These sections are especially useful for giving students a view of finance from the smaller firm's standpoint.

5. *Running Glossary*
A brief definition of important terms appears in the margin of the text. In addition, the key terms in each chapter are boldfaced as they are discussed.

6. *Self-Test Problems*
A set of fairly rigorous self-test problems with detailed solutions is given at the end of the more difficult quantitative chapters. These problems serve (a) to test the student's ability to set up problems for solution and (b) to explain the solution set-up for those who need help.

CHANGES IN THE SECOND EDITION

1. All sections of the book were updated to reflect current interest rates, tax laws, mergers, and so forth as they exist in early 1988.

2. Material on the credit decision has been refined, and the cumbersome equations associated with Chapter 11 have been streamlined.

3. Our section on risk in the first edition has been expanded into a new Chapter 15, Risk and Return.

4. The material on long-term debt securities in Chapter 17 has been expanded to include zero coupon bonds, junk bonds, and floating rate bonds. The chapter also includes an expanded section on preferred stock and its valuation.

5. Chapter 18 now contains a discussion of the valuation of supernormal or nonconstant growth stock.

6. To reflect our own teaching style, as well as that of most adopters, the chapter on cost of capital (Chapter 19) now precedes the chapter on the selection of the firm's target capital structure (Chapter 20).

7. All elements of the capital structure decision, including business and financial risk, are now included in Chapter 20.

8. We deleted the chapter on bankruptcy from the first edition and placed the most important aspects of the topic in Appendix 20A.

9. The introductory material for each chapter from the first edition, Decisions in Finance, as well as Industry Practice, has been retained and updated with new examples that reflect current business practices and problems that practitioners have addressed. These examples demonstrate to students that an understanding of the material in the chapter is crucial to solving real-world problems. Furthermore, these examples provide an interesting guide that lets students know where we are headed in the chapter.

10. Several changes have been made in the end-of-chapter problems:
a. The problems have been annotated to provide the student with a subtle hint about the concept emphasized in the problem.
b. Most problems have been reworked, many extensively, to provide a challenging exercise for students using the second edition of this text.
c. In addition to the revised problems, the number of problems in each chapter has been increased by approximately 25 percent.
d. Computerized problems have been added to most chapters; a diskette with *Lotus 1-2-3* models for these problems is available to adopters from The Dryden Press. The computerized problems are designed to show students the power of computers in financial analysis, and no knowledge of computers or programming is required to use them. The computer problems are designated by a diskette logo next to the problem number (for example, see Problem 7-16).

ANCILLARY MATERIALS

The package of ancillary materials that accompanies the second edition of *Introduction to Financial Management* provides information specifically designed to enhance the text's usefulness for both the student and the instructor. Materials developed exclusively for the second edition of *Introduction to Financial Management* include the following:

1. *Study Guide.* This supplement outlines the key sections of the text, offers students self-test questions for each chapter, and provides a series of problems and solutions similar to those in the text.

2. *Instructor's Manual.* A complete manual is available to instructors who adopt the book. The *Instructor's Manual* contains (1) answers to all test questions, (2) solutions to all text problems, and (3) extensive lecture notes that focus on more difficult topics and that are keyed to special lecture transparencies.

3. *Test Bank.* A test bank with more than 600 class-tested questions and problems in objective format is now available in book form. Test bank questions are well suited for mid-term and final exams.

4. *Overhead Transparencies.* A set of acetate transparencies is available to instructors who adopt the text from their Dryden Press representative. These transparencies highlight key material in the text and can be used as the basis for lectures to both large and small classes.

5. *Computerized Test Bank.* A computerized version of the test bank will be available to adopters for use on the IBM PC and compatible microcomputers.

6. *Supplemental Problems.* Additional problems, organized according to topic and level of difficulty, are also available to instructors from The Dryden Press.

Additional ancillaries that are compatible with all Dryden financial management texts are the following:

1. *Casebooks.* A revised edition of *Cases in Managerial Finance,* 6th ed. (The Dryden Press, 1987) by Eugene F. Brigham and Roy L. Crum, is well suited for use with this text. In addition, a new edition of Harvard-type cases by Diana Harrington, *Case Studies in Financial Decision Making,* 2nd ed. (The Dryden Press, 1989), also coordinated with this text, is available from The Dryden Press.

2. *PROFIT+.* This software supplement by James Pettijohn of Southwest Missouri State University contains 20 user-friendly programs that include the time value of money, forecasting, capital budgeting, and a new spreadsheet program. The program comes with a user's manual and is available for the IBM PC and compatible microcomputers.

3. *Readings Books.* A number of readings books, including *Issues in Managerial Finance,* 3rd ed. (The Dryden Press, 1987), edited by Ramon E. Johnson, can be used as supplements.

4. *Lotus 1-2-3 Book.* A new book, *Finance with Lotus 1-2-3®: Text, Cases, and Models* (The Dryden Press, 1988), by Eugene F. Brigham, Dana A. Aberwald, and Susan E. Ball, is available to explain how many commonly encountered problems in financial management can be analyzed with electronic spreadsheets.

5. *Spreadsheet Program. Joe Spreadsheet* is a full-feature, *Lotus* compatible, microcomputer spreadsheet that can be purchased from The Dryden Press.

ACKNOWLEDGMENTS

We would like to thank several professors who made a special contribution to the development of the second edition. First, our thanks go to those who authored special sections of the text: Christopher Barry, who authored the small business sections at the end of several chapters, and Roy L. Crum, who co-authored the chapter on international business. We would also like to acknowledge the special critical evaluation and suggestions of Professors Bodie Dickerson of Oregon State University and Joseph H. Black of San Jose State University. Professor Dickerson also assisted in the selection and design of the acetate transparencies, and Professor Black made numerous helpful comments about the end-of-chapter questions and problems. Kimberly McCollough played a major role in revising both the *Study Guide* and the *Test Bank.* Her efforts are greatly appreciated.

In addition, the following professors provided comments and suggestions for improving the second edition:

Frank Aleman
Quinebaug Valley Community
College

Bruce Berlin
Ohio University

Mike Binder
Buena Vista College

Sandra Cece
Triton College

Harlan Cheney
University of D.C.

Terrence Clauretie
Louisiana State University

Bill Colclough
University of Wisconsin — La Crosse

James Collier
Memphis State University

Maurice Corrigan
Post College

E. F. Dunham, Jr.
University of Tampa

Philip Fanara, Jr.
Howard University

Timothy Gallagher
Colorado State University

Joseph Moosally
Mankato State University

Austin Murphy
Oakland University

Antonio Rodriguez
University of Michigan — Flint

Dennis Schlais
California State University — Chico

George Seldat
Southwest State University

Rodney Smith
State University of New York

Les Strickler
Oregon State University

Francis Thomas
Stockton State University

Marvin Travis
Saint Leo College

G. W. Ulseth
Rensselaer Polytechnic Institute

Paul Vanderheiden
University of Wisconsin — Eau
Claire

John Wachowicz
University of Tennessee

Richard Whiston
Hudson Valley Community College

Elizabeth Yelland
North Hennepin Community
College

Terry Zivney
University of Wisconsin —
Milwaukee

The efforts of those who helped with the first edition should also be recognized, and we would like to thank them: Faramarz Damanpour, Zane Dennick-Ream, George L. Granger, David J. Johnston, Donald Nast, Clarence C. Rose, Gary Simpson, Les Strickler, John M. Wachowicz, Jr., James W. Walden, Howard R. Whitney, and Sally Jo Wright.

In addition, thanks are due to those who helped with earlier Brigham texts that served as a model for this book.

To our colleagues at The Dryden Press — especially Ann Heath, Judy Sarwark, and Cate Rzasa — we couldn't have done it without your exceptional patience and guidance.

We want to thank Gini Hartzmark for her valuable work in developing the pedagogy and Judy Lary for her meticulous copyediting.

Finally, to our friends and colleagues at San Jose State, University of Florida, and around the country, thank you for your suggestions and support.

CONCLUSION

Finance is, in a real sense, the cornerstone of the free enterprise system, so good financial management is vitally important to the economic health of business firms and hence to our nation and the world. Because of its importance, finance should be widely and thoroughly understood — but this is easier said than done. The field is relatively complex, and it is undergoing constant changes in response to economic conditions. All this makes finance stimulating and exciting but also challenging and sometimes perplexing. We certainly hope that the second edition of *Introduction to Financial Management* will meet these challenges by contributing to a better understanding of the financial system.

B. J. Campsey
San Jose, California
June 1988

Eugene F. Brigham
Gainesville, Florida
June 1988

About the Authors

B. J. Campsey (Ph.D., University of Texas–Austin; MBA, University of Houston) is Professor of Finance and Associate Dean at San Jose State University, San Jose, California. He has also taught at the University of Virginia and was a Visiting Professor at the University of Texas–Austin and Santa Clara University. He has taught undergraduate and graduate courses in managerial finance and investments. He has served as a consultant for financial and industrial firms as well as having been the Director of Candidate Programs for the Chartered Financial Analysts, 1979–1980.

A native of Fort Worth, Texas, Professor Campsey is a member of the Financial Management Association, the American Finance Association, and the Western Finance Association. His research interests are in managerial finance, investments, and financial education. He has written articles for several professional journals and has served as a consultant for several Silicon Valley firms.

Eugene F. Brigham (Ph.D., California–Berkeley; B.S., North Carolina) is Professor of Finance and Director of the Public Utility Research Center at the University of Florida. He has also taught at California–Berkeley, San Jose State, UCLA, Wisconsin, and Connecticut and has lectured in numerous executive programs in the United States and abroad. He is past president of the Financial Management Association, and he has held offices in a number of other finance organizations.

Professor Brigham has served as a consultant to many firms and government agencies, including AT&T, Texas Power & Light, Commonwealth Edison, Shell Oil, Bank of America, and the Federal Reserve Board. He has published articles on various financial issues in *Financial Management,* the *Journal of Finance,* and other journals, and he has authored or coauthored several leading textbooks and casebooks in finance and managerial economics. Professor Brigham currently teaches graduate and undergraduate courses in financial management.

Careers in Finance

Even though some students take an introductory course in financial management because they wish to pursue a career in some area of finance, most take the course because it is required. Whatever the original motivation for taking the course, many students enjoy the topic's material to the extent that they begin to consider the field of finance as a career opportunity. We are often asked, "What kinds of jobs are available to finance majors?"

The answer is that there is a broad range of job opportunities in the area of finance. If one had to categorize this book, it would be considered a business or managerial finance text. Even so, we will study topics in this text related to the two other major sources of employment for finance students—financial institutions, especially banks, and the investment profession.

Working Capital Management. The bulk of this text is concerned with the duties of a financial manager in a corporate or business setting. Most students entering the finance department of a business begin in some area of working capital management. A typical first assignment would be in the credit department. Here credit analysts review initial credit applications and supervise ongoing accounts for signs of deteriorating creditworthiness. More senior assignments would be concerned with the supervision of the firm's cash account. Here the manager is concerned with the rapid receipt of customer payments, probably through lockbox banking arrangements, and the timely disbursement of funds to creditors. This manager will also be responsible for the maintenance of a positive relationship with all of the company's banks.

Capital Budgeting. As the novice financial manager gains experience, even more challenging job opportunities may be found. For example, in the area of capital budgeting a manager must analyze appropriation requests, forecast cash flows from projected capital budgeting projects, and review the progress of current projects. Such a job requires careful coordination with other functional areas, such as marketing for sales information and production engineering for cost figures. The manager in charge of capital budgeting also must project future financing needs that arise from the acceptance of capital budgeting projects.

The manager of capital budgeting would probably elicit the help of the manager for project finance (titles may vary) in planning a project's financing. Generally, the manager for project finance will be responsible for obtaining the lowest-cost funds within the parameters of the firm's target capital structure. To do so this manager must be familiar with current financial market conditions and have a close working relationship with the firm's investment bankers.

Vice President of Finance. The vice president of finance oversees all of the functions of the subordinate financial managers. If the company is a small one, the vice president of finance will probably perform all the functions that have been discussed. Thus this financial manager must plan for future expenditures, evaluate past decisions, and execute the capital structure, capital budgeting, and dividend policy decisions of the firm.

Banking and Investment. Many of the topics covered in this text are also important in other areas of financial employment. For example, a banker would use the analytical tools discussed in Chapters 7 and 8 to analyze the financial statement of a loan application for creditworthiness. Similarly, the techniques of security valuation covered in Chapters 17 and 18 would be used by investment analysts in brokerage firms.

For further information on career opportunities in finance, see:

Jack S. Rader, *Careers in Finance* (Tampa, Fla.: Financial Management Association, 1983). Your instructor may order copies of this brochure by contacting: Financial Management Association, College of Business Administration, University of South Florida, Tampa, FL 33620.

Frank K. Reilly, "Career Opportunities in Investments," in *Investments,* 2nd ed. (Hinsdale, Ill.: The Dryden Press, 1986).

Contents

Part I

INTRODUCTION

The goal of financial management is to maximize stockholders' wealth. It is a simple goal to state, but this entire book is dedicated to evaluating how alternative decisions will influence the value of the firm. By maximizing the firm's value (and thereby increasing the value of its common stock), the goal of shareholder wealth maximization can be implemented.

Chapter 1 contains an overview of financial management, including the duties of a financial manager and the role of finance in a business organization. The forms of business organization and highlights of current information on the federal income tax system, vital to a vast array of financial decisions, are covered in Chapter 2.

Chapter 1

Defining Financial Management

 DECISION IN FINANCE

The Bendix–Martin Marietta War

On August 25, 1982, Bendix Corporation, a manufacturer of air filters, engine starters, and brakes, made a bid for Martin Marietta, an aerospace company, many of whose products complimented its own. But what Bendix's president, William Agee, couldn't foresee was that he was launching one of the messiest corporate takeovers ever waged.

First, Bendix made its offer to purchase Martin Marietta. Martin Marietta responded by employing the Pacman defense—I'll eat you before you eat me—and made an offer to buy Bendix, which it agreed to drop if Bendix dropped its bid for Marietta. When Bendix forged ahead, Marietta enlisted United Technologies to try to buy Bendix too, and made a deal with United to carve up Bendix should the sale go through. When even that did not scare Bendix off, Marietta set up a "doomsday" defense designed to destroy both companies if Bendix bought Marietta. Carefully showing Bendix that it was disconnecting the fail-safes, Marietta set up a situ-

ation in which it was obliged to buy control of Bendix if Bendix bought control of Marietta.

Bendix, assuming a bluff, gambled and bought $1 billion worth of Marietta stock. When Martin Marietta refused to back down, Bill Agee had no choice but to make a quick deal to sell Bendix *and* Martin Marietta to Allied Corporation, a New Jersey industrial company. Marietta, however, was able to take advantage of a loophole in the securities laws, make a separate peace with Allied, and preserve its own independence.

Although Martin Marietta managed to avoid being devoured by Bendix, it paid a high price for its freedom. It walked away from Bendix with 39 percent of its shares in the hands of Allied Corporation and nearly $1 billion in long-term debt, more than 80 percent of its total capital.

As you read this chapter, think about the kinds of issues that Martin Marietta had to weigh in deciding to fight Bendix. What issues did Bendix have to evaluate each time Marietta escalated the battle? Whose interests was each company protecting?

The resolution to this Decision in Finance is given at the end of the chapter.

3

Finance consists of three interrelated subareas: (1) *money and capital markets,* or macro finance, which deals with many of the topics covered in macroeconomics; (2) *investments,* which focuses on the decisions of individuals and financial institutions as they choose securities for their investment portfolios; and (3) *financial management,* or business finance, which involves decisions within the firm. Each of these areas interacts with the others; therefore, a corporate financial manager must have some knowledge of money and capital markets as well as the way in which individuals and institutions are likely to appraise the firm's securities.

finance

Evaluation and acquisition of productive assets, procurement of funds, and disbursement of profits.

The function of financial management is to plan for, acquire, and utilize funds in a way that maximizes the value of the firm. More specifically, **finance** is concerned with evaluating and acquiring productive assets, procuring the least expensive mix of funds, and disbursing profits in a manner consistent with the best interests of the firm's owners. Of course, this is a vast oversimplification of the duties of a financial manager, since we will need to spend the remaining chapters expanding on this operating definition of finance.

The study of financial management has undergone significant changes over the years. When finance first emerged as a separate field of study in the early 1900s, the emphasis was on legalistic matters such as mergers, consolidations, the formation of new firms, and the various types of securities issued by corporations. Industrialization was sweeping the country, and the critical problem that firms faced was obtaining capital for expansion. The capital markets were relatively primitive, making transfers of funds from individual savers to businesses quite difficult. Reports of earnings and asset values in accounting statements were unreliable, while stock trading by insiders and manipulators caused prices to fluctuate wildly. Consequently, investors were reluctant to purchase stocks and bonds. In such an environment it is easy to see why finance in the early 1900s concentrated so heavily on legal issues relating to the issuance of securities.

The emphasis remained on securities through the 1920s. Radical changes occurred during the depression of the 1930s, however, when an unprecedented number of business failures caused finance to focus on bankruptcy and reorganization, on corporate liquidity, and on government regulation of securities markets. Finance was still a descriptive, legalistic subject, but the emphasis shifted from expansion to survival.

During the 1940s and early 1950s, finance continued to be taught as a descriptive, institutional subject, viewed from the outside rather than from the standpoint of management. However, methods of financial analysis designed to help firms maximize their profits and stock prices were beginning to receive attention.

The evolutionary pace quickened during the late 1950s. Whereas the right-hand side of the balance sheet (liabilities and capital) had received more attention in the earlier era, the major emphasis began to shift to asset analysis. Mathematical models were developed and applied to inventories, cash, accounts receivable, and fixed assets. Increasingly, the focus of finance shifted from the outsider's to the insider's point of view, as financial decisions within the firm were recognized to be the critical issue in corporate finance. Descriptive, institutional materials on capital markets and financing instruments were still studied, but these topics were considered within the context of corporate financial decisions.

The 1960s witnessed a renewed interest in the liabilities-capital side of the balance sheet with a focus on (1) the optimal mix of securities and (2) on the way in which individual investors make investment decisions, or *portfolio theory,* and its implications for corporate finance. Corporate financial management is designed to help general management take actions that will maximize the value of the firm and the wealth of its stockholders; therefore, the soundness of corporate financial decisions depends on how investors are likely to react to them. This was recognized in the 1960s and 1970s, and with this recognition came a merging of investments with corporate finance.

Thus far in the 1980s three issues have received emphasis: (1) inflation and interest rates, (2) deregulation of financial institutions and the accompanying trend away from specialized institutions and toward broadly diversified financial service corporations, and (3) a dramatic increase in the use of computers for analyzing financial decisions. Consideration of inflation is being worked into the fabric of both financial theories and the financial decision process, and it has even led to the creation of new financial institutions and industries—for example, money market funds and interest rate futures markets. Older institutions have been forced into major structural changes, and it is getting harder and harder to tell a bank from a savings and loan, or an insurance company from a brokerage firm. Bank of America owned a stock brokerage firm; Merrill Lynch offers checking account services; and Sears, Roebuck is one of the largest U.S. financial institutions, owning such firms as Allstate Insurance, Coldwell Banker Real Estate, and Dean Witter Reynolds Securities. At the same time, technological developments in the computer hardware and telecommunications areas, and the availability of software packages that make otherwise difficult numerical analyses relatively easy, are bringing about fundamental changes in the way managers manage. Data storage, transmittal, and retrieval techniques are reducing the judgmental aspects of management, as financial managers can often obtain relatively precise estimates of the effects of various courses of action.

INCREASING IMPORTANCE OF FINANCIAL MANAGEMENT

These evolutionary changes have greatly increased the importance of financial management. In earlier times the marketing manager would project sales, the engineering and production staffs would determine the assets necessary to meet these demands, and the financial manager would simply raise the money needed to purchase the plant, equipment, and inventories. This mode of operation is no longer prevalent. Today decisions are made in a much more coordinated manner, with the financial manager having direct responsibility for the control process.

Northeast Utilities can be used to illustrate this change. A few years ago Northeast's economic forecasters would project power demand on the basis of historical trends and then give these forecasts to the engineers, who would proceed to build the new plants necessary to meet the forecasted demand. The finance group simply had the task of raising the capital the engineers told them was needed. However, inflation, environmental regulations, and other factors combined to double or even triple plant construction costs, and this caused a corresponding increase in the need for new capital. At the same time, rising fuel costs caused dramatic increases in electricity prices, which lowered demand and made some of the new construction unnecessary. Thus Northeast found itself building plants that it did not need and unable to raise the capital necessary to pay for them. The price of the company's stock declined from $20 to $5. As a result of this experience, Northeast Utilities (and other utilities and industrial companies) now places a great deal more stress on the planning and control process, and this has greatly increased the importance of the finance staff.

Certainly no business can prosper unless all functions—accounting, finance, marketing, personnel, and so forth—are fully staffed with competent individuals. In times of abundant financial resources, the role of the financial manager whose duty it is to acquire external financing may decline in importance. However, Professor Gordon Donaldson of Harvard contends that ". . . in harder times and with expensive money, the importance of the financial function grows."[1]

The direction in which business is moving, as well as the increasing importance of finance, was described in *Fortune*. After pointing out that more than half of today's top executives had majored in business administration versus about 25 percent a few years earlier, *Fortune* continued:

> Career patterns have followed the educational trends. Like scientific and technical schooling, nuts-and-bolts business experience seems to have become less important. The proportion of executives with their primary experience in production, operations, engineering, design, and R. and D. has fallen from a third of the total to just over a quarter. And the number of top officers with legal and financial backgrounds has increased more than enough to make up the difference. Lawyers and financial men now head two out of five corporations.
>
> It is fair to assume the changes in training, and in the paths that led these men to the top, reflect the shifting priorities and needs of their corporations. In fact, the expanding size and complexity of corporate organizations, coupled with their continued expansion overseas, have increased the importance of financial planning and controls. And the growth of government regulation and

---

[1] "Why the Finance Man Calls the Plays," *Business Week*, April 8, 1972, 54.

of obligations companies face under law has heightened the need for legal advice. The engineer and the production man have become, in consequence, less important in management than the finance man and the lawyer.

Today's chief executive officers have obviously perceived the shift in emphasis, and many of them wish they had personally been better prepared for it. Interestingly enough, a majority of them say they would have benefited from additional formal training, mainly in business administration, accounting, finance, and law.[2]

Although the period of high inflation and tight money of the early 1980s has passed, at least temporarily, the importance of the financial manager has continued as the economy moved through a very sluggish 1987. The economy's slow growth created new problems for the firm and its financial managers. However, these problems can create new opportunities. As one executive noted, "The fastest way to the top in any company is to develop and implement a cure for the company's most severe problem and be widely recognized as the individual responsible for solving the company's toughest problem."[3] Thus, although there is no universal way to the top, in hard times when capital is expensive and scarce, the importance of the finance function grows for the firm.

We have been "beating the drum" for finance, but we hasten to note that there are no unimportant functions in a business firm. Our point, rather, is that there are financial implications in virtually all business decisions, and non-financial executives must know enough about finance to incorporate these implications into their own specialized areas of analysis. The importance of finance to all areas of a business is reflected by the fact that most executive development programs report that their most popular course is "Financial Analysis for the Nonfinancial Executive."

Thus it is becoming increasingly important for people in marketing, accounting, production, personnel, and other areas of business to understand finance in order to do a good job in their own fields. Marketing people, for instance, must understand how marketing decisions affect and are affected by financial decisions. When marketing efforts successfully increase sales, for example, additional funds must be found to support increases in inventory, accounts receivable, plant capacity, and so on. Accountants, to cite another example, must understand how accounting data are used in corporate planning and viewed by investors. The function of accounting is to provide quantitative financial information for use in making economic decisions, whereas the main functions of **financial management** are to plan for, acquire, and utilize funds in order to maximize the efficiency and value of the enterprise.[4]

financial management
The acquisition and utilization of funds to maximize the efficiency and value of an enterprise.

---

[2]C. G. Burck, "A Group Profile of the Fortune 500 Chief Executive," *Fortune,* May 1976, 173.

[3]G. A. Weimer, "Finance Favored as Key to the Executive Boardroom," *Iron Age,* April 16, 1979, 35.

[4]American Institute of Certified Public Accountants, *Statement of the Accounting Principles Board No. 4* (New York, October 1970), 17.

THE PLACE OF FINANCE IN A BUSINESS ORGANIZATION

No single organizational structure will serve for all businesses. A huge, worldwide corporation would need an extremely large finance department. For example, Du Pont's finance department contains 9 divisions with a total of 29 sections, as well as separate areas of investor relations, personnel relations, accounting policy, and international finance. A small firm, of course, would not need as much specialization as a vast, multinational corporation like Du Pont. In fact, in a small firm all the necessary financial functions may be handled by only a few persons whose other duties may include such diverse areas as market planning or production management. The smaller the organization, the more the financial duties will be shared among individual managers or perhaps between the accountant and the president.

A fairly typical picture of the role of finance in the organizational structure of a firm is presented in Figure 1-1. The chief financial officer (CFO), who has the title of vice president–finance, reports directly to the president. The controller and the treasurer are the finance vice president's key subordinates.

The dividing line between the functions of the controller and the treasurer is neither exact nor absolute. The position of the treasurer is most closely associated with the topics discussed in this text. This officer has direct responsibility for planning the capital structure and maintaining relationships with all sources of financing, such as banks, shareholders, and other suppliers of funds. The treasurer's office must also keep in contact with the capital markets, generally through an investment banker.

The treasurer is also responsible for the selection and management of the firm's assets. Financial managers must evaluate all capital projects and determine if the investment opportunities should be undertaken. Furthermore, these projects must be monitored for continuing profitability. The management of working capital, which consists of short-term assets, is no less important. The treasurer must insure that enough cash is on hand to cover all checks and invest any excess in money market securities. Management of accounts receivable and inventory is yet another important function of the treasurer's office (although occasionally the controller handles this asset management task).

In larger firms employee benefits, including the pension fund and insurance section, are handled in the treasurer's office. In smaller firms these services generally are handled externally by independent pension managers or insurance agents.

Thus the traditional duties assigned to the treasurer's office can be briefly summarized as selecting and continually evaluating productive assets, forecasting financial needs arising from current and new operations, financing those operations, and establishing dividend policy for the disbursement of the returns of those operations.

Figure 1-1 **Place of Finance in a Typical Business Organization**

In a typical business organization such as that shown here, most general financial management functions fall to the treasurer. The treasurer is responsible for overall financial planning, selection and management of the firm's assets, and management of working capital, accounts receivable, and inventory. To plan and manage effectively, the treasurer needs constant input from the sales and manufacturing areas of the business. The controller oversees all accounting, auditing, and tax matters of the firm.

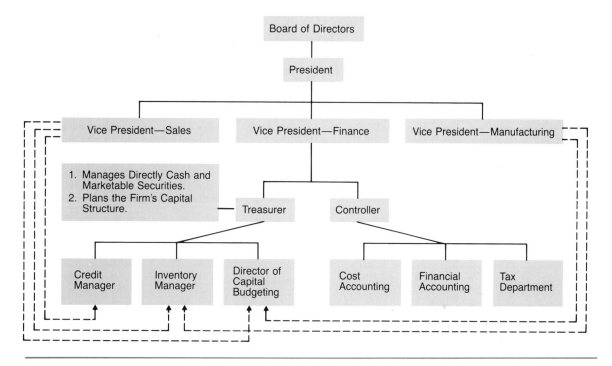

The traditional functions of the controller's office include the generation and interpretation of accounting reports and the monitoring and control of accounts. In other words, the controller generally has responsibility for all elements of accounting and auditing in the firm. Additionally, the controller is often responsible for all tax matters as well as for other information required by government agencies. To a large extent, we leave a discussion of the controller's function to accounting courses.

THE GOALS OF THE FIRM

Decisions are not made in a vacuum—they are made with some objective in mind. *Throughout this book, we operate on the assumption that management's primary goal is to* **maximize the wealth of its stockholders.** As we shall

stockholder wealth maximization

The appropriate goal for management decisions; considers the risk and timing associated with increasing earnings per share in order to maximize the firm's stock price.

see, this translates into *maximizing the price of the common stock.* Firms do, of course, have other objectives — managers, who make the actual decisions, are interested in their own personal satisfaction, in employees' welfare, and in the good of the community and society at large. Still, for the reasons set forth in the following sections, *stock price maximization is probably the most important goal of most business firms,* and it is a reasonable operating objective on which to build decision rules in a book such as this.

Why Managers Try to Maximize Stockholders' Wealth

Stockholders are the owners of the firm and, in theory at least, control management by electing the members of the board of directors, which in turn appoints the management team. Management, in turn, is supposed to operate in the best interest of the stockholders. We know, however, that because the stock of most large firms is widely held, the managers of such firms have a great deal of autonomy. This being the case, might not managements pursue goals other than maximization of stockholder wealth? For example, some argue that a well-entrenched management in a large corporation could work to keep stockholder returns at a fair or reasonable level and then devote part of its efforts and resources to public service activities, to employee benefits, to higher management salaries, or to golf.

Similarly, a firmly entrenched management might avoid risky ventures, even when the possible gains to stockholders are high enough to warrant taking the gamble. The theory behind this argument is that stockholders are generally well diversified, holding portfolios of many different stocks, so if one company takes a chance and loses, the stockholders lose only a small part of their wealth. Managers, on the other hand, are not so well diversified. A manager's salary represents his or her largest wealth asset, even if such factors as stock options are considered. Thus a potential setback, which might result in the manager's demotion or dismissal, is probably more devastating to the manager than it would be to a diversified stockholder. Accordingly, corporate managers may be less motivated to take risks that, if successful, would benefit stockholders (and to some extent managers, if they own or have options to own the firm's stock) by increasing the value of the firm's stock. Managers might also receive a bonus as part of their reward for success in a risky venture. However, if the venture is unsuccessful, it might result in the manager's rebuke, demotion, or even removal from the firm. Therefore, some maintain that managers are not well compensated for their successes and incur disproportionate penalties for their failures. If this is true, would a manager risk his or her job just to maximize the stockholders' wealth, or might the manager be satisfied in providing a less risky but still acceptable rate of return for the stockholder?

It is extremely difficult to determine whether a particular management team is trying to maximize shareholder wealth or is merely attempting to keep stockholders satisfied while pursuing other goals. For example, how can we tell whether or not voluntary employee or community benefit programs are in the long-run best interests of the stockholders? Are relatively high executive salaries really necessary to attract and retain excellent managers, who, in turn, will keep the firm ahead of its competition? When a risky venture is turned down, does this reflect management conservatism, or is it a correct judgment regarding the risks of the venture versus its potential rewards?

It is impossible to give definitive answers to these questions. Although several studies have suggested that managers are not completely stockholder-oriented, the evidence is cloudy. It is true that more and more firms are tying management's compensation to the company's performance, and research suggests that this motivates managers to operate in a manner consistent with stock price maximization.[5] In recent years, tender offers and proxy fights have removed a number of supposedly well-entrenched managements; the recognition that such actions can take place has probably stimulated many other firms to attempt to maximize share prices.[6] Finally, a firm operating in a competitive market, or almost any firm during an economic downturn, will be forced to undertake actions that are reasonably consistent with shareholders wealth maximization. Thus, although managers may have other goals in addition to stock price maximization, there are reasons to view this as the dominant goal for most firms.[7]

What Can Managers Do to Maximize Stock Prices?

Assuming that the financial manager's goal is to maximize the shareholders' wealth, what decisions are important in this task? The financial manager must determine, along with the rest of the management team, the investment, financing, and dividend policies of the firm. These decisions, however, often have many ramifications. For example, management must consider not only the timing and risk of the income stream from the investment, but also the form of the returns. Will **profit maximization** result in stock price maximi-

profit maximization The maximization of the firm's net income; does not consider risk or timing of earnings and thus is not an appropriate standard for financial decisions.

---

[5]Wilbur G. Lewellen, "Management and Ownership in the Large Firm," *Journal of Finance,* May 1969, 299–322. Lewellen concludes that managers seem to make decisions that are largely oriented toward stock price maximization.

[6]A *tender offer* is a bid by one company to buy the stock of another company, whereas a *proxy fight* involves an attempt to gain control by getting stockholders to vote a new management group into office. Both actions are facilitated by low stock prices, so self-preservation can lead management to try to keep the stock values as high as possible.

[7]To insure that a manager acts in the best interest of the shareholders, the firm must incur agency costs to monitor management's actions. For a brief summary of the agency problem, see Eugene F. Brigham, *Fundamentals of Financial Management,* 4th ed. (Hinsdale, Ill.: The Dryden Press, 1986), 9–15. A more complete overview of agency theory may be found in Michael C. Jensen and William H. Meckling, "Theory of the Firm: Managerial Behavior, Agency Costs, and Ownership Structure," *Journal of Financial Economics,* October 1976, 350–360.

earnings per share (EPS)
The net income of the firm divided by the number of shares of common stock outstanding.

zation, or should the financial manager be concerned with some other form of return, such as **earnings per share (EPS)**?

Suppose that Caprock Petroleum has one million shares outstanding and earns $2 million, or $2 per share, and that you own 100 shares of the stock. Now suppose the company sells another one million shares and invests the funds received in assets that produce $1 million of income. Total income will have risen to $3 million, but earnings per share will have declined from $2 to $3,000,000/2,000,000 shares, or $1.50. Your earnings will now be only $150, down from $200. You (and the other original stockholders) will have suffered an earnings dilution, even though total corporate profits have risen. Therefore, other things held constant, *if management is interested in the well-being of its stockholders, it should concentrate on earnings per share rather than on total corporate profits.*

Will maximization of expected earnings per share always maximize stockholder welfare? The answer is *no:* other factors such as timing and risk must also be considered. Think about the *timing of the earnings.* Suppose Caprock has one project that will cause earnings per share to rise by $0.20 per year for five years, or $1.00 in total, whereas another project has no effect on earnings for four years but increases earnings by $1.25 in the fifth year. Which project is better? The answer depends on which project adds the most to the value of the stock, which in turn depends on the time value of money to investors. In any event, timing is an important reason to concentrate on wealth as measured by the price of the stock rather than on earnings alone. We consider the important topic of the time value of money in Chapter 13.

Still another issue relates to **risk**. Suppose one project is expected to increase earnings per share by $1.00, whereas another is expected to raise earnings by $1.20 per share. The first project is not very risky; if it is undertaken, earnings will almost certainly rise by about $1.00 per share. The other project is quite risky, so although our best guess is that earnings will rise by $1.20 per share, we must recognize the possibility that there may be no increase whatsoever. Depending on how averse stockholders are to risk, the first project may be preferable to the second.

The riskiness inherent in projected earnings per share also depends on *how the firm is financed.* As we shall see, a large number of firms go bankrupt every year, and the greater the use of debt, the greater the threat of bankruptcy. Consequently, *although the use of debt financing may increase projected EPS, debt also increases the riskiness of these projected earnings.*

Yet another issue is the matter of paying dividends to stockholders versus retaining earnings and plowing them back into the business, thereby causing the earnings stream to grow over time. Stockholders like cash dividends, but they also like the growth in EPS that results from putting earnings back into the business. The financial manager must decide exactly how much of current earnings should be paid out as dividends rather than retained and reinvested.

risk
The probability that actual future earnings will be below the expected earnings.

AN IMPORTANT MESSAGE TO HOLDERS OF DEBT SECURITIES OF

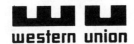

western union

Western Union has improved the terms of the preferred securities being offered to you in exchange for your existing debt holdings in the Company. The Boards of the Telegraph Company and the Corporation strongly urge you to tender your debt securities and allow the Reorganization Plan to proceed.

DIVIDEND INCREASES

The initial dividend on the Class A Senior Preferred Shares being offered for your debt securities has been increased from $13.50 to $15.00 per year.

The annual dividend on the Class B Preferred Shares being offered for your debt securities has been upped from $2.50 to $3.00.

TERMS OF CONVERSION IMPROVED

The conversion terms of the Class B Preferred Shares have been adjusted to provide that the conversion price will be reset six months earlier, on July 1, 1989, and that the minimum conversion price will be $3.00 rather than $4.25 as previously proposed, thus potentially enhancing your equity participation in Western Union's future. Additional Common Shares issuable by reason of this change will reduce the number of Common Shares to be issued to Mr. LeBow.

We urge you to consider these improvements and to follow the Board's recommendation and promptly tender your securities for exchange.

TIME IS RUNNING OUT

The Company is currently in a precarious financial position. It will be unable to meet its existing debt service requirements over any extended period of time. The management of the Company believes that the plan of restructuring provides the only alternative available which will allow the Company to avoid filing under Chapter 11 of the Federal Bankruptcy Code.

CREDIT AGREEMENT EXPIRED

Western Union's agreement with its bank lenders expired on November 13, 1987, and has not been extended. The Corporation is therefore currently in default under its credit agreements and the banks are entitled to demand immediate repayment of all outstanding loans and to realize on the security therefor. In addition, this default could result in a default under substantially all of Western Union's other indebtedness, and, should this happen, the holders of such debt would be entitled to demand immediate repayment. In this event, Western Union would likely be forced to file for protection under Chapter 11 of the Bankruptcy Code.

INTEREST PAYMENTS SUSPENDED

Interest payments due on November 15 on Western Union's 7.90% Debentures and due on December 1 on its 9¼% Debentures and 15% Notes have been deferred in order to conserve cash. An event of default will occur under these securities if such interest payments are not made within thirty days of the due date (in the case of the Debentures) and five days of the due date (in the case of the Notes).

POTENTIAL BANKRUPTCY

A bankruptcy filing would have serious consequences for the holders of the Company's debt securities. Interest payments would be suspended on the date of the filing. Since bankruptcy proceedings may last years, debtholders might have to wait a substantial period of time before learning what they will receive with respect to their claims. It is likely that the Company's relationships with its suppliers, employees and customers would be seriously disrupted by a bankruptcy proceeding, significantly impairing the value of the Company's business and the assets available to all securityholders.

THE NEW WESTERN UNION

The restructuring transactions are intended to do more than just restore Western Union to financial viability. Upon completion of the Offer and the acquisition of Worldcom, we expect Western Union to emerge as a leading carrier of electronic messages worldwide. The cost savings generated by this consolidation are expected to greatly enhance the Company's prospects for profitability, although there can be no assurance that such cost savings or profitability can be achieved. The securities being offered to you pursuant to the Offer will provide you with an equity participation in the Company while providing a current return on your investment. The Board believes that the planned restructuring offers the Company the best chance available for it to provide value to its securityholders, and urges you to carefully consider the Exchange Offer and tender your securities for exchange.

THE BOARD'S RECOMMENDATION

The Boards of Directors of both the Telegraph Company and the Corporation approved the Plan of Reorganization and the terms of the Revised Exchange Offer after careful consideration and close consultation with the Company's financial advisor and Bennett S. LeBow. The consideration being offered in the Revised Exchange Offer is intended to increase the likelihood that the Plan will be consummated. Both Boards unanimously recommend that you accept the Revised Offer and tender your securities for exchange.

The Offer is a vital and necessary component of the Company's planned restructuring. It must be accepted by the holders of at least 80% of the Company's outstanding debt securities or the entire restructuring may not be consummated.

YOUR CONSENT IS CRUCIAL

We hope that, after carefully reviewing the Offer, you will accept the Board's recommendation and tender your securities for exchange. It is also important that you execute a consent to the proposed amendments to the indenture under which your securities were issued.

These amendments must be approved or the plan of restructuring will not be consummated, and Western Union will likely be forced to file for protection under Chapter 11 of the Bankruptcy Code. Approval of the amendments requires the consent of the holders of two-thirds of the outstanding principal amount of each debt security, so your consent is crucial.

The Exchange Offer and solicitation of consents will expire on Tuesday, December 15, 1987. Since time is short, it is imperative that you act promptly. If you have any questions or require assistance in consenting or completing the paperwork for the exchange, please contact the Information Agent:

237 Park Avenue
New York, New York 10017
(800) 365-5500/(800) 221-3343
In New York State: (212) 619-1100

Banks and Brokerage Firms please call:
(212) 883-8900

This advertisement is neither an offer to exchange nor a solicitation of an offer to exchange any securities. The Exchange Offer is made solely by the Prospectus and Solicitation dated October 26, 1987, the Supplement thereto dated November 20, 1987, and the related Consents and Letters of Transmittal all of which can be obtained from the Information Agent. The Exchange Offer is not being made to, consents are not being solicited from, and The Western Union Telegraph Company will not accept tenders or consents from, holders of Old Debentures in any jurisdiction in which the Exchange Offer, the acceptance thereof, or the solicitation or giving of consents, would not be in compliance with the securities and blue sky laws of such jurisdiction.

December 4, 1987

In this public notice to shareholders drafted by The Carter Organization, Western Union encourages its holders of debt securities to exchange them for preferred shares of Western Union. The board of directors of the financially troubled company had constructed a comprehensive plan of recapitalization of which the tender is an important part: ". . . the planned restructuring offers the Company the best chance available to provide value to its securityholders. . . ."

INDUSTRY PRACTICE

The Joys and Woes of Managing an LBO

Leveraged buyouts, or LBOs, are a creature of the 1980s, part of the wave of innovative financing strategies recently concocted by fast-track Wall Street financiers. An LBO is a take-over of a company using borrowed funds, most often using the company's own assets as security for the loans taken out by the acquiring firm. The loans are repaid out of the cash flow of the acquired company. Management may also use this technique to retain control by converting a company from a public asset whose shares are publicly traded to a privately held one.

Richard Ward of California-based U.S. Natural Resources Company belongs to a tiny minority of chief executives. He has served as chief executive of the firm since 1977. During his tenure as CEO, the firm reverted from a publicly to a privately owned firm. What's the difference? "It is more satisfying to run a private company," he says. "No doubt about that."

The recent wave of leveraged buyouts — more than a hundred in just the past five years — has created a new breed of executives who have managed both kinds of companies. And Ward's appraisal is widely shared in this select group. Says W. W. Clements, who was chairman of Dr. Pepper Co. in both its public and private guises: "I think we are better off private." And James Wilcock, who was CEO of publicly owned Joy Manufacturing Co. before running Pace Industries, a Pittsburgh-based LBO, exults, "I have not yet discovered a single drawback to being private."

Because LBOs are a phenomenon of the 1980s, very few executives have sat in both

kinds of chairs. Unlike the traditional large private company, which usually still has a founder or family member looking over the CEO's shoulder, the LBO manager deals with the company that arranged the buyout and these are specialists in finance rather than operations. To find out more about the pleasures and pains of managing a private versus a public company, DUN'S BUSINESS MONTH recently surveyed a wide array of such executives, located with the help of executive recruiters, Canny, Bowen, Inc. The differences turned out to be surprising.

There is freedom that these CEOs had only dreamt of in the past. The freedom to make decisions that will benefit the company long-term. Freedom from board members who second-guess their operating decisions. And freedom from the prying eyes of the Securities and Exchange Commission, securities analysts and the financial press.

The worst burden of being public is the eternal pressure for short-term results that distorts decision-making, the CEOs contend. As a spokesman for Mary Kay Ash, and her son R. Rogers, president and CEO, who are in the process of buying out public shareholders in Mary Kay Cosmetics Co. explained: "Being public puts a premium on short-term plans. There's that pressure for consistent return, quarter by quarter. That's not always in the best interest of the company, long-term."

"Sometimes the solution that is best for the company is not one that will appeal to the public," Pace's Wilcock observes. For example, he says, "If you need to take a big write-off, you should do it and not have to answer for it." John Puth, CEO of privately owned Imperial Clevite, originally the industry group of Gould Inc., contends that it is easier for a private company to report a down quarter. "What our owners and I aim for is meeting a plan, not meeting last year's numbers," he says.

Source: Excerpted from "The Joys and Woes of Managing an LBO," *Dun's Business Month,* September 1985. Reprinted with permission, *Business Month* magazine. Copyright © 1985 by *Business Month* Corporation, 38 Commercial Wharf, Boston, MA 02110.

As a result, Dr. Pepper's Clements believes that a private company can plan more appropriately for the long term. "We can put our money where we think it will do us the most good in the long run," he maintains.

Puth thinks, however, that recently the tough economic climate is forcing Wall Street to pay less attention to quarterly declines in earnings. He cites the minimal impact of IBM's most recent quarterly earnings on its market price. "The pressure on companies is becoming less," he says, "because it is a rare company that can boost earnings every quarter."

The LBO CEO's control over long-run decision-making is a natural outgrowth of his relationship with the LBO board. The typical public company director may be a retired CEO or a current chief operating executive of another company, who frequently forces a CEO to justify his decisions say the top honchos. In contrast, LBO directors, who are also owners, are interested only in the numbers. U.S. Natural Resources' Ward says they watch cash flow rather than earnings per share, since cash flow is the key to the success of any LBO.

G. Ronald Morris, CEO of PT Components, a maker of power transmissions, says that Kohlber, Kravis & Roberts Co., who arranged the LBO never interfered with him in any way in four years of private ownership. The operating responsibilities were 100% on the shoulders of the executives who had tremendous autonomy. "It is a relief to know that no one is second-guessing you," he recalls wistfully. (The company went public again in March to expand its capital base.)

The vast majority of the CEOs are also relieved that they no longer have to operate in a fishbowl. A publicly owned company, of course, has to report quarterly to the SEC and so to the world. And then there are painful annual meetings. None of the CEOs miss the cacaphony of complaints from stockholders who carp that executives compensation is excessive, perks too pervasive and dividends too paltry.

After only nine months at Pace, Wilcock says what impresses him most is the minimum amount of public reporting he has to do. "You don't have to keep stockholders constantly advised of what you are doing. That is a tremendous load off your mind."

Wilcock is firmly convinced that the CEOs of big public companies spend altogether too much time and money cultivating the analysts. He calculates that private ownership saves at least $700,000 to $800,000 a year. Besides eliminating the need for an investor relations executive and airline trips to see analysts, he saves the legal, accounting and public relations costs of SEC-mandated filings.

And privacy has competitive advantages, too, Wilcock notes. "Competitors can't begin to find out as much about us as they could if we were public," he says.

But do all the joys of private ownership make for the best management? Manfred Steinfield, CEO of Shelby Williams Industries, a maker of furniture for hotels and fast food outlets that has been both private and public since he founded it in 1954, argues that public companies are generally better run than private ones. An executive who runs a public company, Steinfield maintains, must be a better manager, because he has to worry about how sales and earnings will stack up every ninety days and, to produce satisfactory results, he has to do more planning and budgeting. "Having to report," he says, "forces you to make decisions, whereas, if you are private, you can say 'Let's wait another month and see what happens.' And you can say it again a month later."

Albert J. Dunlap, one of the proclaimed management winners in the world of LBOs, also finds outside critics serve a purpose. Recruited as CEO of Lily-Tulip Inc. in 1982, when the company was private — and in deep financial trouble — he slashed costs, fired a lot of executives and made Lily the industry's low-cost producer. In March 1984, with its finances in much better shape, the company went public again.

Dunlap says the need to communicate with the financial community takes about 25% of his time. But that exposure to Wall Street analysts can be helpful, "when one of them makes a good suggestion," he says. "It makes you go back and take a second look at your operations and perhaps make changes. It is like having an outside consultant who keeps you sharp and protects you from thinking you know it all."

And there are more serious drawbacks to being private. There is the remorseless pressure of the big debt acquired in taking the company private through an LBO. Dunlap recalls his arrival at embattled Lily-Tulip: "I had to act quickly to reduce the debt, to the exclusion of everything else. So I put in fourteen and fifteen hour days. It requires enormous self-confidence, and you always accept a certain level of risk." Adds Will & Baumer's Nybo: "In an LBO, there is continuous pressure because you have absolutely no room for error."

If the company has a liquidity problem, so does the CEO. The sponsors of an LBO do not have conventional stock options to use as management motivators. So they have to devise compensation packages that will provide incentives in other ways. For one thing, they generally offer bigger salaries, and more frequent raises, than the CEO would be likely to get in a public company. And they make sure that he has a large block of stock in the concern. Over the years, if the company prospers, the CEO may get rich. But without a public market, that wealth exists only on paper. He can cash in his stockholding merges, goes public, or leaves and sells out.

For this reason, many CEOs anticipate going public again as soon as the company is back in good financial shape. Wilcock, for example, does not expect Pace to stay private forever. "If we can get our debt down," he says, "we will probably go public eventually. And our managers will get the big payoff that they deserve."

The CEOs of private companies also have to forego many privileges that are taken for granted in a public company — the wide recognition, the heady publicity, private planes and limousines (most private companies are on too tight a budget to afford such comforts) and other glamorous perks.

On the whole, though, the men who run private companies are far from envious of their counterparts in the public companies. Privacy is a rare commodity these days, and given the opportunity, they intend to make the most of it.

---

dividend policy
Determination of percentage of current earnings to be paid out as dividends to stockholders.

This is called the **dividend policy** decision. The optimal dividend policy is the one that maximizes the firm's stock price. We see, then, that the firm's stock price is dependent on the following factors:

1. Projected earnings per share
2. Riskiness of projected earnings
3. Timing of the earnings stream
4. Manner of financing the firm
5. Dividend policy

Every important corporate decision should be analyzed in terms of its effect on these factors and hence on the price of the firm's stock. For example, a coal company may be considering opening a new mine. If the mine is opened, can it be expected to increase EPS? Is there a chance that costs will exceed estimates, that prices and output will fall below projections, and that EPS will be reduced because the new mine was opened? How long will it take for the new mine to start showing a profit? How should the capital required to open the mine be raised? If debt is used, how much will this increase the firm's riskiness? Should the firm reduce its current dividends and use the cash thus saved to finance the project, or should it finance the mine with external capital? Financial management is designed to help answer such questions as these, plus many more.

Social Responsibility

Another issue that deserves consideration is **social responsibility**: Should businesses operate strictly in the stockholders' best financial interest, or is the firm in some sense responsible for the welfare of society at large? In tackling this question, consider first those firms whose **profits** and **rates of return** on investment are close to **normal** (that is, close to the average for all firms). If some companies attempted to be social do-gooders, thereby increasing their costs over what they otherwise would have been, and if the other businesses in the same industry did not follow suit, the socially oriented firms probably would be forced to abandon their efforts. Thus socially responsible acts that raise costs would be difficult, if not impossible, in industries subject to keen competition.

> **social responsibility**
> The concept that businesses should be responsible to some degree for the welfare of society at large.

> **normal profits/rates of return**
> Those profits close to the average of all firms within an industry.

What about firms with profits above normal levels—could they not devote resources to social projects? Undoubtedly they can; many large, successful firms do engage in community projects, employee benefit programs, and the like to a greater degree than would appear to be called for by pure profit or wealth maximization goals.[8] Still, publicly owned firms are constrained in such actions by capital market factors. Suppose a saver who has funds to invest is considering two alternative firms. One firm devotes a substantial part of its resources to social actions, whereas the other concentrates on profits and stock prices. Many investors are likely to shun the socially oriented firm, thus putting it at a disadvantage in the capital market. After all, why should the stockholders of one corporation subsidize society to a greater extent than stockholders of other businesses? For all these reasons, even highly profitable firms (unless they are closely held rather than publicly owned) are generally constrained against taking unilateral cost-increasing social actions.

Does all this mean that firms should not exercise social responsibility? Not at all—it simply means that most cost-increasing actions may have to be put on a *mandatory* rather than a voluntary basis, at least initially, to insure that the burden of such actions falls uniformly across all businesses. Thus such social benefit programs as fair hiring practices, minority training programs, product safety, pollution abatement, antitrust actions, and the like are more

---

[8]Even firms such as these often find it necessary to justify such programs at stockholder meetings by stating that they contribute to long-run profit maximization.

likely to be effective if realistic rules are established initially and then are enforced by government agencies. It is critical that industry and government cooperate in establishing the rules of corporate behavior and that firms follow the spirit as well as the letter of the law in their actions. In such a setting, the rules of the game become constraints. Throughout this book, we shall assume that managers are stock-price maximizers who operate subject to a set of socially imposed constraints.

Stock Price Maximization and Social Welfare

If firms attempt to maximize stock prices, is this good or bad for society? In general, it is good. Aside from such illegal actions as attempting to form monopolies, violating safety codes, and failing to meet pollution control requirements—all of which are constrained by the government—*the same actions that maximize stock prices also benefit society*. First, stock price maximization requires efficient, low-cost operations that produce the desired quality and quantity of output at the lowest possible cost. Second, stock price maximization requires the development of products that consumers want and need. Additionally, the profit motive leads to new technology, new products, and new jobs. Finally, stock price maximization requires efficient and courteous service, adequate stocks of merchandise, and well-located business establishments because these things are all necessary to make sales, and sales are certainly necessary for profits. Therefore, the types of actions that help a firm increase the price of its stock are also directly beneficial to society at large. This is why profit-motivated enterprise economies have been more successful than other types of economic systems. Since financial management plays a crucial role in the operation of successful firms, and since successful firms are absolutely necessary for a healthy, productive economy, it is easy to see why finance is important from a social standpoint.

The Economic Environment

Although managers can take actions that affect the values of their firms' stocks, there are additional factors that influence stock prices. Included among them are external constraints, the general level of economic activity, taxes, and conditions in the stock market. Figure 1-2 diagrams these general relationships. Working within the set of external constraints shown in the box at the extreme left, management makes a set of long-run strategic policy decisions that chart a future course for the firm. These policy decisions, along with the general level of economic activity and the level of corporate income taxes, influence the firm's expected profitability, the timing of its earnings, the eventual transfer of earnings to stockholders in the form of dividends, and the degree of uncertainty (or risk) inherent in projected earnings and dividends. Profitability, timing, and risk all affect the price of the firm's stock, but so does another factor, the state of the stock market as a whole, for all stock prices tend to move up and down together to some extent.

Figure 1-2 **Summary of Major Factors Affecting Stock Prices**

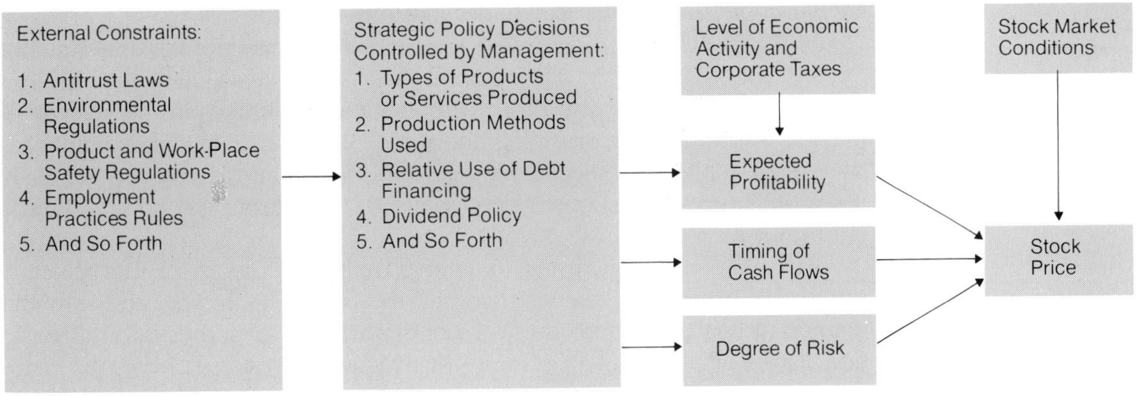

External Constraints:

1. Antitrust Laws
2. Environmental Regulations
3. Product and Work-Place Safety Regulations
4. Employment Practices Rules
5. And So Forth

Strategic Policy Decisions Controlled by Management:

1. Types of Products or Services Produced
2. Production Methods Used
3. Relative Use of Debt Financing
4. Dividend Policy
5. And So Forth

Level of Economic Activity and Corporate Taxes

Stock Market Conditions

Expected Profitability

Timing of Cash Flows

Degree of Risk

Stock Price

ORGANIZATION OF THIS BOOK

This introductory chapter has described, in broad terms, the duties of the financial manager and the goals of the firm. Someone once said, "Any road will do if you don't know where you're going." We have therefore carefully charted our destination—the goal of shareholder wealth maximization—and attempted to indicate how this goal influences the duties and actions of the financial manager. The next chapter explores both the types of business organization under which firms can be structured and the federal tax system.

The chapters in Part II investigate the economic environment in which the financial manager operates. First, the general purpose of financial markets—to transfer savings to firms and individuals with attractive investment opportunities—is analyzed. Then, the principal institution in financial markets, the commercial bank, is described. Finally, the role of interest rates in the economy is explored.

Part III deals with financial statements and financial forecasting. Because both long- and short-term plans are analyzed in terms of future financial statements, it is important to understand how these statements are developed and used by managers and other interested parties, such as creditors and investors. We first review how these statements are constructed, then concentrate on analyzing reports of past operations and on projecting financial statements into the future under different strategic plans and operating conditions.

In Part IV we move into the execution phase of the financial management process. Here current, ongoing operations are examined. From accounting we know that assets which are expected to be converted to cash within a year, such as inventories and accounts receivable, are called *current assets* and that liabilities which must be paid off within a year are called *current liabilities.* The management of current assets and current liabilities is known as *working capital management,* and Part IV deals with this topic.

In the first chapter of Part V we introduce the concept of the time value of money. This chapter plays a key role in most of the subsequent chapters. The first application of the time value of money concept comes in the analysis of fixed asset acquisitions, or capital budgeting. Since major capital expenditures take years to plan and execute, and since decisions in this area are generally not reversible and affect operations for many years, their effect on the value of the firm is obvious.

Part VI focuses on raising long-term capital. Questions of the principal sources and forms of long-term capital, the cost of each type, and how the method of financing affects the value of the firm are all addressed in this section. Part VI also describes the means by which the investor evaluates the firm's debt and equity instruments. The interrelationships among value, cost of capital, capital structure, and dividend policy serve to integrate the book and show how the parts meld into a cohesive whole.

Finally, in Part VII, we consider some subjects that, although important, are best studied within the basic framework of the preceding material presented in the text. Included in this section are mergers and acquisitions, leasing, and international financial management.

SUMMARY

This chapter has provided an overview of financial management. It began with a brief review of the evolution of finance as an academic discipline, tracing developments from 1900 to the present. Next the place of finance in the firm was examined, and we saw that the financial manager has been playing an increasingly important role in the organization. We also considered the goals of financial management and concluded that the key goal in most publicly owned firms is stock price maximization. Managers do have other goals, both personal and social, but in a competitive economy, where managers serve at the pleasure of stockholders, stock price maximization must be the dominant goal.

Financial capital is the major resource for any firm. The duty of the financial manager is to implement the acquisition, allocation, and management of this resource. Therefore, finance permeates all segments of the firm's activities. Because of its broad impact, managers, marketers, and long-range planners, along with chief executive officers (CEOs), must be aware of how their functions influence financial requirements. Thus all managers in the firm must understand the finance function.

SMALL BUSINESS

Resources and Goals in the Small Firm

This book is about financial management, and its concepts apply both to large corporations and to small businesses. The context in which financial management is carried out, however, is quite different in a small business than in a large firm. In these Small Business sections, we will discuss aspects of financial management that differ for or that deserve special mention with respect to small firms.

Small business is vital to America. More than 98 percent of all nonfarm businesses in the United States are considered small by the standards of the Small Business Administration (SBA). The SBA estimates that more than half of this country's innovations in products and services since World War II have been developed by independent small business entrepreneurs. Even more striking is the fact that the majority of new jobs created in the past decade have not been created by corporate giants but by new and growing small businesses.

Thus the financial management of the small firm is an important subject. In beginning this study, the special characteristics of small firms must be borne in mind. Two key characteristics of small firms are: they suffer from resource poverty; and their goals are complex.

Resource Poverty

Imagine the scenario in a large firm when a decision needs to be made about building a new plant. The chief executive officer (CEO) calls on a financial vice president and asks her to organize the financial analysis. She goes to the manager in charge of financial analysis in the particular division considering the expansion, and he in turn organizes a team to conduct the analysis. The team employs twenty to thirty recent MBAs or BBAs who will do the number-crunching, and they will depend on engineering and marketing staffs to provide them with the input data they need. The vice president of finance will call on an investment banker, who will be asked to recommend the best ways to get funds—new equity issue, new debt issue, private security sales, a large banking relationship, and so on. The investment banker will probably organize a team of three or four experienced professionals (earning an average of more than $100,000 per year each) who will work on the plan and prepare recommendations. In short, in a large corporation, there are plenty of people to share the work, and the public security markets are available to fund the projects.

This is not the way it is in a small firm. Suppose that John Thompson, owner of 75 percent of Board Products, Inc., is interested in expanding his company's production line. He ponders the proposal for a while, gets a bid on the project, and consults his banker, who says she's very busy now but she will get back to him. Meanwhile, John is in the process of hiring three new laborers and a secretary and is preparing for a meeting with a potential client. He is tired from having pushed for the past three weeks to get the financial statements and paperwork for the quarterly tax payments completed. John has little time and almost no help in his effort to consider the financial aspects of the production line decision. Because he has no training in capital budgeting, he conducts a seat-of-the-pants analysis and decides to go ahead with the project. Later, it turns out that many details he forgot to include have made the project unworkable. His gut feelings were wrong.

Thompson's case is not unusual. Small business is characterized by resource poverty. In small firms, one or two key individuals often end up taking on far more responsibility than they can reasonably handle. Thompson, for example, may think that other priorities in the business are too important to allow him to spend time putting together a budget or to check regularly to see how well the company is doing against such a budget. He may argue, "I have a pretty good feel for how we're doing cash-wise, and I really don't have the time to go into any more detail. Making budgets doesn't make money."

Not only is management spread thin in small firms, but it is also frequently true that smaller firms cannot acquire new funds needed for business expansion, or they can obtain funds only under very stringent conditions. Until Board Products achieves a fairly substantial size (say, $15 million or so in sales), the company is not likely to be able to sell stock or bonds successfully in public markets. Furthermore, if the company did have a public stock offering, it would be very expensive for the firm compared to the cost of a similar stock issuance by a larger firm. Thus Board Products may have only very limited access to public capital markets. Banks also may be reluctant to loan Board Products much money because the firm lacks a track record.

Small firms are limited both in their access to managerial talent and in their ability to muster adequate financial resources. It is no wonder that small firms often fail either because of poor (or overworked) management or because of undercapitalization.

Goals in the Small Firm

Small businesses' goals also may differ from those of big firms. We pointed out earlier that share price maximization is taken to be the goal of all publicly held firms. John Thompson, however, provides a good example of an owner whose life is tied up in his company. He depends on the firm for his livelihood, and he has staked his future on the success of the company. His personal wealth portfolio probably is not at all diversified; perhaps he has put everything he owns into the company.

Thompson might have a very different attitude toward risk-taking in his firm than would a typical investor in a public company. Such an investor is likely to hold a number of other investments, all contributing to a well-diversified portfolio of holdings, and the investor's personal income may come from a job in an altogether separate industry.

The owner-manager of the small firm is, of course, keenly interested in the value of the company itself; after all, it is probably the most valuable asset the individual owns. In fact, the owner-manager may be considering "taking the firm public" or having it merge with a larger firm some day, and he or she hopes that this would occur at the highest price possible.

Nevertheless, the owner-manager has complex motives. One of them might be the desire to be his or her own boss, even if it means not allowing the firm to progress as rapidly as it otherwise could. There is a value to being in control, a value that is recognized in the finance literature, but that value is extremely difficult to quantify. As a result, small business owners may be observed taking actions that make no sense when considered against a value maximization standard but that are reasonable on the basis of other objectives.

To the extent that the goals of the small firm differ from value maximization, some of the prescriptions in this text may not be entirely applicable. Most of the concepts will be useful for the small business, even if its objectives are different, but they may need to be modified. In any event, these brief Small Business sections will serve as a vehicle for exploring special issues of importance to small firms.

RESOLUTION TO DECISION IN FINANCE

The Bendix–Martin Marietta War

Thomas G. Pownall became chairman of Martin Marietta just months before Bendix launched its fateful bid for control of his company. When it was all over, Pownall was still the boss, but he found himself at the helm of a company that was floundering under the burden of a monstrous debt. Wall Street analysts were pessimistic about the company's future.

Five years later Martin Marietta was back on top, posting record profits and looking forward to a rosy future. Although Pownall attributes his company's good fortunes more to luck than genius, those same analysts are giving him a hefty share of the credit. Pownall managed to unload Marietta's debt much faster than anyone could have predicted. He restructured the company, eliminating less profitable divisions. Using some creative financial strategies, including a debt-for-stock swap and the issuance of an unusual kind of preferred stock that was both convertible and exchangeable, Marietta was able to re-

duce its debt from $1.3 billion following the takeover attempt to $224 million in 1986. It also managed to buy back all of its shares from Allied within one year, nine years ahead of schedule.

And what about Bendix president Bill Agee? Although many would view that setting out to buy a company and ending up selling your own company under duress would not strike most people as a triumph, Bill Agee disagrees. A few days after Bendix had agreed to be taken over by Allied, he and his wife, Mary Cunningham Agee, sat in their New York City hotel suite sipping champagne to celebrate their victory in the Bendix-Martin Marietta war. After all, Allied had paid an average of $80 per share for Bendix stock that had never been sold above $67.50 before.

"In the eyes of everything that is important to me," said Bill Agee, "my God, my company, my family—I think I'm a hero. . . . Maximizing returns for investors, that's what they always preach in Business 101, even if not everyone always practices it. Well, that's what we did. I'm proud of it."

Source: John C. Perham, "Martin Marietta's Stunning Comeback," *Dun's Business Month,* March 1986, 50–52.

QUESTIONS

1-1   Would the normal rate of return on investment be the same in all industries? Would normal rates of return change over time? Explain.

1-2   Would the role of the financial manager be likely to increase or decrease in importance relative to other executives if the rate of inflation increased? Explain.

1-3   Should stockholder wealth maximization be thought of as a long-run or a short-run goal; that is, if one action would probably increase the stock price from a current level of $20 to $25 in 6 months and then to $30 in 5 years, but another action would probably keep the stock price at $20 for several years but then increase it to $40 in 5 years, which action would be better? Can you think of actual examples that might have these general tendencies?

1-4   What is the difference between stock price maximization and profit maximization? Would profit maximization ever not lead to stock price maximization?

1-5   If you were running a large, publicly owned corporation, would you make decisions to maximize stockholders' welfare or your own? What are some actions stockholders could take to insure that your interests and theirs coincided?

Chapter 2

How Business Is Organized and Taxed

 DECISION IN FINANCE

Big Fix for Texas Taxes

Imagine you are CEO of a large corporation with headquarters in Houston. You are approached by the governor to serve on a special task force composed of business and government leaders and charged with performing a complete overhaul of the tax code of the state of Texas. It's a great honor and a unique opportunity to serve your state as well as to represent the interests of business. Of course you say yes. But then what?

The panel is composed of seven business and financial executives, all tax-policy novices (yourself included), as well as four members of the Texas legislature, the state comptroller, and the chief budget officer. You start by reading up on taxes, perusing the works of tax scholars,

even reading textbooks. You listen to expert testimony and hear all sorts of suggestions from citizen taxpayers at public hearings held around the state.

Designing an equitable tax system that will foster growth, attract business to the state, and fund state services is no simple task, and your task force is starting from scratch. How much of the state's revenue should be raised through a sales tax? How much of the tax burden should be borne by business? by property owners? Should Texas, one of only ten states that presently has no state income tax, adopt one?

As you read this chapter, think about these issues. Imagine how the final form of the state tax code will affect your corporation. Think about how a new tax code could be designed to maximize the value of your firm. How could a new tax code benefit all Texas businesses?

See end of chapter for resolution.

Financial management cannot be studied in a vacuum — if the value of a firm is to be maximized, the financial manager must understand the legal and economic environment in which financial decisions are made. This requires a consideration of the forms of business organizations and the types of securities firms issue. Further, value depends on the *usable income* available to invest, and this means the *after-tax income* as reported to investors. Accordingly, this chapter presents some background information on forms of business organization and on the federal income tax system.

ALTERNATIVE FORMS OF BUSINESS ORGANIZATION

There are three major forms of business organization: the sole proprietorship, the partnership, and the corporation. In terms of numbers, about 80 percent of business firms are operated as sole proprietorships, whereas the remainder are divided equally between partnerships and corporations. By dollar value of sales, however, about 80 percent of business is conducted by corporations, about 13 percent by sole proprietorships, and about 7 percent by partnerships. Therefore, because most business is conducted by corporations, both large and small, we shall concentrate on them in this book. Still, it is important to understand the differences among the three forms, as well as their advantages and disadvantages.

Sole Proprietorship

proprietorship
A business owned by one individual.

A **proprietorship** is a business owned by one individual. To go into business as a single proprietor is very simple — one merely begins business operations. However, most cities require even the smallest establishments to be licensed, and occasionally state licenses are required as well.

The proprietorship has two important advantages for small operations. First, it is easily and inexpensively formed, since no formal charter for operations is required and it is subject to few government regulations. Second, the business pays no corporate income taxes. As we shall see, however, this is not always a net advantage, because all earnings of the firm, whether they are reinvested in the business or withdrawn, are subject to personal income taxes.

The proprietorship also has three important limitations: (1) it is difficult for a proprietorship to obtain large sums of capital; (2) the proprietor has unlimited personal liability for business debts and can lose assets beyond those invested in the company; and (3) the life of a business organized as a proprietorship is limited to the life of the individual who created it. For these three reasons, the individual proprietorship is restricted primarily to small business operations. Businesses are frequently started as proprietorships and then converted to corporations if and when their growth causes the disadvantages of the proprietorship form to outweigh its advantages.

Partnership

A **partnership** exists whenever two or more persons associate to conduct a business. Partnerships may operate under different degrees of formality, ranging from informal, oral understandings to formal agreements filed with the secretary of the state in which the firm does business. In a partnership, each partner contributes a certain amount of funding to support the business and does a certain amount of the work needed to run it. Of course, each partner then is entitled to a comparable share of the business's profits or losses. Although partnerships are responsible for only a small fraction of the dollar volume of American business, they are common in small professional firms, such as medicine, law, accounting, and, recently, consulting.

The major advantage of a partnership is its low cost and ease of formation. The disadvantages are similar to those associated with proprietorships: (1) unlimited liability, (2) limited life of the organization, (3) difficulty of transferring ownership, and (4) difficulty of raising large amounts of capital. The tax treatment of a partnership is similar to that for a proprietorship, and when compared to that of a corporation, this can be either an advantage or a disadvantage, depending on the situation. This point is discussed later in the chapter.

Regarding liability, the partners must risk their personal assets as well as their investments in the business, for under partnership law the partners are liable for the business's debts. This means that if any partner is unable to meet his or her pro rata claim in the event the partnership goes bankrupt, the remaining partners must take over the unsatisfied claims, even having to draw on their own personal assets when no other sources are available.

Some of the problems of a general partnership, which we have just described, may be reduced by the formation of a **limited partnership.** In a limited partnership certain partners are designated *general partners* and others *limited partners.* The general partners have the same unlimited liability as with any general partnership, but the limited partners' liability extends only to the amount of their investment in the partnership. Limited partners are often termed *silent partners* because they have no active voice in management. Limited partnerships are quite common in the area of real estate investment, but they have not worked well in many other types of business ventures. They constitute only a small fraction of all partnership businesses.

The first three disadvantages of a general partnership — unlimited liability, impermanence of the organization, and difficulty of transferring ownership — combine to cause the fourth, the difficulty partnerships have in attracting substantial amounts of capital. This is no particular problem for slow-growing businesses, but if a company's products really catch on so that it needs to raise large amounts of capital to expand and thus to capitalize on its opportunities, the capital attraction situation truly becomes a drawback. Thus companies such as Hewlett-Packard and Apple Computer generally begin life as proprietorships or partnerships but at some point find it necessary to convert to corporations.

partnership
An unincorporated business owned by two or more persons.

limited partnership
An unincorporated business owned both by general partners having unlimited liability and by other partners having liability limited to their investment in the firm.

Corporation

A **corporation** is a legal entity created by a state. It is separate and distinct from its owners and managers. This separateness gives the corporation three major advantages: (1) it has an *unlimited life* — it can continue after its original owners and managers are dead; (2) it permits *easy transferability of ownership interest,* because ownership interests can be divided into shares of stock, which are transferred far more easily than partnership interests; and (3) it permits *limited liability.* To illustrate, if, on the one hand, you invested $10,000 in a partnership and the partnership went bankrupt owing a considerably larger sum of money, you could be assessed for a share of these debts. Thus an investor in a partnership is exposed to unlimited liability. On the other hand, if you invested $10,000 in the stock of a corporation, your potential loss on the investment would be $10,000 — your liability would be limited to the amount of your investment in the business.[1]

Whereas a proprietorship or a partnership can commence operations without much paperwork, setting up a corporation is a bit more involved. The incorporators must prepare a *charter* and a set of *bylaws.* The **charter** includes the following information: (1) name of proposed corporation, (2) type of activities it will pursue, (3) amount of capital stock, (4) number of directors, and (5) names and addresses of directors. The charter is filed with the secretary of the state in which the firm will be headquartered, and when it is approved, the corporation is officially in existence.

The **bylaws** are a set of rules drawn up by the founders of the corporation to aid in governing the internal management of the company. Included are such points as (1) how directors are to be elected (all of them elected each year or, say, one third each year); (2) whether the existing stockholders will have the first right to buy any new stock the firm issues; (3) what provisions there are for management committees (such as an executive committee or a finance committee) and their duties; and (4) what procedures there are for changing the bylaws themselves, should conditions require it. Lawyers have standard form charters and bylaws in their word processors, and they can set up a corporation with little effort. For about $500 — less if you find a hungry young lawyer fresh out of law school — a business can be incorporated.

The value of any business other than a very small one probably will be maximized if it is organized as a corporation. The reasons are as follows:

1. Limited liability reduces risk to investors, and the lower the risk, other things held constant, the higher the value of the firm.

2. Value is dependent on growth opportunities, which in turn are dependent on a firm's ability to attract capital. Because corporations can attract capital

---

[1]In the case of small corporations, the limited liability feature is often a fiction, because bankers and credit managers frequently require personal guarantees from the stockholders of small, weak businesses.

more easily than unincorporated businesses, they have superior growth opportunities.

3. The value of an asset also depends on its **liquidity,** which means the ease of selling the asset and converting it to cash. Because an investment in the stock of a corporation is much more liquid than a similar investment in a proprietorship or partnership, this too means that the corporate form of organization can enhance the value of a business.

4. Corporations are taxed differently than proprietorships and partnerships. In some instances the tax laws favor corporations. This point is discussed in the next section of the chapter.

Since most firms are indeed managed with value maximization in mind, it is easy to see why most business is conducted by corporations.

liquidity
The ability to sell an asset at a reasonable price on short notice.

THE FEDERAL INCOME TAX SYSTEM

The value of any financial asset, such as a share of stock, a bond, or a mortgage, and the values of most real assets, such as plants or even whole firms, depend on the stream of cash flows produced by the asset. Cash flows from an asset consist of *usable* income plus depreciation. Depreciation will be discussed later in the chapter, but usable income means income *after taxes*. Proprietorship and partnership income must be reported and taxed as personal income to the owners, whereas most corporations must first pay taxes on their own income, and stockholders must then pay taxes on corporate after-tax income distributed to them as dividends. Therefore, both *personal* and *corporate* income taxes are important in the determination of cash flows from an asset.

In October of 1986, President Reagan signed a sweeping new tax law that changed the United States' tax system in fundamental ways. We incorporated the major provisions of the new tax law into this chapter and throughout the book. Most parts of the new tax law take effect in 1987, but to reduce adverse effects on individuals and corporations who had laid plans on the basis of the old law, parts of the new law will be phased in over a two- to three-year transition period. During that period, certain provisions will be blends of the new and the old provisions. For example, the federal tax rate on the top increments of individuals' income under the old law was 50 percent, and it will be 28 percent once the new law is fully implemented. During 1987, however, the rate for most wealthy individuals was 38.5 percent. To avoid unnecessary detail, we will, for the most part, focus on the tax system as it will exist once the 1986 changes have been fully implemented.

You should also note that the details of our tax laws are changed fairly often—indeed, a nontrivial change has occurred, on average, every 1½ years since 1913, when our federal income tax system began. Further, because certain parts of the tax system are tied to the inflation rate, changes automatically occur each year, depending on the rate of inflation during the previous year. Therefore, even though this chapter will give you a good knowledge of the basics of the tax system, you should consult current rate schedules and other data as published by the Internal Revenue Service (and available in U.S. post offices) before you file your personal or business tax return.

Federal income tax rates for individuals go up to 33 percent, and when state and city income taxes are included, the marginal tax rate on an individual's income can approach 40 percent. Business income is also taxed heavily. The income from partnerships and proprietorships is reported by the individual owners and consequently is taxed at rates going up to 40 percent, whereas corporate profits are subject to federal income tax rates of up to 39 percent. Just as with individuals, state and local taxes will raise the overall percentage of income proprietorships, partnerships, and corporations pay in taxes. Because of the magnitude of the tax bite, taxes play an important role in many financial decisions.

Taxes are so complicated that university law schools offer master's degrees in taxation to practicing lawyers, many of whom also have CPA licenses. In a field complicated enough to warrant such detailed study, we can cover only the highlights. This is really enough, though, because business people and investors should and do rely on tax specialists rather than trust their own limited knowledge. Still, it is important to know the basic elements of the tax system as a starting point for discussions with tax experts.

Individual Income Taxes

Individuals pay taxes on wages and salaries, on investment income (dividends, interest, and profits from the sale of securities), and on the profits of proprietorships and partnerships. The U.S. tax rates are **progressive** to some extent, which means that the higher the income, the larger the percentage paid in taxes.[2] Table 2-1 gives the tax rates for single individuals and married couples filing joint returns under the rate schedules that will take effect in 1988. Here are the highlights of the table:

1. Taxable income is defined as gross income minus exemptions and a set of deductions that are spelled out in the instructions to the tax forms people must file. In 1987, each taxpayer receives an exemption of $1,900 for each dependent, including the taxpayer, which reduces taxable income. This exemption rises to $2,000 in 1989, and thereafter it will be indexed to rise with inflation. However, high income taxpayers must pay a surtax which takes away the value of the personal exemptions. Also, certain expenses such as

progressive tax
A tax that requires a higher percentage payment on higher incomes. The personal income tax in the United States, which goes from a rate of 0 percent on its lowest increments to 28 percent on the highest increments, is progressive.

taxable income
Gross income minus allowable deductions as set forth in the Tax Code.

---

[2]Before the 1986 Tax Code revisions, rates were more steeply progressive, going from 11 percent to 50 percent, but higher-income taxpayers were able to use a variety of tax shelters that lowered effective tax rates substantially. Indeed, many people had incomes in the millions and paid no taxes. The 1986 changes eliminated most tax shelters and, in reality, did little to affect the progressivity of our tax system.

Table 2-1 **Individual Tax Rates for 1988**

If Your Taxable Income Is	You Pay This Amount on the Base of the Bracket	Plus This Percentage on the Excess over the Base	Average Tax Rate (on Top of Bracket)
Single Individuals			
Up to $17,850	$ 0	15%	15.0%
$17,850–$43,150	2,678	28	22.6
$43,150–$100,480	9,762	33	28.5
Over $100,480	28,680	28	28.0

If Your Taxable Income Is	You Pay This Amount on the Base of the Bracket	Plus This Percentage on the Excess over the Base	Average Tax Rate (on Top of Bracket)
Married Couples Filing Joint Returns			
Up to $29,750	$ 0	15%	15.0%
$29,750–$71,900	4,462	28	22.6
$71,900–$171,090	16,264	33	28.6
Over $171,090	48,997	28	28.0

Notes:

a. The tax rates are for 1988 and beyond. However, the income ranges at which the 28 percent rate takes effect, and also the ranges for the surtax, are scheduled to be indexed with inflation beyond 1988, so they will change from those shown in the table.

b. Technically, a surtax of 5 percent is imposed on income in the range $43,150 to $100,480 for single individuals and in the range $71,900 to $171,090 for married couples. This surtax is designed (1) to eliminate the effects of the 15 percent rate on the first increments of income and (2) to eliminate the benefits of the personal exemption. The surtax ceases when the personal exemption has been fully offset, and hence the dollar amount at which the marginal rate drops back to 28 percent depends on the number of exemptions claimed. The amounts shown above assume one exemption for a single individual and two exemptions for a married couple. Different tables, similar to the one we present but with different numbers of exemptions, are available from the Internal Revenue Service.

c. It appears from the last column that the average rate rises above 28 percent. What really is happening is that additional income equal to the personal exemption discussed in note b is being taxed, and that tax is added in when calculating the average rate on the taxable income.

mortgage interest paid, state and local taxes paid, and itemized charitable contributions can be deducted and used to reduce taxable income.

2. The **marginal tax rate** is the tax on the last unit of income. Marginal tax rates begin at 15 percent, rise to 28 percent, then to 33 percent, and finally fall back to 28 percent and remain constant thereafter.

marginal tax rate
The tax applicable to the last unit of income.

3. One can calculate average tax rates from the data in the table. For example, if Diane Malone, a single individual, had a taxable income of $30,000, her tax bill would be ($17,850)(0.15) + ($30,000 − $17,850)(0.28) = $2,678 + $3,402 = $6,080. Her **average tax rate** would be $6,080/$30,000 = 20.3% versus a *marginal rate* of 28 percent. If Diane received a raise of $1,000, bringing her income to $31,000, she would have to pay $280 of it as taxes, so her after-tax raise would be $720.

average tax rate
Taxes paid divided by taxable income.

bracket creep
A situation that occurs
when progressive tax
rates combine with infla-
tion to cause a greater
portion of each taxpay-
er's real income to be
paid as taxes.

4. As indicated in the footnote to the table, current legislation provides for tax brackets to be indexed to inflation to avoid the **bracket creep** which occurred during the 1970s and which de facto raised tax rates substantially.[3]

Taxes on Dividend and Interest Income. Dividend and interest income received by individuals from corporate securities is taxed at rates going up to 33 percent. Because corporations pay dividends out of earnings that have already been taxed, there is *double taxation* of corporate income.

It should be noted that under U.S. tax laws, interest on most state and local government bonds, called *municipals* or *"munis,"* is not subject to federal income taxes. Thus investors get to keep all of the interest paid on municipal bonds but only a fraction of the interest paid on bonds issued by corporations or by the U.S. government. This means that a lower-yielding muni can provide the same after-tax return as a higher-yielding corporate bond. For example, a taxpayer in the 33 percent marginal tax bracket who could buy a muni that yielded 9 percent would have to receive a before-tax yield of 13.43 percent on a corporate or U.S. Treasury bond to have the same after-tax income:

$$\frac{\text{Equivalent pre-tax yield}}{\text{on taxable bond}} = \frac{\text{Yield on muni}}{1 - \text{Marginal tax rate}}$$

$$= \frac{9\%}{1 - 0.33} = 13.43\%.$$

This exemption from federal taxes stems from the separation of federal and state powers, and its primary purpose is to help state and local governments borrow at lower rates than would otherwise be available to them.

Capital Gain versus Ordinary Income. Assets such as stocks, bonds, and real estate are defined as *capital assets*. If you buy a capital asset and later sell it for more than your purchase price, the profit is defined as a **capital gain;** if you suffer a loss, it is called a **capital loss.** An asset sold within 6 months of the time it was purchased produces a *short-term gain or loss,* whereas one held for more than 6 months produces a *long-term gain or loss.* Thus, if you

capital gain or loss
The profit (loss) from
the sale of a capital asset
for more (less) than its
purchase price.

---

[3]For example, if you were single and had a taxable income of $17,850, your tax bill would be $2,678. Now suppose inflation caused prices to double and your income, being tied to a cost of living index, rose to $35,700. Because our tax rates are progressive, if tax brackets were not indexed, your taxes would jump to $7,676. Your after-tax income would thus increase from $15,172 to $28,024, but, because prices have doubled, your real income would decline from $15,172 to $14,012 (calculated as one-half of $28,024). You would be in a higher tax bracket, so you would be paying a higher percentage of your real income in taxes. If this happened to everyone, and if Congress failed to change tax rates sufficiently, real individual incomes would decline because the federal government would be taking a larger share of the national product. This has been called the federal government's "inflation dividend." However, since tax brackets are indexed, if your income doubled because of inflation, your tax bill would double, but your after-tax real income would remain constant at $15,172. Bracket creep was a real problem during the 1970s and early 1980s, but indexing has put an end to it.

buy 100 shares of GE stock for $70 per share and sell it for $80, you make a capital gain of 100 × $10, or $1,000. However, if you sell the stock for $60, you will have a $1,000 capital loss. If you hold the stock for more than 6 months, the gain or loss is long-term; otherwise, it is short-term. If you sell the stock for $70, you make neither a gain nor a loss; you simply get your $7,000 back and pay no taxes on it.

From 1921 through 1986, long-term capital gains were taxed at substantially lower rates than ordinary income. For example, in 1986 long-term gains were taxed at only 40 percent of the tax rate on ordinary income. However, the tax law changes that took effect in 1987 eliminated this differential, and capital gains income is now taxed as if it were ordinary income.

There was a great deal of controversy over the elimination of the preferential rate for capital gains. It was argued that if capital gains were taxed at favorable rates, businesses would retain a higher percentage of their incomes in order to provide their stockholders with capital gains as opposed to highly taxed dividend income, and this earnings retention would stimulate investment and economic growth. The proponents of the capital gains differential lost the argument in 1986, but the law retained all the language dealing with capital gains specifically to make it easier to reinstate the differential if economic conditions suggest that it is needed to encourage growth.

When capital gains were taxed at favorable rates, this had implications for dividend policy (it favored lower payouts and higher earnings retention), and it also favored stock investments over debt investments because part of the income from stock normally came from favorably-taxed capital gains. Thus one can anticipate certain changes in corporate financial policy as a result of the elimination of the differential. Also, because the differential may be reinstated, it is important that you at least know what it is.

Corporate Income Taxes

The corporate tax structure, shown in Table 2-2, is relatively simple. To illustrate, if a firm had $100,000 of taxable income, its tax bill would be:

$$\text{Taxes} = 0.15(\$50,000) + 0.25(\$25,000) + 0.34(\$25,000)$$
$$= \$7,500 + \$6,250 + \$8,500$$
$$= \$22,250,$$

and its average tax rate would be $22,250/$100,000 = 22.25\%$.

For $200,00 of income, the tax bill would be:

$$\text{Taxes} = 0.15(\$50,000) + 0.25(\$25,000) + 0.34(\$25,000) + 0.39(\$100,000)$$
$$= \$7,500 + \$6,250 + \$8,500 + \$39,000$$
$$= \$61,250.$$

The average tax rate for this level of income is 30.63%, calculated as
$$\$61,250/\$200,000 = 30.63\%.$$

Table 2-2 **Corporate Tax Rates**

If a Corporation's Taxable Income Is	It Pays This Amount on the Base of the Bracket	Plus This Percentage on the Excess over the Base	Average Tax Rate (on Top of Bracket)
Up to $50,000	$ 0	15%	15.0%
$50,000 to $75,000	7,500	25	18.3
$75,000 to $100,000	13,750	34	22.3
$100,000 to $335,000	22,250	39	34.0
Over $335,000	113,900	34	34.0

Notes:
a. The rates shown here are for 1988 and beyond.
b. For income in the range of $100,000 to $335,000, a surtax of 5% is added to the base rate of 34%. This surtax, which eliminates the effects of the lower rates on income below $75,000, results in a marginal tax rate of 39% for income in the $100,000 to $335,000 range.

For $400,000 of income, the tax bill would be:

$$\text{Taxes} = 0.15(\$50,000) + 0.25(\$25,000) + 0.34(\$25,000)$$
$$+ 0.39(\$235,000) \text{ at } 0.34(\$65,000)$$
$$= \$7,500 + \$6,250 + \$8,500 + \$91,650 + \$22,100$$
$$= \$136,000,$$

with the average tax rate equal to $136,000/$400,000 = 34%.

Indeed, for all income over $335,000, one can disregard the surtax and simply calculate the corporate tax rate as 34 percent of all taxable income. Thus the corporate tax is progressive up to $335,000 of income, but it is constant thereafter.[4]

Interest and Dividend Income Received by a Corporation. Interest income received by a corporation is taxed as ordinary income at regular corporate tax rates. However, 80 percent of the dividends received by one corporation from another is excluded from taxable income, whereas the remaining 20 percent is taxed at the ordinary tax rate. Thus a corporation earning more than $335,000 and paying a 34 percent marginal tax rate would pay $(0.2)(0.34) = 0.068 = 6.8\%$ of its dividend income as taxes, so its effective tax rate would

---

[4]Before 1987, many large, profitable corporations paid zero income taxes. The reason this happened was: (1) expenses, especially depreciation, are defined differently for the purpose of calculating taxable income than for reporting earnings to stockholders, so some companies reported positive profits to stockholders but losses — hence no taxes — to the Internal Revenue Service; and (2) some companies that did have tax liabilities used various tax credits, including the investment tax credit (discussed later in the chapter) to offset taxes that would otherwise be payable. This situation will be drastically curtailed in the future.

be 6.8 percent. If this firm had $10,000 in pre-tax dividend income, its after-tax dividend income would be:

$$\text{After-tax income} = \text{Before-tax income} - \text{Taxes}$$

$$= \text{Before-tax income} - (\text{Before-tax income})(\text{Effective tax rate})$$

$$= \text{Before-tax income}(1 - \text{Effective tax rate})$$

$$= \$10,000(1 - 0.068)$$

$$= \$10,000(0.932) = \$9,320.$$

If the corporation passes its own after-tax income on to its stockholders as dividends, the income is ultimately subjected to *triple taxation:* (1) the original corporation is first taxed, (2) the second corporation is then taxed on the dividends it received, and (3) the individuals who receive the final dividends are taxed again. This is the reason for the 80 percent exclusion on intercorporate dividends.

Notice that if a corporation has surplus funds which can be invested in marketable securities, the tax factor favors investment in stocks, which pay dividends, rather than in bonds, which pay interest. For example, suppose IBM had $100,000 to invest, and it could buy bonds that paid interest of $10,000 per year or stock that paid dividends of $10,000. If IBM were in the 34 percent tax bracket, its tax on the interest, if it bought bonds, would be 0.34($10,000) = $3,400 and its after-tax income would be $6,600. If it bought stock, its tax would be 0.34[(0.2)($10,000)] = $680 and its after-tax income would be $9,320. Other factors might lead IBM to invest in bonds, but the tax factor certainly favors stock investments when the investor is a corporation.

Interest and Dividends Paid by a Corporation. A firm's operations can be financed with either debt or equity capital. If it uses debt, it must pay interest on this debt, whereas if it uses equity, it will pay dividends to the equity investors (stockholders). The interest paid by a corporation is deducted from its operating income to obtain its taxable income, but dividends paid are not deductible. Therefore, a firm needs $1 of pre-tax income to pay $1 of interest, but if it is in the 34 percent bracket, it needs

$$\frac{\$1}{1 - \text{Tax rate}} = \frac{\$1}{0.66} = \$1.5152$$

of pre-tax income to pay $1 of dividends.

To illustrate, Table 2-3 shows the situation for a firm whose assets produced $1 million of earnings before taxes. If the firm were financed with debt, requiring $1 million in interest payments, its taxable income would be zero, taxes would be zero, and the lenders would receive the entire $1 million. If the firm had no debt, however, and thus was entirely equity financed, all $1 million of the operating income would be taxable income. If the firm's tax rate

Table 2-3 **Cash Flows to Investors under Debt and Equity Financing**

	Under Debt Financing	Under Equity Financing
Before-tax income	$1,000,000	$1,000,000
Interest	1,000,000	0
Taxable income	$ 0	$1,000,000
Taxes (34%)	0	340,000
After-tax income	$ 0	$ 660,000
Income to debt investors	$1,000,000	
Income to equity investors		$ 660,000
Advantage to debt	$ 340,000	

were 34 percent, the firm's tax liability would be $1,000,000(0.34) = $340,000. Thus the firm's stockholders would receive only $660,000 versus the $1 million received by the lenders.

Although we have not evaluated the financial risk of a loan that requires a $1 million interest payment, this example emphasizes that interest is a tax-deductible expense that has a profound effect on the way businesses are financed, because the U.S. tax system favors debt financing over equity financing. This point is discussed in more detail in Chapters 19 and 20.

Corporate Capital Gains. Before the 1986 Tax Code revisions, corporate long-term capital gains were taxed at rates lower than ordinary income, just as with individuals. Under current law, however, corporations' capital gains are taxed at the same rates as their operating income.

Corporate Loss Carry-Back and Carry-Forward. Ordinary corporate operating losses can be carried back **(carry-back)** to each of the preceding 3 years or forward **(carry-forward)** for the following 15 years and used to offset taxable income in those years. For example, an operating loss in 1988 could be carried back and used to reduce taxable income in 1985, 1986, and 1987, or carried forward and used in 1989, 1990, and so on to the year 2003. The loss must be applied first to the earliest year, then to the next earliest year, and so on until losses have been used up or the 15-year limit has been reached.

To illustrate, Wildcat Drilling Supply had a $1 million *pre-tax* profit in 1985, 1986, and 1987, but it then had a bad year in 1988 and lost $7 million. Wildcat would use the carry-back feature to recompute taxes for 1985, using $1 million of the $7 million in 1988 operating losses to reduce the 1985 pre-tax amount to zero. This would permit the company to recover the amount of taxes paid in 1985, so in 1989 Wildcat could receive a refund of its 1985 taxes because of the loss experienced in 1988. Because $6 million of unrecovered losses would still be available, Wildcat would repeat this procedure for 1986 and 1987. Thus in 1989 it would receive a refund for taxes paid on $3 million

**tax loss carry-back
and carry-forward**
Losses that can be carried backward or forward in time to offset taxable income in a given year.

of income from 1985 through 1987. Wildcat would still have $4 million of unrecovered losses that it could carry forward and use annually, subject to the 15-year limit. The purpose of carry-back, carry-forward provisions is, of course, to avoid penalizing corporations whose incomes fluctuate considerably from year to year.

Improper Accumulation to Avoid Payment of Dividends. Corporations could refrain from paying dividends to enable their stockholders to avoid personal income taxes on dividends. To prevent this, the Tax Code contains an **improper accumulation** provision, which states that earnings accumulated by a corporation are subject to penalty rates *if the purpose of the accumulation is to enable stockholders to avoid the personal income tax.* A cumulative total of $250,000 (the balance sheet item "retained earnings") is by law exempted from the improper accumulation tax. This is a benefit primarily to small corporations.

> **improper accumulation**
> Retention of earnings by a business for the purpose of enabling stockholders to avoid personal income taxes.

Note, however, that the improper accumulation penalty applies only if the retained earnings in excess of $250,000 are *shown to be unnecessary to meet the reasonable needs of the business.* A great many companies do indeed have legitimate reasons for retaining more than $250,000 of earnings. For example, earnings may be retained and used to pay off debt, to finance growth, or to provide the corporation with a cushion against possible cash drains caused by losses. How much a firm should properly accumulate for uncertain contingencies is a matter of judgment. We shall consider this matter again in Chapter 21, which deals with corporate dividend policy.

Consolidated Corporate Tax Returns. If a corporation owns 80 percent or more of another corporation's stock, it can aggregate income and file one consolidated tax return; thus the losses of one company can be used to offset the profits of another. (Similarly, one division's losses can be used to offset another division's profits.) No business ever wants to incur losses (you can go broke losing $1 to save 34¢ in taxes), but tax offsets do make it more feasible for large, multidivisional corporations to undertake risky new ventures or ventures that will suffer losses during a development period.

DEPRECIATION

Suppose a firm buys a milling machine for $100,000 and uses it for 5 years, after which it is scrapped. The cost of the goods produced by the machine must include a charge for the machine, and this charge is called *depreciation.* Because depreciation reduces profits as calculated by the accountants, the higher a firm's depreciation charges, the lower its reported net income. Depreciation is not a cash charge, however, so higher depreciation levels do not reduce cash flows. Indeed, higher depreciation levels *increase* cash flows, because the greater the firm's depreciation, the lower its tax bill.

Companies generally calculate depreciation one way when figuring taxes and another way when reporting income to investors. Most use the *straight line* method for stockholder reporting (or book purposes), and they use the fastest rate permitted by law for tax purposes.

Congress changes the permissible tax depreciation methods from time to time. Before 1954 the straight line method was required for tax purposes, but in 1954 *accelerated* methods (double declining balance and sum-of-years'-digits) were permitted. Then, in 1981, the old accelerated methods were replaced by a simpler procedure known as the **Accelerated Cost Recovery System** (**ACRS**, which is pronounced "acres"). The ACRS system was changed again in 1986 as a part of the Tax Reform Act. Our discussion of depreciation is based on ACRS as it was modified in 1986.

Tax Depreciation Life

For tax purposes, the cost of an asset is expensed gradually over its depreciable life. Historically, an asset's depreciable life was determined by its estimated useful economic life; it was intended that an asset would be fully depreciated at approximately the same time that it reached the end of its useful economic life. However, ACRS totally abandoned that practice — it set simple guidelines that created several classes of assets, each with a more-or-less arbitrarily prescribed life called a *recovery period* or *class life.* These recovery periods are designed to be shorter than the economically productive life of the assets. Under the original ACRS method, the majority of business assets had a 3- to 5-year recovery period (or depreciable life). The new recovery periods under the Tax Reform Act of 1986 are less generous — most assets have slightly longer recovery periods. Most depreciable business assets placed in service in 1987 and after will have a 5- to 7-year recovery period.

Even with the slightly longer recovery period for assets placed in service in 1987 and after, the major effect of the ACRS system has been to shorten the period over which assets may be depreciated, thus giving businesses larger tax deductions and thereby increasing cash flows available for reinvestment. Table 2-4 describes class lives and asset types under the 1986 Tax Reform Act. The first column in Table 2-4 shows the ACRS class life, whereas the second column describes the types of assets that fall into each category. With the straight line method, a uniform annual depreciation charge is allowed; the annual depreciation charge is equal to the cost of the asset divided by the years of the asset's class life. The ACRS recovery allowances as set by Congress always equal or exceed the straight line rates. Therefore, a firm will always obtain a faster depreciation write-off if it uses the ACRS recovery allowances than if it uses straight line, when an option exists.[5]

---

[5]As a benefit to very small companies, the Tax Code also permits companies to *expense,* which is equivalent to depreciating over one year, up to $10,000 of equipment. Thus, if a small company bought one asset worth up to $10,000, it could write the asset off in the year it was acquired. We shall disregard this provision throughout the book.

Accelerated Cost Recovery System (ACRS)
A depreciation system that allows businesses to write off the cost of an asset over a period much shorter than its operating life.

Table 2-4 **Class Lives and Asset Types for ACRS under the 1986 Tax Reform Act**

Class Life	Type of Property
3-year	Computers and equipment used in research
5-year	Automobiles, tractor units, light-duty trucks, computers, and certain special manufacturing tools
7-year	Most industrial equipment, office furniture, and fixtures
10-year	Certain longer-lived types of equipment
27.5-year	Residential rental real property such as apartment buildings
31.5-year	All nonresidential real property, including commercial and industrial buildings

Computing ACRS Depreciation

Under earlier depreciation methods, the rate at which the value of an asset actually declined was estimated, and this rate was then used as the basis for tax depreciation. Thus different assets were depreciated along different paths over time. For most assets placed in service after December 31, 1986, a 200 percent declining balance depreciation method (with certain modifications discussed later) is used. For assets placed in service between 1981 and 1986, depreciation rates or *recovery allowance percentages* were published. Although there are no official recovery percentages at this time, we have prepared the recovery allowances in Table 2-5 based on the prescribed depreciation methods. Using these rates, the yearly recovery allowance or depreciation expense is determined by multiplying the asset's *depreciable basis* by the applicable recovery allowance percentage.

Half-Year Convention. The ACRS recovery percentages as shown in Table 2-5 employ the **half-year convention** — that is, it is assumed that all assets are put into service at mid-year and hence generate a half-year's depreciation, irrespective of when they actually go into service.[6] Because an asset is considered to have been placed in service at mid-year, a half-year's depreciation remains at the end of the cost recovery period. Thus the recovery period for 5-year property begins at mid-year and is completed 5 years later. The effect of this convention is that the firm must wait an extra year to fully depreciate an asset; thus the actual write-off periods are 4, 6, 8, and 11 years, as seen in the

half-year convention
A feature of ACRS in which all assets are assumed to be put into service at mid-year and thus allowed a half-year's depreciation.

---

[6]Care must be taken in order to qualify for the half-year convention, however. If the firm purchases more than 40 percent of its depreciable assets in the final quarter of the tax year, the assets will be depreciated using a new "mid-quarter" convention rather than the usual mid-year convention.

Table 2-5 **Recovery Allowances for Personal Property under the Tax Reform Act of 1986**

Ownership Year	Class of Investment			
	3-Year	5-Year	7-Year	10-Year
1	33%	20%	14%	10%
2	45	32	25	18
3	15	19	17	14
4	7	12	13	12
5		11	9	9
6		6	9	7
7			9	7
8			4	7
9				7
10				6
11				3
	100%	100%	100%	100%

Notes:

a. Congress developed recovery allowances based on a 200 percent declining balance method with a switch to straight line depreciation when it becomes advantageous to the firm. Using the 10-year class assets as an example, the recovery allowances were computed as follows: First, the straight line allowance would be 10 percent per year, so the 200 percent declining balance multiplier is $2.0 \times 10\% = 20\%$. However the half-year convention assumes the asset is placed in service at mid-year, so the ACRS allowance is 10 percent (one-half of 20%). For Year 2, 90 percent of the asset's depreciable basis remains to be depreciated, so $0.20(90\%) = 18.0\%$. By Year 3, $10\% + 18\% = 28\%$ of the possible depreciation has been taken, leaving 72%, so $0.2(72\%) = 14.4\%$ and is rounded to 14%, and so on. After 5 years, straight line depreciation exceeds the declining balance depreciation, so the switch to straight line is automatically made. Since the asset was placed in service at mid-year (the half-year convention) and the asset is to be depreciated over 10 years, one-half year's depreciation remains to be taken in the 11th year. We rounded the Table figures to the nearest whole number.

b. Other recovery periods exist for other types of assets. For example, residential rental property (apartments) is depreciated over a 27.5 year life, while commercial and industrial structures are depreciated over 31.5 years.

recovery percentages in Table 2-5.[7] The half-year convention also applies if the straight line option is used, with half of one year's depreciation taken in the first year, and the remaining half-year's depreciation in the year following the end of the class life.

depreciable basis
The portion of an asset's value that can be depreciated for tax purposes.

Depreciable Basis. The **depreciable basis** is an important element of ACRS, because each year's allowance (depreciation expense) depends on the asset's basis. An asset's basis is determined by the cost of the asset plus any costs required to place the asset in operation, such as transportation and installation charges. Salvage value of the asset, if any, is *not* considered in determining the asset's basis. Thus all assets are depreciated as if they will have no salvage value

[7]Because our purpose is to teach finance and not taxation, we will ignore the somewhat cumbersome half-year's depreciation at the end of the asset's life in most examples and problems. Thus, if we were illustrating the depreciation of a 3-year asset, the recovery allowances would be as follows: Year 1 — 33%, Year 2 — 45%, and Year 3 — 22%. This simplifying assumption will be noted wherever it is used.

INDUSTRY PRACTICE

Tax Reform

In September 1986, Congress passed a law that fundamentally overhauled the United States' tax system. Although the tax code has changed often over the years, this tax reform legislation was the most sweeping in recent history. In its broad outlines, the bill provided tax cuts totaling a whopping $300 billion over five years and reduced deductions by an equal amount. The law slashed the top tax rates paid by corporations and individuals and shifted the burden of taxation more heavily to business.

The new law should be beneficial to the economy in the long run. It encourages investment for economic reasons rather than for tax advantages and provides many individuals with more income to spend or save. But for almost all corporations, this latest dose of tax reform is just like all the rest — a new welter of rules to be mastered in order to keep tax bills to the legal minimum.

Even though corporate executives certainly are interested in a healthy economy, their main concern is with how a piece of legislation affects their particular business or industry. With a tax law as broad and complex as this latest one, implications for any individual business may be difficult to sort out. Sometimes it is the smallest print that has the biggest impact.

The new law raises the amount that businesses pay in taxes by almost $110 billion over five years while it cuts the amount individuals pay by an equal amount. Accountants estimate that more than a third of the boost in the corporate tax bill will come from often obscure accounting changes. Major industry groups such as auto, steel, and retailing end up handing a big chunk of their new tax savings right back to Uncle Sam.

For example, until 1986, retailers whose customers purchased goods on revolving charge accounts paid taxes only on the payments they had actually received. The new law forces retailers to pay taxes on a portion of the installment payments they are due to receive in the future. Another accounting provision requires some manufacturers and companies in heavy industry to capitalize (defer) some of their inventory, construction, and development costs into the future, thereby reducing deductions and increasing taxes paid. Manufacturers that hold large inventories are hardest hit by this accounting rule.

"Smokestack" industries seem to be most adversely affected by the new law, whereas consumer goods manufacturers and service providers get a shot in the arm from the boost in consumer spending. However, the winners and losers are not that easy to identify. Obviously, the ways in which people choose to spend any increase in disposable income will determine how many industries, especially those facing higher taxes, fare. Heavily capitalized businesses tend to pay more taxes but they too may be helped by increases in consumer spending. For example, a profitable airline that has spent heavily on new aircraft and equipment has a higher tax bill under the new law, but it benefits if a boost in consumer income causes an increase in air travel.

Other ways the new tax law effects business are equally hard to foresee. For example, two major elements of the new law tend to cancel each other out: the repeal of the investment tax credit and the reduction in tax rates. How specific businesses are affected varies widely from company to company and depends on myriad accounting rules and interpretations.

Applying the new law to General Motors' 1985 tax return provides a good illustration. Analysts at Goldman Sachs estimate that under the new law, GM would have saved $601 million as a result of the lower tax rate paid by corporations. However, GM would have been denied an investment tax credit of $509 million. At Ford, however, the balance would tip in the other direction. Ford would have gained $226 million from the lower tax rate but would have been denied $345 million worth of investment tax credits.

Although tax law changes leave corporate executives anxiously speculating how their balance sheets will be affected, some members of the business community aren't losing any sleep over them. Legions of lawyers, accountants, and business publishers who crank out thousands of pages on taxation every year don't expect to be hurting for business any time soon. There has never been an income-tax change that has actually reduced the number of rules and regulations, and this one is no exception. Tax experts predict that the confusion generated as businesses adapt to the new system should keep them gainfully employed for many years to come.

when they are retired from service. If the asset can be sold at retirement, its salvage value is considered to be a recapture of depreciation and is taxed as ordinary income.

investment tax credit (ITC)

A specified percentage of the cost of new assets that businesses can at times deduct as a credit against their income taxes.

Investment Tax Credit. An **investment tax credit (ITC)** provides for a direct reduction of taxes, and its purpose is to stimulate business investment. ITCs were first introduced in the Kennedy administration in 1961, and they have been put in and taken out of the tax system depending on what Congress thinks about the need to stimulate business investment versus the need for federal revenues. Prior to the 1986 Tax Reform Act, the credit applied to depreciable personal property with a life of 3 or more years, and it amounted to 6 percent of short-lived assets and 10 percent of longer-lived assets. The tax deduction was determined by multiplying the cost of the asset by the applicable percentage. Even though ITCs were eliminated by the tax revisions in 1986, you should be aware of what ITCs are, because there is a good chance that they will be reinstated at some future date.

CASH FLOW ANALYSIS

As noted earlier, management's primary goal is stock price maximization. As we shall see, a stock's value is based on the *present value of the cash flows* that investors expect the stock to provide in the future. Although any individual investor could sell the stock and receive cash for it, the **cash flow** provided by the stock itself is its expected future dividend stream, and that dividend stream provides the fundamental basis for the stock's value.

cash flow

The actual net cash, as opposed to accounting net income, that flows into (or out of) a firm during some specified period.

accounting profit

A firm's net income as calculated on its income statement.

Because dividends are paid in cash, a company's ability to pay dividends depends on its projected cash flows. Cash flows are generally correlated with **accounting profit,** which is simply net income as calculated on the income statement. Companies with relatively high accounting profits generally have relatively high cash flows, but the relationship is not precise. Therefore, investors are concerned about cash flow projections as well as profit projections.

It should also be noted that firms can be thought of as having two separate but related bases of value—*existing assets,* which provide profits and cash flows, and *growth opportunities,* or the chance to make new investments that will increase future profits and cash flows. Further, the ability to take advantage of growth opportunities often depends on the availability of the cash needed to buy new assets, and the cash flow from existing assets is often the primary source for the funds needed for profitable new investments. This is another reason for both investors and managers to be concerned about cash flows as well as profits.

For our purposes, it is useful to divide cash flows into two classes: *operating cash flows* and *other cash flows.* **Operating cash flows** are those that arise from normal operations, and they are, in essence, the difference between sales revenues and cash expenses plus taxes paid. Other cash flows arise from the issuance of stock, from borrowing, or from the sale of fixed assets, as illustrated by CBS's recent sale of its toy division for $200 million. Our focus here is on operating cash flows.

operating cash flows
Those cash flows that arise from normal operations; the difference between sales revenues and cash expenses plus taxes paid.

Operating cash flows can differ from accounting profits (or net income) for two primary reasons:

1. All the taxes reported on the income statement may not have to be paid during the current year, or, under certain circumstances, the actual cash payments for taxes may exceed the tax figure deducted from sales to calculate net income. The reasons for these tax cash flow differentials are discussed in detail in accounting courses.

2. Sales may be on credit and hence do not represent cash, and some of the expenses (or costs) deducted from sales to determine profits may not be cash costs. Thus operating cash flows could be larger or smaller than accounting profits during any given year. We consider the cash flow implications of credit sales in a later chapter, whereas the effects of the major noncash expense, depreciation, are discussed in the next section.

Depreciation and Cash Flows

Table 2-6 shows how depreciation affects operating cash flows. Column 1 reproduces Gaylord Distribution Systems' 1987 income statement as it would be reported to the firm's stockholders. Column 2 of Table 2-6 shows the same income statement on a cash flow basis, assuming (1) that all sales were for cash, (2) that taxes and all costs except depreciation were paid in cash during 1987, and (3) that no buildups occurred in inventories or other assets. How much cash was generated from operations? In Table 2-6 we see that the answer is $19.3 million, and it can be found either by developing a cash flow statement, as in Column 2, or from the regular income statement by adding net income and depreciation. Assuming that sales were all for cash, the firm took in $401 million of cash money. Its costs other than depreciation were $360.3 million, and these expenses were paid in cash, leaving $40.7 million. Depreciation is not a cash charge—the firm does not pay out the $4.9 million of

Table 2-6 **Gaylord Distribution Systems Accounting Profits and Cash Flows for 1987 (Millions of Dollars)**

	Accounting Profits (1)	Operating Cash Flows (2)
Sales	$401.0	$401.0
Cost of goods sold (excluding depreciation)	280.7	280.7
Other operating expenses	79.6	79.6
Depreciation	4.9	n.a.
Total costs	$365.2	$360.3
Sales minus costs	$ 35.8	$ 40.7
Interest expense	12.6	12.6
Net before taxes	$ 23.2	$ 28.1
Taxes	7.9	7.9
Net before preferred stock dividends	$ 15.3	$ 20.2
Preferred dividends	0.9	0.9
Net available to common stock	$ 14.4	$ 19.3
Add back depreciation	4.9	n.a.
Cash flow	$ 19.3	$ 19.3

depreciation expenses — so $40.7 million of cash money is still left after depreciation. Taxes and interest, however, are paid in cash; thus $12.6 million for interest and $7.9 million for taxes must be deducted from the $40.7 million cash earnings before interest and taxes (EBIT), leaving a cash flow from operations of $20.2 million. Finally, $0.9 million of cash is paid out as dividends. The result is a net cash flow of $19.3 million. This is the same number we calculated in Column 1 by adding $14.4 million of net income and $4.9 million of depreciation expense. Thus, because depreciation is a noncash charge, it is added back to net income to calculate the approximate net cash flow from operations.

SUMMARY

This chapter presented some background information on forms of business organization and income taxes for both individuals and businesses. First, we saw that firms may be organized as *proprietorships,* as *partnerships,* or as *corporations.* The first two types are easy and inexpensive to form. However, corporations have major advantages in terms of risk reduction, ability to raise capital, and investment liquidity, and these features make it possible to maximize the value of any business except a very small one by using the corporate form of organization. Accordingly, corporations are the dominant form of business organization.

The value of any asset is dependent on the effective income it produces for its owner. *Effective income* means *after-tax income.* Because corporate in-

RESOLUTION TO DECISION IN FINANCE

Big Fix for Texas Taxes

The scenario of the imaginary Texas CEO is not as far fetched as one might think. The Texas legislature, which has struggled ineffectually for some time to overhaul the state's antiquated and poorly functioning tax code, commissioned a business-government tax task force in April 1987. The group has been given carte blanche to recommend a new tax system for Texas.

The state has been burdened by what the select committee's executive director describes as "a 1960s tax base working in a 1980s economy." Texas's top-heavy revenue system derives two-thirds of its funds from only three sources: a hefty 8 percent sales tax that impacts most heavily on middle-income citizens and the poor, a gasoline tax, and a production tax on oil and natural gas. The system, dependent as it is on a healthy oil and natural gas industry to generate revenue, has been limping along since oil prices began fluctuating in 1982.

The select committee hopes that its new tax plan will correct many of the inequities in the present tax system. Although individuals now bear a relatively small tax burden, the state's sales tax is highly regressive. Heavy manufacturing, public utilities, and the petroleum industry now foot the bulk of the state's corporate tax bill, whereas the service sector of the economy pays little or no tax. To make matters worse, a state court has ruled unconstitutional the property-tax system that funds the public schools.

The select committee is said to be considering a state income tax, and it is also studying Michigan's value-added tax as a model. Michigan, a state whose economy, like Texas, is greatly affected by the health of a single industry, adopted a value-added tax more than a decade ago in an effort to improve revenue stability. Replacing a handful of different business taxes, this "single business tax" is unrelated to profits but taxes instead the "value added" to a product in the form of material, labor, and so on at each stage of the production process.

The select committee has set high goals for itself, hoping to compile a report that not only makes specific recommendations but also sets forth a rationale for taxation that will influence legislators for decades to come. Even though the committee is not due to hand down its report until 1989, according to Bill Alloway, director of the Texas Association of Taxpayers, "They're dramatically elevating the tax IQ of the state of Texas."

Source: Adapted from Eugene Carlson, "Texas Tackles a Big Problem: How to Repair Its Tax Code," *The Wall Street Journal,* December 1, 1987, p. 37.

come is taxed at federal tax rates going up to 39 percent, and because personal income is subjected to additional federal tax rates of up to 33 percent, the tax consequences of various decisions have a most important effect on a firm's value. It is not necessary to memorize everything about taxes — indeed, this would be impossible. However, you should understand the basic differences between corporate and personal taxes, should know that interest is a tax deduction to the payer of the interest, should know how tax depreciation is determined, and so on. These matters will come up throughout the book as we examine various types of financial decisions.

The U.S. tax laws permit fixed assets to be depreciated over time, and the annual depreciation expense is a tax deduction. The current depreciation system is called the *Accelerated Cost Recovery System (ACRS)*. As we shall see in Chapter 14, where we discuss capital budgeting cash flow estimation, tax depreciation rules have a major effect on the profitability of capital investments.

Finally, a distinction was made between accounting profits (net income) and cash flows. Both concepts are important. Reported profits give investors an idea about how profitable the company has been during some past period and hence how well it may be expected to do in the future, whereas operating cash flows give both investors and managers an idea of how much cash the business is generating and thus has available for distribution to its owners or for reinvestment in profitable new projects.

QUESTIONS

2-1 What are the three principal forms of business organization? What are the advantages and disadvantages of each?

2-2 Suppose you owned 100 shares of General Motors stock and the company earned $6 per share. Suppose further that GM could either pay all its earnings out as dividends (in which case you would receive $600) or retain the earnings in the business, buy more assets, and cause the price of the stock to go up by $6 per share (in which case the value of your stock would rise by $600).
   a. How would the tax laws influence what you, as a typical stockholder, would want the company to do?
   b. Would your choice be influenced by how much other income you had?
   c. How might the corporation's decision with regard to dividend policy influence the price of its stock?

2-3 What does *double taxation of corporate income* mean?

2-4 If you were starting a business, what tax considerations might cause you to prefer to set it up as a proprietorship or a partnership rather than as a corporation?

2-5 Explain how the federal income tax structure affects the choice of financing (debt versus equity) used by U.S. business firms.

2-6 Explain the half-year convention and how it is used in current depreciation (cost recovery) computations.

2-7 Explain how the federal government can (and from time to time does) influence the level of business activity by adjusting the Investment Tax Credit.

2-8 For someone planning to start a new business, is the average or the marginal tax rate more relevant?

PROBLEMS

(Note: By the time this book is published, Congress may have changed tax rates and other provisions of the current law. As noted in the chapter, such changes occur fairly often. Also, note that many of the provisions of the 1986 Tax Act are phased in over varying lengths of time. Work all the problems on the assumption that all aspects of

the 1986 Act have been fully implemented, even though transition rates actually may apply to the year in question, and assume that the tax rates and other provisions as set forth in the text are still current.)

2-1 **Corporate tax liability.** In 1988 Reno Industries had $200,000 in taxable income.
   a. What federal income tax will the firm pay?
   b. What is the firm's average tax rate?
   c. What is the firm's marginal tax rate?

2-2 **Corporate tax liability.** Austin Sound Company had a 1988 income of $250,000 from operations after all operating costs but before (1) interest charges of $10,000, (2) dividends paid of $20,000, and (3) income taxes. What is the firm's income tax liability?

2-3 **Corporate tax liability.** Cupertino Computers had $200,000 of taxable income from operations in 1988.
   a. What is the company's federal income tax bill for the year?
   b. Assume Cupertino Computers receives an additional $20,000 of interest income from some bonds it owns. What is the tax on this interest income?
   c. Now assume that the firm does *not* receive the interest income but does receive an additional $20,000 as dividends on some stock it owns. What is the tax on this dividend income?

2-4 **Loss carry-back, carry-forward.** Alamo Steel has made $200,000 before taxes during each of the last 15 years, and it expects to make $200,000 a year before taxes in the future. However, this year (1988) Alamo incurred a loss of $1,200,000. Alamo will claim a tax credit at the time it files its 1988 income tax returns and will receive a check from the U.S. Treasury. Show how it calculates this credit, and then indicate Alamo's tax liability for each of the next 5 years. To ease calculations, assume a 30 percent tax rate on *all* income.

2-5 **Personal taxes.** Katharine Chapman of San Francisco has the following situation for the year 1988: salary of $60,000; dividend income of $10,000; interest on GMAC bonds of $5,000; interest on state of California municipal bonds of $10,000; proceeds of $22,000 from the sale of 100 shares of IBM stock purchased in 1982 at a cost of $9,000; and proceeds of $22,000 from the November 1988 sale of 100 shares of IBM stock purchased in October 1988 at a cost of $21,000. Katharine gets one exemption ($1,950), and she has allowable itemized deductions of $5,000; these amounts will be deducted from her gross income to determine her taxable income.
   a. If she files an individual return, what is Katharine's tax liability for 1988?
   b. What are her marginal and average tax rates?
   c. If she had some money to invest and was offered a choice of either California bonds with a yield of 9 percent or more GMAC bonds with a yield of 11 percent, which should she choose and why?
   d. At what marginal tax rate would Katharine be indifferent to the choice between California and GMAC bonds?

2-6 **Depreciation.** Mountain View Industries purchased two new assets in 1988. The first is a 3-year class asset and the other is classified as a 5-year asset for ACRS depreciation (cost recovery) purposes. The assets each cost $100,000 and may be depreciated under the ACRS 200 percent declining balance method. [*Note:* For ease of computation, assume that 22.0 percent of the 3-year asset's value is recovered (depreciated) in the third year and that 17.0 percent of the 5-year asset's value will be recovered in year 5.]

a. What depreciation expense will the company report for tax purposes over the next 5 years, if each asset has *no* expected salvage value?

b. How would your answer in part a change if each asset had a $20,000 expected salvage value?

2-7 **Depreciation.** Quantum Systems (QS) will commence operations on January 2, 1988. It expects to have sales of $200,000 in 1988, $250,000 in 1989, and $400,000 in 1990. QS also forecasts that operating expenses excluding depreciation will total 60 percent of sales in each year during this period and that it will have interest expenses of $12,000 in 1988, $15,000 in 1989, and $20,000 in 1990. QS will make an investment in fixed assets of $100,000 on January 2, 1988. These assets will be depreciated over their 3-year class life using the ACRS 200 percent declining balance method. [*Note:* For ease of computation, assume that 22 percent of the asset's value will be depreciated in 1990, with no remaining depreciation in 1991. Use the corporate tax rates from Table 2-2.]

a. What is the depreciation expense in each year (1988 through 1990) on the 3-year class life equipment?

b. What is QS's tax liability in each year from 1988 to 1990?

c. What is QS's cash flow in each year from 1988 to 1990?

2-8 **Form of organization.** John Murphy has published a weekly advertising supplement for years. He has operated his business as a sole proprietorship for several years, but projected changes in his business's income have led him to consider incorporating.

Murphy is married and has two daughters. His family's only income, an annual salary of $40,000, is from operating the business. (The business actually earns more than the $40,000, but Murphy reinvests the additional earnings in the business.) He itemizes deductions, and he is able to deduct $6,100. The deductions, combined with his four personal exemptions for 4 × $1,950 = $7,800, giving him a taxable income of $40,000 − $6,100 − $7,800 = $26,100. (Disregard the increase in personal exemptions in 1989.) Of course, his actual taxable income, if he does not incorporate, would be higher by the amount of reinvested income. Murphy estimates that his business earnings before salary and taxes for the period 1988 through 1990 will be as follows:

Year	Earnings before Salary and Taxes
1	$50,000
2	70,000
3	90,000

a. What would Murphy's total taxes (corporate plus personal) be in each year from 1988 to 1990 under:

1. A corporate form of organization? (1988 tax = $5,415)

2. A proprietorship? (1988 tax = $6,241)

b. Should Murphy incorporate? Discuss.

Part II

THE FINANCIAL ENVIRONMENT

The financial manager does not make decisions in a vacuum. Part II of this text describes the financial environment in which we all work.

The job of financial intermediaries is to efficiently transfer funds from surplus economic units to deficit economic units. Chapter 3 introduces the processes and the institutions involved in successfully converting savings to productive investments. Although large business firms deal with a variety of financial intermediaries, all businesses utilize at least some of the services provided by one type of intermediary — the commercial bank, which is discussed in Chapter 4. The chapter also describes the means by which the Federal Reserve System influences the economy. The economic health of the country is measured by interest rates; Chapter 5 examines the components which determine those rates.

Chapter 3

Financial Markets

Is Wall Street Losing Its Grip on Corporate America?

Business had been booming on Wall Street. The bull market had been running for so long that it seemed as if people had forgotten what it was like for almost any deal to go sour. Wall Street was thick with young millionaires. Then came the crash. On Monday, October 19, 1987, the market took a plunge that shook Wall Street like an earthquake. The Dow Jones Industrial Average, which tracks 30 blue chip stocks and is considered to be the pulse of the stock market, did a spectacular 508-point nosedive. In one stomach-churning day, the advances of the preceding years were vaporized, along with many investors' profits. The aftershocks sent over-the-counter stocks tumbling, along with stock markets around the globe. It seemed that panic, like data, could be transmitted electronically in the blink of an eye.

The effects of the crash were immediately apparent everywhere on Wall Street. Investment firms slashed their staffs, froze salaries, abandoned marginally profitable businesses, and trimmed their expenses. E.F. Hutton, the brokerage firm, was backed into a shotgun wedding

with its former rival, Shearson Lehman Brothers, and other companies put consolidation plans into the works.

But aside from the impact of the crash on Wall Street, what was its effect on Main Street Corporate America? The years leading up to the crash had spawned a strong symbiotic relationship among the stock market, investment banks, and corporations. Although it was, at times, an antagonistic alliance, many American corporations profited from their relationship with Wall Street. Financial wizards created a dazzling assortment of innovative financing vehicles that allowed corporations to raise money in new ways. Stocks, issued at a moment's notice, provided instant cash that could be further stretched with new debt offerings. Corporate raiders made millions buying companies whether they wanted to be bought or not. Suddenly, on October 19th, all that changed. Or did it?

As you read this chapter, think about the ways that the crash might affect American corporations in the long run. How might the ways that corporations raise money be affected? What might be the effect on the market for new stocks?

See end of chapter for resolution.

The duties of a financial manager, discussed in Chapter 1, can be distilled (with some imagination, perhaps) into two basic decisions that concern (1) the firm's investment in assets and (2) how those assets are to be financed. In this chapter we discuss the means by which necessary funds are made available to businesses and, specifically, the role of the stock and bond markets in raising money for business.

THE ROLE OF FINANCIAL MARKETS

At the risk of oversimplification, it can be said that financial markets exist to convert savings into productive investments. In other words, without financial markets, each economic unit[1] would have to be self-supporting. An individual business could not invest in additional assets unless they were financed with the firm's own current savings. Thus, without financial markets, every opportunity to invest would depend on the individual economic unit's ability to save.

Unfortunately, most economic units that have productive investment opportunities often do not have all the savings required to finance their projects. For example, suppose Potomac Electric Power Company forecasts an increase in the demand for power in the Washington, D.C. area and decides to build a new power plant. Because it almost certainly will not have the $2 billion necessary to pay for the plant, it will have to raise this capital in the market. Or suppose Mr. Jones, the proprietor of a Birmingham hardware store, decides to expand into appliances. Where will he get the money to buy the initial inventory of TV sets, washers, and freezers? Similarly, if the Smiths want to buy a home that costs $90,000, but they have only $20,000 in savings, how can they raise the additional $70,000? Also, if the city of Sacramento wants to borrow $20 million to finance a new sewage plant, and if the federal government needs $140 billion to cover its projected 1990 deficit, they each need sources for raising this capital.

On the other hand, because some individuals and firms have incomes that are greater than their current expenditures, they have funds available to invest. For example, Edgar Rivers has an income of $46,000 but his expenses are only $40,000, and in 1987 General Motors Corporation had accumulated about $2.5 billion of excess cash that it could make available for investment.

Entities wanting to borrow money are brought together with those having surplus funds in the *financial markets.* Note that "markets" is plural — there are a great many different financial markets, each one consisting of many institutions, in a developed economy such as ours. Each market deals with a somewhat different type of security, serves a different set of customers, or operates in a different part of the country. The following are some of the major types of markets:

---

[1]The most important economic units within the domestic economy are business firms, individuals (often referred to as households), and governments (local, state, and national). Although our comments are directly concerned with business firms, the statements are valid for the other economic units as well.

Physical Asset Markets and Financial Asset Markets. These terms must be distinguished. Physical assets (also called "tangible" or "real" assets) include wheat, autos, real estate, computers, machinery, and so on. Financial assets are stocks, bonds, notes, mortgages, and other *claims on assets*.

Spot Markets and Futures Markets. These are terms that refer to whether the assets are being bought or sold for "on the spot" delivery (literally, within a few days) or for delivery at some future date, such as six months in the future. The futures markets (which include the options markets) are growing in importance, but a detailed discussion of these specialized markets is beyond the scope of this text.

Money Markets. These markets are for short-term (less than one year) debt securities. The New York **money market** is the world's largest, and it is dominated by the major U.S. banks, although branches of foreign banks are also active there. London, Tokyo, and Paris are other major money market centers.

money market
The financial market in which funds are borrowed or loaned for less than one year.

Capital Markets. These are markets for long-term debt and corporate stocks. The New York Stock Exchange, which handles both the stocks and the bonds of the largest corporations, is a prime example of a **capital market.** The stocks and bonds of smaller corporations are handled in other segments of the capital market.

capital market
The financial market for long-term debt (one year or longer maturity) and equity securities.

Mortgage Markets. These markets deal with loans on residential, commercial, and industrial real estate, and on farmland.

Consumer Credit Markets. These involve loans on automobiles and appliances, as well as loans for education, vacations, and so on.

World, National, Regional, and Local Markets. Depending on an organization's size and scope of operations, it may be able to borrow all around the world or it may be confined to strictly local, even neighborhood, markets.

Primary Markets. These are markets in which newly issued securities are bought and sold for the first time. If AT&T were to sell a *new* issue of common stock to raise capital, it would be a **primary market** transaction.

primary markets
The markets in which newly issued securities are bought and sold for the first time.

Secondary Markets. These are the markets in which existing, outstanding securities are bought and sold. The New York Stock Exchange is a **secondary market** for securities because it deals in "used" as opposed to newly issued stocks and bonds. The firm receives no money when its stock sells in the secondary market, yet the existence of the secondary market insures an active market for the stock if more is issued.

secondary markets
The markets in which stocks are traded after they have been issued by corporations.

Although savings must equal investment, financial markets allow the savings and investment process to be separated. Thus savers do not necessarily have to have their own productive investment opportunities. Because savings and investment are rarely equal for individual economic entities, a healthy economy is vitally dependent on efficient transfers of funds from savers to firms and individuals who need capital; that is, the economy depends on *efficient financial markets*. Without transfers, the economy simply could not function. Potomac Electric could not raise capital, so the citizens in the Washington, D.C. area would not have enough electricity; the Smith family would not have adequate housing; Edgar Rivers would have no place to invest his savings; and so on. Obviously, a country's level of productivity, and hence its standard of living, would be much lower. It is therefore essential that financial markets function efficiently — not only quickly but also at a low cost.[2]

THE ROLE OF FINANCIAL INTERMEDIARIES

We have indicated that savings must equal investment, but we have not indicated how the process is implemented. Basically, the transfer of funds from saving units to those units with productive opportunities but not enough savings to initiate the investment process (we call these deficit economic units "borrowers") is facilitated by **financial intermediaries.** Financial intermediaries include commercial banks, savings and loan associations, credit unions, pension funds, life insurance companies, and mutual funds. These intermediaries aid the capital allocation process in several ways.

financial intermediaries
Specialized financial firms that facilitate the transfer of funds from savers to those who need capital.

By way of explanation, let's consider an economy devoid of financial intermediaries. Further, let's assume that a businesswoman, Ms. Rossi, has discovered a cure for the common cold but requires $400,000 to obtain the proper productive assets for manufacture and distribution of the product. She must find someone with savings to invest in her project.[3]

Ms. Rossi has several problems if no financial intermediaries exist. First, she must find someone with savings. Through family and friends, she finds a saver, Mr. Chapman. Ms. Rossi's problems are not over, however. In persuading Mr. Chapman to invest, Ms. Rossi will encounter several obstacles. First, Mr. Chapman may not have enough savings to cover the entire $400,000 investment; therefore, Ms. Rossi must search for more investors. Second, Mr. Chapman realizes that by putting all of his money into a single project, he is facing more risk than he would if he diversified by investing in several projects.[4] With this higher risk Mr. Chapman may require a greater return than Ms. Rossi wishes to pay. Third, Mr. Chapman may need to withdraw his funds for retirement or a financial emergency before the project is completed, causing

---

[2]When organizations such as the United Nations design plans to aid developing nations, just as much attention must be paid to the establishment of cost-efficient financial markets as to electrical power, transportation, communications, and other infrastructure systems. Economic efficiency is simply not possible without a good system for allocating capital within the economy.

[3]For the purposes of our example, the investment may be in the form of either an equity share or a loan.

[4]We discuss diversification and how it reduces risk in Chapter 15.

INDUSTRY PRACTICE

It's War on Insider Trading

No one on Wall Street ever flew as high or crashed as hard as Ivan F. Boesky. On November 15, 1986, Boesky, America's richest and best-known risk arbitrageur, agreed to pay $100 million in penalties to settle Securities and Exchange Commission (SEC) charges of insider trading. In addition, he agreed to plead guilty to one felony count carrying a prison term of one to five years and is barred from the securities industry for life. Boesky's fall from the pinnacle of wealth and power on Wall Street sent tremors through the financial world. The SEC's continuing investigation of insider trading is expected to bring down the careers and reputations of several other major Wall Street players. As a result, public confidence in securities markets has surely been diminished, and increased regulation of financial activity seems likely.

Boesky amassed one of Wall Street's most spectacular fortunes by acting as a risk arbitrageur. Arbitrageurs bid for announced takeover targets that they believe are undervalued in the marketplace relative to the price they will eventually fetch if a proposed transaction is consumated. Theoretically, arbitrageurs provide liquidity to the marketplace and assume risks that the rest of the market will not accept by gambling on the outcome of a business transaction in progress.

Their central role in the market for stocks involved in takeover attempts puts arbitrageurs in a unique position to profit from privileged information about the likely outcome of a particular deal. Dennis B. Levine, a 33-year-old

Sources: "End of Ivan Boesky Leads to Broader Probe of Inside Information," *Wall Street Journal,* November 17, 1986; "Disputes Arise over Value of Laws on Insider Trading," *Wall Street Journal,* November 17, 1986; and Ivan Boesky, *Merger Mania* (New York: Holt, Rinehart & Winston, 1985).

mergers and acquisitions specialist at Drexel Burnham Lambert, Inc., recruited Boesky to an insider trading scheme by first offering him free information about deals in which Levine was involved. Levine has admitted passing on information about merger negotiations in progress between ITT and Sperry, Coastal's bid for American Natural Resources, and a leveraged buyout of McGraw-Hill. Over time, the contacts between Levine and Boesky turned into a torrent, with Levine's telephone records showing hundreds of calls to Boesky, sometimes as many as 20 a day.

Had the relationship stopped there, lawyers say, the government might have had difficulty proving an insider trading case against Boesky. The SEC acknowledges, at least at the outset, that Levine didn't tell Boesky the sources of his information. Boesky, as an arbitrageur, didn't breach any privileged relationships with insiders. He might have argued that he didn't know he was receiving information Levine had stolen from his employer or had obtained from others who had stolen information. Moreover, stock trades by Boesky, who routinely speculated in the stocks of rumored and real takeover targets, wouldn't necessarily have corroborated claims made by Levine of trading on inside information.

But according to the SEC, Boesky was evidently so impressed by the quality of Levine's information that he entered into an explicit profit-sharing agreement with him. He promised to pay 5% of the profits from information that triggered a purchase of securities and from those profits earned on stock positions influenced by information obtained by Levine. In reaching this agreement, Levine made explicit what was already obvious — Boesky was getting inside information.

The two pledged themselves to secrecy and Boesky, using his vast capital and Levine's information, embarked on a highly profitable stock-buying spree. For example, the SEC alleges that Boesky made $9.2 million in profits from transactions in just three stocks — Nabisco, Houston Natural Gas, and FMC — involved in takeovers or restructuring. He also profited from trading Boise Cascade, General Foods, Union Carbide, and others. In all, the SEC says Boesky made more than $50 million in unlawful profits. His illicit earnings dwarf the unlawful profits earned by others accused of insider trading, including Levine.

The Boesky scandal renews controversy about the role of insider trading laws in securities markets. Although no one disputes that Boesky violated the law, some lawyers and economists wonder whether the vagueness of those laws and the SEC's aggressive enforcement of them doesn't act to inhibit the flow of information necessary for those markets to operate optimally. They worry that any legislation enacted in response to the Boesky affair may hamper the competitive interaction of traders, investors, and market makers, which gives the United States the greatest securities markets in the world. While only a handful of scholars advocate a repeal of insider trading laws, even the laws' supporters are sometimes troubled by the vagueness of the legal definition of insider trading.

As it now stands, in order for someone to be guilty of insider trading, he or she must receive or convey information in a violation of confidentiality. In addition, the individual must have acted with the intent to defraud and must have profited directly from the use of the ill-gotten

information. The rules, however, are fuzzy about some types of activity. For example, suppose an arbitrageur calls executives at two companies he suspects are merging. It would be illegal for either executive to impart the information that a transaction was pending, but it probably wouldn't be illegal for the executives' assistants to let slip the fact that their bosses have been involved in meetings all night — a valuable clue. But suppose the arbitrageur sends flowers to the assistants or promises to buy them dinner; that would fall into a legal gray area. However, if an arbitrageur pays the assistants, he's definitely over the line.

Some experts fear that the laws' ambiguity poses problems for securities professionals who want to obey the law and are confused about what types of actions are prohibited. They also worry that the laws' fuzziness creates obstacles for prosecutors bringing cases against inside traders. Securities analysts who call corporate executives with legitimate questions sometimes believe that fears about possible insider trading prevent them from getting revealing answers.

The Boesky case doesn't appear to have broken any new legal ground because Boesky's apparent offer to pay for inside information made it a blatant violation of the law. However, by exposing such a complicated and sensitive case, the SEC not only demonstrated its sleuthing tenacity but clearly served notice that the focus of its crackdown on insider trading has moved from the cabdrivers, printers, and assorted small fry on the periphery of Wall Street to the traders, investment bankers, and lawyers centrally positioned in the takeover game.

refinancing problems for Ms. Rossi. Any or all of these problems — search for investors, divisibility of savings (a saver may wish to invest more or less than a project requires), risk (which will drive up the investor's required return), and liquidity — may end the investment project before it begins. We see, then, that if productive investments cannot be financed, economic growth could stagnate.

Figure 3-1 **Diagram of the Capital Formation Process**

There are three traditional ways of transferring capital between savers and those who need funds. Direct transfers without intermediaries are possible, but they lack efficiency and security. Investment banking houses serve as intermediaries in indirect transfers and thus technically do not create their own financial claims. Financial intermediaries actually create new financial products such as checking and saving accounts, mutual fund shares, and insurance policies. The intermediary uses savers' funds to purchase borrowers' financial claims such as stock, bonds, and mortgages. The financial products offered by intermediaries are more compatible with savers' needs for safety, liquidity, or maturity.

1. Direct Transfers

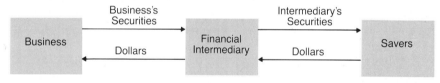

2. Indirect Transfers through Investment Bankers

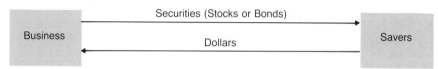

3. Indirect Transfers through a Financial Intermediary

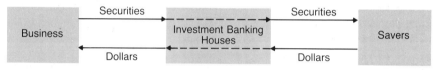

In a developed economy such as the United States', many of the problems encountered by entrepreneurs like Ms. Rossi are alleviated by financial intermediaries. Of course, not all transactions, even in a complex, developed economy, require the services of an intermediary. Transfers of capital between savers and those who need funds can take place in three different ways, as diagrammed in Figure 3-1:

1. *Direct transfers* of money and securities, as shown in the top section, occur when a business sells its stocks or bonds directly to savers, without going through any type of intermediary.

2. Transfers may take place through an *investment banking house,* such as Merrill Lynch, which serves as a middleman and facilitates the issuance of securities. Although they may serve as financial intermediaries in many respects, technically investment bankers are not intermediaries because they do not create their own financial claims. The businesses' securities and the savers' money merely pass through the investment banking house.

3. The bottom section of Figure 3-1 shows that transfers may occur through a *financial intermediary,* such as a bank or mutual fund, which obtains funds from savers and then issues its own securities in exchange. For example, a saver may give dollars to a bank, receiving from it a certificate of deposit, and the bank may then lend the money to a small business in the form of a mortgage loan. Thus intermediaries create new forms of capital — in this case a certificate of deposit, which is more liquid than a mortgage. This transformation of one financial claim into another that better meets the risk and return needs of the saver increases general market efficiency.

For simplicity, our example assumes that the entity in need of capital is a business, and specifically a corporation, although it is easy to visualize the demander of capital as a potential home purchaser, a government unit, and so on.

Direct transfers between businesses and savers are possible and do occur on occasion, but generally it is more efficient for a business to obtain the services of a specialized financial institution called an **investment banking house.** Merrill Lynch, Solomon Brothers, and E. F. Hutton are examples of financial service corporations that offer investment banking services. Such organizations (1) help corporations design securities with the features that will be most attractive to investors, (2) buy these securities from the issuing corporation, and then (3) resell them to savers in the primary markets. Thus the investment bankers are middlemen in the process of transferring capital from savers to businesses.

The financial intermediaries shown in the third section of Figure 3-1 do more than simply transfer money and securities between firms and savers — these intermediaries literally create new financial products. For example, an individual saver may not have the capital or the inclination to finance a new home mortgage for a borrower. A direct loan of this type would be quite risky, since the borrower could default and since, once the loan was made, the savings that were lent could not be withdrawn and would not be repaid for many years. However, a saver who deposits money in a savings and loan association is actually making an indirect loan to a home buyer. By opening a savings account instead of loaning money as an individual, the saver enjoys several advantages: he or she does not have to evaluate borrowers; the money is available on demand; and it is insured, within limits, by a government agency. Thus intermediaries repackage the original financial claims of borrowers into financial claims on themselves. Financial obligations of intermediaries are also called "indirect securities," because they represent a rearrangement of the borrower's original promise to pay into one that is more compatible with the saver's needs for safety, return, liquidity, and maturity. These indirect claims include checking accounts, mutual fund shares, money market accounts, passbook savings, and life insurance policies.

investment banking house
A financial institution that underwrites and distributes new investment securities and helps businesses obtain financing.

In addition, the cost of the intermediary's funds to the borrower will be lower than if a direct loan from the original saver could be negotiated. Because intermediaries are generally large institutions, they gain economies of scale in analyzing the creditworthiness of potential borrowers, in processing and collecting loans, and in pooling risks, thus helping individual savers avoid "putting all their financial eggs into one borrower's basket." These factors allow intermediaries to lend at lower rates than can individual savers. Further, intermediaries are better able to attract funds, since a system of specialized intermediaries can enable savings to do more than just draw interest. Thus people can put money into banks and get both interest and a convenient way of making payments (checking), put money in life insurance policies and receive both interest and financial protection in the event of early death, and so on.

In the United States and other developed nations, a large group of specialized, highly efficient financial intermediaries has developed. The situation is, however, changing rapidly, and different types of institutions are performing services that formerly were reserved for others, causing institutional distinctions to become blurred. Still, there is a degree of institutional identity, and the following are the major classes of intermediaries:

Commercial Banks. These are the traditional "department stores" of finance, serving a wide variety of savers and those with needs for funds. In fact, commercial banks continue to expand into an ever widening range of services, including stock brokerage and insurance. Historically, the commercial bank has been the major financial institution that handled checking accounts and that through the Federal Reserve System expanded or contracted the money supply. Today, however, some of the other institutions discussed here also provide checking services and significantly influence the effective money supply. Because commercial banks and the Fed play such an important role in the overall economy, their functions are discussed separately in Chapter 4.

Savings and Loan Associations (S&Ls). Traditionally serving individual savers as well as residential and commercial mortgage borrowers, S&Ls take the savings of many small savers, then lend the money to home buyers and other types of borrowers. The savers are provided a degree of liquidity that would be absent if they bought the mortgages or other securities directly. Therefore, one major economic function of the S&Ls is to "create liquidity" that would otherwise be lacking. Also, the S&Ls have more expertise in analyzing credit, setting up loans, and making collections than individual savers could possibly have; hence the S&Ls reduce the cost and increase the feasibility of making real estate loans. Finally, they hold large, diversified portfolios of loans and other assets and thus spread risks in a manner that would be impossible if small savers were making direct loans. Because of these factors, savers benefit by being able to invest their savings in more liquid, better managed, and less risky accounts, whereas borrowers benefit by being able to obtain more capital, and at lower costs, than would otherwise be possible.

Mutual Savings Banks. Operating primarily in the northeastern states, these banks accept savings primarily from individuals and lend mainly on a long-term basis to home buyers and consumers. Mutual savings banks are very similar to S&Ls.

Credit Unions. These are cooperative associations whose members have a common bond, such as being employees of the same firm. Members' savings are loaned only to other members, generally for automobile loans, home improvements, and the like. Credit union loans often are the least expensive source of funds available to an individual borrower.

Pension Funds. These are retirement plans funded by corporations or government agencies for their workers and administered primarily by the trust departments of commercial banks or by life insurance companies. Pension funds invest primarily in bonds, stocks, mortgages, and real estate.

Life Insurance Companies. These take savings in the form of annual premiums, invest the funds received in stocks, bonds, real estate, and mortgages, and then make payments to the beneficiaries of the insured parties. In recent years, life insurance companies have also offered a variety of tax-deferred savings plans designed to provide benefits to the participants when they retire.

mutual fund
Corporation that invests the pooled funds of savers, thus obtaining economies of scale in investing and reducing risk by diversification.

money market fund
A mutual fund that invests in short-term, low-risk securities and that allows investors to write checks against their accounts.

Mutual Funds. These are corporations that accept dollars from savers and then use these dollars to buy stocks, long-term bonds, or short-term debt instruments issued by businesses or government units. These organizations pool funds and thus reduce risks by diversification. They also gain economies of scale, which lower the costs of analyzing securities, managing portfolios, and trading in stocks and bonds. Different **mutual funds** are designed to meet the objectives of different types of savers. Hence there are bond funds for those who desire safety; stock funds for savers who are willing to accept substantial risks in the hope of very high returns; and still other funds that are used as interest-bearing checking accounts (the **money market funds**). There are literally hundreds of different mutual funds with dozens of different goals and purposes.

Historically, the financial institutions have been heavily regulated, with the major purpose of this regulation being to insure the safety of the institutions for the protection of their savers. However, this regulation — which has taken the form of prohibition of nationwide branching, restrictions on the types of assets the institutions can buy, ceilings on the interest rates they can pay, and limitations on the types of services they can provide — has tended to impede the free flow of capital from surplus to deficit areas and thus has hurt the efficiency of the capital markets. Recognizing this fact, Congress has authorized some important changes, and more will be coming along.

The major result of the developing changes is a blurring of the distinctions among the different types of institutions. Indeed, the trend in the United States today is toward huge **financial service corporations,** which own banks, S&Ls, investment banking houses, insurance companies, pension plan operations, and mutual funds and which have branches across the country and, indeed, around the world. Sears, Roebuck is, interestingly, one of the largest (if not *the* largest) financial service corporation. It owns Allstate Insurance, Dean Witter (a leading brokerage and investment banking firm), Coldwell Banker (the largest real estate brokerage firm in the United States), a huge credit card business, and a host of other related businesses. Other financial service corporations, most of which started in one area and have now diversified to cover the full financial spectrum, include Transamerica, Merrill Lynch, American Express, Citicorp, and Prudential.

financial service corporations

Institutions whose services include a wide variety of financial operations, usually including banks, S&Ls, investment banking, insurance, pension plans, and mutual funds.

THE STOCK MARKET

As noted earlier, secondary markets are the markets in which outstanding, previously issued securities are traded. By far the most active market — and the one of most importance to financial managers — is the *stock market.* It is here that the price of each stock, and hence the value of a business firm, is established. Since the primary goal of financial management is to contribute to the maximization of the firm's stock price, a knowledge of the market in which this price is established is clearly essential for anyone involved in managing a firm.

The Stock Exchanges

There are two basic types of stock markets — the **organized security exchanges,** which are typified by the **New York Stock Exchange (NYSE)** and the **American Stock Exchange (AMEX),** and the less formal over-the-counter markets. The organized exchanges have actual physical market locations, and because they are easier to describe and understand, we shall consider them first.

organized security exchanges

Formal organizations having tangible, physical locations and that conduct auction markets in designated ("listed") securities.

New York Stock Exchange; American Stock Exchange

The two major U.S. security exchanges.

The organized security exchanges are tangible, physical entities. Each of the larger ones occupies its own building, has specifically designated members, and has an elected governing body — its board of governors. Members are said to have "seats" on the exchange, although everybody stands up. These seats, which are bought and sold, represent the right to trade on the exchange. As recently as 1979, seats on the NYSE sold for as little as $40,000. Until June 1986, the highest price ever recorded for the purchase of a seat on the NYSE was $575,000; less than one year later, in April 1987, the cost of membership had increased to $1.1 million. However, the price of membership fluctuates with market trends. By May 1987, a seat on the exchange was offered for sale at $1,050,000, but the best offer was only $625,000.

Most of the larger investment banking houses operate *brokerage departments* that own seats on the exchanges and designate one or more of their officers as members. The exchanges are open on all normal working days, with

The trading floor of the New York Stock Exchange is the central location where registered members of the exchange meet to buy and sell shares for customers.

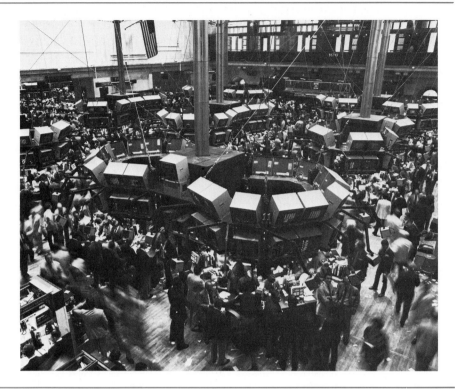

Courtesy of the New York Stock Exchange, Edward C. Topple, photographer.

the members meeting in a large room equipped with telephones and other electronic equipment that enable each brokerage house member to communicate with the firm's offices throughout the country.

Like other markets, security exchanges facilitate communication between buyers and sellers. For example, Merrill Lynch (the largest investment banking firm) might receive an order in its Atlanta office from a customer who wants to buy 100 shares of General Motors stock. Simultaneously E. F. Hutton's Denver office might receive an order from a customer wishing to sell 100 shares of GM. Each broker communicates by wire with the firm's representative on the NYSE. Other brokers throughout the country are also communicating with their own exchange members. The exchange members with *sell orders* offer the shares for sale, and they are bid for by the members with *buy orders*. Thus the exchanges operate as *auction markets*.

The Over-the-Counter Market

over-the-counter market
A large collection of brokers and dealers, connected electronically by telephones and computers, that provides for trading in unlisted securities.

In contrast to the organized security exchanges, the **over-the-counter market** is a nebulous, intangible organization. An explanation of the term over-the-counter will help clarify exactly what this market is. The exchanges operate as auction markets — buy and sell orders come in more or less simultaneously, and the exchanges are used to match these orders. But if a stock is traded less frequently, perhaps because it is the stock of a new or a small firm, few buy and sell orders come in, and matching them within a reasonable length of time would be difficult. To avoid this problem, brokerage firms maintain an inventory of the stocks. They buy when individual investors wish to sell, and sell when investors want to buy. At one time the inventory of securities was kept in a safe, and when bought and sold, the stocks were literally passed over the counter.

Today over-the-counter markets are defined as all facilities that provide for security transactions not conducted on the organized exchanges. These facilities consist primarily of (1) the relatively few dealers who hold inventories of over-the-counter securities and who are said to "make a market" in these securities, (2) the thousands of brokers who act as agents in bringing these dealers together with investors, and (3) the computers, terminals, and electronic networks that facilitate communications between dealers and brokers. The dealers who make a market in a particular stock continually quote a price at which they are willing to buy the stock (the **bid price**) and a price at which they will sell shares (the **asked price**). These prices, which are adjusted as supply and demand conditions change, can be read off computer screens all across the country. The spread between bid and asked prices represents the dealer's profit.

bid price
The price a broker or dealer in securities will pay for a stock.

asked price
The price at which a broker or dealer in securities will sell shares of stock out of inventory.

In terms of numbers of issues, the majority of stocks are traded over-the-counter. However, because the stocks of larger companies are listed on the exchanges, it is estimated that two-thirds of the dollar volume of stock trading takes place on the organized security exchanges.

Some Trends in Security Trading Procedures

From the NYSE's inception in the 1800s until the 1970s, the majority of all stock trading occurred on the Exchange and was conducted by member firms. The Exchange established a set of minimum brokerage commission rates, and no NYSE member firm could charge a commission lower than the set rate. However on May 1, 1975, the Securities and Exchange Commission, with strong prodding from the antitrust division of the Justice Department, forced the NYSE to abandon its fixed commissions. Commissions declined dramatically, falling in some cases as much as 80 percent from former levels. These changes were a boon for the investing public but not for the brokerage industry. A number of "full service" brokerage houses went bankrupt, and others were forced to merge with stronger firms. Many Wall Street experts predict that, once the dust settles, the number of brokerage houses will have declined from literally thousands in the 1960s to perhaps 20 large, strong, nationwide companies, all of which are units of diversified financial services corporations.

Stock Market Reporting

Information on transactions both on the organized exchanges and in the over-the-counter market is contained in daily newspapers as well as in specialized business publications such as *Investor's Daily* and *The Wall Street Journal.*

Table 3-1 **Stock Market Transactions, May 5, 1987**

| 52 Weeks | | | | Yld. | P/E | Sales | | | | Net |
High	Low	Stock	Div.	(%)	Ratio	(100s)	High	Low	Close	Change
				— A — A — A —						
33⅝	20⅛	AAR s	.50	1.7	20	381	29⅜	27¾	29	− ¼
37	21⅞	ADT	.92	2.9	18	317	31⅜	30⅜	31¼	+1¼
41½	23⅝	AFG	.12e	.3	11	1129	38¾	38	38½	+ ⅝
42	16¾	AGS		...	21	864	42	40½	41½	+ ⅝
13¾	6¾	AMCA		...	...	12	7½	7½	7½	...
9⅜	4⅞	AM Intl		...	...	1507	6⅝	6⅜	6½	− ¼
33¾	24½	AM Int pf	2.00	7.5	...	29	26⅝	26½	26½	− ¼
62⅛	47¼	AMR		...	12	7845	55⅞	54	55⅞	+2½
12⅜	8	ARX s		...	12	76	10¼	10	10¼	+ ⅛
73½	28¾	ASA	2.00a	3.1	...	740	66½	65⅛	65½	− ¾
20	9¾	AVX		1.7	96	202	19⅛	18½	19⅛	+ ¾
67	41	AbtLb s	1.00	1.6	25	7345	61⅜	59⅝	61⅜	+1⅞

Source: *The Wall Street Journal,* May 6, 1987, p. 58.

Although it is not within the domain of this text to delve deeply into the matter of financial reporting — that is more properly the field of investment analysis — it is useful to understand what information is available on the financial pages and how it is presented.

Table 3-1 represents a section of the stock market page for stocks listed on the New York Stock Exchange taken from *The Wall Street Journal* published on Wednesday, May 6, 1987. For each listed stock it provides specific data on the trading that took place on the previous day (Tuesday, May 5th in this case), as well as other more general information. Similar information is available on stocks listed on the other organized exchanges as well as those sold over-the-counter. Stocks listed on the NYSE are arrayed in alphabetical order from AAR Industries to the Zweig Fund; the data in Table 3-1 were taken from the top of the page. The two columns on the left show the highest and lowest selling prices for the stocks during the last 52 weeks. For example, AAR Industries, the first stock listed, has traded in a range from 33⅝ to 20⅛ (that is, from a high of $33.625 to a low of $20.125) during the last year. The figure just to the right of the company's abbreviated name is the dividend; AAR has a current indicated dividend of $0.50 per share and a **dividend yield** of 1.7 percent in 1987. Next comes the ratio of the stock's price to its annual earnings (the P/E ratio). Although controversy exists among analysts about the intrinsic value of the P/E ratio as an analytical tool, its existence on the financial page allows the computation of the firm's approximate earnings. In this case, AAR's earnings per share for the period are approximately $1.45. The P/E ratio is followed by the volume of trading for the day; 38,100 shares of AAR's common stock traded on May 5, 1987. Following the trading volume come the high and low prices for transactions and the stock's closing price on that trading day.

dividend yield
A stock's current dividend divided by the stock price.

Thus, on May 5, 1987, AAR's common stock sold as high as $29.375 and as low as $27.75. The day's last transaction, called the closing price, occurred at $29. The last column gives the change from the closing price on the previous day. Because AAR was down $0.25, the previous close must have been $29.25 on May 4, 1987.

The stock market page also provides other information about equity instruments. For example, the *s* following AAR, ARX, and AbtLb (Abbott Laboratories) indicates that these firms had a stock split or a stock dividend of 25 percent or more within the last 52 weeks. Quotations for other types of equity instruments, such as preferred stock, warrants, and rights issues, are also listed on this page. For example, in addition to its common stock, AM International has a quotation for an issue of preferred stock which pays a dividend of $2. Preferred stock is discussed in detail in Chapter 17.

Bond Markets

Corporate bonds are traded much less frequently than common stock, and more than 95 percent of the bond trading that does occur takes place in the over-the-counter market. The reason is that bonds are more likely than common stock to be owned by and traded among large financial institutions such as life insurance companies and pension funds, which deal in very large blocks of securities. It is relatively easy for the over-the-counter bond dealers to arrange the transfer of large blocks of bonds among the relatively few holders of the bonds. It would be impossible to conduct similar operations in the stock market among the literally millions of large and small stockholders.

Information on bond trades in the over-the-counter market is not published. However, a representative group of bonds is listed by the bond division of the NYSE and is traded on that exchange. Information on NYSE bond trades is published daily, and it reflects reasonably well the conditions in the larger over-the-counter market.

Table 3-2 presents a section of the bond market page in the May 6, 1987, issue of *The Wall Street Journal,* reporting the bond trades of May 5, 1987. A total of $43 million in bonds, representing 815 issues, were traded on that date, but we show only those of Alabama Power Company. Bonds can have any denomination, but most have a par (or maturity) value of $1,000. All of Alabama Power's bonds have a par value of $1,000; this is how much the company borrowed and how much it must repay when the bond matures. Because other denominations are possible, however, for trading and reporting purposes bond prices are quoted as a percentage of par. Looking at the first bond listed, we see that there is a 9 after the company's name to indicate that the bond is of the series that pays 9 percent interest; thus it pays 0.09($1,000) = $90 of interest per year.[5] Nine percent is defined as the bond's **coupon rate.** The

coupon rate
The stated, or nominal rate of interest on a bond.

---

[5]The Alabama Power bonds, like most in the United States, pay interest semiannually; therefore the company would send a check for $45 every six months to the holder of one of the 9s of 2000.

Table 3-2 **NYSE Bond Market Transactions, May 5, 1987**

Bonds	Cur Yld	Vol	High	Low	Close	Net Chg.
AlaP 9s2000	9.4	4	96	96	96	...
AlaP 7⅞s02	9.3	25	85	84⅝	84⅝	− 1⅜
AlaP 9¾s04	9.8	5	100	98	100	+ ¾
AlaP 8⅞06	9.6	10	92¼	92⅛	92⅛	...
AlaP 8¾07	9.7	4	90¼	90¼	90¼	−1
AlaP 9¼07	9.6	10	96¾	96¾	96¾	+ 1⅜
AlaP 9½08	9.8	5	96½	96½	96½	− ⅝
AlaP 9⅝08	9.8	11	97¾	96	97¾	+ 1¼
AlaP 12⅝10	11.8	44	106¾	106⅝	106⅝	+ ⅛

Notes:
1. *The Wall Street Journal* lists only those Alabama Power bonds that were actually traded on the NYSE on May 5, 1987. Since the company has a total of 31 separate bond issues, several did not trade that day.
2. All the Alabama Power bonds that traded on May 5, 1987, originally sold with 30-year maturities.
Source: *The Wall Street Journal*, May 6, 1987, p. 48.

current yield
The annual interest payment of a bond divided by its market price.

2000 indicates that the first bond must be repaid in the year 2000; it is not shown in the table, but this bond was issued in 1970 and hence had a 30-year maturity when it was issued. The 9.4 in the second column is the bond's **current yield,** which is the annual interest payment divided by the bond's closing price: Current yield = $90/$960 = 9.375%, rounded to 9.4%. Only 4 of these bonds traded on May 5, 1987. Because the prices shown are expressed as a percentage of par, the high, low, and close of 96 means that the price of the bond remained unchanged throughout the day at $960 (96 percent of $1,000 par). As with common stock, the net change column refers to the change in price from the closing on the previous trading day.

Alabama Power has been growing, and it has been selling bonds almost every year to finance its growth. As we see in Chapters 5 and 17, interest rates vary over time, and companies generally set their coupon rates at levels that reflect the going rate of interest. If rates were set lower, investors simply would not buy the bonds, and the company could not borrow the money it needed. The fact that the coupon rates shown in the table rise as we move down the list indicates the general rise in interest rates after 1970.

Bond prices reflect how much investors are willing to pay for bonds, given their riskiness, as well as the interest they pay and interest rates available elsewhere in the economy. Alabama Power's 9s of 2000 were worth $1,000 when they were issued in 1970, but people were not willing to pay $1,000 in the spring of 1987 for a bond that would provide only $90 of interest per year when $1,000 would purchase a newer bond that would pay $100 or more in interest annually. Thus the 9s of 2000 have fallen in price from $1,000 when issued in 1970 to $960 in 1987 because competitive interest rates have risen.

We will discuss interest rates in Chapter 5 and how investors determine the price of these debt instruments in Chapter 17.

Regulation of Security Markets

Sales of new and existing securities on the organized exchanges as well as through the over-the-counter markets are regulated by the **Securities and Exchange Commission (SEC)** and, to a lesser extent, by each of the 50 states. The actions of investment bankers are also prescribed by the SEC. Certain rules apply to the issuance of new securities, whereas other rules apply to existing securities traded in the secondary markets.

1. **Elements in the Regulation of New Issues by the SEC:**

    a. The SEC has jurisdiction over all interstate offerings to the public in amounts of $1,500,000 or more.

    b. Securities must be registered with the SEC at least 20 days before they are publicly offered. The **registration statement** provides financial, legal, and technical information about the company. A **prospectus** summarizes this information for use in selling the securities. SEC lawyers and accountants analyze both the registration statement and the prospectus. If the information is inadequate or misleading, the SEC will delay or stop the public offering.

    c. After the registration has become effective, the securities may be offered, but any sales solicitation must be accompanied by the prospectus. Preliminary or "red herring" prospectuses may be distributed to potential buyers during the 20-day waiting period, but no sales can be finalized during this time. The red herring prospectus contains all the key information that will appear in the final prospectus except the price.

    d. If the registration statement or prospectus contains misrepresentations or omissions of material facts, any purchaser who suffers a loss may sue for damages. Severe penalties may be imposed on the issuer, its officers, directors, accountants, engineers, appraisers, underwriters, and all others who participated in the preparation of the registration statement.

2. **Elements in the Regulation of Outstanding Securities:**

    a. The SEC regulates all national securities exchanges. Companies whose securities are listed on an exchange must file reports similar to registration statements with both the SEC and the stock exchange and must provide periodic reports as well.

    b. The SEC has control over corporate **insiders.** Officers, directors, and major shareholders of a corporation must file monthly reports of changes in their holdings in the corporation's stock. Any short-term profits from such transactions are payable to the corporation. The prohibition against trading on information which is not available to the public goes beyond those directly connected to the firm. Anyone who obtains information not available to the public from a corporate insider is prohibited from acting on this information to gain profits. The insider trading scandals in 1986

Securities and Exchange Commission (SEC)
The U.S. government agency that regulates the issuance and the trading of stocks and bonds.

registration statement
A statement of facts filed with the SEC about a company planning to issue securities.

prospectus
A document describing a new security issue and the issuing company.

insiders
Officers, directors, major stockholders, or others who may have access to information not available to the public about the company's operations.

and 1987 prove that the SEC is very thorough in finding those who attempt to make profits by trading on inside information.

c. The SEC has the power to prohibit manipulation by such devices as pools (aggregations of funds used to affect prices artificially) or wash sales (sales between members of the same group to record artificial transaction prices).

d. The SEC has control over the proxy machinery and practices.

e. Control over the flow of credit into security transactions is exercised by the Board of Governors of the Federal Reserve System. The Fed exercises this control through a **margin requirement,** which stipulates the percentage of the purchase price of the security that must be supplied from equity sources. Thus, if the margin requirement is 60 percent, the purchaser must initially supply 60 percent of the security's financing, and the remaining 40 percent (1 − the margin requirement) may be borrowed. The margin requirement has been 50 percent since 1974. A decline in the stock's price can result in inadequate coverage, forcing the stockbroker to issue a margin call, which in turn requires investors either to put up more money or to have their margined stock sold to pay off their loans. Without a margin requirement to ensure significant equity in any investment, such forced sales could further depress stock prices, setting off a disastrous downward spiral. Before the Great Crash of 1929, no equity margin was required to purchase stock, so many investors used 100 percent debt to obtain their securities. When prices fell, these investors were unable to cover their debt, forcing the sale of their securities at successively lower and lower values. Thus, without the stabilizing influence of a margin requirement, the spiral of lower prices and margin calls was an important contributor to the 1929 stock market crash.

margin requirement
Minimum percentage of equity that must be used to purchase a security.

3. State Regulations:

a. States have some control over the issuance of new securities within their boundaries. This control is usually exercised by a "corporation commissioner" or an official with a similar title.

b. State laws relating to security sales are called **Blue Sky Laws** because they were put into effect to keep unscrupulous promoters from selling securities that offered the blue sky but actually had little or no asset backing.

Blue Sky Laws
State laws that prevent the sale of securities that have little or no asset backing.

In general, government regulation of securities trading is designed to insure that investors receive information that is as accurate as possible, that no one artificially manipulates (that is, drives up or down) the market price of a given stock, and that corporate insiders do not take advantage of their position to profit in their companies' stocks at the expense of other stockholders. Neither the SEC nor the state regulators can prevent investors from making foolish decisions or from having bad luck, but they can and do help investors obtain the best data possible for making sound investment decisions.

MARKET EFFICIENCY

During the last decade and a half, financial research has centered on the question of capital market efficiency. These studies of efficiency have been concerned with how effectively stock prices reflect value. Efficiency in this context refers to the ability of stock prices to (1) react quickly to new information and (2) reflect, at any point in time, all available information about the securities.

Requirements for an **efficient capital market** are relatively few and realistic in today's investment world. First and perhaps foremost, there must be a reasonably large number of profit-seeking individuals engaged in security analysis who operate independently from one another. Second, the investors should have quick and full access to any news about present and potential investments. Announcements of new information will be disseminated as soon as the news breaks; thus new information will come to the market in a random fashion. Finally, the efficient market hypothesis assumes that investors are rational in that they will act quickly to adjust security prices in light of new information.

One of the critical requirements for an efficient market is the free flow of reliable information to analysts and investors. The SEC and other government agencies have labored to insure that accurate information is quickly disseminated and that no special interest group is able to profit from special access to nonpublic information. The majority of academic studies, found in summary form in most textbooks on security analysis, agree that financial markets, although not perfect, are very efficient. An efficient market is therefore one in which security prices adjust rapidly to new information, reflecting all available information including the risk associated with a particular security.

The basic nature of all financial decisions is the trade-off between possible risk and expected return. In an efficient market, securities will be priced to reflect the risks involved, with higher-risk issues providing the larger expected returns (as illustrated by Figure 3-2). This suggests that the proposed trade-off between risk and return should prevail in a rational economic environment. If investors are unwilling to accept financial risk, they should invest in low return but riskless Treasury bills. If they desire higher returns, however, they must be willing to accept greater levels of risk. Thus, as investors move from the riskless Treasury bills to riskier securities, they accept more risk in the expectation of receiving higher returns.

Studies of the realized returns of securities in the capital markets have supported the concept of a trade-off between risk and return. In one such study by Ibbotson and Sinquefield,[6] which covered the investment period from 1927 to 1981, the securities with the least risk (Treasury bills) were found to have provided the lowest rate of return, whereas the class of securities with

efficient capital market
Market in which securities are fairly priced in the sense that the price reflects all publicly available information on each security.

[6]Roger G. Ibbotson and Rex A. Sinquefield, *Stocks, Bonds, Bills, and Inflation: The Past and the Future* (Charlottesville, Va.: Financial Analysts Research Foundation, 1982).

Figure 3-2 **Risk and Expected Returns on
Different Classes of Securities**

The risk/return trade-off in the financial markets is shown in this figure. An investor
willing to invest in the most risky security, common stock, has the potential to earn
the highest rate of return. Investing in the least risky security, Treasury bills, will
provide the lowest return. This risk/return trade-off hypothesis has been empirically
demonstrated in a study by Ibbotson and Sinquefield covering 55 years.

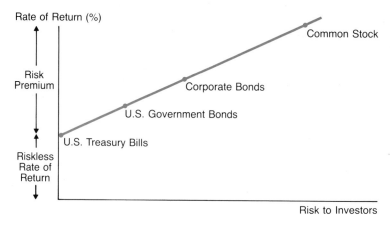

the most risk (common stock) provided the highest rate of return.[7] Therefore,
because of the efforts of the SEC, which insures that financial information is
quickly and accurately provided, and the competition among many analysts,
financial markets appear to be efficient in pricing securities relative to their
risk.

---

[7]A word of caution is probably necessary at this point. Remember that this and other studies
were based on past data for many securities over long periods of time. A selected high-risk
security may not provide superior returns over any time period. After all, if high-risk securities
always provided the highest returns, there would be no risk.

SMALL BUSINESS

Venture Capital Finance: Money and Help

A small business manager who believes his or her business has the potential for fast growth to a substantial size may want to consider enlisting venture capital support. Many small business owners think of venture capital as nothing more than a source of financing, and one that is not very appealing. Some believe that the venture capitalist will try to steal a large share of the business for a small investment. For that reason, venture capitalists are sometimes mistakenly called "vulture capitalists."

What does venture capital add to a small firm with high potential? A high-quality venture capital partner early in the life of a small business will greatly increase the business's chances of becoming successful. The reason is that venture capitalists offer more than money: they offer a broad range of experience in working with companies that have achieved exactly what the small business owner is seeking. They have helped other companies develop markets, control their finances, attract and keep personnel, and prepare themselves for a public offering of stock or a sellout to a larger firm.

One of the most successful venture deals ever occurred when Technology Venture Investors (TVI) invested $500,000 in Microsoft in 1981. Microsoft, the highly successful software company, did not need financing at all. It accepted the equity investment so that it could obtain the benefit of TVI's help in designing the right strategy for the firm. In return, TVI got a small piece of Microsoft's equity. With that help, Microsoft became the darling of Wall Street in a public stock offering in 1985.

Thus, a venture capital partner is more than a mere source of financing. The small business owner, therefore, must look well beyond the surface to find a good venture capital partner. Perhaps most importantly, there should be a good fit between the two parties. They should get along well and be motivated by similar goals for the firm.

What Venture Capital Is

A recent PhD dissertation describes venture capital as "capital bundled with consulting." When a firm and a venture capital team come to terms, several benefits should be achieved. In essence, the venture capital team becomes a part of the firm. First, it invests its money to receive a share of the business or a stake in future revenues or profits. Next, the venture capitalist probably will place on the young firm's board of directors someone who brings expertise that the firm is lacking. Of course the board member will look out for the interests of the venture capitalist, but he or she also will help management find key employees, possibly including a CEO, and will serve as a consultant to the company—a consultant motivated by a share of the firm.

Venture capital, then, offers financing and more. It includes management expertise and consulting, assistance with finding key employees, assistance with planning the direction of the firm and its strategies, and assistance in avoiding the pitfalls that cause so many promising young companies to fail. It frequently also includes a commitment to provide later rounds of financing that are commonly needed after a venture gets off the ground; such agreements are subject to management achieving targets in sales or profits.

How Venture Capital Is Found

To attract venture capital, the company must start with a well-developed business plan. Because venture capitalists often see hundreds of business plans a year, the plan must effectively sell the company without going into excessive detail. Brevity ensures that the plan gets read. If key factors can't be covered briefly, they should be relegated to appendices or exhibits so that the general theme can be seen without them.

Once the business plan has been prepared and critiqued by successful business people, it can be distributed. Some venture capitalists specialize in true start-ups, but most will want to see that the idea or product has been developed at least to the stage that it can be market-tested. If the firm has a track record of profitable operations for several years and is ready to move ahead to the next growth level, so much the better.

Frustrating as it may seem, a business plan will not stir the interest of every venture capitalist. A new entrepreneur should expect to send the plan to numerous parties before even an interview may be granted.

Many states now have venture capital fairs at which entrepreneurs can present their proposals to a room full of potential investors. If those are available in the area — or even outside the area — they are well worth attending.

Why Proposals Fail

Venture capital proposals are rejected for many reasons. The most common is that the firm's proposal doesn't fit the capitalist's interests. Venture capital firms often specialize in certain fields and will not fund proposals outside of those fields. For example, some will fund only electronics, and some, as a matter of policy, will not consider electronics; some focus on start-ups, whereas others will not deal with start-ups.

The two other most common reasons that proposals fail are financial and managerial. Venture deals are inherently very risky; a large proportion of them fail completely, in spite of careful screening. Therefore, a deal cannot promise merely a healthy rate of return, it must promise a return consistent with very high risk. Venture deals are often expected to satisfy hurdle rates of 15 to 25 percent over safe, short-term investments. Thus, if the deal promises a "secure" income, venture capital isn't the right source of financing.

Venture capitalists and others who study small businesses find that poor-quality management is one of the most important causes of business failure. As a result, the venture capitalist will probe deeply to find out who is on the management team, what their experience is, what their strengths are, how committed they are, and how well they work with others. Management problems often constitute the pivotal factor in the decision to fund or not fund the deal.

The Nature of the Deal

Venture capitalists encounter many deals, and they see many failures. Therefore, they can be expected to deal in no-nonsense, hard-nosed terms. Because they realize that even a well-researched proposal has a high likelihood of failing, they must do extremely well on those deals that do succeed. As a result, venture capitalists will ask for a sufficient piece of the business to earn them a high rate of return if the business succeeds. Many owners are reluctant to accept such terms. However, the owner who wants to be greedy with the company would be well advised to remember the examples of successful entrepreneurs. Mitch Kapor of Lotus Development Corporation, for example, might today own 100 percent of a very small business (or a bankrupt one) rather than a minority share of a business worth hundreds of millions of dollars. He could not have achieved the dominance of the software market that he did achieve without the money and able assistance of Ben Rosen and the Sevin-Rosen venture team.

In addition to wanting a sizable piece of the deal's profits, venture projects are also financed through convertible debt. The convertible debt is better than straight equity for the venture capitalist, because it provides protection on the downside and it allows the venture capitalist to share (by conversion) on the upside.

The deal that is struck may contain a provision for the removal of current management. Such a provision is anathema to an entrepreneur who can't imagine being removed from a company of his or her own creation, but it is there for a good reason. If this management cannot achieve the goals that have been agreed to, it is better *for all parties concerned* to get someone who can. The provision is tough, but it is often essential to the success or failure of a proposal.

The Venture Team Must Also Sell

The venture capitalist doesn't make all the decisions about whether or not to "do a deal"; he or she must also sell the entrepreneur on the venture team. The venture capitalist should start out the first meeting with a capsule of the team's experience and with a set of references. Just as the venture capitalist will check numerous references and background information on

the entrepreneur, the entrepreneur should very carefully check the venture capitalist's background. Has this individual or team been successful in helping companies grow to the public offering or acquisition stage in the past? What do former clients think about the venture capitalist's contribution to the success of the venture? The entrepreneur may also call up others in the venture capital community for references, or may ask a banker to do some checking for him or her.

Venture capital is risk capital. For it to succeed in helping a young firm grow and flourish, there must be an excellent fit between the entrepreneur and the venture firm.

SUMMARY

Financial markets exist in a dynamic economy because the savings of individual economic units and their investment opportunities are seldom equal. Because few economic units are fully self-supporting, financial markets must transfer savings from surplus units to deficit units that have productive investment opportunities.

Financial intermediaries facilitate the transfer of funds from savers to the firms and individuals who need capital. Financial intermediaries perform several services, including (1) bringing savings and deficit units together and (2) reducing the saver's risk by converting the ultimate borrower's financial promises into the intermediary's own financial claims, which are more consistent with the saver's requirements for investment amount, risk (including liquidity), and return.

For business firms, retained earnings represent corporate savings from year to year. When these savings are insufficient for investment needs, corporations must either sell more equity or borrow from lenders in the money or capital markets.

The capital market is the market wherein long-term debt and equity capital is acquired. Although some direct financing exists, most transactions take place on either the organized exchanges or in the over-the-counter market. Primary market sales raise new capital, and sales in the secondary market provide a source of liquidity for current investors.

The money market is the short-term component of the financial system. The chief financial intermediary in this market is the commercial bank, and in the next chapter we investigate the role of banks in the financial system. We also examine the Federal Reserve System's attempts to control the economy by manipulation of the money supply, principally through the banking system.

RESOLUTION TO DECISION IN FINANCE

Is Wall Street Losing Its Grip on Corporate America?

Although all the ramifications may not yet be clear, the stock market crash certainly acted to change Wall Street's relationship with thousands of companies—a relationship that had become a major force in the American economy. Some on Wall Street still eagerly assert that the crash did little to diminish their role in the financing of Corporate America. "Wall Street's relationship with Corporate America could be closer than ever," speculates Robert S. Pirie, the president of Rothschild Inc., an investment bank. "The easy-money days are behind us; Corporate America will need Wall Street as never before" to find new ways of raising capital. Chrysler Corporation Treasurer Frederic Zuckerman may not share Mr. Pirie's optimism about Wall Street's vital role, but he certainly agrees that it is going to be much more difficult for companies to raise money than it has been in the past. According to Zuckerman, the days when a financial officer, when asked to line up money for a major project, could "step up and say to his chairman, 'Piece of cake'" are definitely over.

There are clear signs that while money is in short supply, Corporate America may be looking away from Wall Street and back to more traditional sources, such as commercial banks and insurance companies, when it comes time to raise capital.

Source: Steve Swartz and Bryan Burrough, "The Aftermath: Crash Could Weaken Wall Street's Grip on Corporate America," *The Wall Street Journal,* December 29, 1987, 1, 4.

In the 1980s, during the stock market's heyday, investment banks filled their coffers by working both sides of the street. They fueled the corporate takeover boom by helping raiders unseat managements and break up companies. But they also helped corporations defensively restructure to help ward off unwelcome takeover attempts. They counseled American companies to take on extra debt, sell valuable assets, and concoct lucrative compensations packages, called golden parachutes, for executives facing dismissal in the course of a takeover.

The crash almost certainly marked the beginning of a slowdown in takeover activity. Says Donald G. Drapkin, vice chairman of Revlon Group Inc., the acquisitive consumer-goods concern, "The financing environment is very difficult. The initial-public-offering market is dead. . . . Investment bankers are petrified." Of course, with stock prices way down, a few cash-rich raiders may find a legion of takeover bargains.

Although investment bankers may bemoan a falloff in mergers and acquisitions, many corporate executives are hoping that takeover activity will slow way down and stay that way. They say that they would like to foster long-term growth rather than fret over next quarter's earnings. They want to worry about their bottom lines instead of whether they should restructure their companies to ward off unwelcome suitors. "Corporate America has got to get back to its knitting," asserts Texas entrepreneur H. Ross Perot. To that many corporate executives say, "Amen."

QUESTIONS

3-1   What would happen to the standard of living in the United States if people lost faith in the safety of our financial institutions? Explain.

3-2   How does a cost-efficient capital market hold down the prices of goods and services?

3-3   In what way does the secondary market contribute to the efficient functioning of the primary market?

3-4   What is the financial intermediary's primary role in the economy?

3-5   What are the most important services provided by financial intermediaries?

3-6   What would happen to required rates of return if no financial intermediaries existed?

PROBLEMS

3-1   **Stock quotations.** Look up IBM's common stock in *The Wall Street Journal* or another appropriate financial publication.
   a. On what exchange is the stock listed?
   b. What is the dividend per share based on the latest quarterly payment?
   c. What is the stock's dividend yield?
   d. What is the price/earnings ratio, based on the closing price, and the most recent 12 months' earnings per share?
   e. Based on the P/E multiple, what is the most recent 12 months' earnings per share for the firm?
   f. How many shares were sold on the trading day you investigated?
   g. How much did the stock's price rise or fall from the close of the previous day's trading?
   h. Is the stock's closing price closer to the stock's high or low for the year?

3-2   **Bond quotations.** Look up General Motors Acceptance Corporation's bonds in *The Wall Street Journal* or another appropriate financial publication. The firm's bonds are identified by "GMA" in *The Wall Street Journal*'s bond listings. Specifically, answer the following questions based on GMA's 8⅞99 bond. (*Note:* If this bond is not listed in *The Wall Street Journal* when you are working on this problem, choose another GMA bond with a similar coupon and maturity.)
   a. On what exchange is the bond listed?
   b. In what year will the bond mature?
   c. How much interest will the investor receive during the year?
   d. If an investor purchased the bond at the end of the trading day, what price would be paid?
   e. What was the bond's price at the close of the previous day's trading?
   f. Was the bond selling above, below, or at par?
   g. If General Motors Acceptance Corporation were to sell a new issue of bonds, approximately what coupon rate would be required for the issue to sell at par?

Chapter 4

The Commercial Banking System

 DECISION IN FINANCE

A New Chairman for the Fed

When Paul A. Volcker reached into his pocket on June 1, 1987, and pulled out a tightly worded letter of resignation addressed to President Reagan, he ended an eight-year reign as chairman of the Federal Reserve Bank. Although his decision to step down was certainly based on numerous factors, many Fed watchers believe that mounting opposition from Reagan-appointed members of the Federal Reserve Board of Governors prompted Volcker to refuse a third term of office. The five other members are fiercely independent and not shy about voicing their economic views, which were often in opposition to the chairman's. The Board, dominated by pro-growth supply-siders, sees less inflationary threat from robust growth in the money supply than Mr. Volcker. But, having achieved his heroic stature at the Fed as an inflation fighter, Volcker was careful not to step down until he could be certain that his successor would carry on his highly effective crusade against inflation. When he and the President

met to discuss possible candidates for the chairmanship, economist Alan Greenspan's name was at the top of both their lists.

A conservative, chronically gloomy forecaster with a reputation for always putting the most pessimistic interpretation on any data, Greenspan is a rabid anti-inflationist. Not nearly as flamboyant as the 6'7", cigar-chomping Volcker, Greenspan took office in the fall of 1987, expecting to enjoy a long and quiet honeymoon period. But Greenspan was quickly put to the test. On October 19, or "black Monday," as it was quickly dubbed, the stock market plummeted a record 508 points in a single, nearly catastrophic day of trading.

As you read this chapter, think about the kinds of decisions that Alan Greenspan and the Fed's Board of Governors routinely must make. How do the Fed policies affect the country's economy? What might be the effects of a change in leadership at the Fed for American corporations? What actions might the Federal Reserve Board take in the wake of a financial crisis like "black Monday"?

See end of chapter for resolution.

In the previous chapter we evaluated the role of financial intermediaries, especially those who serve to channel long-term funds from ultimate lenders to ultimate borrowers. As important as these intermediaries are, if the single most important financial intermediary was to be identified, it would be the commercial bank. Unlike the financial intermediaries discussed in Chapter 3, commercial banks tend to lend for periods of one year or less, although they also provide intermediate-term loans of from three to five years and in some cases even longer.

Beyond a discussion of the commercial banking system's role as a critical component in providing needed financing for business, this chapter emphasizes the attempts of the Federal Reserve System (Fed) to regulate the economy, which it does largely through the banking system. We therefore review the tools available to the Fed for influencing the availability and cost of money and credit in the national economy. Our discussion of interest rate determination will continue in Chapter 5.

THE BANKING SYSTEM

The commercial banking system is the largest of all financial intermediaries. In fact, the financial assets of the banking system are almost as large as the assets of all other financial intermediaries combined. Furthermore, the bulk of all deposits in the U.S. financial system reside in commercial banks.

Especially since the passage of the Depository Institutions Deregulation and Monetary Control Act of 1980, banks have become virtual financial supermarkets, offering savings certificates, IRA and Keogh retirement plans, trust and leasing departments, and, of course, a wide variety of short- and medium-term loans for individuals, businesses, and state and federal governments. Banks are also important providers of mortgage loans.

Nevertheless, banks probably enjoy their lofty status in our financial system not so much because of this impressive array of services, but because of two other very important factors. First, the commercial bank is important to the economy because demand deposits are money, and the bank can create demand deposits through the extension of credit in the form of loans. Recently other financial intermediaries have gained the right to expand money and credit, but these efforts are *quite* limited when compared to the banking system. Second, banks are important because the Federal Reserve System works principally through the banking system to affect the money supply and, therefore, interest rates.

Sources and Uses of Bank Funds

A review of a typical commercial bank's balance sheet (see Table 4-1) provides information about the sources of bank funds and the uses to which those funds are put.[1]

---

[1]Although this presentation of the items that compose a bank's balance sheet is not technical, some readers may wish to refer to Chapter 6, Examining a Firm's Financial Data, before continuing with this chapter.

Table 4-1 **Balance Sheet of a Typical Commercial Bank**

Assets		Liabilities and Capital	
Cash	11.3%	Demand deposits	20.8%
Investments	23.8	Savings deposits	15.2
Loans	58.2	Time deposits	36.5
Other assets	6.7	Borrowed funds	18.3
Total assets	100.0%	Other liabilities	2.9
		Capital	6.3
		Total liabilities and capital	100.0%

Demand deposits, at one time the major source of bank funds, are deposits made by individuals, businesses, and government units that are available on demand, usually through a check. Thus demand deposits are the major source of liquidity for all economic units.

Today the most important sources of bank funds are savings and time deposits. *Passbook savings accounts* are deposits evidenced by entries in a passbook. Although banks retain the legal right to require 30 days' notice of withdrawal, they seldom insist on advance notice, allowing funds to be withdrawn on demand. In fact, a variation of the passbook account, the **NOW (Negotiable Order of Withdrawal) account,** allows withdrawals by check.

A **certificate of deposit (CD)** is a receipt for funds deposited in an institution for a specified time and interest rate. Generally, the interest rate on CDs increases with the term to maturity. Certificates of deposit were known but not widely used until Citibank of New York announced in 1961 that it would issue CDs in negotiable form. The negotiability feature allows the funds to be utilized before maturity. These CDs were specifically designed to attract business funds and other deposits in large denominations beginning at $100,000. Other certificates in much smaller denominations are available to individuals and other small savers. Unlike the larger $100,000 CDs, these savings certificates are not redeemable prior to maturity.[2]

In addition to deposits, banks may choose to finance a part of their assets with borrowed funds. A portion of these borrowings may be from the Federal Reserve System itself. As we shall see, however, banks are restricted as to the purpose and term of loans from the Fed. Therefore, a large proportion of bank borrowing takes place in the **federal funds market,** which essentially involves a bank with excess reserves lending funds to a bank that has a temporary need for reserves.

A bank's **capital account** is similar to a business firm's net worth or common stock equity account. This account reveals the owners' contribution to the bank's financing, both through the purchase of the common stock and through

demand deposits
Noninterest-bearing transaction deposits at commercial banks that are available on demand, usually through a check.

NOW (Negotiable Order of Withdrawal) account
A form of savings account that allows withdrawal by check.

certificate of deposit (CD)
A time deposit evidenced by a negotiable (for large-denomination CDs, generally $1 million or more) or nonnegotiable (usually denominations under $100,000) receipt issued for funds left with the financial institution for a specified period of time; rates of interest generally depend on the amount of deposit and time to maturity.

federal funds market
The market in which depository institutions lend reserve funds among themselves for short periods of time.

capital account
The account that represents a bank's total assets minus its liabilities.

---

[2]If a saver must redeem a certificate, the interest rate paid reverts to the passbook level minus an early-withdrawal penalty, generally three months' interest.

INDUSTRY PRACTICE

The Changing Face of Banking

Banking used to be a pretty cushy business — bankers hours . . . lots of special attention from the government . . . not much competition. Bankers could turn a nice profit by charging a healthy premium for funds loaned out while paying pittance for deposits. Until recently, bankers had little to fear but other bankers. But not anymore.

Commercial banks are overrun by competitors. Foreign banks, most notably the Japanese, are taking a bigger and bigger piece of the banking pie. New financial instruments concocted by Wall Street wizards and fierce competition from auto finance firms have kept some of the banks best customers, both large and small, out of the bank entirely. To make matters worse, overloaded foreign borrowers are balking at repaying their loans, cutting painfully into banks' profits.

Although banks used to be able to count on friendly protection from Congress, their old ally has turned on them of late. With the economies of many Third World nations staggering under the burden of their debts to U.S. banks, legislators are pressing banks to grant concessions to debtor countries. On the other hand, Washington is dragging its feet on whether or not to modify the 55-year-old restrictions of the Glass-Steagall Act. This legislation, which separates commercial and investment banking activities, effectively bars banks from such lucrative financial activities as insurance, securities underwriting, and mutual funds. As one would expect, banks and other proponents of bank expansion into Wall Street's exclusive domain assert that increased competition would only foster increased market efficiency. Meanwhile, Wall Streeters howl in protest and Washington wrings its hands and sits on the fence.

If Congress won't let banks compete more freely, bankers could take drastic measures. Some bankers are threatening open revolt, vowing to give up their bank charters altogether so that they can branch out into more profitable businesses. Even Alan Greenspan, chairman of the Federal Reserve Bank, says that banks must be allowed to move into other businesses to stay healthy. Critics argue that U.S. banks are too fragile to compete in such risky ventures as insurance and securities underwriting.

It is clear that something needs to be done. While the economy enjoyed a long period of healthy expansion, bank profits remain flat. Worse, nearly 20 percent of all banks insured by the Federal Deposit Insurance Corporation reported losses in 1986. The FDIC's chairman, L. William Seidman, predicts a rise in the number of bank failures as well.

Some of the problems can be blamed on oil-induced economic woes, but according to a study of U.S. banking by the Federal Reserve Bank of New York, there has been a general decline in bank profitability irrespective of geographic location. Big banks seem to be the worst hit. The oversupply of banks means that there are just too few borrowers relative to the number of lenders. At the same time, fierce competition from foreign banks and Wall Street has stolen a huge segment of the banks' business.

Meanwhile, banking costs have shot up. Before 1981 the rate of interest that banks paid depositors was regulated by Congress. Since then, the ceiling has been lifted and banks have to compete with money market funds by paying higher interest rates to lure depositors.

Source: Sarah Bartlett, "Are Banks Obsolete?" *Business Week,* April 6, 1987, 74–82; and Robert E. Norton, "Unleashing Banks on Wall Street," *Fortune,* September 29, 1986, 99–101.

But although banks are competing with a host of less heavily regulated financial institutions, they pay a hefty premium for the privilege of being banks. The rule of thumb is that for a bank to cover reserves, deposit insurance, and other regulated requirements, it needs to build in an extra 1.25 percentage points into the rate of a loan. The competition incurs none of these costs.

Corporate America, once the bankers' bread-and-butter customer, is now taking its business elsewhere. Less heavily regulated foreign banks can usually offer lower rates, whereas Wall Street has made it easier for major companies to raise money by selling commercial paper through the public markets. Just a few years ago U.S. banks dominated the list of the top ten worldwide; today, only one U.S. bank is on that list.

What is the American banker to do? Bankers are lobbying fiercely to be allowed to enter into other lucrative markets. In the meantime, many banks are trying to sell investment services such as merger advice or are financing leveraged buyouts. Other banks are cutting back, leaving foreign markets where they can no longer effectively compete.

All in all, the once staid U.S. banking industry finds itself in a maelstrom of change. How it weathers the conflicting forces of increased competition, losses from soft foreign loans, and changing regulatory constraints will determine whether U.S. banks will remain viable or become increasingly obsolete.

the undistributed profits which are retained by the bank. The total assets of the bank minus all liabilities equals the bank's capital.

The bank's capital provides a cushion to protect depositors from losses. Losses to banks generally occur from loans that cannot be repaid or from poor investments. These losses cannot be borne by depositors (customer deposits are liabilities to the bank), so they are charged against the bank's capital. Thus, if a bank had 60 percent capital, up to 60 percent of the bank's loans could be uncollectible and there would still be sufficient funds to pay depositors. Of course, banks do not have capital accounts equaling 60 percent of assets. The typical commercial bank has only 5 to 7 percent of its assets financed by the capital account. Thus the traditional banker's conservatism is well founded because loans or investments can decline by only 5 to 7 percent before the bank becomes insolvent. This low level of bank capitalization has also led banking to be among the most regulated of all industries. Yet, for all their regulation, the environment of the eighties has not been kind to banks. As Table 4-2 indicates, the largest quarterly losses in the history of banking have occurred during the decade of the eighties. The losses occurred in relation to loans from developing nations, the oil industry, and agriculture.

On the left-hand side of the balance sheet, the first asset one encounters is cash. Actually the account includes more than just vault cash. Part of the **cash account** includes "items in process of collection," which is the value of checks drawn on other banks but not yet collected. The cash account also includes funds that are required by law to be kept on deposit at the district Federal Reserve Bank.

cash account
The account that represents a bank's vault cash, float, and funds required to be kept on deposit with the Federal Reserve.

Table 4-2 **Largest Quarterly Loan Losses by Commercial Banks**

	Loss (in millions)	Quarter
Citicorp*	$2,500	2nd 1987
Chase Manhattan*	1,400	2nd 1987
Continental Illinois	1,160	2nd 1984
BankAmerica	640	2nd 1986
BankAmerica	338	2nd 1985
InterFirst (Dallas)	281	2nd 1986
InterFirst (Dallas)	249	2nd 1983
First City (Houston)	232	1st 1986

*Estimate
Source: *The Wall Street Journal*, May 20, 1987, 1; *San Francisco Chronicle*, May 28, 1987, 27.

Of the three components of the cash account, actual cash kept at the bank for daily transactions would be the smallest amount for most banks. First, banks are able to maintain relatively small amounts of vault cash because normal transactions generally result in approximately the same amount of cash deposits as cash withdrawals. Second, like other businesses, banks wish to keep their funds invested in productive, high-return assets. Excess cash is therefore channeled into more productive loans and investments.

A second use of funds is the purchase of securities for investment purposes. These securities are required by law to be of the highest investment quality. Typically, the majority of these securities are issued by the state and other political subdivisions in the bank's geographic area. U.S. Treasury securities also account for a large proportion of the bank's investment portfolio.

Investments provide a rate of return for a bank, but that is not their principal role. Banks are required by law to hold reserves equal to a certain percentage of their deposits. These required reserves must be kept as vault cash or as deposits at the district Federal Reserve Bank. The bank's investment portfolio provides liquidity in case more required reserves are needed. The investments must be of high quality so that they may be converted into cash quickly, with little chance of loss. The primary business of banks is to lend money in support of economic growth in their area. Fortunately, loans also represent an investment of funds with the highest rate of return. If there is not enough demand for loans or if the quality of demand is low, however, banks turn to investment in securities as a source of revenue.

Banks are the major source of short-term credit for the business sector. Historically, banks have preferred to make self-liquidating loans. In our agrarian past a farmer would borrow money to buy seed and upon harvest would repay the loan with the proceeds of the crop's sale. A modern equivalent of a self-liquidating loan would be a merchant's borrowing to increase inventory before Christmas. After Christmas the merchant would repay the loan from the proceeds of the holiday sales. These short-term loans were the historical rule

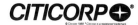
for banks because their primary source of funds was short-term demand deposits. However, with the greater proportion of funds now coming from time and savings deposits, banks are increasingly willing to provide intermediate, 3- to 7-year term loans. Some loans, such as real estate loans, are for even longer periods.

Approximately 80 to 85 percent of a bank's revenue is generated from interest on loans. Much of the remainder accrues from investment in state, local, and federal government securities. Service charges and earnings on other assets provide a small but growing source of revenue for the bank.

Demand Deposit Creation

In the United States the most important form of money is demand deposits, not currency. This means that commercial banks are at the heart of the nation's financial system. This status is not simply due to their role as conservators of the financial system's demand deposits but, rather, to the banking system's ability to create money.

As we shall see later in this chapter, the Fed requires a bank to maintain a stated portion of its demand, time, and savings deposits on reserve at the Fed or in vault cash. This means, of course, that the bank is not required to keep the remaining deposited funds at the bank and that these funds may be lent to others. For example, if the overall reserve requirement were 25 percent, a $1,000 deposit would result in a required reserve of $250 against the deposit liability. However, $750 of the deposit would be considered to be excess or free reserves, and it could be lent or invested by the bank. It is through its loans and secondarily through its investments that the bank makes a profit.

By lending excess reserves, banks create money. Assume for a moment that there are currently no excess reserves in the banking system and that the Fed's reserve requirement for deposits is 15 percent.[3] Suppose further that a customer deposits $1,000 in the bank. For that single transaction the bank's balance sheet would be increased by $1,000, as follows:

Assets		Liabilities	
Reserves	$1,000	Customer deposits	$1,000

Because the bank must maintain only 15 percent of the deposit as required reserves, $850 represents excess reserves. Since banks are in business to make a profit, they will wish to lend the money. Of course, the bank does not lend cash; rather, it simply credits the account of the borrower with $850. Thus the bank has created money through the granting of the loan, and its balance sheet will appear as follows:

Assets		Liabilities	
Reserves	$1,850	Customer deposits	$1,850

This is the first stage of a potentially large deposit-expansion process. At each stage in the process, both total loans and total deposits for the banking system increase by an amount equal to the excess reserves before the loans

---

[3]Actually, reserve requirements depend on the size and type of deposits at a commercial bank. See Table 4-4 on page 88 for a more complete explanation.

Table 4-3 **Deposit Expansion — Commercial Banking System**

		New Loans	Reserves Required	Reserves Excess	Total Demand Deposit
New demand deposit: $1,000			$ 150	$850	$1,000
Expansion stage:	1	$ 850	128	722	1,850
	2	722	108	614	2,572
	3	614	92	522	3,186
	4	522	78	444	3,708
	5	444	67	377	4,152
	6	377	57	320	4,529
	7	320	48	272	4,849
	8	272	41	231	5,121
	.	.	.	.	.
	.	.	.	.	.
	.	.	.	.	.
Final stage of expansion		$5,667	$1,000	$ 0	$6,667

were made. The increase in required reserves based on the deposit expansion of $850 is $128. Thus:

Total reserves gained from initial deposit		$1,000
Required reserves for initial deposit	$150	
Required reserves for first loan	$128	
Excess reserves after first loan		$ 722

Now these excess reserves of $722 may be lent to another customer seeking to borrow from the bank.

When the borrowed funds are used for purchases, the borrower will write a check that may be deposited in another bank. However, the movement of excess reserves from one bank to another will not end the expansion process in the system. Whichever bank receives the deposit also acquires an equal amount of reserves, of which all but 15 percent will be excess. In theory this process can continue through several stages until there are no excess reserves remaining.

The process of deposit expansion is presented in Table 4-3. It is theoretically possible for the commercial banking system to expand the original $1,000 deposit into $5,667 in loans, since banks need to maintain only 15 percent of each deposited dollar in reserves. We can determine the maximum possible expansion in deposits by using the following ratio:

$$\text{Total deposit expansion} = \frac{\text{Initial demand deposit}}{\text{Reserve requirement}}.$$

In our example:

$$\text{Total deposit expansion} = \frac{\$1,000}{0.15} = \$6,667,$$

which includes the $5,667 in loans and the initial $1,000 deposit.

Realistically, however, several factors prevent the full limit of credit expansion. First, if customers decide to keep portions of their newly created demand deposits in the form of cash rather than in the bank, there will be less available excess reserves to lend. Second, the bank may decide, as a matter of policy, to keep some excess reserves in the bank in case of unexpected contingencies. These excess reserves would be invested in high-quality, short-term marketable securities. The securities, often called **secondary reserves,** provide the bank with both income and liquidity. Third, the bank may have excess reserves that it wishes to lend but cannot find sufficiently qualified borrowers. Any or all of these factors create "leakages" that reduce the deposit-expansion potential within the commercial banking system.

secondary reserves
Excess reserves invested by banks in marketable securities.

THE FEDERAL RESERVE SYSTEM

Since commercial banks are at the center of the nation's financial system, a number of regulatory agencies have been developed to control the banking system and its ability to create credit. The most important of these is the **Federal Reserve System.** The Fed attempts to influence the ability of banks to create credit (and hence influence the money supply) principally by increasing or reducing the reserves available to the banking system. Later in the chapter we shall review the three major tools that the Fed may use to exercise control over reserves.

Federal Reserve System
The central banking system in the United States; the chief regulator of the banking system.

Organization and Structure

The Federal Reserve Act of 1913 allowed the country to be divided into 12 Federal Reserve Districts. The districts' operations are conducted through a Federal Reserve Bank located in each district. These banks are located in Boston, New York, Philadelphia, Cleveland, Richmond, Atlanta, Chicago, St. Louis, Minneapolis, Kansas City, Dallas, and San Francisco. Branches of the district banks are located in 24 additional cities.

The real decision-making authority in the Federal Reserve System is given to its **Board of Governors** in Washington, D.C. The seven members of the Board are appointed by the President and confirmed by the Senate. Even so, the framers of the Federal Reserve Act wished to keep the Board as free from political influence as possible. The seven Board members are appointed for terms of fourteen years, and their terms are arranged so that one expires every two years. Thus it would, in theory, take a President almost a full two terms to appoint a majority to the Board. However, resignations or deaths can create a faster turnover on the Board. For example, President Carter appointed five

Board of Governors of the Federal Reserve System
Seven-member decision-making authority of the Fed.

members of the Board in slightly more than three years. Thus, although the Fed has legal independence from the executive and legislative branches of government, great influence is still exerted on the Fed's policies by the political sector of the government.[4]

Another component of the Federal Reserve System is the organization of member banks. All national banks are legally required to be members of the System. In addition, approximately 10 percent of all state banks voluntarily joined the Federal Reserve System. One reason that more state banks did not join the System is that the Fed's reserve requirements generally were higher than the state-imposed reserve requirements. The **Depository Institutions Deregulation and Monetary Control Act of 1980** opened the Fed's services to all depository institutions for a fee. The same legislation removed the impediment of differing state and federal reserve requirements. After an initial phase-in period, the reserve requirements became the same for all depository institutions regardless of membership in the Federal Reserve System.

Another important element of the Federal Reserve System is the **Federal Open Market Committee (FOMC),** which has responsibility over **open-market operations.** Open-market operations are the purchases and sales of U.S. Government securities conducted through the Federal Reserve Bank of New York. As we shall see, open-market operations are the most effective monetary tool available to the Fed. Thus the FOMC is at the heart of the Fed's power. It consists of twelve members—the seven members of the Board of Governors and representatives from five of the twelve Federal Reserve District Banks. One of the five is always the president of the Federal Reserve Bank of New York, because this bank is responsible for the transaction of the open-market operations. The other four members rotate among the presidents of the remaining eleven Federal Reserve Districts.

Tools of Monetary Policy

The Board of Governors of the Federal Reserve System cannot dictate its monetary objectives to the banking system. By affecting reserves in the system, however, it influences the money supply and hence interest rates.[5] The principal tools of control are changes in the reserve requirements, changes in the discount rate, and open-market operations. Reserve requirements refer to the percentage of each type of deposit that deposit institutions must hold as reserves. Discount policy refers to the terms under which deposit institutions may borrow from the Fed. Open-market operations involve the purchase or sale of U.S. Government securities.

Depository Institutions Deregulation and Monetary Control Act of 1980
Act that eliminated many of the distinctions between commercial banks and other depository institutions.

Federal Open Market Committee (FOMC)
Committee of the Federal Reserve System that has responsibility over open-market operations.

open-market operations
The purchase and sale of U.S. Government securities by the Federal Reserve System.

---

[4]Even though the designers of the Fed attempted to shield it from political influence, it is difficult to believe the members of the Board of Governors are immune to political pressures. After all, Nixon designed plays for then Redskins coach George Allen; and it's an even bet that other presidents will provide subsequent Redskin coaches with some strategy in the future.

[5]The interrelationship of reserves, money supply, and interest rates is not a simple one and is open to much debate and controversy. The interested reader should refer to any of the many excellent money and banking or economics texts for further details.

Reserve Requirements

The Federal Reserve System requires all depository institutions to hold reserves against their deposits. The way in which these reserves are determined changed in February 1984. Previously, banks were required to compute their reserve positions based on a weekly average determined from average deposits two weeks earlier. Because of the delay, the system was called the *lagged reserve requirement.*

required reserves
The minimum reserves that a bank must hold as vault cash or reserve deposits with the Federal Reserve.

Under the new system, called the *contemporaneous reserve requirement,* the amount of **required reserves** will be based on the two-week average of checking account deposits ending on the second Monday of the period. Banks must settle their reserve requirements every other Wednesday, as before. However, with contemporaneous reserves the maintenance period begins after two days rather than after two weeks, as was done before.

The new system applies only to checking accounts. Other nontransaction deposit accounts continue to have their reserves computed on a lagged basis. Two-thirds of the nation's 40,000 depository institutions are exempt from the contemporaneous reserve requirement because of their small size. Nevertheless, 96 percent of all checking account deposits will still be covered by the new method.

It would appear that the reserve requirement could serve as a powerful direct tool in the management of banks' reserve position. In truth, however, the reserve requirement is seldom used. From 1963 to the implementation of the Monetary Control Act, reserve requirements on demand deposits were changed only five times, and those on savings deposits were changed twice. A summary of reserve requirements as of May 1987 is presented in Table 4-4.

Table 4-4 **Reserve Requirements of Depository Institutions**

Type of Deposit, and Deposit Interval	Depository Institution Requirements after Implementation of the Monetary Control Act	
	Percent of Deposits	**Effective Date**
Net Transaction Accounts		
$0 million–$36.7 million	3	12/30/86
More than $36.7 million	12	12/30/86
Nonpersonal Time Deposits		
By original maturity		
Less than 1½ years	3	10/6/83
1½ years or more	0	10/6/83
Eurocurrency Liabilities		
All types	3	11/13/80

Source: *Federal Reserve Bulletin,* May 1987, p. A7.

The major tools of the Federal Reserve System are used to influence depository institution reserves. Yet the Fed appears to be less willing to fully utilize a tool that directly changes required reserves. Why? Basically, the Fed's reluctance to use reserve requirements as an active tool of monetary policy stems from the fact that it is too powerful an instrument to be used in fine tuning the economy. Consider the effect of an increase in the reserve requirements in a tight money period. Even a 1 percent increase in the reserve requirements would increase required reserves by hundreds of millions of dollars. Furthermore, just as we have noted with the multiple expansion of credit when reserves increase, a decrease in excess reserves could further reduce demand deposits by a multiple many times larger than the original 1 percent decline in reserves as banks are forced to call in outstanding loans. Such a radical decline in money and credit would be potentially damaging to the economic system. Thus the potential effect of even a modest change in the reserve requirements makes it a tool that is seldom used by the Federal Reserve System.

The Discount Rate

The **discount rate** is the rate of interest that the Fed charges to institutions that borrow reserves. Institutions may find themselves temporarily short of reserves when there has been a large or unexpected shift in reserves, perhaps due to a large withdrawal. Institutions may also borrow from the Fed during times of tight money to relieve temporary reserve imbalances.

discount rate
The interest rate charged by the Fed for loans of reserves to depository institutions.

It is important to note that the Federal Reserve System views these loans as a temporary mechanism for the adjustment of the specific institution's reserve position. The Fed discourages the use of these funds for profit making. Moreover, these borrowings are considered to be a privilege and not a right. Thus the Fed can and does exert pressure on institutions to curtail their borrowings. Although the privilege of borrowing offers a safety valve to relieve temporary strains on reserves, there are strong incentives to repay borrowings quickly. For example, if a particular institution shows a borrowing pattern that is characterized by frequent or continuing indebtedness over an extended period, the Fed may press for repayment, even if it means that the bank must call in some loans or liquidate some investments. Therefore, banks are reluctant to use the Fed for other than temporary needs. In fact, some banks, particularly large banks, avoid the Fed altogether as a source of temporary credit.

When the Federal Reserve System was established in 1913, the discount rate was considered to be the principal instrument of monetary control authorized by Congress. Such has not been the case, however. As Figure 4-1 shows, the discount rate has lagged behind other short-term rates, such as the Treasury bill rate. The discount rate often follows movement in the prime rate as well. For example, the prime rate rose on three separate occasions in the late spring of 1987, from 7.5 percent in early April to 8.25 percent in late May, yet

90

Figure 4-1 **The Discount Rate and the Treasury Bill Rate, 1975–1987**

The Federal Reserve System makes loans to banks to correct temporary imbalances in their required reserves at a rate of interest known as the discount rate. First envisioned as a major instrument of monetary control, the Fed's discount rate has proven instead to lag behind other short-term rates. This figure, for example, shows how the Treasury bill rate led the discount rate from 1975 to 1987.

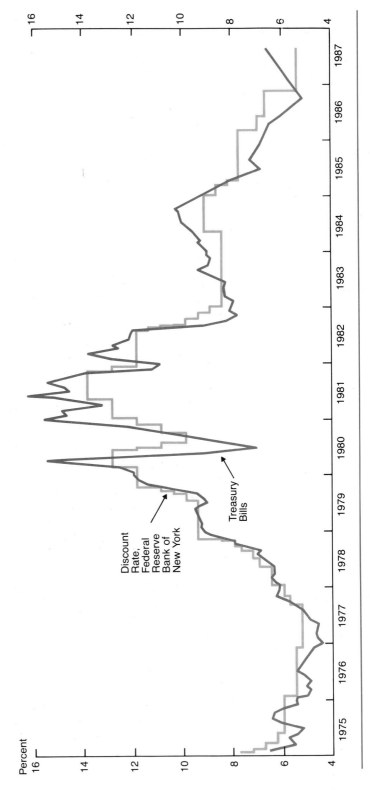

Source: Economic Indicators, September 1987, 30.

the discount rate remained at 5.5 percent during the period. Obviously, an effective instrument of monetary policy would lead, not follow, market rates.

Even though the discount rate is not the active tool of monetary policy that the Fed's founders envisioned it to be, announcements of changes in the discount rate have an important psychological effect in the financial community. Increases in the discount rate are thought to signal a movement toward tight money policies, for example. If such an announcement causes financial institutions to become more stringent in loan policies or causes businesses to reconsider expansion plans, the discount rate, in a roundabout fashion, has done part of its job.

Open-Market Operations

The ability to change both reserve requirements and the discount rate remains important to Federal Reserve monetary policy. However, the infrequency of change in the reserve requirements and the lagging nature of the discount rate indicate that they are not the most important tools in the Fed's arsenal. The purchase and sale of U.S. Government securities, called open-market operations, is the most useful instrument of monetary policy available to the Federal Reserve. Unlike changes in the reserve requirements, which could trigger massive changes in bank reserves, securities may be bought and sold in any quantity to fine-tune the economy. Changes in the discount rate may have little effect on bank reserves because a bank may seek funds elsewhere, but open-market operations are an effective means of increasing or decreasing bank reserves, even if the bank does not directly participate in the securities transaction, since the bank's customers write or receive checks that affect reserves when the securities are bought or sold.

Assume that the Federal Open Market Committee (FOMC) has determined that an expansion in the money supply is desirable to stimulate a depressed economy. The FOMC will direct the Federal Reserve Bank of New York to buy government securities through government securities dealers.[6] The Federal Reserve Bank pays for its purchases with a check drawn on itself. The securities dealer deposits the check in a bank, which now has an increase in excess reserves. It is important to note that this increase in reserves does not take away from the reserves of any other bank; rather it comes from funds that the Fed has created by drawing a check on itself. This action obtains the desired results in two ways. First, as the Fed purchases securities, demand will exceed supply and the price of securities will rise. The increase in price has the effect of reducing the securities' yield.[7] This interest rate effect will spread to other sectors of the financial markets, reducing yields on other interest-bearing securities, including the rates charged for loans. Concurrently, the bank will wish

---

[6]The Fed does not buy or sell securities directly from individuals or banks. The government securities dealers supply the securities to the general public and banks.

[7]The inverse relationship between prices and rates of return will be discussed in Chapter 17.

to lend the excess reserves, which were generated by the government securities dealer's deposit of the Fed's check. To stimulate borrowing, the bank will further lower the interest rate it charges on loans. Thus the purchase of government securities by the Fed has increased the money supply and put in motion events which will serve to lower interest rates. These lower interest rates will encourage additional borrowing and spending, providing benefit to the depressed economy.[8]

During a period of excessive expansion or inflation, the FOMC will sell securities to reduce bank reserves. Of course, as the supply of securities increases relative to demand, the securities' price will fall, resulting in an increase in interest rates. This is only the first stage in the Fed's attempt to slow economic growth, however. As the government securities dealers' checks for the purchased securities clear, banks will lose reserves. The effect of reserve deficiencies for individual banks will quickly spread through the banking system. Banks may attempt to replenish reserves by borrowing through the interbank federal funds market. As the demand for excess reserves increases, the rate charged for these funds will increase and the reserves will become less easily obtained. Banks will be forced to sell securities and reduce their loan portfolios to generate needed reserves. The sale of securities by banks, along with those sold by the Fed, further increases interest rates, since an oversupply relative to demand depresses their price. Because banks have fewer excess reserves, the availability of credit is affected, further increasing interest rates. Thus the sale of securities by the Fed reduces the ability of banks to lend to some and results in higher interest rates, which discourages others from borrowing. The resulting reduction in debt-financed spending is desirable for an economy faced with excessive, inflationary expansion.

SUMMARY

This chapter has concentrated on the largest of all financial intermediaries, the commercial banking system. The banking system's power to create money via the creation of demand deposits sets banks apart from most intermediaries. The shift in their sources of funds from shorter-duration demand deposits to longer-term time and savings deposits has allowed banks to increase the maturity schedule of their loans. Short-term loans of less than a one-year maturity still dominate the banks' loan portfolios, however.

The Federal Reserve System attempts to influence the economic health of the nation principally through affecting the reserves of commercial banks. Its central instrument of monetary policy is open-market operations. Purchases of U.S. Government securities by the Fed have an expansionary effect on the money supply, whereas sales of securities have a restraining effect. The Fed does not change the reserve requirements often because open-market operations accomplish the same purpose without the potentially severe conse-

---

[8]The Federal Reserve must take care not to overstimulate the economy through excessive creation of credit, which can lead to expectations of greater inflation.

SMALL BUSINESS

Building a Banking Relationship

For many small businesses, a good banking relationship can mean the difference between failure and survival. The banker is important for two reasons. The most obvious one is that the banker may loan the business money for working capital, expansion, equipment, and so on, that will allow the firm to continue to grow. The less obvious reason is that the banker may be a valuable source of financial advice for the inexperienced small business owner. Once the bank has loaned the business money, it is in both the bank's and the business's interest for the company to survive. Thus a good banker will take a genuine interest in the firm and will care about how it is doing.

Even though the banker is interested in the firm's survival, the bank is also likely to be more risk-averse than the business, because the bank shares in the firm's downside risk but not in its upside potential. If the firm fails, the entrepreneur and the bank both lose their investment. If things go well, the banker gets back only the loan money plus interest, but the entrepreneur has potential for unlimited success. The entrepreneur, therefore, may be willing to take great risks in the hopes of great rewards, whereas the banker may want to play it safe.

There is a possibility, then, of a conflict of interest between the banker and the entrepreneur. Because of that conflict, the bank will often impose restrictions on how the firm can use its revenues or profits, how much the firm can pay the entrepreneur in salary, and other matters. The bank probably will require some or all of the business's assets as collateral to insure the loan. Nevertheless, the banker will be concerned about and watchful for the one thing the entrepreneur most wants to avoid — the failure of the business. To that end, the banker will follow the firm's financial health very closely, and that watchful eye can be of great benefit to the entrepreneur.

Many small businesses do not have personnel with financial expertise. The banker may serve in an advisory capacity and make up for some of those gaps in knowledge. As long as the entrepreneur realizes that the advice is somewhat prejudiced by the banker's risk aversion, such advice can be extremely helpful.

Finding the Right Banker

Often the small business owner may not know where to begin to find the right banker. Stretched for funds, she or he goes to the nearest bank and asks for money to fund an idea or proposal. If the bank is largely a retail bank with little expertise in commercial accounts, one of two negative events may occur:

1. The banker turns down the loan, failing to see that the proposal is in fact a good one; or

2. The banker makes a loan that shouldn't have been made, the proposal cannot return the funds, and the entrepreneur ends up worse off than before the loan was made.

In either case, both of these events are avoidable.

The right banker satisfies at least three conditions. First, the banker should understand the type of business the entrepreneur has. Second, the banker is interested in the business and will commit to follow it closely. Third, the banker is experienced and understands the pitfalls that wipe out small firms. In addition, the bank itself should be adequately capitalized to offer funds at the level at which the business needs them and should provide other services (such as cash management or factoring) that the business may need to use.

It is important that the banker and entrepreneur are able to communicate well. If they can't, their relationship will not be optimal for either side.

The Approach

The first meeting between the banker and entrepreneur should not involve a very detailed discussion of the firm's financial statements. Rather, it should be a get-acquainted session in which the banker learns about the business and the entrepreneur learns about the bank and banker. At that first meeting, the entrepreneur should leave the business's historical financial statements with the banker for review.

By not immediately delving into problems and projections at the first meeting, the two people have an opportunity to become acquainted without pressure. Also, at such a meeting the entrepreneur may create the impression that she or he is in control of the business rather than being excessively anxious to resolve some financial crisis.

The second meeting (if there is one) should begin with a discussion of the historical financial statements and then should lead to a presentation of projections. Together the banker and entrepreneur will discuss the business's financing needs. The banker, if an effective one, will have some suggestions that will improve the projections in some way.

How the Banker Evaluates

Bankers are trained to use the five Cs when evaluating a loan proposal. These comprise the following:

- Character
- Capacity (to manage)
- Cash flow
- Collateral
- Conditions

The *character* factor considers whether or not the entrepreneur is a person who takes obligations seriously, is honest, and is straightforward. The second management factor, *capacity,* questions whether this manager can handle the business.

The next three Cs deal with financial issues. The banker first will ask, "Can the firm generate the *cash flow* to repay this loan or, if it is a re-

volving line, to service the debt and keep it current?" Many loans are made to finance specific assets, such as equipment or receivables, and those are matched against *collateral.* Is the bank protected by the value of the collateral? Finally, many loans that are perfectly viable under one set of economic *conditions* may not be feasible under others. In the oil belt, for example, bankers are reluctant to loan funds against oil revenues whenever such revenues are especially unpredictable.

Points from a Credit Department Manager

The credit department manager of a large commercial bank was interviewed to obtain his point of view about establishing a banking relationship with a small business. He summarized the points he teaches new officers to consider when reviewing a proposal to grant credit.

First, he tells officers to simply ask "Why do you need the money?" He wants to know not only how the funds will be used, but also why the company cannot generate funds itself. This is not to imply that the bank is taking the arrogant view that "We only loan money to people who don't need it." Rather, the credit manager wants to be sure that the entrepreneur understands the business well enough to know the answers.

Next, the manager tells officers to carefully investigate how the loan will be repaid. If the funds will come from operating cash flows, how realistic are the projections? If it is a seasonal working capital line, what is the company's track record on managing inventory and receivables? If it is not seasonal, is the firm sufficiently profitable to handle the debt from operating profits?

The banker realizes that some working capital in a growing business is essentially permanent. His next concern is whether or not management is truly in control of the business and if the financing can be supported by assets (see the discussion of factoring receivables in Chapter 12's Small Business section).

The final question the credit manager asks, which he considers to be the most important of all, is: "What are your biggest problems?" The manager should explain that he isn't looking for firms that have no problems; he realizes that every firm has problems. He is really trying to find out whether the entrepreneur is:

1. perceptive and in control of the business; and

2. frank and candid, willing to talk honestly about the business's problems.

The credit department head explained that a good small business person will perceive problems. If the entrepreneur isn't aware of them, they can lead to business failure; if they are known, the problems perhaps can be solved. It is especially important that the entrepreneur understands cash flows.

Frankness was the key. The business person's willingness to openly share concerns was thought by that credit department head to be the bank's greatest protection against "surprises."

Conclusion

For a small business, a good banking relationship can mean the difference between success and failure. Establishing that relationship is important. Both sides are better off if the relationship can be an open one in which the banker and the business owner understand each other and communicate honestly with each other in dealing with the difficult problems of the small but growing firm.

quences of changes in reserve requirements. Similarly, the Fed does not rely on discount rates as a major instrument of monetary policy. In part, the discount rate is a less effective tool because banks can avoid borrowing at the Fed by borrowing in the federal funds market.

The ability of the Fed to increase or decrease bank reserves is only a part of the equation in the determination of interest rates. In the next chapter we explore how interest rates are determined.

QUESTIONS

4-1   What are the three principal tools that the Federal Reserve System uses in affecting the nation's money supply?

4-2   When the Fed buys government securities, is it attempting to increase or decrease the money supply?

4-3   Why is the Fed reluctant to use the reserve requirement as an active tool in monetary policy?

4-4   From the standpoint of a commercial bank's balance sheet, evaluate the following statement: "One financial unit's asset is another's liability."

4-5   If the primary goal of the financial manager is to maximize shareholder wealth, what is the bank manager's primary goal?

4-6   Why do banks attempt to minimize their investment in excess reserves?

4-7   What are the characteristics of securities that banks would obtain for their investment portfolios?

RESOLUTION TO DECISION IN FINANCE

A New Chairman for the Fed

The Federal Reserve System is the government's most important instrument for regulating the U.S. banking system. Although its mandate is to create an environment for sustained economic growth by regulating the commercial banks' ability to create credit, the effects of its policies and actions are felt well beyond the confines of the banking system. The Fed is one of the cornerstones of the U.S. economy and an important actor in international finance.

As such, much of the responsibility for cleaning up after the debacle of "black Monday" fell to Chairman Greenspan and the Fed. The 61-year-old Greenspan, who brought little experience in the complexities of central banking with him to the job, earned high marks for his handling of the crisis. He and other Fed officials responded quickly to the stock market collapse and used the full powers of the Fed to keep the market crash from spiraling out of control.

In this case, Greenspan's chronic pessimism paid off handsomely. Shortly after taking office, Greenspan quietly launched a crisis-manage-

ment project to spot weaknesses in the U.S. economy and generate alternatives to a variety of financial catastrophe scenarios ranging from bank failures to a collapse of the stock market. Therefore, officials at the Fed weren't caught unprepared by the events of October 19.

In the aftermath of the crash, the Fed acted quickly to insure that the banking system would have enough money to avoid a shortage of credit, which would cause a rise in short-term interest rates that might lead to a recession. It also countered inflationary pressures that were pressing interest rates upward.

Having weathered his first major crisis well, Chairman Greenspan still faces many challenges. An adroit politician, he has worked to garner the support of other Board members in an effort to avoid the conflicts that plagued his predecessor. But, as a political team player, he still must deal with critics who question his ability to act independently from the Reagan administration. With the onslaught of election year pressures, many observers fear that Greenspan will be compelled to push the Fed into policies that foster short-term growth versus solid progress against inflation in order to enhance the Republican's record. In any event, Greenspan is sure to be making Fed policy and headlines, at least until his term of office expires in 1991.

Source: Blanca Riemer, "What's in Store at the Fed," *Business Week,* June 15, 1987; Mike McNamee, "Alan Greenspan Is Headed for a Quiet Honeymoon," *Business Week,* August 3, 1987; and Alan Murray, "Passing the Test: New Fed Chairman Greenspan Wins a Lot of Praise on Handling of Stock-Market Crash," *The Wall Street Journal,* November 25, 1987.

4-8   Why have banks, among financial institutions, historically been the major suppliers of short-term funds to borrowers?

4-9   What is the importance of the Depository Institutions Deregulation and Monetary Control Act of 1980? (Note: This question requires investigation of sources outside this text.)

PROBLEMS

4-1   **Open market operations.** The Fed buys $5 million in government securities.
  a. Will the money supply expand or contract?
  b. If the reserve requirement is 10 percent, what is the potential increase (decrease) in demand deposits?

4-2   **Open market operations.** The Fed sells $8 million in government securities.
  a. Will the money supply expand or contract?
  b. If the reserve requirement is 12.5 percent, what is the potential increase (decrease) in demand deposits?

4-3   **Comparative financial statements.** Obtain the financial statement of a local bank. Compare the bank's balance sheet with that of a manufacturer (or see Carter Chemical Company's balance sheet in Chapter 6). What major differences are apparent?

Chapter 5

Interest Rates

DECISION IN FINANCE

When Interest Rates Go Up, What Happens to Bond Prices?

Most people wouldn't think that Merrill Lynch & Co. has an image problem. After all, the giant brokerage house is one of the nation's largest and, thanks to its ads featuring a longhorn bull, one of the most widely recognized. In the investment banking business, however, retail clout isn't necessarily the ticket to prestige. Recently, Merrill Lynch has been trying to shake off its "broker to the masses" image and move up to the first echelon of sophisticated investment banks. Toward that end, the firm has recently made impressive gains in underwriting and has moved dramatically into Wall Street's most volatile markets, such as high-yield junk bonds and mortgage securities.

To make big gains in volatile markets, Merrill Lynch has had to take big risks, especially in the fledgling mortgage-backed securities market. In essence this market acts to transform the mortgage market into a pseudo-bond market. The classic 30-year fixed rate mortgage is essentially a stream of monthly payments. In the mortgage-backed securities market, government agencies pool similar mortgages written by banks and savings and loans and sell securities backed by these mortgages. Large investors then buy a slice of that steady cash flow in the form of

See end of chapter for resolution.

mortgage-backed securities, thereby providing fresh funds to be used for more capital lending.

The enormous mortgage-backed securities market is highly volatile, hypersensitive to even small fluctuations in the interest rate. This is because homeowners can pre-pay their loans when interest rates head down or hold onto their fixed rate loans longer when interest rates rise. Because mortgage holder behavior is unpredictable, the key to valuing these securities is being able to guess how quickly borrowers will pre-pay their loans.

On April 8, 1987, Merrill Lynch entered the mortgage securities market with a $1.7 billion issue of stripped securities called IOs (interest-only) and POs (principal-only). These securities are a particularly risky form of mortgage-based securities in which the interest and principal portions of the securities are traded separately. Prior to April 8, interest rates had been slowly rising but their future direction was unclear.

As you read this chapter, try to think of factors that you would take into account if you were in charge of pricing Merrill Lynch's offering of IOs and POs. If interest rates went up, what would likely happen to the price of mortgage-backed securities? How could Merrill Lynch act to protect itself against undue losses due to interest rate fluctuations?

interest rate
The price paid by borrowers to lenders for the use of funds.

Capital in a free economy is allocated through the price system. The **interest rate** is the price paid to borrow capital, whereas in the case of equity capital, investors' returns come in the form of dividends and capital gains. The factors that affect the supply of and demand for investment capital, and hence the cost of funds, are discussed in this chapter.

THE COST OF FUNDS

production opportunities
The return available within an economy from investment in productive (cash-generating) investments.

time preferences for consumption
The preferences of consumers for current consumption as opposed to saving for future consumption.

The two most fundamental factors affecting the cost of funds are **production opportunities** and **time preferences for consumption.** To see how these factors operate, visualize an isolated island community where people live on fish. They have a certain stock of fishing gear that permits them to survive reasonably well, but they would like to have more fish. Now suppose Mr. Crusoe were to have a bright idea for a new type of fishnet that would enable him to double his daily catch. However, it would take him a year to perfect his design, build his net, and learn how to use it efficiently, and Mr. Crusoe would be likely to starve before he could put his new net into operation. Therefore he might suggest to Ms. Robinson, Mr. Friday, and several others that if they would give him one fish each day for a year, he would return two fish a day during all of the next year. If someone accepted the offer, the fish which Ms. Robinson or one of the others would give to Mr. Crusoe would constitute *savings;* these savings would be *invested* in the fishnet; and the extra fish caught would constitute a *return on the investment.*

Obviously, the more productive Mr. Crusoe thought the new fishnet would be, the higher his expected return on the investment would be and the more he could offer to pay Ms. Robinson or the others for their savings. In the example we assumed that Mr. Crusoe would be able to pay, and would offer, a 100 percent rate of return—he offered to give back two fish for every one he received. Quite possibly he could have decided to offer only 1.5 fish next year for every one he received this year, which would be a 50 percent rate of return to Ms. Robinson or the other potential savers. Mr. Crusoe might even be able to attract savings for less. How attractive Mr. Crusoe's offer appeared to potential savers would depend in large part on their *time preferences for consumption.* For example, Ms. Robinson might be thinking of retirement, and she might be willing to trade fish today for fish in the future on a one-for-one basis. On the other hand, Mr. Friday might have a wife and several children and need his current fish, so he might be unwilling to lend a fish today except in exchange for three fish next year. Mr. Friday would be said to have a high time preference for consumption and Ms. Robinson a low time preference. Note also that if the entire population were living at the subsistence level, time preferences for current consumption would necessarily be high, aggregate savings would be low, interest rates would be high, and capital formation would be difficult.

In a more complex society there are many businesses like Mr. Crusoe's, many products, and many savers like Ms. Robinson and Mr. Friday. Further-

INDUSTRY PRACTICE

In Japan We (Must) Trust

For Peoria, Illinois, 1987 started out strong. After years of retrenching at Peoria's largest employer, Caterpillar Tractor Company, residents finally felt the start of a rebound. More people began taking out loans to buy houses and to expand businesses. "Things were really picking up, but then interest rates jumped," says Peoria Savings & Loan President Roger Kilpatrick. "Since then demand for new loans has been off 20% to 25%."

Peoria wasn't alone. In April 1987, mortgage rates nationwide spurted into double digits, sending housing starts tumbling to their lowest levels in four years. The unexpected rate increase produced horrendous losses on Wall Street in bond and mortgage securities trading. More broadly, the jump pushed down economic growth to a 2.6 percent annual pace in the second quarter of 1987, from 4.4 percent the previous three months.

What caused the spike in rates? People pontificate about reemerging inflation and government and trade deficits — the usual suspects. Forget all that: The rise wasn't made in Washington or Wall Street. It was made in Tokyo. Behind today's slumping bond market and rising interest rates lies Japan's skittishness about the dollar.

During the past few years it has become clear that Japanese banks and life insurance companies have come to dominate bond markets around the globe. In the summer of 1987, Japan's foreign assets surpassed $450 billion. Its foreign investments could reach $700 billion by 1990. By moving even a small part of this money from one country to another, Japanese investors spur economic activity at one spot on the globe, squelch it somewhere else.

Unlike OPEC funds, which are usually stashed timidly in banks, the huge Japanese cash pile is mostly invested in bonds. That's important because a bond market determines rates for business loans, mortgages, and consumer credit.

Even as rates were climbing in Peoria, the Japanese were buying bonds in Britain and Germany, pushing down European rates. The Japanese made it cheaper to borrow in Munich but dearer in Milwaukee. The power center of world finance is shifting from the canyons of Wall Street to Tokyo's financial district, a clutch of perhaps a hundred modern buildings standing across the moat from the Imperial Palace.

Up until 1987, big Japanese life insurance companies and banks had been docile investors in the U.S.: They would buy Treasury bonds and hold them until maturity. But in 1985 and 1986, as the dollar fell 45 percent against the yen, Japanese institutions incurred more than $10 billion in foreign exchange losses on their vast holdings of U.S. Treasury bonds. Shareholders and policyholders began asking uncomfortable questions.

Once burned, twice shy. In early 1987, with the U.S. trade and budget deficits gaping, Japanese banks and life insurance companies lost confidence in the greenback. They didn't want any more foreign exchange losses. They virtually stopped buying U.S. Treasury bonds, triggering a decline in the dollar and a spike in interest rates. And that's what caused homebuying to slow in Peoria.

The view from Tokyo, if anything, suggests that the dollar will continue to fall against the yen and continue to put upward pressure on U.S. interest rates. Investment managers at Japan's largest financial institutions seem uniformly bearish on the dollar and U.S. bonds. Why so bearish on the dollar? To a man, Japanese money managers cite the U.S. inflation rate,

Source: Adapted by permission from Edward A. Finn, Jr., "In Japan We (Must) Trust," *Forbes,* September 21, 1987, 32–34. © Forbes Inc., 1987.

which is running at 5 percent plus, nearly four points above Japan's. On top of that, they worry that Washington will continue to flounder in its efforts to cut the budget deficit.

Noting the rise in U.S. Treasury rates, Richard Koo, senior economist at Nomura Securities, says, "Think of that jump as tuition for America. Now you have learned how dependent you are on foreign capital." It is a lesson we will learn again and again as long as our actions are limited by our position as an international debtor.

more, people use money as a medium of exchange rather than barter with fish. Still, the interest rate paid to savers depends in a basic way on (1) *the rate of return producers can expect to earn on invested capital* and (2) *consumers' and savers' time preferences for current versus future consumption.* Producers' expected returns set an upper limit on how much they can pay for savings, whereas consumers' time preferences for consumption establish how much consumption they are willing to defer and hence how much they will save at different levels of interest offered by producers.[1]

INTEREST RATES

As we discuss in Chapter 19, the firm's cost of capital is determined by the rate of return required by its debt and equity investors. That return is dependent, in part, on factors specific to the firm itself: its financing, product innovation, competition, and management skills, to name a few. However, the firm's cost of capital is not determined only by factors that apply exclusively to the firm; cost considerations are broader and include the general level of interest rates in the economy. The basis for interest rates in the economy is shaped by market forces — the supply and demand for funds, risks such as inflation, and investor expectations about the future. The way in which the economic forces combine to determine market interest rates is analyzed in the following sections.

Figure 5-1 graphs the production/consumption situation in a supply/demand framework. Savers will save more if producers offer higher interest rates on savings, and producers will borrow more if savers accept a lower return on their savings. There is an equilibrium rate, k, which produces a balance between the aggregate supply of and demand for capital in the economy. The equilibrium rate of return is that rate which is required to induce savers to invest and, simultaneously, it is the rate which borrowers are willing to pay. This rate, k, is not static; it changes over time, depending on conditions. For

---

[1]The term *producers* is really too narrow. A better word might be *borrowers,* which would include home purchasers, people borrowing to go to college, or even people borrowing to buy autos or to pay for vacations, in addition to business borrowing.

Figure 5-1 **Supply of and Demand for Savings**

This figure shows how the supply/demand system works to determine the rate of
interest (k) on savings. The investment curve indicates that borrowers (producers)
will try to attract more savings from savers as interest rates decrease. Conversely, the
savings curve shows that savers will try to save more only as interest rates increase.
These conflicting desires of savers and borrowers come together at some equilibrium
point, k, creating a balance between supply of and demand for savings. At that point,
savings will equal investment (S = I).

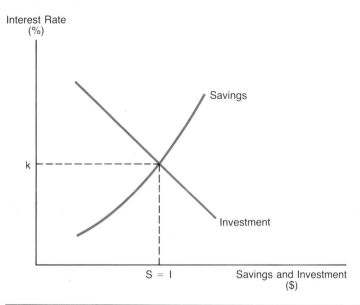

example, if a major technological breakthrough occurs and raises the rate of
return on producers' investment, the investment curve in Figure 5-1 will shift
to the right, causing both k and S = I to increase. Similarly, if consumers'
attitudes change and they become more thrifty, the savings curve will shift to
the right, causing k to decline but S = I to increase.

There are many capital markets in the United States. In addition, U.S. firms
raise and invest capital throughout the world, and foreign firms also borrow
and lend capital in the United States. There are markets in the United States
for real estate loans; farm loans; business loans; federal, state, and local government loans; and consumer loans. Within each category, there are regional
markets as well as different submarkets. For example, in real estate there are
separate markets for first and second mortgages and for loans on owner-occupied homes, apartments, office buildings, shopping centers, vacant land, and
so on. Within the business sector, there are dozens of types of debt as well as
several sharply differentiated markets for common stocks. There is a price for

each type of capital, yet, even with all the differentiation in the capital markets, rates in the various capital markets are interrelated. Thus, when the interest rate on business loans increases, the interest rate on owner-occupied homes will also increase.

The price for each type of capital changes over time as shifts occur in supply and demand conditions. Figure 5-2 shows how long- and short-term interest rates to business borrowers have varied since the 1950s. Short-term interest rates are more volatile than long-term rates. This is because short-term rates are responsive to current economic conditions, whereas long-term rates primarily reflect long-run expectations for the economy, especially inflation. Thus short-term rates are especially prone to rise during booms and then to fall during recessions (indicated by the shaded areas in Figure 5-2). As a result, short-term rates are sometimes above and sometimes below long-term rates. The relationship between long- and short-term rates, which is called the *term structure of interest rates,* is discussed later in this chapter.

When the economy is expanding, firms need capital, and this demand for funds pushes interest rates up. Also, because inflationary pressures are stronger during business booms, the Federal Reserve tends to tighten the money supply at such times, which also exerts upward pressure on rates. Conditions are reversed during recessions: slack business reduces the demand for credit, the Fed increases the money supply, and the result is a drop in interest rates. In addition, inflationary pressures are normally weakest during recessions, and this too helps to keep interest rates down.

These tendencies do not hold exactly, and the early part of the 1974–1975 recession is a case in point. The price of oil increased dramatically in 1974, exerting inflationary pressures on other prices and raising fears of serious, long-term inflation. These fears pushed interest rates to high levels. Investors "looked over the valley" of the 1974–1975 recession, forecast a continued problem with inflation, and demanded an inflation premium that kept long-term rates high by historical standards.

The relationship between inflation and long-term interest rates is highlighted in Figure 5-3, which plots rates of inflation along with long-term interest rates. Before 1965, when the average rate of inflation was about 1 percent, interest rates on AAA-rated bonds generally ranged from 4 to 5 percent. As the war in Vietnam accelerated in the mid-1960s, the rate of inflation increased and interest rates began to rise. The inflation rate dropped after 1970, and so did long-term interest rates. However, the 1973 Arab oil embargo was followed by a quadrupling of oil prices in 1974, causing a spurt in the price level that in turn drove interest rates to new record highs in 1974 and 1975. Inflationary pressures eased in late 1975 and 1976 but then rose again after 1976. In 1980 inflation rates hit the highest level on record, and fears of a renewal of double-digit inflation kept long-term interest rates at relatively high levels. As confidence built that inflation was under control, interest rates declined. In the second quarter of 1987, however, inflation fears again began to increase interest rates.

Figure 5-2 **Long- and Short-Term Interest Rates, 1953–1987**

This figure depicts the fluctuation of long- and short-term interest rates over the past 35 years and shows how these rates have responded to business recessions. Recessions have caused sharp drops in short-term rates because of Federal Reserve intervention and falling demand for money. Long-term rates are much less affected by recessions, since these rates are based on long-range expectations that are not significantly changed by relatively temporary recessions.

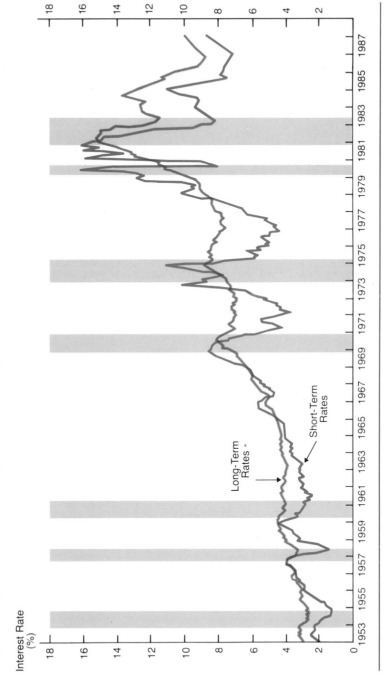

Interest Rate
(%)

Long-Term
Rates

Short-Term
Rates

Note:
The shaded areas designate business recessions. Short-term rates are measured by four- to six-month loans to very large, strong corporations, and long-term rates are measured by AAA corporate bonds.
Source: *Federal Reserve Bulletin,* various issues.

106

Figure 5-3 **Relationship between Annual Inflation Rates and Long-Term Interest Rates**

There is a close, although not perfect, correlation between interest rates and rates of inflation, as shown in this figure. Over a 35-year period, the two rates tended to fluctuate together. The inflation premium built into long-term interest rates is based on expectations of future inflation, with these expectations arising largely from past and present experiences of inflation rates.

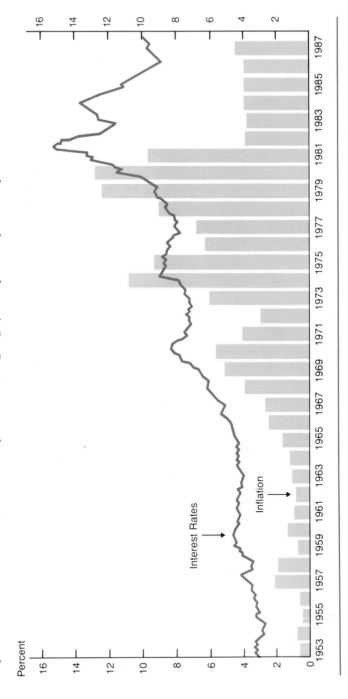

Notes:
1. Interest rates are those on AAA long-term corporate bonds.
2. Inflation is measured as the annual rate of change in the consumer price index (CPI).

THE DETERMINANTS OF MARKET INTEREST RATES

In general, the nominal interest rate on a debt security, k, is composed of a pure rate of interest, k*, plus risk premiums that reflect inflation, default, liquidity (or marketability), and maturity (or interest rate risk). This relationship can be expressed as follows:

$$k = k^* + IP + DP + LP + MP.$$

Here,

  k = stated, or nominal, rate of interest.[2]

  k* = pure rate of interest; pronounced "k-star."

  IP = inflation risk premium.

  DP = default risk premium.

  LP = liquidity risk premium.

  MP = maturity risk premium.

We discuss the components whose sum makes up the stated or nominal rate in the following sections.

The Pure Rate of Interest

The **pure rate of interest, k*,** is defined as the equilibrium interest rate on a riskless security if no inflation is expected. The pure rate is also called the *real, risk-free rate,* and it may be thought of as the rate of interest on short-term U.S. Treasury securities (which have little risk) in an inflation-free world. The pure rate is not static; it changes over time depending on economic conditions, especially (1) the rate of return corporations and other borrowers can expect to earn on productive assets and (2) people's time preferences for current versus future consumption. Borrowers' expected returns on real asset investment set an upper limit on how much they can afford to pay for borrowed funds, whereas savers' time preferences for consumption establish how much consumption they are willing to defer and hence the amount of funds they will lend at different levels of interest. It is difficult to measure k* precisely, but most experts think that in the United States it has fluctuated in the range of 2 to 4 percent in recent years.

pure rate of interest, k*
The risk-free rate of interest. It is that rate of return that would cause investors to postpone current consumption, if no risks existed in the financial environment.

---

[2]The term *nominal* as it is used here means the *stated* rate as opposed to the *real* rate, which is adjusted for inflation. If you bought a 10-year Treasury bond in March 1987, the stated or nominal rate would be about 7.3 percent, but if inflation averages 4 percent over the next 10 years the real rate would be about 7.3% − 4.0% = 3.3%.

Inflation Risk Premium

inflation

An increase in the volume of money and credit relative to the available supply of goods, resulting in a rise in the general level of prices.

Inflation has a major impact on interest rates; it can erode the purchasing power of the dollar and lower the real rate of return on investments. To illustrate its effects, suppose you saved up $1,000 and invested it in a Treasury bond which matures in 1 year and which pays 5 percent interest. At the end of the year, you would receive $1,050 — your original $1,000 plus $50 of interest. Now suppose the rate of inflation during the year was 10 percent, and it affected all items equally. If beer had cost $1 per bottle at the start of the year, it would cost $1.10 at the end. Therefore, you could have bought $1,000/$1 = 1,000 bottles at the beginning of the year, but only $1,050/$1.10 = 955 bottles at the end. In *real terms,* you would be worse off; you would have received $50 of interest, but it would not be sufficient to offset inflation. You would have been better off having bought and held 1,000 bottles of beer (or some other storable asset such as land, timber, apartment buildings, wheat, or gold) than having bought bonds.

inflation risk premium (IP)

A premium for anticipated or expected inflation that investors add to the pure rate of return.

Investors are well aware of all of this, so when they lend money, they add an **inflation risk premium (IP)** to the rate they would have charged in the absence of inflation. For a riskless default-free U.S. Treasury bill (T-bill), the actual interest rate charged, $k_{T\text{-bill}}$, would be the pure rate of interest, k^*, plus the inflation premium (IP):

$$k_{T\text{-bill}} = k^* + IP.$$

Therefore, if the pure rate of interest for riskless default-free investments were $k^* = 3.5\%$, and if inflation were expected to be 5 percent (and hence IP = 5%) over the next year, the rate of interest on 1-year T-bills would be 8.5 percent. On May 1, 1987, the expected 1-year inflation rate was about 3.5 percent and the yield on 1-year T-bills was 6.8 percent, which implies that the pure rate of interest on that date was about 3.3 percent.

It is important to note that the rate of inflation built into interest rates is the *rate of inflation expected in the future,* not the rate experienced in the past. Thus, the latest reported figures might show an annual inflation rate of 4 percent, but that is for the *past* period, and if people on the average expect a 6 percent inflation rate for the future, then 6 percent would be built into the interest rate as the inflation risk premium (IP). Note also that the inflation rate reflected in the interest rate on any security is the *average rate of inflation expected over the security's life.* Thus the inflation rate built into a 1-year bond is the expected inflation rate for the next year, but the inflation rate built into a 30-year bond is the average rate of inflation expected over the next 30 years.

If you turn once again to Figure 5-2, you will note the high correlation between inflation and interest rates over the years. The relationship is not perfect, however, because it is built on expectations. Studies have shown that inflation expectations for the future are closely related to recent inflation rates. In 1974–1975 and again in the late 1970s to 1980, when high inflation rates were unusual for the United States, investors' forecasts of inflation were too low and inflation was greater than interest rates. Therefore, investors' purchasing power eroded as price increases exceeded the rate of return they earned on their investments. Because of these experiences with high inflation, the rates in the early to mid-1980s remained high relative to current inflation as investors' fear of renewed high inflation kept the inflation risk premium (at least with hindsight) artificially high.

Inflation risk premiums are based on forecasts that are closely related to, although not perfectly correlated with, recent inflation experience. Therefore, if the inflation rate reported for the past few months increased, people would tend to raise their expectations for future inflation, and this change in expectations would cause an increase in interest rates.

Default Risk Premium

The risk that a borrower will *default* on a loan, which means that the borrower cannot pay either the interest or principal, also affects the market interest rate of a security; thus the greater the potential for default, the higher the interest rate lenders will charge. Because Treasury securities have no default risk, they carry the lowest interest rates on taxable securities in the United States. For corporate bonds, the higher the bond's rating, the lower its default risk and, consequently, its interest rate. The **bond ratings** range from AAA, which is the rating for the financially strongest firms, down to D, which is the rating applied to companies already in bankruptcy. The following are some representative interest rates on long-term bonds during January 1987:[3]

bond ratings
Ratings assigned to bonds based on the probability of their firms' default. Those bonds with the smallest default probability are rated AAA and carry the lowest interest rates.

Security	Rate	Default Risk Premium
U.S. Treasury	7.6%	
AAA corporate	8.4	0.8%
AA corporate	8.9	1.3
A corporate	9.2	1.6
BAA corporate	9.7	2.1

The difference between the interest rate on a Treasury security and that of a corporate bond *with similar maturity, liquidity, and other features* is defined as the **default risk premium (DP).** Therefore, if the previously listed bonds are otherwise similar, the default risk premium is relatively low for AAA corporate bonds (DP = 8.4% − 7.6% = 0.8%), but the default risk premium is higher for the higher risk BAA corporate bonds (DP = 9.7% − 7.6% = 2.1%). Default risk premiums vary somewhat over time, but the January 1987 figures are representative of levels in recent periods.

default risk premium (DP)
The difference between the interest rate on a Treasury bond and that on a corporate bond.

Liquidity Risk Premiums

A highly **liquid asset** is one that can be sold at approximately its intrinsic value and thus converted into spendable cash on short notice. Active markets, which provide liquidity, exist for government securities, for the stocks and

liquid asset
An asset that can be readily converted to spendable cash.

---

[3]*Federal Reserve Bulletin,* April 1987, p. A24.

liquidity risk premium (LP)
A premium added to the equilibrium interest rate on a security that cannot be converted to cash on short notice.

bonds of the larger corporations, and for the securities of certain financial intermediaries. If a security is *not* liquid, investors will add a **liquidity risk premium (LP)** when they establish the market interest rate on the security. It is very difficult to measure liquidity premiums, but a differential of at least one and probably two percentage points exists between the least liquid and most liquid financial assets of similar default risk and maturity.

Maturity Risk Premium

U.S. Treasury securities are free of default risk in the sense that one can be virtually certain that the federal government will pay interest on its bonds and also will pay them off when they mature; therefore, the default risk premium on Treasury securities is essentially zero. Further, active markets exist for Treasury securities, so their liquidity premiums also are close to zero. Thus, as a first approximation, the rate of interest on a Treasury bond should be equal to the pure rate, k*, plus the inflation risk premium, IP. An adjustment is needed, however. The prices of long-term bonds decline sharply whenever interest rates rise, and since interest rates can and do rise occasionally, all long-term bonds, even Treasury bonds, have an element of risk called **interest rate risk.** As a general rule, the bonds of any organization, from the U.S. government to Eastern Airlines, have more interest rate risk the longer the maturity of the bond.[4] Therefore, a **maturity risk premium (MP),** which is higher the longer the years to maturity, must be included in the required interest rate.

interest rate risk
The risk of capital losses to which investors are exposed due to changing interest rates.

maturity risk premium (MP)
A premium for the risk to which investors are exposed due to the length of a security's maturity.

The effect of maturity risk premiums is to raise interest rates on long-term bonds relative to those on short-term bonds. This premium, like the others, is extremely difficult to measure, but (1) it seems to vary over time, rising when interest rates are more volatile and uncertain and falling when they are more stable, and (2) in recent years, the maturity risk premium on 30-year T-bonds generally appears to have been in the range of one to two percentage points.

reinvestment rate risk
Risk that a decline in interest rates will lead to lower income when short-term bonds mature and funds are reinvested.

We should mention that whereas long-term bonds have interest rate risk, short-term bonds have a **reinvestment rate risk.** When short-term bonds mature and the funds are reinvested, or "rolled over," a decline in interest rates would mean reinvestment at a lower rate and hence a decline in interest income. To illustrate, suppose you had $100,000, invested it in 1-year T-bonds, and lived on the income. In 1981, when short-term rates were about 15 percent, your income would have been about $15,000. However, your income would have declined to about $9,000 by 1983 and to just under $7,000 by 1987. Had you invested your money in long-term bonds, your income (but not the value of your principal) would have been stable. Thus, although the principle

---

[4]For example, if you had bought a 30-year Treasury bond for $1,000 in 1972, when the long-term interest rate was 7 percent, and held it until 1981, when long-term T-bond rates were about 14.5 percent, the value of your bond would have declined to about $513. That would represent a loss of almost half your money, and it demonstrates that long-term bonds, even U.S. Treasury bonds, are not riskless. However, had you invested in short-term bills in 1972 and subsequently reinvested your principal each time the bills matured, you would have still had $1,000. This point will be discussed in detail in Chapter 17.

is preserved, the interest income provided by short-term bonds varies from year to year, depending on reinvestment rates.

THE TERM STRUCTURE OF INTEREST RATES

A study of Figure 5-2 reveals that at certain times, such as 1987, short-term interest rates were lower than long-term rates, whereas at other times, such as 1979 and 1980, short rates were higher than long rates. The relationship between long and short rates, which is known as the **term structure of interest rates,** is important to corporate treasurers who must decide whether to borrow by issuing long- or short-term debt. It is also important to investors who must decide whether to buy long- or short-term bonds. Thus it is important to understand (1) how long- and short-term rates are related to each other and (2) what causes shifts in their relative positions.

To begin, we can look up in a source such as *The Wall Street Journal* or the *Federal Reserve Bulletin* the interest rates on bonds of various maturities at a given point in time. For example, Figure 5-4 presents interest rates for Treasury issues of different maturities on two dates. The set of data for a given date, when plotted on a graph such as that in Figure 5-4, is defined as the **yield curve** for that date. The yield curve changes over time as interest rates rise and fall. In March 1980, short-term rates were higher than long-term rates, so the yield curve on that date was *downward sloping.* However, in April 1987, short-term rates were lower than long-term rates, so the yield curve at that time was *upward sloping.* Had we drawn the yield curve during January 1982, it would have been essentially horizontal, for long-term and short-term bonds on that date had about the same rate of interest. (See Figure 5-2.)

Figure 5-4 shows yield curves for U.S. Treasury securities, but we could have constructed them for corporate bonds — for example, we could have developed yield curves for IBM, General Motors, Eastern Airlines, or any other company that borrows money over a range of maturities. Had we constructed such curves and plotted them on Figure 5-4, the corporate yield curves would have been above those for Treasury securities on the same date because of the addition of default risk premiums, but they would have had the same general shape as the Treasury curves. Also, the more risky the corporation, the higher its yield curve; thus Eastern, which in the spring of 1986 was on the verge of bankruptcy, would have had a yield curve significantly higher than that of IBM, which is an extremely strong company.

In a stable economy such as the United States had in the 1950s and early 1960s, in which (1) inflation fluctuated in the 1 to 3 percent range, (2) the expected future rate of inflation was about equal to the current rate, and (3) the Federal Reserve did not actively intervene in the markets, all interest rates were relatively low, and the yield curve generally had a slight upward slope to reflect maturity effects. People often define such an upward-sloping yield curve as a **"normal" yield curve,** and a yield curve which slopes downward as an **inverted,** or **"abnormal," yield curve.** Thus, in Figure 5-4 the yield curve for March 1980 was inverted, but the one for April 1987 was normal.

term structure of interest rates
The relationship between yields and maturities of securities.

yield curve
A graph showing the relationship between yields and maturities of securities.

"normal" yield curve
An upward-sloping yield curve.

inverted ("abnormal") yield curve
A downward-sloping yield curve.

Figure 5-4 **U.S. Treasury Bond Interest Rates on Different Dates**

This figure shows the actual yield curves for various term Treasury bonds in two recent years. In 1987 investors expected inflation to rise from the then-current 4 percent; this produced an upward-sloping yield curve, meaning long-term bonds offered a higher interest rate than did short-term bonds. In 1980, however, inflation was expected to decline, creating a downward-sloping yield curve; that is, in 1980 the Treasury was not able to sell long-term bonds at the same high rate at which it was selling short-term bonds. The 1987 situation was favorable to the long-term saver, whereas the situation in 1980 favored the short-term saver.

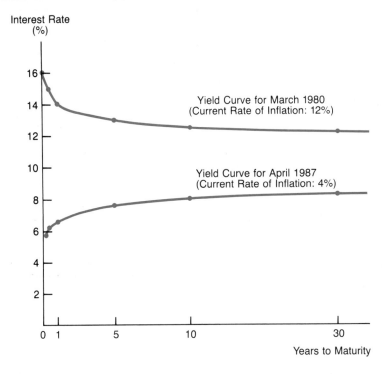

Term to Maturity	Interest Rate	
	March 1980	**April 1987**
3 months	16.0%	5.8%
6 months	15.0	6.2
1 year	14.0	6.5
5 years	13.5	7.6
10 years	12.8	8.0
30 years	12.3	8.3

Term Structure Theories

Several theories have been used to explain the shape of the yield curve. The three major ones are the *market segmentation theory*, the *liquidity preference theory*, and the *expectations theory*.

Market Segmentation Theory. Briefly, the **market segmentation theory** states that each lender and each borrower has a preferred maturity. For example, a person borrowing to buy a long-term asset like a house, or an electric utility company borrowing to build a power plant, would want a long-term loan. However, a retailer borrowing in September to build its inventory for Christmas would prefer a short-term loan. Similar differences exist among savers; a person saving up to take a vacation next summer would want to lend in the short-term market, but someone saving for retirement 20 years hence should probably buy long-term securities.

    The thrust of the market segmentation theory is that the slope of the yield curve depends on supply/demand conditions in the long-term market relative to those in the short-term market. Thus, according to this theory, the yield curve could at any given time be either upward sloping or downward sloping. An upward-sloping yield curve would occur when there was a large supply of funds relative to demand in the short-term market but a relative shortage of funds in the long-term market. Similarly, a downward-sloping curve would indicate relatively strong demand in the short-term market compared to that in the long-term market.

market segmentation theory
The theory that each borrower and lender has a preferred maturity and that the slope of the yield curve depends on the supply of and demand for funds in the long-term market relative to the short-term market.

Liquidity Preference Theory. The **liquidity preference theory** states that long-term bonds normally yield more than short-term bonds for two reasons. First, investors generally prefer to hold short-term securities, because such securities are more liquid in the sense that they can be converted to cash with little danger of loss of principal. Investors will, therefore, accept lower yields on short-term securities. Second, borrowers react in exactly the opposite way; they generally prefer long-term debt, because short-term debt subjects them to a greater danger of having to repay the debt under adverse conditions. Accordingly, borrowers are willing to pay a higher rate, other things held constant, for long-term funds than for short-term funds. Taken together, these two sets of preferences — and hence the liquidity preference theory — imply that under normal conditions the yield curve should be upward sloping.

liquidity preference theory
The theory that lenders prefer to make short-term loans rather than long-term loans, and hence they will lend short-term funds at lower rates than long-term funds.

Expectations Theory. The **expectations theory** states that the yield curve depends on expectations about future inflation rates. Specifically, k_t, the nominal interest rate on a U.S. Treasury bond that matures in t years, is found as follows:

$$k_t = k^* + IP_t.$$

expectations theory
The theory that the shape of the yield curve depends on investors' expectations about future inflation rates.

Here k^* is the real, risk-free interest rate and IP_t is an inflation premium which is equal to the average rate of inflation over the t years before the bond matures.[5]

Now note that (1) the Treasury can borrow on a short-term basis such as 90 days, on a long-term basis such as 30 years, or anywhere in between, and (2) the inflation premium built into any bond's interest rate is the *average inflation rate* over the bond's life, or its *term to maturity*. Therefore, it is appropriate to add a subscript, t, to the inflation premium, depending on its maturity. Thus $IP_t = IP_3$ is the inflation premium for a 3-year bond, and it is equal to the average inflation rate expected over the next 3 years.

To illustrate, suppose that in late December 1988 the real rate of interest was $k^* = 2\%$, and expected inflation rates for the next 3 years were as follows:

	Expected Annual (1-Year) Inflation Rate	Expected Average Inflation Rate During the Indicated Period	
1989	9%	9 ÷ 1	= 9.0%
1990	6%	(9 + 6) ÷ 2	= 7.5%
1991	3%	(9 + 6 + 3) ÷ 3	= 6.0%

Given these expectations, the following pattern of interest rates would be expected to exist:

	Real Rate (k^*)		Inflation Premium, Which Is Equal to the Average Expected Inflation Rate (IP_t)		Treasury Bond Rate $(k_{T\text{-bond}})$
1-year bond	2%	+	9.0%	=	11.0%
2-year bond	2%	+	7.5%	=	9.5%
3-year bond	2%	+	6.0%	=	8.0%

Had the pattern of expected inflation rates been reversed, with inflation expected to rise from 3 percent to 9 percent, the following situation would have existed:

1-year bond	2%	+	3.0%	=	5.0%
2-year bond	2%	+	4.5%	=	6.5%
3-year bond	2%	+	6.0%	=	8.0%

These hypothetical data are plotted in Figure 5-5. The lines represent yield curves and the graphs depict the term structure of interest rates. Whenever the annual rate of inflation is expected to decline, the yield curve points down. Conversely, if inflation is expected to increase, the yield curve points up.

---

[5]Our discussion of expectations theory centers on Treasury bonds, which are default free. In an attempt to center our discussion on the effects of expected inflation, we have chosen to ignore liquidity and maturity risks at this time. Perhaps a better, although slightly more complicated, presentation would include the effects of liquidity and maturity risks and would center on the real, default-free interest rate rather than the pure rate of interest that we have used.

Figure 5-5 **Hypothetical Example of the Term
Structure of Interest Rates**

The inflation premium built into the interest rate for any security is the average inflation rate expected over the life, or term to maturity, of the security. The term structure of interest rates is depicted by the hypothetical yield curves shown in this figure. If inflation is expected to decline, short-term securities will yield more than long-term securities, as shown in yield curve a. Conversely, if inflation is expected to increase, as in yield curve b, short-term securities will yield less than long-term securities.

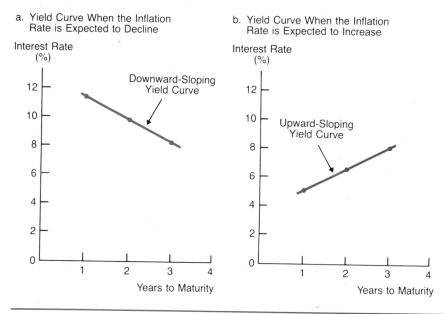

Various tests of these theories have been conducted, and they indicate that all three theories have some validity. Thus the shape of the yield curve at any given time is affected by supply/demand conditions in the long- and short-term markets, liquidity preferences, and expectations about future inflation. One factor may dominate in one economic period, another in other periods, but they all affect the structure of interest rates.

OTHER FACTORS THAT INFLUENCE INTEREST RATE LEVELS

In addition to inflationary expectations, liquidity preferences, and normal supply/demand fluctuations, other factors influence the general level of interest rates and the shape of the yield curve. The three most important ones are Federal Reserve policy, the level of the federal budget deficit, and the level of business activity.

Federal Reserve Policy

As you probably learned in Chapter 4 or in your studies of economics, (1) the money supply has a major effect on both the level of economic activity and the rate of inflation, and (2) in the United States the Federal Reserve System controls the money supply. If the Fed wants to stimulate the economy, it increases the money supply growth rate. The initial effect of such an action is to cause interest rates to decline, but the action also may lead to an increase in the expected rate of inflation, which in turn pushes interest rates up. The reverse holds if the Fed tightens the money supply.

To illustrate, in 1981 inflation was quite high, so the Fed tightened up the money supply. The Fed deals primarily in the short-term end of the market, so this tightening had the direct effect of pushing short-term interest rates up sharply. At the same time, the very fact that the Fed was taking strong action to reduce inflation led to a decline in expectations for long-run inflation, which led to a drop in long-term bond yields. Short-term rates decreased shortly thereafter.

During periods when the Fed is actively intervening in the markets, the yield curve will be distorted. Short-term rates will be temporarily "too high" if the Fed is tightening credit and "too low" if it is easing credit. Long-term rates are not affected as much by Fed intervention, except to the extent that such intervention affects expectations for long-term inflation.

Federal Deficits

If the federal government spends more than it takes in from tax revenues, it runs a deficit, and that deficit must be covered either by borrowing or by printing money. If the government borrows, this injects more demand into the market for the available supply of credit, and that pushes up interest rates. If it prints money, that increases expectations for future inflation, which also drives up interest rates. Thus the larger the federal deficit, other things held constant, the higher the level of interest rates. Whether long- or short-term rates are affected more depends on how the deficit is financed, so we cannot state, in general, how deficits will affect the slope of the yield curve.

Business Cycles

Figure 5-2, presented earlier, can be examined to see how business conditions influence interest rates. The following are the key points revealed by the graph:

1. Because inflation has generally been increasing since 1953, the tendency has been toward higher interest rates.

2. Until 1966, short-term rates were almost always below long-term rates. Thus in those years the yield curve was almost always "normal" in the sense that it was upward sloping, as the liquidity preference theory suggests it should be if inflation rates are stable.

3. The shaded areas in the graph represent recessions, during which the demand for money falls and, at the same time, the Federal Reserve tends to increase the money supply in an effort to stimulate the economy. As a result, there is a tendency for interest rates to decline during recessions.

4. During recessions short-term rates experience sharper declines than long-term rates. This occurs because (1) the Fed operates mainly in the short-term sector and hence its intervention has a major effect here and (2) long-term rates reflect the average expected inflation rate over the next 20 to 30 years, and this expectation generally does not change much even when the current rate of inflation is low because of a recession.

INTEREST RATE LEVELS AND STOCK PRICES

Interest rates have two effects on corporate profits. First, because interest is a cost, the higher the rate of interest, the lower a firm's profits, other things held constant. Second, interest rates affect the level of economic activity, and business profits are affected by economic activity. Interest rates obviously affect stock prices because of their effects on profits, but, perhaps even more important, their effect is caused by competition in the marketplace between stocks and bonds. If interest rates rise sharply, investors can get a higher return on their money in the bond market, which induces them to sell stocks in order to transfer funds from the stock market to the bond market. Such transfers in response to rising interest rates obviously depress stock prices. Of course, the reverse occurs if interest rates decline. Indeed, the bull market of 1985 to 1987, when the Dow Jones Industrial Index rose from 1100 to 2400, was due almost entirely to the sharp drop in long-term interest rates.

The experience of Commonwealth Edison, the electric utility serving the Chicago area, can be used to illustrate the effects of interest rates on stock prices. In 1984 Commonwealth's stock sold for $21 per share, and because the company paid a $3 dividend, the dividend yield was $3/$21 = 14.3%. Commonwealth's bonds at the time yielded about 14.3 percent, so if someone had $100,000 and invested it in either the stock or the bonds, his or her annual income would have been about $14,300. (The investor might also have expected the stock price to grow over time, providing some capital gains, but that point is not relevant for the example.)

By early 1987, all interest rates were much lower, and Commonwealth's bonds were yielding only 9.5 percent. If the stock still yielded 14.3 percent, investors could switch $100,000 out of the bonds and into the stock and, in the process, increase their annual income from $9,500 to $14,300. Many people did exactly that—as interest rates dropped, orders poured in for the stock, and its price was bid up. Currently, Commonwealth's stock sells for $33, up over 50 percent from the 1984 level, and the dividend yield (9.2%) is very close to the bond yield (9.5%).

INTEREST RATES AND BUSINESS DECISIONS

The yield curve for April 1987, shown earlier in Figure 5-4, indicates how much the U.S. government had to pay in 1987 to borrow money for 1 year, 5 years, 10 years, and so on. A business borrower would have had to pay somewhat more, but assume for the moment that we are back in 1987 and that the yield curve for that year also applies to your company. Now suppose your company has decided to build a new plant with a 30-year life which will cost $1 million and to raise the $1 million by selling an issue of debt (or borrowing) rather than by selling stock. If you borrowed in 1987 on a short-term basis — say, for one year — your interest cost for that year would be only 6.5 percent, or $65,000, whereas if you used long-term (30-year) financing, your cost would be 8.3 percent, or $83,000. Therefore, at first glance it would seem that you should have used short-term debt.

However, this could prove to be a horrible mistake. If you use short-term debt, you will have to renew your loan every year, and the rate charged on each new loan will reflect the then-current short-term rate. Interest rates could return to their March 1980 levels, so by 1989 you could be paying 14 percent, or $140,000, per year. These high interest payments would cut into and perhaps eliminate your profits. Your reduced profitability could easily increase your firm's risk to the point where your bond rating would be lowered, causing lenders to increase the risk premium built into the interest rate they charge you, which in turn would force you to pay even higher rates. These very high interest rates would further reduce your profitability and would worry lenders even more, making them reluctant to renew your loan. If your lenders refused to renew the loan and demanded payment, as they have every right to do, you might have trouble raising the cash. If you had to make price cuts to convert physical assets to cash, you might incur heavy operating losses or even bankruptcy.

On the other hand, if you used long-term financing in 1987, your interest costs would remain constant at $83,000 per year, so an increase in interest rates in the economy would not hurt you. You might even be able to buy up some of your bankrupted competitors at bargain prices — bankruptcies increase dramatically when interest rates rise, primarily because many firms do use short-term debt.

Does all this suggest that firms should always avoid short-term debt? Not necessarily. If the Reagan administration's economic program continues to work, inflation will remain low in the next few years, and so will interest rates. If you had borrowed on a long-term basis for 8.3 percent in April 1987, your company would be at a major disadvantage if its debt was locked in at 8.3 percent while its competitors (who used short-term debt in 1987 and thus rode interest rates down in subsequent years) had a borrowing cost of only 6 or 7 percent. On the other hand, Reagan's program (or his successor's) might not continue to work, and large federal deficits might drive inflation and interest rates up to new record levels. In that case, you would wish you had borrowed on a long-term basis in 1987.

Financing decisions would be easy if we could predict future interest rates accurately. Unfortunately, predicting future interest rates with consistent accuracy is somewhere between difficult and impossible — people who make a living by selling interest rate forecasts say it is difficult; many others say it is impossible.

Even if it is difficult to predict future interest rate *levels,* it is easy to predict that interest rates will *fluctuate* — they always have, and they always will. This being the case, sound financial policy calls for using a mix of long- and short-term debt, as well as equity, in such a manner that the firm can survive in most interest rate environments. Further, the optimal financial policy depends in an important way on the nature of the firm's assets; the easier it is to sell off assets and thus to pay off debts, the more feasible it is to use large amounts of short-term debt. This makes it more feasible to finance current assets than fixed assets with short-term debt. We will return to this issue later in the book, when we discuss working capital management.

SUMMARY

This chapter has described how interest rates are determined and some of the ways in which interest rates affect business decisions.

The pure, interest rate (k^*) is determined as a joint product of (1) the rate of return on investment available to producers and (2) consumers' time preferences for current consumption as opposed to saving for future consumption. To establish the interest rate for a given loan, we must add to the pure interest rate risk premiums which reflect (1) expected inflation over the life of the loan (IP), (2) the default risk inherent in the loan (DP), (3) the degree of liquidity of the loan (LP), and (4) the maturity of the loan (MP):

$$k = k^* + IP + DP + LP + MP.$$

Interest rates fluctuate over time. Long-term rates change primarily because of changes in the rate of expected inflation, whereas short-term rates reflect both expected inflation and Federal Reserve intervention in the markets.

The yield curve describes the relationship between long- and short-term interest rates. When inflation is expected to continue at the current rate, the yield curve tends to slope upward because of maturity effects; such a curve is called "normal." However, in recent years the yield curve has been "abnormal," or inverted, about as often as it has been normal.

RESOLUTION TO·DECISION IN FINANCE

When Interest Rates Go Up, What Happens to Bond Prices?

Although in its infancy, the mortgage-backed securities market is enormous. In 1986, the trading volume in mortgage-backed securities topped $2.5 billion. Yet, some analysts worry that the market for these securities may have grown faster than investors' understanding of how it functions. Merrill Lynch's experience should only add to the analysts' concern.

When interest rates go up, bond prices go down. It's a fundamental law of the financial world. But even financial giants such as Merrill Lynch find mortgage-backed securities hard to figure out. Stripped securities can be even more confusing since the interest-only (IO) portions and the principal-only (PO) portions are traded separately. When interest rates are declining, homeowners rush to prepay their high-interest mortgages at lower rates. The investor who holds high-yield mortgage-backed bonds stands the risk that part of the mortgage pool making up that bond will be paid off early. Conversely, when rates are going up, borrowers hang on to their mortgages, dragging out the average time it takes for the principal to be paid. The end result is a highly volatile market in which the value of mortgage-backed securities can gyrate wildly depending on the timing of homeowners' payments.

When Merrill Lynch entered the mortgage securities market with a $1.7 billion issue of IOs and POs on April 8, 1987, interest rates had already begun to rise a few days earlier. However, Merrill Lynch apparently mispriced its offering, setting the price of IOs at least 10% too low and its POs about 10% too high. As a result, when interest rates surged, investors snapped up the IOs leaving Merrill Lynch with a huge $900 million stock of unsold POs.

Merrill Lynch's blunder garnered the firm little sympathy on Wall Street because most firms are careful to sell off IOs and POs in equal proportions so that the remaining unsold securities are hedged. That way they can protect themselves against holding only one side of a stripped issue should interest rates set securities prices gyrating wildly.

Merrill Lynch's management is quick to point out that the sharp upturn in interest rates in the spring of 1987 caused bond-trading losses up and down Wall Street. Furthermore, it blames much of its loss on unauthorized trading by one of its mortgage securities traders who subsequently was fired. However, analysts are reluctant to accept these explanations for one of the largest trading losses in Wall Street history (totally more than $275 million). In the end, however, Merrill Lynch may have lost more than money with its belly flop in mortgage-backed securities; it may have lost a shot at a most coveted first-tier investment banking berth—at least for now.

Sources: *Wall Street Journal*, May 6, 1987, p. 1. *Wall Street Journal*, May 11, 1987, p. 4. "How Wall Street Is Driving the Mortgage Market," Christopher Farell, *Business Week*, May 4, 1987, pp. 108–109. "The Big Loss at Merrill Lynch: Why It Was Blindsided," Ellen Spragins, *Business Week*, May 18, 1987, pp. 112–113.

QUESTIONS

5-1 Suppose interest rates on residential mortgages of equal risk were 14 percent in California and 16 percent in New York. Could this differential persist? What forces might tend to equalize rates? Would differences in borrowing costs for businesses of equal risk located in California and New York be more or less likely than residential mortgage rate differentials? Would differentials in the cost of money for New York and California firms be more likely to exist if the firms being compared were very large or if they were very small?

5-2 Which fluctuates more, long-term or short-term interest rates? Why?

5-3 You think that the economy is just entering a recession. Your firm must raise capital immediately, and debt will be used. Would it be better to borrow on a long-term or a short-term basis? Explain.

5-4 Suppose the population of Area A is relatively young, whereas that of Area B is relatively old. Everything else about the two areas is equal.
  a. Would interest rates be the same or different in the two areas? Explain.
  b. Would trends toward nationwide branching by banks and S&Ls and toward the development of diversified financial corporations affect your answer to Part a?

5-5 Suppose a new and much more liberal Congress and administration were elected, and their first order of business was to change the Federal Reserve System and force the Fed to greatly expand the money supply. What effect would this have
  a. On the yield curve at the present time?
  b. On the yield curve that would probably exist two or three years in the future?

5-6 The federal government (1) encouraged the development of the S&L industry; (2) forced the industry to make long-term, fixed interest rate mortgages; and (3) restricted the S&Ls' capital largely to deposits that were withdrawable on demand or very short notice.
  a. Would S&Ls be better off in a world with a "normal" or an inverted yield curve? Explain.
  b. If federal actions such as deficit spending and expansion of the money supply produced a sharp increase in inflation, why might it necessitate a federal bailout of the S&L industry?

5-7 Assume that the yield curve is horizontal. You and other investors now receive information that suggests the economy is headed into a recession. You and most other investors think that the Fed will soon relax credit and that this will lead to a decline in short-term interest rates. Over the long run (the next 5, 10, or 15 years) people expect a fairly high rate of inflation, and they expect that this will keep long-term rates fairly high. Explain what all of this will probably do to the yield curve. Use a graph to illustrate your answer.

5-8 Suppose interest rates on Treasury bonds rose from 12 percent to 17 percent. Other things held constant, what do you think would happen to the price of an average company's common stock?

5-9 Why are Treasury bills popular short-term investments for corporations and commercial banks?

5-10 The curve describing the relationship between interest rates and term to maturity is known as the _____ curve. Other things held constant, how would each of the following factors affect the slope and the general position of this curve? Indicate by a ($+$) if it would lead to an upward shift in the curve, a ($-$) if it would cause the curve to shift downward, or a (0) if it would have no effect or an indeterminate effect on the slope or position of the curve.

	Effect on the Yield Curve	
	Slope	**Position**
a. Investors perceive the risk of default to increase on securities with longer maturities; that is, they become increasingly uncertain about the more distant future.	————	————
b. Future interest rates are expected to fall.	————	————
c. The Federal Reserve pumps a large amount of money into the banking system.	————	————
d. Business firms begin a massive inventory build-up.	————	————
e. An inexpensive and efficient method of harnessing nuclear power is developed. This development leads to a decline in the expected rate of inflation.	————	————

SELF-TEST PROBLEM

ST-1 Assume that it is now January 1, 1988. The rate of inflation is expected to average 5 percent throughout 1988. However, increased government deficits and renewed vigor in the economy are then expected to push inflation rates higher. Investors expect the inflation rate to be 6 percent in 1989, 7 percent in 1990, and 8 percent in 1991. The real rate of interest, k^*, is currently 3 percent. Assume that no maturity or liquidity risk premiums are required on bonds with 5 years or less to maturity. The current interest rate on 5-year T-bonds is 10 percent.

a. What is the average expected inflation rate over the next 4 years?

b. What should be the prevailing interest rate on 4-year T-bonds?

c. What is the implied expected inflation rate in 1992, or Year 5?

PROBLEMS

5-1 **Yield curves.** Suppose you and most other investors expect the rate of inflation to be 10 percent next year, to fall to 5 percent during a recession in the following year, and then to run at a rate of 8 percent thereafter. The real rate, k^*, is 2 percent. Maturity risk premiums on Treasury securities rise from zero on very-short-term bonds (those that mature in a few days) by 0.30 percentage points for each year to maturity up to a limit of 1.5 percentage points on 5-year or longer T-bonds.

a. Calculate the interest rates on 1-, 2-, 3-, 4-, 5-, 10-, and 20-year Treasury securities, and plot the yield curve.

b. Now suppose AT&T, an AAA-rated company, has bonds with the same maturities as the Treasury bonds. As an approximation, plot an AT&T yield curve on the same graph with the Treasury bond yield curve. (Hint: Think about the risk premium on AT&T's long-term versus its short-term bonds.)

5-2   **Yield curves.** Look in *The Wall Street Journal* or some other paper which publishes interest rates on U.S. Treasury securities. Identify some Treasury bonds which mature at various dates in the future, record the years to maturity and the interest rate for each, and then plot a yield curve. (Note: Some of the bonds — for example, the 3 percent issue which matures in February 1995 — will show very low yields. Disregard them — these are "flower bonds," which can be turned in and used at par value to pay estate taxes, so they always sell at close to par and have a yield which is close to the coupon yield, irrespective of the going rate of interest. Also, the yields quoted in the *Journal* are not for the same point in time for all bonds, so random variations will appear. An interest rate series that is purged of flower bonds and random variations, and hence one that provides a better picture of the true yield curve, can be obtained from the *Federal Reserve Bulletin.*)

5-3   **Risk premiums.** Look in *The Wall Street Journal.* Examine the interest rates for comparable maturity dates of U.S. Treasury securities and government agency securities.
    a. Which group of securities carries the slightly higher interest rate?
    b. Why do you think this relationship exists?

5-4   **Expected interest rates.** Assume that the pure rate of interest is 3 percent and that the maturity and liquidity risk premiums are zero. If the nominal rate of interest on 1-year Treasury bonds is 11 percent and the rate on 2-year Treasury bonds is 13 percent, what rate of inflation is expected during Year 2? Comment on why the average rate over the 2-year period differs from the 1-year rate expected for Year 2.

ANSWER TO SELF-TEST PROBLEM

ST-1   **a.** Average = (5% + 6% + 7% + 8%)/4 = 26%/4 = 6.50%
    b. $k_{T\text{-bond}}$ + k* + I = 0.03 + 0.065 = 0.095 = 9.50%
    c. If the 5-year T-bond rate is 10 percent, the inflation rate is expected to average approximately 10% − 3% = 7% over the next 5 years. Thus the Year 5 implied inflation rate is 9.0 percent:

$$7\% = (5\% + 6\% + 7\% + 8\% + I_5)/5$$

$$35\% = 26\% + I_5$$

$$I_5 = 9\%.$$

Part III

FINANCIAL STATEMENTS AND FINANCIAL PLANNING

A company's financial statements tell an important story about the firm. The financial manager or financial analyst must be able to interpret these statements in order to completely understand them. Chapter 6 discusses the four basic financial statements—the *income statement,* the *balance sheet,* the *statement of retained earnings,* and the *statement of cash flows.* Financial analysis, explored in Chapter 7, allows the analyst to evaluate the firm's financial strengths and weaknesses. Management may then utilize this knowledge to plan for future financial challenges. Predicting future business conditions is an important requisite to effective financial management. Chapter 8 provides useful tools for making projections of future financial statements. Managers use these financial projections to plan and evaluate future operating alternatives.

Chapter 6

Examining a Firm's Financial Data

Campbell Soup Company
used its annual report to
proclaim 1986 "The Year
of Soup" explaining that
"1986 was the year that
Campbell Soup Company
began transforming
soup—an old food
favorite—into a modern
day, life-style product.
And in doing so
transformed itself."
Campbell sales rose to
$4.4 billion in 1986, a 10
percent increase over the
previous year.

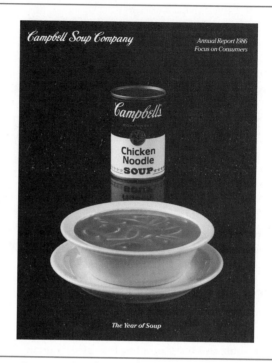

Source: Courtesy of Campbell Soup Company.

Any analysis of a firm, whether by management or investors, must include an examination of the company's financial data. The most obvious and readily available source of these financial data is the company's *annual report*. In this chapter we examine the *basic financial data* that are available in the firm's annual report. In following chapters we discuss the *techniques of financial analysis* used to evaluate financial data in the determination of the firm's relative riskiness, profit potential, and general managerial competence.

THE ANNUAL REPORT

annual report

A report, issued annually
by corporations to their
stockholders, containing
basic financial statements
and management's opin-
ion of operations and fu-
ture prospects.

Of the various reports corporations issue to their stockholders, the **annual report** is by far the most important. Two types of information are given in this report. First, there is a verbal statement that describes the firm's operating results during the past year and discusses new developments that will affect future operations. Second, the report presents four basic financial statements — the *income statement,* the *balance sheet,* the *statement of retained earnings,* and the *statement of cash flows.* Taken together, these statements give an accounting picture of the firm's operations and financial position. Detailed data are provided for at least the two most recent years, along with historical summaries of key operating statistics for the prior five to ten years.

The quantitative information and the verbal information are equally important. The financial statements report *what has actually happened* to earnings and dividends over the past few years, whereas the verbal statements represent an attempt to explain *why things turned out the way they did.* For example, suppose earnings dropped sharply last year. Management may report that the drop resulted from a strike at a key facility at the height of the busy season, but then will go on to state that the strike has now been settled and that future profits are expected to bounce back. Of course, this return to profitability may not occur, and investors will want to compare management's past statements with subsequent results. In any event, the information contained in the annual report is used by investors to *form expectations* about future earnings and dividends and about the riskiness of these expected cash flows. Therefore the annual report is obviously of great interest to investors.

THE INCOME STATEMENT

An **income statement** summarizes a firm's revenues and expenses over an accounting period — generally one year. Table 6-1 presents an income statement as it might appear in an annual report. This financial statement records the 1986 and 1987 profits and disbursements of Carter Chemical Company, a major producer of industrial and consumer chemical products.

    Reported at the top of the statement are net sales, from which various costs, including income taxes, are subtracted to obtain net income available to common shareholders. Although this is the general form for income statements, several variations exist. For example, rather than deducting all operating costs from sales, as in Table 6-1, some income statements deduct cost of goods sold from sales to produce gross profits. Gross profits are then reduced by all operating expenses to obtain operating profits.

    The most important continuing source of revenue for a business is *sales* or *operating revenues.* For a manufacturer like Carter, the sales account is the accumulation of total units sold multiplied by their respective prices.

income statement
A statement summarizing the firm's revenues and expenses over an accounting period.

Operating Costs and Expenses

In a typical manufacturing firm, the operating costs and expense accounts include all costs required to obtain raw materials and convert them into finished products, the costs of selling, and the costs associated with overseeing operations. *Cost of goods sold* represents costs associated with raw materials acquisition and direct production costs. Sales expenses for salaries, travel, commissions, promotion, and advertising generally are the most important items in *selling expenses.* Staff and executive salaries and office expenses are the major items in *general and administrative expenses.* Of course, expenses attributable to assets used in the production, selling, and supervision processes must be accounted for through these direct costs, through *depreciation,* or through *lease payments.*

Table 6-1 **Carter Chemical Company: Income Statement for Year Ending December 31 (Millions of Dollars, except Per-Share Data)**

	1987	1986
Net sales	$3,000	$2,850
Costs and expenses:		
Labor and materials	$2,544	$2,413
Depreciation	100	90
Selling	22	20
General and administrative	40	35
Lease payments on buildings	28	28
Total costs	$2,734	$2,586
Net operating income, or earnings before interest and taxes (EBIT)	$ 266	$ 264
Less interest expense:		
Interest on notes payable	$ 8	$ 2
Interest on first mortgage bonds	40	42
Interest on debentures	18	3
Total interest	$ 66	$ 47
Earnings before tax	$ 200	$ 217
Combined state and federal income tax (at 40%)	80	87
Net income after taxes available to common stockholders	$ 120	$ 130
Disposition of net income		
Dividends to common stockholders	$ 100	$ 90
Addition to retained earnings	$ 20	$ 40
Per share of common stock		
Earnings per share (EPS)[a]	$ 2.40	$ 2.60
Dividends per share (DPS)[a]	$ 2.00	$ 1.80

[a]Fifty million shares are outstanding: see Table 6-2. Calculations of EPS and DPS for 1987 are as follows:

$$EPS = \frac{\text{Net income after tax}}{\text{Shares outstanding}} = \frac{\$120,000,000}{50,000,000} = \$2.40.$$

$$DPS = \frac{\text{Dividends paid to common stockholders}}{\text{Shares outstanding}} = \frac{\$100,000,000}{50,000,000} = \$2.00.$$

Even though the computation of these expenses appears to be unambiguous, several of them have a wide latitude of expression. Great discretion is allowed managers in calculating depreciation and valuing inventory (as part of cost of goods sold).[1] Because these calculations have a notable effect on reported income, you may wish to review alternative means of calculating depreciation in Chapter 2.

---

[1]These are not the only areas of managerial discretion in financial reporting. Such items as the determination of pension fund liabilities and the decision between expensing or capitalizing certain costs also have an important effect on reported profits.

INDUSTRY PRACTICE

Going with the Flow

These days, Wall Street analysts aren't just looking at a company's reported earnings to get their finger on the company's financial pulse. Instead, they're increasingly interested in the flow . . . the company's cash flow, that is. Cash flow is the hot new financial barometer, and everyone — analysts, investors, and takeover specialists — is studying what it has to say about a company's financial health and earning power.

Cash flow has sometimes been called "owners earnings," which is a good way to think about what cash flow says about a company. After all, owners of private companies aren't much interested in reported profits; when all is said and done, reported profits have to be shared with the IRS. Instead, their focus is on bringing in enough cash to pay workers, pay the bank for money borrowed, and keep the business going and growing. An entrepreneur is not interested in traditionally reported profit figures but instead goes with the flow.

Cash flow can be measured in several different ways. A market analyst and a corporate raider would be interested in different measures of cash flow. Generally, however, a good measure of a company's cash flow includes net income plus charges such as depreciation, amortization, and depletion, which reduce net income but don't take money out of the corporate kitty.

Although a handful of gadfly market analysts have been touting the virtues of cash flow analysis for years, it has only recently come into vogue. Enactment of the Accelerated Cost Re-

covery System in 1981 let companies depreciate assets much more quickly than before. Even though ACRS was designed to encourage capital spending, money plowed into new plant and equipment cuts into reported earnings. With sluggish reported earnings but a thriving American business climate, Wall Street began looking for another measure of future corporate earning power.

Some investment experts dismiss cash flow figures as a passing fad or a way to gloss over poor earnings and to justify too-high stock prices. However, although it is the traditional indicator of corporate performance, reported earnings can be distorted by accounting rules, the tax codes, and financing decisions. Cash flow analysis, its proponents claim, can cut through those distortions and provide a clearer picture of a company's financial health and earnings potential.

Cash flow analysis has found strong backing, especially among takeover specialists who seek to exploit the discrepancy between strong cash flow figures and mediocre earnings as a lever for acquisition bids. These leveraged buyouts are financed by borrowing funds, using the value of the firm to be acquired as collateral. The collateral value of the target company is based on the value of the company's physical assets and its projected cash flow.

Still, some long-time cash flow mavens like Tom Nourse, a San Diego-based analyst who provides cash flow analyses to institutional investors and who publishes an investment newsletter, are afraid that today's takeover specialists and investors may be distorting the true meaning of cash flow figures. Nourse contends that "properly measured over a period of time, comparative cash flow is a better determinant of value [than earnings]," but he adds that many cash flow proponents are taking an overly sim-

Source: Elizabeth Kaplan, "Wall Street Zeros in on Cash Flow," *Dun's Business Month,* July 1985, 40–41; Jeffrey Laderman, "The Savviest Investors are Going with the Flow," *Business Week,* September 7, 1987, 92–93; and Joseph Duncan, "That Puzzling Profit Performance," *Dun's Business Month,* September 1985, 38.

plistic view of the numbers and ignoring future reinvestment needs. One of the problems, says Jim Chanos, an analyst with Deutsche Capital, is that takeover specialists and investors alike are treating depreciation as if it were "a mere accounting convention." The problem, of course, is that in the real world outside the accountants' office, when an asset is fully depreciated, it must be replaced.

Nourse counsels against accepting "wildly optimistic" projections made about companies based on cash flow numbers. He says that it's not just the quantity of cash flow but the quality

as well that is telling about a company. "If most of the cash flow is coming from depreciation, it's not as good as a company where most is coming from income," says Nourse.

Maybe that's why the Financial Accounting Standards Board prohibits public companies from reporting cash flow per share the same way they report earnings per share. Where the cash flow comes from is just as important as how much there is. Still, the same thing can be said about reported earnings. These days a savvy balance sheet analyst will want to know about both.

Remaining Disbursements

The *earnings before interest and taxes,* or *operating profits,* are further reduced by interest payments on debt — which must be paid whether the company is profitable or losing money. Payment of principal is not indicated on the income statement but is reported, as we shall see, on the balance sheet.

All firms have a partner, some might say an "uninvited" partner, who demands a predetermined percentage of the profits. This partner is, of course, the U.S. government, which requires that a portion of the firm's profits be paid in the form of income taxes. State and local governments require tax payments as well. Certain accounting conventions allow the firm to postpone these tax payments.

The Bottom Line

Financial managers often refer to net income as "the bottom line," pointing out that of all the items on the income statement, net income draws the greatest attention. A manager once noted, "Net income is so important that we underline it twice!"

The firm's net income is either paid to the shareholders in the form of dividends or retained by the firm to support its growth. These divisions are reported in total dollars. The dividends to shareholders are reported on a per-share basis, as well. Similarly, net income is also reported on a per-share basis. Carter earned $2.40 per share in 1987, down from $2.60 in 1986, but it raised the dividend from $1.80 to $2.00.

THE BALANCE SHEET

The income statement reports on operations *over a period of time* — for example, during the calendar year 1987. The **balance sheet,** on the other hand, may be thought of as a snapshot of the firm's financial position *at a point in time* — for example, on December 31, 1987.

    The left-hand side of Carter's balance sheet, which is shown in Table 6-2, shows the firm's assets, and the right-hand side of the statement shows claims against the assets. These claims against assets are divided into two types — those claims that arise from the investment of funds by the owners of the firm, which constitutes the firm's **equity,** and those claims that arise from the debt the firm owes the nonowners of the firm. Because these debts must be repaid, they constitute the firm's **liabilities.**

balance sheet
A statement of the firm's financial status at a specific point in time.

equity
Financing supplied by the firm's owners.

liabilities
All the legal claims held against the firm by non-owners.

Assets

The **assets** are listed in the order of their liquidity, or the length of time it typically takes to convert them to cash. The current assets, or working capital, of the firm consist of assets that are normally converted into cash within one year. Temporary stores of liquidity are *cash* and *marketable securities.* Examples of securities used for temporary investment purposes are identified in Chapter 10. *Inventories* include raw materials used in the production process,

assets
All things to which the firm holds legal claim.

Table 6-2 **Carter Chemical Company:**
Balance Sheet as of December 31
(Millions of Dollars)

Assets	1987	1986	Claims on Assets	1987	1986
Cash	$ 50	$ 55	Accounts payable	$ 60	$ 30
Marketable securities	0	25	Notes payable	100	60
Accounts receivable	350	315	Accrued wages	10	10
Inventories	300	215	Accrued federal income taxes	130	120
Total current assets	$ 700	$ 610	Total current liabilities	$ 300	$ 220
Gross plant and equipment	$1,800	$1,470	First mortgage bonds	$ 500	$ 520
Less depreciation	500	400	Debentures	300	60
Net plant and equipment	$1,300	$1,070	Total long-term debt	$ 800	$ 580
			Stockholders' equity:		
			Common stock (50,000,000 shares,		
			$1 par)	$ 50	$ 50
			Additional paid-in capital	100	100
			Retained earnings	750	730
			Total stockholders' equity (common net		
			worth)	$ 900	$ 880
Total assets	$2,000	$1,680	Total claims on assets	$2,000	$1,680

work in process, and finished goods awaiting sale. *Accounts receivable* result when the firm sells a product on credit. When the customer pays, the account receivable is converted to cash.

Assets with a useful life of more than one year are referred to as *fixed assets.* These assets typically include the plant, equipment, office furniture, and other assets which may be used repeatedly in the production process. With extended usage these assets will eventually wear out. *Depreciation* was at one time supposed to reflect the decline in an asset's useful productive value. However, because depreciation is a noncash expense which postpones the firm's taxes, the actual relationship between an asset's productive value and its book value is low. In fact, since the introduction of the Accelerated Cost Recovery System (ACRS) method of depreciation in 1981, the economic or productive life of an asset is no longer tied to its tax life; an asset's tax life is generally shorter than its economic or productive life. We have discussed the implications of depreciation for the firm's profits in Chapter 2.

Liabilities

A liability is a claim against the assets of the firm. On the balance sheet, these liabilities are listed in the order in which they mature and must be repaid. Current liabilities are those debts that mature within one year.

Accounts payable represent the amount the company owes to business creditors for purchases of goods on open account. Each of these purchases is recorded on the seller's balance sheet as an account receivable. *Notes payable* are more formal evidence of short-term debt owed to banks or other lenders. *Accruals* are current expenses which have not yet been paid as of the date of the balance sheet. *Accrued wages* and *accrued federal income taxes* are payable on a periodic basis — weekly or monthly for wages and quarterly for taxes. These accounts build as the wage and tax liabilities increase during the period. Once paid, they are reduced by the amounts paid, and then they begin to built again as the process resumes.

Long-term liabilities are debt obligations with more than a single year remaining until maturity. The debt may have been incurred from any source, such as from financial intermediaries or through the sale of bonds. Table 6-2 indicates Carter Chemical Company has two bonds outstanding, a *first mortgage bond* issue and a *debenture* issue.[2]

The bond's principal may be repaid either at maturity in a lump sum or in periodic repayments. The provision for the orderly repayment of a bond issue is known as a *sinking fund.* Carter is required to pay off $20 million each year. Accordingly, its outstanding mortgage bonds declined by $20 million from December 31, 1986 to December 31, 1987. The current portion of the long-term debt is included in notes payable here, although in a more detailed balance sheet it would be shown as a separate item.

---

[2]We discuss differences in bond indentures (debt contracts) in Chapter 17.

Stockholders' Equity

The **stockholders' equity,** or **net worth,** represents the owners' claim against the assets of the firm. This claim differs significantly from the claims of nonowners. For one thing, the claim does not mature and thus never needs to be paid off. Second, the equity amount is not a set amount; rather, it is a residual. That is,

$$\text{Assets} \quad - \quad \text{Liabilities} \quad = \quad \text{Stockholders' equity}$$
$$\$2,000,000,000 - \$1,100,000,000 = \quad \$900,000,000.$$

Suppose assets decline in value; for example, suppose some of the firm's inventory is obsolete and is written off. Because liabilities remain constant, the value of the net worth declines. Therefore, the risk of asset-value fluctuations is borne entirely by the stockholders. Note, however, that if asset values rise, these benefits accrue exclusively to the stockholders.

The equity section of the balance sheet is divided into three accounts — *common stock, paid-in capital,* and *retained earnings.* The first two accounts arise when the firm issues new common stock to raise capital. A **par value** is generally assigned to common stock — Carter's stock has a par value of $1. Now suppose Carter were to sell 1 million additional shares at a price of $30 per share. The company would raise $30 million, and the cash account would go up by this amount. On the right-hand side of the balance sheet, the transaction would be reflected by an increase of $1 per share, or a total increase of $1 million in the common stock account. The remaining $29 per share would be added to the **paid-in capital** account. This account is occasionally referred to by its more descriptive title, *capital in excess of par.* The results of a sale of new common stock are as follows:

	Before Sale of Stock
Common stock (50,000,000 shares, $1 par)	$ 50,000,000
Paid-in capital	100,000,000
Retained earnings	750,000,000
Total stockholders' equity	$900,000,000

	After Sale of Stock
Common stock (51,000,000 shares, $1 par)	$ 51,000,000
Paid-in capital	129,000,000
Retained earnings	750,000,000
Total stockholders' equity	$930,000,000

Thus, after the sale, common stock would show $51 million, paid-in capital would show $129 million, and there would be 51 million shares. Naturally, the retained earnings account is not affected by the sale of new common stock.

The common stock and paid-in capital accounts provide information about external sources of equity funds. Self-generated, or internal, equity comes from the undistributed profits of the firm. The retained earnings account is built up over time by the firm "saving" a part of its net income rather than paying all

stockholders' equity (net worth)
The capital supplied by stockholders — capital stock, paid-in-capital, and retained earnings. *Common equity,* or *stockholders' equity,* is that part of the total net worth belonging to the common stockholders.

par value
The nominal or face value of a stock or bond.

paid-in capital
The funds received in excess of par value when the firm sells stock.

of its earnings out as dividends.[3] Thus, since its inception, Carter has retained, or plowed back, a total of $750 million — $20 million was added in the last year.

The breakdown of the equity accounts is important for some purposes but not for others. For example, a potential stockholder would want to know if the company had actually earned the funds reported in its equity accounts or if the funds had come mainly from selling stock. A potential creditor, on the other hand, would be more interested in the amount of money the owners had put up than in the form in which they put it up. In the remainder of this chapter, we generally aggregate the three equity accounts and call this sum *common equity* or *net worth.*

THE CASH FLOW CYCLE

As a company like Carter Chemicals goes about its business, it makes sales, which lead to a reduction of inventories, to an increase in cash, and, if the sales price exceeds the cost of the item sold, to a profit. If the item is sold on credit rather than for cash, the transaction is slightly more complicated. The inventory account is reduced and accounts receivable are increased; then, when the customer pays, accounts receivable are reduced and the cash account is increased. These transactions cause the balance sheet to change, and they also are reflected in the income statement. It is important that you understand that (1) businesses deal with *physical* units like autos, computers, and chemicals; (2) physical transactions are translated into dollar terms through the accounting system; and (3) financial analysis is designed to examine the accounting numbers in order to measure how efficient the firm is at making and selling physical goods and services. In other words, financial analysis helps determine how good the company is at taking resources in the form of labor and materials and converting them into some product or service that people want and are willing to pay for.

Several factors make financial analysis difficult. One is accounting. Different methods of inventory valuation and depreciation can lead to differences in reported profits for otherwise similar firms, and a good financial analyst must be able to adjust for these differences if he or she is to make valid comparisons between companies. Another factor involves timing. An action is taken at one point in time, but even though its full effects are not felt until some later period, the effects of the action need to be evaluated before its final results are known.

To understand how timing influences the financial statements and hence financial analysis, one must understand the **cash flow** cycle within a firm, as set forth in Figure 6-1. Here rectangles represent balance sheet accounts (as-

cash flow
The actual net cash, as opposed to accounting net income, that flows into or out of the firm during some specified period; equal to net income after taxes plus noncash expenses, including depreciation.

---

[3]A word of caution is in order here. The retained earnings account does *not* represent a pool from which funds may be withdrawn. The retained earnings account simply indicates the source, corporate savings, from which some of the firm's assets were originally procured.

Figure 6-1 **Cash and Materials Flows within the Firm**

The focal point of a firm's cash flow cycle is its cash account, whose balance is influenced by the firm's other accounts (rectangles) and activities (circles). The lower portion of this diagram shows how the cash account is increased through stock issues and borrowing. The cash is then used to purchase raw materials and acquire fixed assets, both of which feed into the production of goods and eventually replenish the cash account through sales. Note that cash flows continuously through this cycle, so that lags in any one portion will influence all portions and will ultimately affect the cash account.

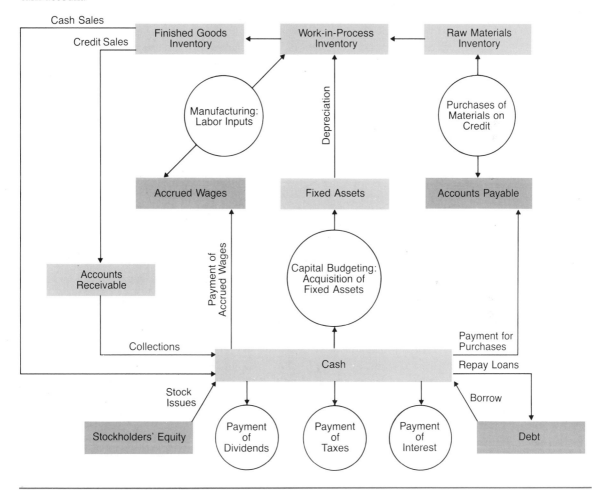

sets and claims against assets) and circles represent actions taken by the firm. Various transactions cause changes in the accounts. The purchase of raw materials inventory reduces cash, whereas the collection of accounts receivable increases cash. The diagram is by no means a complete representation of the cash flow cycle; to avoid undue complexity, it shows only the major flows.

The cash account is the focal point of the figure. Certain events, such as collecting accounts receivable or borrowing money from the bank, will cause the cash account to increase, whereas the payment of taxes, interest, and so on will cause the cash account to decline. Similar comments could be made about all the balance sheet accounts — their balances rise, fall, or remain constant depending on events that occur during the period under study, which for Carter is December 31, 1986, through December 31, 1987.

Projected sales increases may require the firm to raise cash by borrowing from its bank or selling new stock. For example, if the firm anticipates an increase in sales, it will (1) expend cash to buy or build fixed assets, (2) step up purchases, thereby increasing raw materials inventories and accounts payable, (3) increase production, which causes an increase in accrued wages and work-in-process, and (4) eventually build up its finished goods inventory. Some cash will have been expended, lowering the cash account, and the firm will have obligated itself to expend still more cash to pay off its accounts payable and accrued wages. These events will have occurred *before* any cash has been generated. Even when the expected sales do occur, there will still be a lag in the generation of cash until receivables are collected. For example, if Carter grants credit for 30 days, it will be about 30 days after the sale is made before cash comes in. Depending on how much cash the firm had at the beginning of the buildup, on the length of its production-sales-collection cycle, and on how long it can delay payment of its own payables and accrued wages, the firm may have to obtain substantial amounts of additional cash by selling stock or bonds or by borrowing from a bank or other financial institution.

If the firm is profitable, its sales revenues will exceed its costs, and its cash inflows will eventually exceed its cash outlays. However, even a profitable firm can experience a cash shortage if it is growing rapidly. It may have to pay for plant, materials, and labor before cash from the expanded sales starts flowing in. For this reason, rapidly growing firms often require large bank loans or capital from other sources.

An unprofitable firm will have larger cash outlays than inflows. This, in turn, will typically cause a slowdown in the payment of accrued wages and accounts payable, and it may also lead to heavy borrowings. Thus liabilities build up to excessive levels in unprofitable firms. Similarly, an overly ambitious expansion plan will be reflected in an excessive buildup of inventories and fixed assets, whereas a poor credit and collection policy will produce bad debts and reduced profits that first show up as high accounts receivable. Financial analysts are well aware of these relationships, and they use the analytical techniques discussed in the remainder of this chapter and in the next chapter to help discover problems before they become too serious.

statement of retained earnings

A statement reporting that portion of earnings not paid out in dividends. The figure that appears on the balance sheet is the sum of retained earnings for each year of the company's history.

THE STATEMENT OF RETAINED EARNINGS

Changes in the equity accounts between balance sheet dates are reported in the **statement of retained earnings;** Carter's statement is shown in Table 6-3. The company earned $120 million during 1987, paid out $100 million in

Table 6-3 **Carter Chemical Company: Statement of Retained Earnings for Year Ending December 31, 1987 (Millions of Dollars)**

Balance of retained earnings, December 31, 1986	$730
Add: Net income, 1987	120
Less: Dividends to stockholders	(100)
Balance of retained earnings, December 31, 1987	$750

dividends, and plowed $20 million back into the business. Thus the balance sheet item "retained earnings" increased from $730 million at the end of 1986 to $750 million at the end of 1987.

Note that the balance sheet account "retained earnings" represents a *claim against assets,* not assets per se. Furthermore, firms retain earnings primarily to expand the business; this means investing in plant and equipment, inventories, and so on, *not* in a bank account. Thus retained earnings as reported on the balance sheet do not represent cash and are not available for the payment of dividends or anything else.[4]

THE STATEMENT OF CASH FLOWS

The graphic analysis given in Figure 6-1 is converted to numerical form and reported in annual reports as the **statement of cash flows,** often called the *sources and uses of funds statement.* This statement is designed to show how funds were obtained and how they were used. It helps answer questions such as these: Was the expansion program financed by sale of debt or equity? How much of its required capital has the firm been able to generate internally? Has the firm been building up its liquid assets, or is it becoming less liquid? Is output from the new plant selling, or are inventories building up? Are customers paying on time, or are accounts receivable building up? Because information such as this is useful both for investment analysis and for corporate planning, the statement of cash flows is an important part of the annual report.

statement of cash flows
A statement reporting the firm's sources of financing and the uses of those funds during an accounting period.

The Role of Depreciation

Before we discuss the statement of cash flows in detail, we should pause to consider one of its most important elements — **depreciation.** First, what is depreciation? In effect, it is an annual charge against income that reflects a rough estimate of the dollar cost of the capital equipment used in the production process. For example, suppose a machine with an ACRS class life of 5

depreciation
An annual noncash charge against income that reflects a rough estimate of the dollar cost of equipment used in the production process.

---

[4]Recall from your accounting courses that the amount recorded in the retained earnings account is *not* an indication of the amount of cash the firm has. That amount (as of the balance sheet date) is found in the cash account — an asset account. A positive number in the retained earnings account indicates only that, in the past, according to generally accepted accounting principles, the firm has earned an income and its dividends have been less than that reported income.

Table 6-4 **Carter Chemical Company:**
Cash Flows vs. Reported Income for 1987
(Millions of Dollars)

	Income Statement (1)	Cash Flows (2)
Sales	$3,000	$3,000
Costs and expenses		
All costs except depreciation	2,634	2,634
Depreciation (D)	100	—
Earnings before interest and taxes (EBIT)	$ 266	$ 366
Interest expense	66	66
Earnings before taxes	$ 200	$ 300
Taxes	80	80
Net income (NI)	$ 120	N.A.
Cash flow: CF = NI + D = $120 + $100 =	$ 220	$ 220

N.A. = Not Applicable

years and a zero expected salvage value was purchased in 1987 for $500,000. This $500,000 cost is not expensed in the purchase year but, rather, is charged against production over the machine's 5-year depreciable life. If the depreciation expense were not taken, profits would be overstated and taxes would be too high. This point has been illustrated in Chapter 2. The annual depreciation allowance is deducted from sales revenues, along with such other costs as labor and raw materials, to determine income. However, depreciation is not a cash outlay; funds were expended back in 1987, so the depreciation charged against the income in years 1987 through 1991 is not a cash outlay, as are labor or raw materials charges. _Depreciation is a noncash charge_.

This point is illustrated with data for Carter Chemical Company in Table 6-4. Here Column 1 shows an abbreviated version of Carter's income statement, whereas Column 2 shows the statement on a cash flow basis. Assume for the moment that (1) all sales are for cash, (2) all costs except depreciation were paid during 1987, and (3) no buildups occurred in inventories or other assets. How much cash would have been generated from operations? From Column 2 we see that the answer is $220 million. The sales are all for cash, so the firm took in $3 billion in cash money. Its costs other than depreciation were $2,634 million, and these were paid in cash, leaving $366 million. Again, depreciation is _not_ a cash charge — the firm does not pay out the $100 million of depreciation expenses — so $366 million of cash money is still left after depreciation. Taxes and interest, however, are paid in cash, so $66 million for interest and $80 million for federal and state income taxes must be deducted from the $366 million EBIT cash flow, leaving a net cash flow from operations of $220 million. As shown in Column 1, this $220 million is, of course, exactly equal to profit after tax plus depreciation: $120 million plus $100 million equals $220 million. Therefore, because depreciation is a noncash charge, it is added back to net income to approximate cash flows from operations, and it is included as a source of funds in the statement of cash flows, as discussed in the next section.

Before leaving the subject of depreciation, we should sound a word of caution. Depreciation does not *really provide* funds; it is simply a noncash charge. Hence it is added back to net income to obtain an estimate of the cash flow from operations. If the firm made no sales, however, depreciation certainly would not provide cash flows. To see this point more clearly, consider the situation of Communications Satellite Corporation (Comsat), which derives its income principally from two satellites, one positioned over the Atlantic and one over the Pacific. Comsat's cash flows are approximately equal to its net income plus its depreciation charges. Yet, if its two satellites stopped working, sales would vanish, and although accountants might still calculate depreciation, this depreciation would provide no cash flows (except possibly some tax loss carry-backs).

Preparing the Statement of Cash Flows

The statement of cash flows is designed to answer at a glance these three questions: (1) Where did the firm get its funds during the year? (2) What did it do with its available funds? (3) Did operations during the year tend to increase or decrease the firm's liquidity as measured by its cash and marketable securities balances?[5]

The starting point in preparing a statement of cash flows is determining the change in each balance sheet item and then recording it as either a source or a use of funds in accordance with the following rules:

Sources:

1. *Increase in claims* (that is, an increase in a liability or capital account). Borrowing from a bank is an example.

2. *Decrease in an asset account.* Selling some fixed assets or reducing inventories are examples.

Uses:

1. *Decrease in a claim against assets.* Paying off a loan is an example.

2. *Increase in an asset account.* Buying fixed assets or building inventories are examples.

---

[5]There are several different formats for presenting the statement of cash flows, which used to be called a statement of changes in financial position. The older format focused on net working capital (current assets minus current liabilities). The cash flow approach is now used since it provides information in the most useful way for financial analysts.

Table 6-5 **Carter Chemical Company: Changes in Balance Sheet Accounts during 1987 (Millions of Dollars)**

	Dec. 31, 1987	Dec. 31 1986	Change Source	Use
Cash	$ 50	$ 55	$ 5	$
Marketable securities	0	25	25	
Accounts receivable	350	315		35
Inventories	300	215		85
Gross plant and equipment	1,800	1,470		330
Accumulated depreciation[a]	500	400	100	
Accounts payable	60	30	30	
Notes payable	100	60	40	
Accrued wages	10	10		
Accrued taxes	130	120	10	
Mortgage bonds	500	520		20
Debentures	300	60	240	
Common stock	50	50		
Paid-in capital	100	100		
Retained earnings	750	730	20	
Totals			$470	$470

[a]Depreciation is a "contra-asset," not an asset. Hence an increase in depreciation is a source of funds.

Thus sources of funds include bank loans and retained earnings, as well as money generated by selling assets, collecting receivables, and even drawing down the cash account. Uses include acquiring fixed assets, building up inventories, and paying off debts.

Table 6-5 shows the changes in Carter Chemical Company's balance sheet accounts during the calendar year 1987, with each change designated as a source or a use. Sources and uses *each* total $470 million. Note that the table does not contain any summary accounts, such as total current assets or net plant and equipment. If we included summary accounts in Table 6-5 and then used these accounts to prepare the statement of cash flows, we would be double counting.

The data contained in Table 6-5 are next used to prepare the formal statement of cash flows, or sources and uses of funds statement. The one contained in Carter's annual report is shown in Table 6-6. Note that every item in the "change" columns of Table 6-5 is carried over to Table 6-6 except for retained earnings. The statement of cash flows reports net income as a source and dividends as a use rather than netting these items out and simply reporting the increase in retained earnings. Cash and marketable securities are combined in Table 6-6. Like most large companies, Carter Chemicals regards its marketable securities as cash equivalents, so with regard to cash flows, they are not distinguished.

Table 6-6 **Carter Chemical Company:**
1987 Statement of Cash Flows
(or Sources and Uses Statement)
(Millions of Dollars)

Sources:

Net income	$120
Depreciation[a]	100
Increase in accounts payable	30
Increase in accrued taxes	10
Total sources from operations	$260

Uses:

Increase in accounts receivable	$ 35
Increase in inventories	85
Increase in fixed assets	330
Total uses in operations	$450
Net funds from operations	($190)[b]

Financing Activities:

Increase in notes payable	$ 40
Increase in debentures	240
Repayment of mortgage bonds	(20)
Net funds from financing	$260
Less: Common dividends	100
Increase or (decrease) in cash and marketable securities	($ 30)

[a]Depreciation is a *contra-asset,* not an asset. Hence, an increase in depreciation is a source of funds. You might wish to refer to Chapter 2 for a further discussion of why depreciation is regarded as a source of funds.
[b]Recall that parentheses denote negative numbers here and throughout the book.

Table 6-6 pinpoints the sources and uses of Carter Chemical's funds, where the term "funds" is defined as cash and marketable securities. The top part of the table shows funds generated by and used in operations. For Carter Chemical, operations provided $260 million but required the use of $450 million, so $190 million of net new money was required to support operations. By far the heaviest use of funds was to increase fixed assets.

Carter Chemical's financing activities included borrowing from banks (notes payable) and the sale of debentures while it paid off part of its mortgage bonds. In net, Carter raised $260 million from the financial markets in 1987. Carter also paid $100 million in common stock dividends during the year.

When all of these sources and uses are totaled, we see that Carter had a $30 million shortfall during 1987. It met that shortfall by selling its marketable securities for a total of $25 million and reducing its cash balance by $5 million, as seen in Table 6-5.

Carter Chemical Company is a strong, well-managed company, and its statement of cash flows shows nothing unusual or alarming. It does show a $190 million net cash drain from operations but that is entirely attributable to its expansion of net fixed assets. If the company chooses to cut back on its fixed asset expansion, it would generate positive cash flows. Thus, the cash outflow from operations does not appear likely to continue, thereby bleeding the company to death.

SUMMARY

In order to analyze any firm properly, managers and investors must be able to understand the company's financial data. The most obvious source of data for a publicly traded company is its annual report. This report contains four basic statements: the *income statement,* the *balance sheet,* the *statement of retained earnings,* and the *statement of cash flows.*

The income statement provides a detailed view of the flow of funds, both revenues and expenses, over the most recent accounting period. The focus of the income statement is the residual earnings available to stockholders after all financing and operating costs have been deducted and the claims of the federal and state government (uninvited) partners have been satisfied. The income statement indicates the amount of current earnings that is paid to owners in the form of dividends or reinvested to finance future operations.

The income statement provides a view of the firm over a period of time, whereas the balance sheet indicates the status of the firm at a specific point in time. The balance sheet describes the assets controlled by the firm and how those assets were financed. The financing of the firm is divided between contributions of owners and those of the firm's creditors.

Changes in the equity accounts between balance sheet dates are reported in the statement of retained earnings. Since many firms generate the majority of equity funds internally through undistributed profits, this statement is an important source of information on continuing equity financing.

The statement of cash flows restates information from the income statement and balance sheet. This statement answers the simple but critical questions, "Where did the money come from?" and "Where did the money go?" Thus it provides information about the sources of financing and the uses of those funds over the reporting period.

In the next chapter we explore methods that are available to further analyze the firm's financial data.

QUESTIONS

6-1   What four statements are contained in most annual reports?

6-2   Is it true that if a typical firm reports $20 million of retained earnings on its balance sheet, that firm's directors could declare a $20 million cash dividend without any qualms whatsoever?

6-3   What is the relationship between each rectangle in Figure 6-1 and each individual source and use in a statement of cash flows?

RESOLUTION TO DECISION IN FINANCE

Letters from Chairman Buffett

Of all the documents that large companies publish, none receives so much attention as the annual report to shareholders. At some companies — such as General Electric — top executives begin work on the report as much as six months before its publication. And most hire professional designers and writers to insure that the final product will look sharp and read well.

Obviously, so much fuss would hardly be necessary if the only goal of an annual report were to inform shareholders about financial results. But, in fact, most big companies have turned their annual report into flashy management showcases. In slick magazine format, using four-color photos, feature stories, and elaborate graphics, each firm tells the story its chairman would like to see told. To get the desired results, most annual reports are now produced by the director of public relations instead of the chief financial officer.

Because of their puffery, annual reports have lost credibility with serious seekers of financial information. Instead, Wall Street analysts and other sophisticated investors prefer more straightforward financial disclosure documents, such as 10-Ks, proxies, 8-Ks, and 13-Ds, all of which contain more detailed and unadorned information and must by law be filed with the Securities and Exchange Commission.

Of course, a company's philosophy and personality do count, and few other documents can offer better insight into these intangibles than an annual report. Most financial experts believe,

however, that companies owe it to their investors to distinguish between the fanfare and the facts. They want to see more annual reports that realistically examine management's conduct of business affairs and factually discuss projects that will improve corporate welfare in the future. They'd like to see annual reports become the equivalent of management report cards, detailing strengths and weaknesses and plans for improvement. Given such information, they claim, shareholders would be better equipped to make intelligent investment decisions.

Chairman Warren Buffett's letters, although probably a bit too subjective for financial reporting purists, represent a giant step in the desired direction. In fact, Berkshire Hathaway's annual reports contain no photographs, colored ink, bar charts, or graphs, freeing readers to focus on the company's financial statements and Buffett's interpretation of them. Some CEOs might contend that such a bare-bones approach is too dull for the average stockholder and, further, that some readers may actually be intimidated by the information overload. But Buffett would no doubt counter that, whatever its shortcomings, his approach shows much greater respect for shareholders' intelligence and capacity to understand than does the average annual report.

A. A. Sommer, Jr., who chaired an SEC panel formed in 1976 to study disclosure practices, says that his group agreed that letters like Buffett's were important. But, he says, "Warren's letters are unique. Few CEOs are as smart in as many ways as Warren. It would be awfully hard to require that kind of discussion from all CEOs." In other words, it takes a chairman with interesting ideas to write an interesting chairman's letter.

Sources: "Letters from Chairman Buffett," *Fortune,* August 22, 1983, 137–141; "Annual Reports Get an Editor in Washington," *Fortune,* May 7, 1979, 210–222; "Annual Reports: The Rites of Spring," *Wall Street Journal,* March 12, 1984, 26.

PROBLEMS

6-1   **Balance sheet construction.** Arrange these income statement items in their proper order:

Labor and material expense	Net income
Depreciation	Lease payments on buildings
Earnings before interest and taxes	Sales
Selling and administrative expense	Federal tax
Earnings before taxes	Interest payments

6-2   **Income computation.** Ashley's Card Shop, Inc. sold 40,000 cards at $1.00 each this month. The cards cost 75 cents wholesale. Ashley's newspaper and radio advertising expenses are $1,000 monthly. Mr. and Mrs. Ashley work in the shop and pay themselves a combined monthly salary of $3,500. The monthly rent payment for the shop is $2,300, and the depreciation on the store fixtures is $700 per month. The tax rate is 30 percent. What is the store's profit or loss for the month?

6-3   **Income computation.** McIntire Construction Company had total revenue of $375,000 last year. For the period, labor costs were $140,000; material costs were $60,000; depreciation expense was $25,000; administrative expenses were $70,000; interest on its loan was $10,000; and the principal repayment on the loan was $5,000. The firm's marginal tax rate is 35 percent.
a. What is the firm's reported net income?
b. Where does the principal repayment appear on the income statement?

6-4   **Income computation.** Romero Resources' retained earnings account on its 1986 balance sheet was $1,000,000, and the account equaled $1,200,000 at the end of 1987.
a. If the firm paid no dividends (zero dividend payout) in 1987, what was Romero's reported net income after taxes (retained earnings) for 1987?
b. If, unlike part a, Romero paid 20 percent of net income to its shareholders in the form of common stock dividends, what was the firm's reported net income after dividends (retained earnings) for the 1987 period?
c. If, unlike parts a or b, Romero retained 60 percent of earnings (net income), what was the firm's reported net income after dividends (retained earnings) for the period?

6-5   **Categorizing balance sheet accounts.** Balance sheet items may be categorized as follows:

Current assets (CA)	Long-term debt (LTD)
Fixed assets (FA)	Common stock equity (CSE)
Current liabilities (CL)	

Categorize each of the following accounts:

____Debt maturing in less than one year	____Cash
____Accounts receivable	____Common stock
____Debt maturing in more than one year	____Short-term notes payable
____Paid-in capital	____Retained earnings
____Mortgage bond	____Accruals
____Inventory	____Plant and equipment
____Accounts payable	____Short-term marketable securities

6-6   **Net worth accounts.** New Mexico Gas and Electric has the following net worth section reported on its balance sheet:

Common stock ($2 par)	$10,000,000
Paid-in capital	12,000,000
Retained earnings	53,000,000
Total shareholders' equity	$75,000,000

The company is planning to sell an issue of $8,500,000 in equity at $8.50 per share. Fill in the following net worth section to reflect the sale of the new equity:

Common stock ($2 par)	$_____
Paid-in capital	_____
Retained earnings	_____
Total shareholders' equity	$_____

6-7   **Net worth accounts.** Shortly after the sale of the stock, New Mexico Gas and Electric (from Problem 6-6) reported that net income for the year was $38,500,000. The company announced that it would pay dividends totaling $25,000,000.
   a. What was the firm's earnings per share?
   b. What was the firm's dividends per share?
   c. Complete the following net worth section to reflect the stock sales and the effect of the firm's earnings and dividend payment:

Common stock ($2 par)	$_____
Paid-in capital	_____
Retained earnings	_____
Total shareholders' equity	$_____

6-8   **Income computation.** Clary's, Inc. had $8,750,000 in retained earnings on December 31, 1986. The firm paid $700,000 in dividends during 1987 and reported retained earnings on December 31, 1987, to be $9,362,500. What was Clary's reported net income for 1987?

6-9   **Balance sheet effects.** What effect would each of the following events have on a firm's balance sheet?
   a. Purchase of a new asset for $4 million cash.
   b. Purchase of a new asset for $4 million financed with 35 percent debt and 65 percent cash.
   c. Sale of $200,000 in merchandise for cash.
   d. Sale of $200,000 in merchandise for credit.
   e. Inventory write-off of $400,000 due to obsolescence.
   f. Payment of $100,000 to trade creditors.

6-10   **Balance sheet effects.** Refer to Tables 6-1 and 6-2 to answer the following questions:
   a. What would Carter Chemical Company's balance sheet item "retained earnings" for 1987 have been if the firm paid $50 million in dividends for the year?
   b. What would Carter's 1987 EPS have been had net income for that year been $140 million rather than $120 million?
   c. Suppose that you knew that Carter's EPS was $2.40 and that net income was $120 million. Could you use this information to determine the number of shares outstanding?

    d. If Carter sold inventories carried at $200 million for only $50 million, what effects would this have on the firm's balance sheet? (Disregard tax effects.)

    e. Carter's accountants find that ACRS depreciation (see Chapter 2) shortens the tax life of assets. This would increase the firm's depreciation expense. How will this action affect the company's cash flows? No calculations are necessary.

6-11 **Sources and uses.** Determine the increase or decrease in net working capital for Missouri Steel last year, given the following information. (Assume no other changes have occurred over the past year.)

Decrease in cash	$180
Decrease in short-term marketable securities	150
Increase in accounts receivable	300
Decrease in accounts payable	120
Increase in accrued wages and taxes	90
Increase in inventories	210
Increase in notes payable	180

6-12 **Statement of cash flows.** The consolidated balance sheets for the Homebuilder's Supply Company at the beginning and end of 1987 follow. The company bought $150 million worth of fixed assets. The charge for depreciation in 1987 was $30 million. Earnings after taxes were $76 million, and the company paid out $20 million in dividends.

    a. Fill in the amount of source or use in the appropriate column.

    b. Prepare a statement of cash flows.

    c. Briefly summarize your findings.

Homebuilder's Supply Company: Balance Sheet, Beginning and End of 1987 (Millions of Dollars)

	Jan. 1	Dec. 31	Change Source	Change Use
Cash	$ 30	$ 14	_____	_____
Marketable securities	22	0	_____	_____
Net receivables	44	60	_____	_____
Inventories	106	150	_____	_____
Total current assets	$202	$224	_____	_____
Gross fixed assets	$150	$300	_____	_____
Less: Depreciation	(52)	(82)	_____	_____
Net fixed assets	$ 98	$218	_____	_____
Total assets	$300	$442	_____	_____
Accounts payable	$ 30	$36	_____	_____
Notes payable	30	6	_____	_____
Other current liabilities	14	30	_____	_____
Long-term debt	16	52	_____	_____
Common stock	76	128	_____	_____
Retained earnings	134	190	_____	_____
Total claims on assets	$300	$442	_____	_____

Chapter 7

Interpreting Financial Statements

 DECISION IN FINANCE

Cooking the Books

Stories of accounting irregularities are commonplace, usually recounting how top management inflated profits or how some low-level employee tried to conceal the way he used corporate funds to line his pockets. But recently, tales of a new brand of financial finagling have made headlines, relating how middle managers faked the numbers to fool the boss. These managers weren't stealing money or taking bribes or kickbacks or anything like that. Rather, they "cooked the books" to make top management believe they were meeting their budgets and doing a good job. For some the payoff from the figure fudging was a bonus or a promotion; for others it was nothing more than keeping their jobs. According to Professor Lee Seidler of New York University, this is a completely new trend of disclosed fraud, whose goal is to improve the manager's position rather than to steal money.

The fraud has hit some of the nation's best-known companies, among them H. J. Heinz Company, PepsiCo, McCormick & Company, and the J. Walter Thompson advertising agency. The scene of the "crime" at PepsiCo was the

company's Mexican and Philippine bottling operations. In November 1982 the company announced that officials there had falsified accounts since at least 1978. The cumulative effect—net income overstated by $92,100,000, or 6.6 percent of total net income for 1978 through the third quarter of 1982. In addition, PepsiCo said that the units' assets were overstated by $79,400,000, mainly due to overvaluing bottle and case inventories. As a result of these and other problems, PepsiCo said 1982 earnings per share would be 25 percent below 1981's restated earnings of $3.22 per share.

Tactics of the deception, which was discovered by local employees and reported to internal auditors at PepsiCo headquarters, included creating false invoices, inflating inventories and receivables, and deferring legitimate expenses to a later period—all designed to boost sales and earnings.

As you read this chapter, consider how falsified sales and earnings reports would affect the analysis of a company's financial statements. Since actual stealing isn't involved in cooking the books, does anyone get hurt? If so, who? What action should PepsiCo have taken when it discovered the deception?

See end of chapter for resolution.

In Chapter 6 we examined the major sources of financial information — the income statement and the balance sheet. We also discussed evaluative statements, such as the statement of cash flows, which aid in the interpretation of the available financial data. In this chapter we continue our discussion of the techniques of financial analysis, specifically ratio analysis, by which firms' relative riskiness, creditworthiness, profit potential, and general managerial competence can be appraised.

IMPORTANCE OF FINANCIAL STATEMENTS

Financial statements report both on a firm's position at a point in time and on its operations over some past period. Their real usefulness, however, lies in the fact that they can be used to help predict the firm's future earnings and dividends, as well as the riskiness of these cash flows. From an equity investor's viewpoint, *predicting the future* is what financial statement analysis is all about. Of course, current debtholders and others who are considering lending to the firm are also concerned with the firm's future, although the firm's debt investors and its equity investors are usually concerned with different aspects of the firm's future. From management's viewpoint, *financial statement analysis is useful both as a way to anticipate future conditions and, more importantly, as a starting point for planning actions that will influence the future course of events for the firm.*

RATIO ANALYSIS

Financial ratios are designed to show relationships among financial statement accounts. Ratios put numbers into perspective. For example, Firm A may have $5,248,760 of debt and annual interest charges of $419,900, whereas Firm B's debt may total $52,647,980 and its interest charges equal $3,948,600. The true burden of these debts, and the companies' ability to repay them, can be ascertained only by comparing each firm's debt to its assets and its interest charges to the income available for payment of interest. Such comparisons are made by **ratio analysis.**

ratio analysis
Analysis of the relationships among financial statement accounts.

A single ratio is relatively useless in making relevant evaluations of a firm's health. To be effectively interpreted, a ratio must be systematically compared in one of the following ways: (1) compared to several ratios in a network such as the Du Pont system of analysis[1] or other logical groupings, (2) compared to the trends of the firm's own ratios, (3) compared to management's goals for key ratios, or (4) compared to selected ratios of other firms in the same industry. When comparing a firm's ratios to those of other companies, care must be taken to select similar firms of corresponding size and industry type to insure the appropriate comparison of financial data. For example, small firms

---

[1]Discussed later in this chapter.

INDUSTRY PRACTICE

New Distortions in Financial Statements

Financial analysts are worried. The growing gap between stagnant accounting practices and the rapidly changing financial world leaves them looking through an increasingly cloudy crystal ball. As accountants struggle to adapt principles that were developed long before today's designer securities and hyperactive financial markets, there is a growing belief that today's financial statements reflect a warped image of financial reality. Even the experts who believe that fears of an accounting apocalypse are exaggerated agree that for an overwhelming number of financial transactions, the rules of accounting are sketchy, dubious, or simply nonexistent.

The situation is most acute for banks and other financial institutions whose voracious appetite for funds continually involves them in new financial instruments and markets. Accounting's harshest critics contend that bank accounting as it stands now is little more than a powder keg of potential liabilities.

Under current accounting practices it is not uncommon for identical transactions to be handled completely differently, depending upon whose financial statement it appears. The resale of bankers acceptances is a good example. Assume that a bank accepts a $50 million obligation; that is, for a fee it guarantees timely payment of a customer's bill for $50 million. The bank then turns around and limits its risk by selling half of the obligation to another bank. Although the original bank remains legally liable for repayment of the full $50 million, some banks carry only a $25 million liability on their balance sheets, whereas others recognize the full amount.

Source: Adapted from Elizabeth Kaplan, "New Distortions in Financial Statements," *Dun's Business Month,* June 1986, 46, 47, and 50.

The Financial Accounting Standards Board (FASB) concedes that Wall Street's dizzying proliferation of exotic financial instruments has left the accounting profession's rule-setting body scrambling to catch up. The FASB is swamped with unresolved issues about new financial instruments and markets, and even when it does tackle a problem, as in the case of bankers acceptances, it often fails to come up with a solution.

The FASB's legendary slowness in responding to new financial developments is a product of its painstaking due-process procedures and the inherently hair-splitting nature of accounting discourse. However, a growing number of accounting experts are convinced that only a quickly implemented, far-reaching overhaul of the current system will avert disaster. Even the government is worried. In an unprecedented step, the Securities and Exchange Commission expressed its alarm. Thus prodded, the FASB voted to formally commit itself to a comprehensive review.

But many experts wonder whether the FASB is capable of responding to the challenges of present-day business innovations. They argue that accountants often cannot escape from the narrow conceptual framework of their profession. Even though the rules of accounting never contemplated some of the new financial instruments, accountants continue to try to extend the old principles to encompass completely new practices.

Compounding the situation are the hosts of Wall Street wizards poised at the ready to capitalize on any loophole that presents itself. Although financial transactions are theoretically motivated by economic considerations, investment bankers concede that there are many deals that are being manufactured in order to get a desired accounting treatment.

One of the more colorful examples of this kind of accounting opportunism involves a set of transactions spawned by FASB Statement 76. This rule allowed companies to erase a debt by setting aside high quality assets (usually government securities) in a trust and dedicating the income to paying off the debt. For a time, a sort of cottage industry for manufacturing gains sprang up as Wall Street opportunists gleefully arranged arbitrage transactions to take advantage of Rule 76. Companies issued cheap debt in the Euromarket and then created special trusts of Treasury securities to pay back the notes. Because Treasury debt, at the time, had higher yields than Eurobonds, under Statement 76 the companies recorded gains through this form of debt extinguishment.

The rule was eventually changed to disallow these practices, but the episode illustrates the FASB's plight. "The FASB is like a fire brigade right now, putting out brush fires while they can't keep ahead of the larger conflagration," says one industry analyst.

At present, the FASB is still struggling to come up with a meaningful agenda for getting the situation under control. However, some observers think that whatever form it takes, a comprehensive overhaul is sure to fan the flames, at least in the short-run. For example, it seems likely that the controversy surrounding mark-to-the-market accounting that last raged during the inflationary seventies is sure to be rekindled.

To summarize the debate, value accounting proponents contend that carrying assets on the books at the price that was originally paid for them is an archaic practice. Securities firms and others currently carry all of their holdings at market value, periodically changing the value of their assets to reflect their current market value — that is, marking to the market. But banks and thrifts only mark to the market the value of the securities in their portfolios. All other assets are carried on the books at their original, historical costs. It is argued that in an era of loan sales and securitization, when many banks originate assets, such as mortgages, only to sell them off, such historical accounting is anachronistic.

Proponents of mark-to-the-market accounting claim that besides portraying a more accurate financial picture, adoption of the new system would clear away much of the accounting clutter that plagues banks and thrifts. "Marking to the market is a terrific discipline," says Edward O'Brien, president of the Securities Industry Association. "You wouldn't have some of these unusual transactions that are designed to take advantage of historical cost accounting."

Bankers, however, recoil at the prospect. If a long-term asset is held to maturity, they argue, fluctuations in market price are irrelevant. Besides, they believe that the use of current value accounting in financial statements would be misleading and create unnecessary complications. Even mark-to-the-market proponents concede problems in valuing loans and potential disruptions in accounting practices if historical cost accounting was completely abandoned. "My concern is that it's a very slippery slope," says John Stewart, a partner with Arthur Anderson & Co. "Once you move to marking to the market, where do you stop?"

However, a more pertinent question for the FASB, as it stands poised at the verge of a major overhaul of the current practice of accounting, might be, "Where do you begin?"

must often rely on trade credit and other short-term liabilities to finance the firm's assets, whereas larger firms have access to the capital markets for financing. This fact may lead to significant differences in liquidity and debt ratios if these firms are compared. Similarly, cross-industry comparisons often lead to incorrect conclusions. Thus an acceptable inventory turnover ratio for a retail jeweler would lead to disaster if adopted by a meat packer.

Analysts who use financial ratios extensively may be characterized as belonging to three main groups: (1) *managers,* who use ratios to help analyze, control, and thus improve the firm's operations; (2) *credit analysts,* such as bank loan officers or credit managers for industrial companies, who analyze ratios to help ascertain a company's ability to pay its debt; and (3) *security analysts,* including stock analysts, who are interested in a company's efficiency and growth prospects, and bond analysts, who are concerned with a company's ability to pay interest on its bonds and with the assets that would be available to bondholders if the company went bankrupt.

Thus each group of analysts has specific areas of interest it wishes to investigate. A bank loan officer would concentrate on the short-term health of a firm, whereas a stock analyst would be more concerned with a firm's long-term prospects. Analysts, then, calculate specific groups of ratios rather than all possible ratios, as their purpose dictates. Therefore, ratios may be categorized into specific task groupings. We have categorized ratios into five groups: (1) liquidity ratios, (2) asset management ratios, (3) debt management ratios, (4) profitability ratios, and (5) market value ratios. Some of the most valuable ratios in each category are discussed and illustrated next, using Carter Chemical Company's financial data that were presented in Tables 6-1 and 6-2.

Liquidity Ratios

One of the financial analyst's first concerns is liquidity: Will the firm be able to meet its maturing obligations? Carter Chemical Company has debts totaling $300 million that must be paid off within the coming year. Can these obligations be satisfied? A full liquidity analysis requires the use of cash budgets (described in Chapter 10); however, by relating the amount of cash and other current assets to the current obligations, ratio analysis provides a quick and easy-to-use measure of liquidity. Two commonly used **liquidity ratios** are presented in the sections that follow.

liquidity ratio
The relationship of a firm's cash and other current assets to its current obligations.

current ratio
The ratio computed by dividing current assets by current liabilities.

Current Ratio. The **current ratio** is computed by dividing current assets by current liabilities. Current assets normally include cash, marketable securities, accounts receivable, and inventories; current liabilities consist of accounts payable, short-term notes payable, current maturities of long-term debt, accrued income taxes, and other accrued expenses (principally wages).

If a company is getting into financial difficulty, it begins paying its bills (accounts payable) slowly, building up bank loans, and so on. If these current liabilities are rising faster than current assets, the current ratio will fall, and this could spell trouble. Accordingly, the current ratio is the most commonly used measure of short-term solvency, because it provides an indicator of the extent to which the claims of short-term creditors are covered by assets that are expected to be converted to cash in a period roughly corresponding to the maturity of the claims.

The calculation of the current ratio for Carter at year-end 1987 follows. (All dollar amounts in this section are in millions.)

$$\text{Current ratio} = \frac{\text{Current assets}}{\text{Current liabilities}} = \frac{\$700}{\$300} = 2.3 \text{ times.}$$

$$\text{Industry average} = 2.5 \text{ times.}$$

Carter's current ratio is slightly below the average for the industry, 2.5, but not low enough to cause concern. It appears that Carter is in line with most other chemical firms. Since current assets are scheduled to be converted to cash in the near future, it is highly probable that they could be liquidated at close to their stated value. With a current ratio of 2.3, Carter could liquidate current assets at only 43 percent of book value and still pay off current creditors in full.[2]

Although industry average figures are discussed later in some detail, it should be stated at this point that an industry average is not a magic number that all firms should strive to maintain. In fact, some very well-managed firms will be above it, and other good firms will be below it. If a firm's ratios are very far removed from the average for its industry, however, the analyst must be concerned about why this variance occurs. Thus a deviation from the industry average should signal the analyst to check further.

Note also that Carter's current ratio declined to 2.3 in 1987 from 2.8 in 1986. Thus the *trend* is poor, and this could indicate potential future difficulties. More will be said about *trend analysis* later in the chapter.

quick (acid test) ratio
The ratio computed by deducting inventories from current assets and dividing the remainder by current liabilities.

Quick (Acid Test) Ratio. The **quick (acid test) ratio** is calculated by deducting inventories from current assets and dividing the remainder by current liabilities. Inventories typically are the least liquid of a firm's current assets and hence are the assets on which losses are most likely to occur in the event of liquidation. Therefore, this measure of the firm's ability to pay off short-term obligations without relying on the sale of inventories is important.

$$\text{Quick (acid test) ratio} = \frac{\text{Current assets} - \text{Inventory}}{\text{Current liabilities}} = \frac{\$400}{\$300}$$

$$= 1.3 \text{ times.}$$

$$\text{Industry average} = 1.0 \text{ times.}$$

The industry average quick ratio is 1.0, so Carter's 1.3 ratio compares favorably with other firms in the industry. If the accounts receivable can be collected, the company can pay off current liabilities even without selling any inventory. Again, however, it should be noted that the trend is downward — 1.3 in 1987 versus 1.8 in 1986.

---

[2]$(1/2.3) = 0.43$, or 43 percent. Note that $(0.43)(\$700) \approx \$300$, the amount of current liabilities.

Asset Management Ratios

The second group of ratios is designed to measure how effectively the firm is managing its assets. In particular, the **asset management ratios** answer this question: Does the total amount of each type of asset as reported on the balance sheet seem reasonable, too high, or too low in view of current and projected operating levels? Carter Chemical Company and other companies must borrow or obtain capital from other sources to acquire assets. If they have too many assets, their interest expenses are too high; hence profits are too low. If assets are too low, operations will not be as efficient as possible.

asset management ratios
Set of several ratios, including inventory utilization, average collection period, and total asset utilization, which are designed to measure how effectively the firm's assets are being managed.

Inventory Utilization. The **inventory utilization** ratio, sometimes called the *inventory turnover ratio,* is defined as sales divided by inventories.

$$\text{Inventory utilization (or turnover)} = \frac{\text{Sales}}{\text{Inventory}} = \frac{\$3,000}{\$300} = 10 \text{ times.}$$

$$\text{Industry average} = 9 \text{ times.}$$

inventory utilization
The ratio of sales divided by inventories; also known as *inventory turnover.*

As a rough approximation, each item on Carter's inventory is sold out and restocked, or "turned over," 10 times per year. Its gross profit is therefore 10 times the difference between its selling prices and the cost of its inventory. Carter's ratio of 10 times compares favorably with an industry average of 9 times. This suggests that the company does not hold excessive stocks of inventory; excess stocks are, of course, unproductive and represent an investment with a low or zero rate of return. This high inventory utilization ratio also reinforces our faith in the current ratio. If the turnover were low—say, 3 or 4 times—we might wonder whether the firm was holding damaged or obsolete materials not actually worth their stated value.

Two problems arise in calculating and analyzing the inventory utilization ratio. First, sales are at market prices; if inventories are carried at cost, as they generally are, it would be more appropriate to use cost of goods sold in place of sales in the numerator of the formula. Established compilers of financial ratio statistics such as Dun & Bradstreet, however, use the ratio of sales to inventories carried at cost. To develop a figure that can be compared with those developed by Dun & Bradstreet, it is therefore necessary to measure inventory utilization with sales in the numerator, as we do here.

The second problem lies in the fact that sales occur over the entire year, whereas the inventory figure is for one point in time. It would be better to use an average inventory.[3] If the firm's business is highly seasonal, or if there has been a strong upward or downward sales trend during the year, it becomes essential to make some such adjustment. To maintain comparability with industry averages, we did not use the average inventory figure.

---

[3]Preferably, the average inventory would be calculated by summing the monthly figures during the year and dividing by 12. If monthly data are not available, one can add the beginning and ending figures and divide by 2; this will adjust for secular trends but not for seasonal fluctuations.

average collection period (ACP)
The ratio computed by dividing average *credit* sales per day into accounts receivable; indicates the average length of time the firm must wait after making a credit sale before receiving payment.

Average Collection Period. The average collection period, which is used to appraise the accounts receivable, is computed by dividing average daily sales into accounts receivable to find the number of days' sales tied up in receivables.[4] This is defined as the **average collection period (ACP)** because it represents the average length of time that the firm must wait after making a sale before receiving cash. The calculations for Carter show an average collection period of 42 days, slightly above the 36-day industry average.

$$\text{Average collection period} = \frac{\text{Receivables}}{\text{Average sales per day}} = \frac{\text{Receivables}}{\text{Annual sales/360}}$$

$$= \frac{\$350}{\$3,000/360} = \frac{\$350}{\$8.333} = 42 \text{ days.}$$

$$\text{Industry average} = 36 \text{ days.}$$

This ratio also can be evaluated by comparison with the terms on which the firm sells its goods. For example, Carter's sales terms call for payment within 30 days, so the 42-day collection period indicates that customers, on the average, are not paying their bills on time. If the trend in the length of the collection period during the past few years has been rising while the credit policy has not changed, this would be even stronger evidence that steps should be taken to expedite the collection of accounts receivable.

fixed assets utilization
The ratio of sales to fixed assets; also known as *fixed assets turnover.*

Fixed Assets Utilization. The **fixed assets utilization** ratio, often called the *fixed assets turnover* ratio, measures the utilization of plant and equipment:

$$\text{Fixed assets utilization} = \frac{\text{Sales}}{\text{Net fixed assets}} = \frac{\$3,000}{\$1,300} = 2.3 \text{ times.}$$

$$\text{Industry average} = 3.0 \text{ times.}$$

Carter's ratio of 2.3 times compares poorly with the industry average of 3 times, indicating that the firm is not using its fixed assets to as high a percentage of capacity as are the other firms in the industry. The financial manager should bear this fact in mind when production people request funds for new capital investments.

A potential problem of major proportion exists when the fixed assets utilization ratio is used for comparative purposes. Inflation has caused the value of many assets that were purchased in the past to be seriously understated. Therefore, if we were comparing an old firm that had acquired many of its fixed assets years ago at low prices with a new company that had acquired its fixed assets only recently, the older firm probably would have a higher com-

---

[4]Because information on the proportion of credit sales to total sales is generally unavailable, total sales may be used as a substitute in the ACP calculation. However, since all firms do not have the same proportion of credit sales to total sales, there is a good chance that the average collection period will be understated if total sales is used rather than credit sales.

puted turnover ratio. This, however, would be more reflective of the problems with the accounting statements than with the newer firm's inefficiency. The accounting profession is trying to devise ways of providing financial statements that are more reflective of current, rather than historic, values. The problem of comparisons would be eliminated if balance sheets were stated on a current basis, but at the moment the problems still exist. Because financial analysts typically do not have the data necessary to make adjustments, they simply recognize that a problem exists and deal with it judgmentally. In Carter's case, the issue is not a serious one because all firms in the industry have been expanding at about the same rate, so the balance sheets of the comparison firms are indeed comparable.

Total Assets Utilization. The **total assets utilization** ratio measures the utilization or turnover of all the firm's assets—it is calculated by dividing sales by total assets.

total assets utilization
The ratio that measures the turnover of all of a firm's assets, computed by dividing sales by total assets.

$$\text{Total assets utilization} = \frac{\text{Sales}}{\text{Total assets}} = \frac{\$3,000}{\$2,000} = 1.5 \text{ times.}$$

$$\text{Industry average} = 1.8 \text{ times.}$$

Carter's ratio is somewhat below the industry average. The company is not generating a sufficient volume of business for the size of its asset investment. Sales should be increased, some assets should be disposed of, or both steps should be taken.

Debt Management Ratios

The extent to which a firm uses debt financing, or **financial leverage,** has three important implications: (1) By raising funds through debt, the owners maintain control of the firm with a limited investment. (2) Creditors look to the equity, or owner-supplied funds, to provide a margin of safety; if the owners have provided only a small proportion of the total financing, the risks of the enterprise are borne mainly by its creditors. (3) If the firm earns more on investments financed with borrowed funds than it pays in interest, the return on the owners' capital is magnified, or "leveraged."

financial leverage
The extent to which a firm uses debt financing.

The first point is obvious, but to better understand how financial leverage affects risk and return, consider Table 7–1. Here we are analyzing two companies that are identical except for the way they are financed. Firm U (for "unleveraged") has no debt, whereas Firm L (for "leveraged") is financed half with equity and half with debt that has an interest rate of 16 percent. Both companies have $100 in assets and $120 in sales. Their ratio of operating income to assets, or the *basic earning power ratio,* is EBIT/Total assets = $30/$100 = 0.30 = 30%. Even though both companies' assets have the same earning power, Firm L provides its stockholders with a return on equity of 22 percent, versus only 15 percent for Firm U. This difference is caused by Firm L's use of debt.

Table 7–1 **Effect of Financial Leverage on Stockholders' Returns**

Firm U
(Unleveraged)

Current assets	$40	Debt	$ 0
Fixed assets	60	Common equity	100
Total assets	$100	Total claims	$100

Sales	$120
Operating costs	90
Operating income (EBIT)	30
Interest	0
Taxable income	30
Taxes (50%)*	15
Net income	$15

$$\text{ROE}_U = \$15/\$100 = 15\%$$

Firm L
(Leveraged)

Current assets	$40	Debt (16%)	$50
Fixed assets	60	Common equity	50
Total assets	$100	Total claims	$100

Sales	$120
Operating costs	90
Operating income (EBIT)	$ 30
Interest	8
Taxable income	$ 22
Taxes (50%)*	11
Net income	$ 11

$$\text{ROE}_L = \$11/\$50 = 22\%$$

*A 50% tax rate is used for ease of calculation.

Financial leverage raises the rate of return to stockholders for two reasons. First, because interest is deductible, the use of debt financing lowers the tax bill and leaves more of the firm's operating income available to its investors. Second, if the firm's basic earning power rate (EBIT/Total assets) exceeds the interest rate on debt, as it generally does, a company can use debt to finance assets, pay the interest on the debt, and have something left over as a bonus for its stockholders. For our hypothetical firms, these two effects have combined to push Firm L's rate of return on equity up to a level almost 50 percent higher than that of Firm U. Thus debt can be used to "leverage up" a firm's rate of return on equity.

However, financial leverage can cut both ways; if the return on assets declines, the leveraged firm's return on equity will fall further and faster. Suppose, for example, that the operating costs for both firms rose to $120 because of inflation, yet competitive pressures during a recession kept them from increasing sales prices. Consequently, in terms of Table 7–1, operating costs would rise to $120 and EBIT would drop to zero for both firms. If we worked through the rest of the table, we would see that Firm U would be in a break-even position, with net income = $0 and ROE = 0%, whereas Firm L would have net income = − $8 and ROE = − 16%. Firm U, because of its strong balance sheet, could ride out the recession and be ready for the next boom. Firm L, on the other hand, would be under great financial pressure. Because of its losses, its cash would be depleted and it would need to raise funds. Running a loss, it would have a hard time selling stock to raise capital, and the losses would also make its debt look risky, which would cause lenders to raise the interest rate. This would amplify L's problems, and the firm might not recover to be around to enjoy the next boom.

We see, then, that firms with relatively low debt ratios have less risk of loss when the economy is in a recession, but they also have lower expected returns when the economy booms. Conversely, firms with high leverage ratios run the risk of large losses, but they also have a chance of earning high profits. The prospects of high returns are desirable, but investors are averse to risk. Decisions about the use of leverage, then, require firms to balance higher expected returns against increased risk.

Determining the optimal amount of debt for a given firm is a complicated process, and we defer a discussion of this topic until Chapter 20, when we will be better prepared to deal with it. For now we will simply consider the ways analysts examine the firm's use of debt in financial statement analysis.

Total Debt to Total Assets. The ratio of total debt to total assets, generally called the **debt ratio,** measures the percentage of total funds provided by creditors. Debt includes current liabilities and all bonds. Creditors prefer low debt ratios, because the lower the ratio, the greater the cushion against creditors' losses in the event of liquidation. The owners, on the other hand, may seek high leverage either to magnify earnings or because selling new stock means giving up some degree of control.

debt ratio
The ratio of total debt to total assets.

$$\text{Debt ratio} = \frac{\text{Total debt}}{\text{Total assets}} = \frac{\$1,100}{\$2,000} = 55\%.$$

$$\text{Industry average} = 40\%.$$

Carter's debt ratio is 55 percent; this means that creditors have supplied more than half the firm's total financing. Since the average debt ratio for this industry — and for manufacturing generally — is about 40 percent, Carter would find it difficult to borrow additional funds without first raising more equity capital. Creditors would be reluctant to lend the firm more money, and management would probably be subjecting the firm to the risk of bankruptcy if it sought to increase the debt ratio still more by borrowing.

times interest earned (TIE)
The ratio of earnings before interest and taxes to interest charges; measures the ability of a firm to meet its annual interest payments.

Times Interest Earned. The **times-interest-earned (TIE)** ratio is determined by dividing earnings before interest and taxes (EBIT) by the interest charges. The TIE ratio measures the extent to which earnings can decline without resultant financial embarrassment to the firm because of an inability to meet annual interest costs. Failure to meet this obligation can bring legal action by the creditors, possibly resulting in bankruptcy. Note that the before-tax profit figure is used in the numerator. Because income taxes are computed after interest expense is deducted, the ability to pay current interest is not affected by income taxes.

$$\text{TIE} = \frac{\text{EBIT}}{\text{Interest charges}} = \frac{\$266}{\$66} = 4 \text{ times.}$$

$$\text{Industry average} = 6 \text{ times.}$$

Carter's interest is covered 4 times, whereas the industry average is 6 times. Thus, the company is covering its interest charges by a minimum margin of safety and deserves only a fair rating. This ratio reinforces the conclusion based on the debt ratio that the company might face some difficulties if it attempts to borrow additional funds.

fixed charge coverage ratio
This ratio expands the times-interest-earned ratio to include all inescapable charges, not just interest expense.

Fixed Charge Coverage. The **fixed charge coverage ratio** is similar to the times-interest-earned ratio, but it is more inclusive because it recognizes that many firms lease assets and incur long-term obligations under lease contracts. Leasing has become widespread in recent years, making this ratio preferable to the times-interest-earned ratio for most financial analysis. Fixed charges include interest plus annual long-term lease obligations, and the fixed charge coverage ratio is defined as follows:

$$\frac{\text{Fixed charge}}{\text{coverage ratio}} = \frac{\text{Earnings before taxes} + \text{Interest charges} + \text{Lease obligations}}{\text{Interest charges} + \text{Lease obligations}}$$

$$= \frac{\$200 + \$66 + \$28}{\$66 + \$28}$$

$$= \$294/\$94 \qquad = 3.1 \text{ times.}$$

$$\text{Industry average} = 5.5 \text{ times.}$$

Carter's fixed charges are covered 3.1 times, as opposed to an industry average of 5.5 times. Again, this indicates that the firm is somewhat weaker than creditors would prefer it to be, and it points up the difficulties that Carter probably would encounter if it attempted to increase its debt.

Profitability Ratios

profitability ratios
The ratios that show the combined effects of liquidity, asset management, and debt management on operating results.

Profitability is the net result of a large number of policies and decisions. Although the ratios examined thus far reveal some interesting things about the way the firm is operating, the **profitability ratios** show the combined effects of liquidity, asset management, and debt management on operating results.

Profit Margin on Sales. The **profit margin on sales,** computed by dividing net income after taxes by sales, gives the profit per dollar of sales.

$$\text{Profit margin} = \frac{\text{Net profit after taxes}}{\text{Sales}} = \frac{\$120}{\$3,000} = 4\%.$$

$$\text{Industry average} = 5\%.$$

Carter's profit margin is somewhat below the industry average of 5 percent, indicating that the firm's sales prices are relatively low or that its costs are relatively high, or both.

Basic Earning Power Ratio. The **basic earning power ratio,** which was discussed earlier in connection with financial leverage, is calculated by dividing the earnings before interest and taxes (EBIT) by total assets.

$$\text{Basic earning power ratio} = \frac{\text{EBIT}}{\text{Total assets}} = \frac{\$266}{\$2,000} = 13.3\%.$$

$$\text{Industry average} = 17.2\%.$$

This ratio is useful for comparing firms in different tax situations and with different degrees of financial leverage. Carter is not getting as much operating income out of its assets as is the average chemical company. This occurs because of its low turnover ratios and also because of its low profit margin on sales.

Return on Total Assets. The ratio of net profit to total assets measures the **return on total assets (ROA).**

$$\text{Return on total assets (ROA)} = \frac{\text{Net profit after taxes}}{\text{Total assets}} = \frac{\$120}{\$2,000} = 6\%.$$

$$\text{Industry average} = 9\%.$$

Carter's 6 percent return is well below the 9 percent average for the industry. This low rate results from three primary factors: (1) the low profit margin on sales, (2) the low utilization of total assets, and (3) Carter's above-average use of debt, which causes its interest payments to be high and its profits to be reduced, and contributes in turn to the low profit margin on sales.

Return on Common Equity. The ratio of net profit after taxes to common equity measures the **return on common equity (ROE).**

$$\text{Return on common equity (ROE)} = \frac{\text{Net profit after taxes}}{\text{Common equity}} = \frac{\$120}{\$900} = 13.3\%.$$

$$\text{Industry average} = 15.0\%.$$

profit margin on sales
Profit per dollar of sales, computed by dividing net income after taxes by sales.

basic earning power ratio
The ratio of operating profits to assets; indicates the power of a firm's assets to generate operating income.

return on total assets (ROA)
The ratio of net income after taxes to total assets.

return on common equity (ROE)
The ratio of net profit after taxes to common equity; measures the rate of return on stockholders' investment.

Carter's 13.3 percent return is below the 15.0 percent industry average, but not as far below as the return on total assets. This results from Carter's greater use of debt, a point analyzed in detail later in the chapter.[5]

Market Value Ratios

market value ratios
The ratios that relate a firm's stock price to its earnings and book value per share.

Market value ratios relate the firm's stock price to its earnings and book value per share. They give management an indication of what investors think of the company's past performance and future prospects. If the firm's liquidity, asset management, debt management, and profitability ratios are all good, its market value ratios will be high, and the stock price probably will be as high as can be expected.

price/earnings (P/E) ratio
The ratio of price to earnings; shows how much investors are willing to pay per dollar of profits.

Price/Earnings Ratio. The **price/earnings (P/E) ratio** shows how much investors are willing to pay per dollar of reported profits. Carter's stock sells for $28.50, so with an EPS of $2.40, its P/E ratio is 11.9.

$$\text{Price/earnings ratio} = \frac{\text{Price per share}}{\text{Earnings per share}} = \frac{\$28.50}{\$2.40} = 11.9 \text{ times.}$$

$$\text{Industry average} = 12.5 \text{ times.}$$

Generally, P/E ratios are higher for firms with high growth prospects but lower for riskier firms. Carter's P/E ratio is slightly below those of other large chemical producers, which suggests that the company is regarded as being somewhat riskier than most, as having poorer growth prospects, or both.

Market/Book Ratio. The ratio of a stock's market price to its book value gives another indication of how investors regard the company. Companies with high rates of return on equity generally sell at higher multiples of book value than those with low returns. Carter's book value per share is $18.00:

$$\text{Book value per share} = \frac{\text{Stockholders' equity}}{\text{Shares outstanding}} = \frac{\$900}{50} = \$18.00.$$

market/book ratio
The ratio of a stock's market price to its book value.

Dividing this value into the market price per share gives a **market/book ratio** of 1.6 times:

$$\text{Market/book ratio} = \frac{\$28.50}{\$18.00} = 1.6 \text{ times.}$$

$$\text{Industry average} = 1.8 \text{ times.}$$

Investors are willing to pay slightly less for Carter's book value than for that of an average chemical company.

---

[5]The fact that Carter's basic earning power and ROE are both 13.3 percent is a coincidence; normally, they differ. Actually, if more decimal places had been shown, the two ratios would have been different from each other.

Figure 7-1 **Rate of Return on Common Equity, 1983–1987**

In addition to comparing ratios to industry averages, it is important to analyze what trends various ratios are taking. By simply plotting Carter's rate of return on common equity for each year, one can determine the trend that the ratio has taken from 1983 to 1987. A potential investor can quickly see that Carter's rate has declined since 1984, whereas the industry rate as a whole has been comparatively steady.

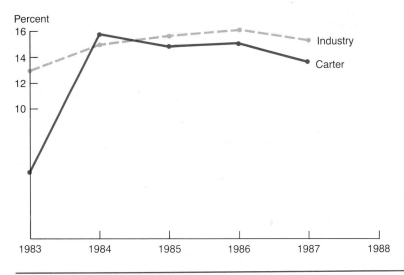

The typical railroad, which has a very low rate of return on assets, has a market/book value ratio of less than 0.5. Very successful firms, such as IBM, achieve high rates of return on their assets, and they have market values well in excess of their book values; IBM's is 2.6 times.

Trend Analysis

It is important to analyze trends in ratios as well as their absolute levels, for the trends give clues as to whether the financial situation is improving or deteriorating. To do a **trend analysis,** one simply graphs a ratio against years, as shown in Figure 7–1. This graph shows that Carter's rate of return on common equity has been declining since 1984, even though the industry average has been relatively stable. Other ratios could be analyzed similarly.

trend analysis
The analysis of a firm's financial ratios over time to determine the improvement or deterioration of a financial situation.

Summary of Ratio Analysis: The Du Pont System

Table 7-2 summarizes Carter Chemical Company's ratios, and Figure 7-2, which is called a *Du Pont chart* because that company's managers developed the general approach, shows the relationships among debt, asset utilization, and profitability ratios. The left-hand side of the chart develops the *profit margin*

Table 7-2 **Summary of Carter Chemical Company's Ratios (Millions of Dollars)**

Ratio	Formula for Calculation	Calculation	Ratio	Industry Average	Evaluation
Liquidity					
Current	$\dfrac{\text{Current assets}}{\text{Current liabilities}}$	$\dfrac{\$\ 700}{\$\ 300}$ =	2.3 times	2.5 times	Good
Quick, or acid test	$\dfrac{\text{Current assets} - \text{Inventory}}{\text{Current liabilities}}$	$\dfrac{\$\ 400}{\$\ 300}$ =	1.3 times	1 time	Good
Asset Management					
Inventory utilization turnover	$\dfrac{\text{Sales}}{\text{Inventory}}$	$\dfrac{\$3,000}{\$\ 300}$ =	10 times	9 times	Good
Average collection period (ACP)	$\dfrac{\text{Receivables}}{\text{Sales/360}}$	$\dfrac{\$\ 350}{\$8.333}$ =	42 days	36 days	Bad
Fixed assets utilization	$\dfrac{\text{Sales}}{\text{Fixed assets}}$	$\dfrac{\$3,000}{\$1,300}$ =	2.3 times	3 times	Bad
Total assets utilization	$\dfrac{\text{Sales}}{\text{Total assets}}$	$\dfrac{\$3,000}{\$2,000}$ =	1.5 times	1.8 times	Bad
Debt Management					
Debt to total assets	$\dfrac{\text{Total debt}}{\text{Total assets}}$	$\dfrac{\$1,100}{\$2,000}$ =	55 percent	40 percent	Bad
Times interest earned (TIE)	$\dfrac{\text{Earnings before interest and taxes}}{\text{Interest charges}}$	$\dfrac{\$\ 266}{\$\ 66}$ =	4 times	6 times	Bad
Fixed charge coverage	$\dfrac{\text{Earnings before taxes} + \text{Interest charges} + \text{Lease obligations}}{\text{Interest charges} + \text{Lease obligations}}$	$\dfrac{\$\ 294}{\$\ 94}$ =	3.1 times	5.5 times	Bad
Profitability					
Profit margin on sales	$\dfrac{\text{Net profit after taxes}}{\text{Sales}}$	$\dfrac{\$\ 120}{\$3,000}$ =	4 percent	5 percent	Bad
Basic earning power	$\dfrac{\text{Earnings before interest and taxes}}{\text{Total assets}}$	$\dfrac{\$\ 266}{\$2,000}$ =	13.3 percent	17.2 percent	Bad
Return on total assets (ROA)	$\dfrac{\text{Net profit after taxes}}{\text{Total assets}}$	$\dfrac{\$\ 120}{\$2,000}$ =	6 percent	9 percent	Bad
Return on common equity (ROE)	$\dfrac{\text{Net profit after taxes}}{\text{Common equity}}$	$\dfrac{\$\ 120}{\$\ 900}$ =	13.3 percent	15 percent	Bad
Market Value					
Price/earnings (P/E)	$\dfrac{\text{Price per share}}{\text{Earnings per share}}$	$\dfrac{\$28.50}{\$\ 2.40}$ =	11.9 times	12.5 times	Bad
Market/book	$\dfrac{\text{Market price per share}}{\text{Book value per share}}$	$\dfrac{\$28.50}{\$18.00}$ =	1.6 times	1.8 times	Bad

on sales. The various expense items are listed, then summed to obtain Carter's total costs. Subtracting costs from sales yields the company's net income, which, when divided by sales, indicates that 4 percent of each sales dollar is left over for stockholders.

The right-hand side of the chart lists the various categories of assets, which are summed and then divided into sales to find the number of times Carter "turns its assets over" each year. Carter's total asset utilization, or turnover, ratio is 1.5 times.

Figure 7-2 **Modified Du Pont Chart Applied to
Carter Chemical Company (Millions of Dollars)**

The Du Pont chart was created to illustrate the relationships among key financial
ratios. The left side of the chart develops a firm's profit margin; the right side
develops its total assets utilization ratio. The profit margin is then multiplied by the
assets utilization ratio to arrive at the rate of return on assets (ROA). The matter of
debt is brought into the chart by multiplying the ROA by the equity multiplier to
arrive at the rate of return on equity (ROE). The ROE could be calculated more
simply, but the Du Pont chart is useful for illustrating how debt, asset utilization, and
profitability ratios interact to determine the ROE.

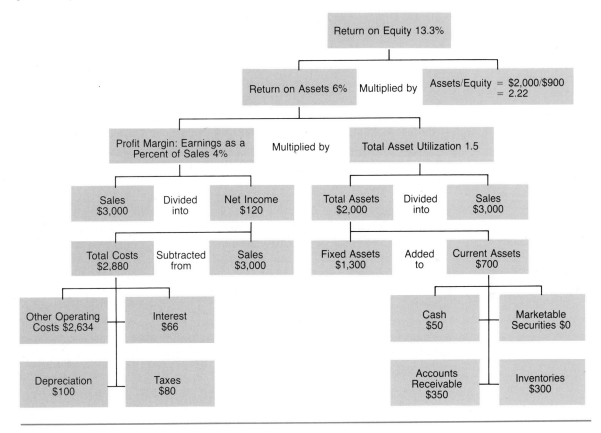

The profit margin times the total asset turnover ratio is defined as the *Du
Pont equation,* which gives the rate of return on assets (ROA):

ROA = Rate of return on assets = Profit margin × Total assets turnover

$$= \frac{\text{Net profit after taxes}}{\text{Sales}} \times \frac{\text{Sales}}{\text{Total assets}}$$

$$= 4\% \times 1.5 = 6\%.$$

Carter makes 4 percent, or 4 cents, on each dollar of sales. Assets were turned over 1.5 times during the year, so Carter earned a return of 6 percent on its assets.

If Carter used only equity, the 6 percent rate of return on assets would equal the rate of return on equity. However, 55 percent of the firm's capital is supplied by creditors. Because the 6 percent return on *total* assets all goes to stockholders, who put up only 45 percent of the capital, the return on equity is higher than 6 percent. Specifically, the rate of return on assets (ROA) must be multiplied by the *equity multiplier,* which is the ratio of assets to common equity, to obtain the rate of return on equity (ROE):

$$ROE = ROA \times \text{Equity multiplier}$$

$$= \frac{\text{Net income}}{\text{Assets}} \times \frac{\text{Assets}}{\text{Common equity}}$$

$$= 6\% \times (\$2,000/\$900)$$

$$= 6\% \times 2.22 = 13.3\%.$$

This 13.3 percent rate of return could, of course, be calculated directly: net income after taxes/common equity = $120/$900 = 13.3 percent. However, the Du Pont equation shows how the rate of return on assets and the use of debt interact to determine the return on equity.

Du Pont system

A system of analysis designed to show the relationships among return on investment, asset turnover, and profit margin.

Management can use the **Du Pont system** to analyze ways of improving the firm's performance. On the left, or profit margin, side of Figure 7-2, marketing people can study the effects of raising sales prices (or lowering them to get greater volume), of moving into new products or markets with higher margins, and so on. Cost accountants can study the expense items and, working with engineers, purchasing agents, and other operating personnel, seek ways of holding down costs. On the turnover, or asset utilization, side, financial analysts, working with both production and marketing people, can investigate ways of reducing the investment in various types of assets. At the same time, the treasurer can analyze the effects of alternative financing strategies, seeking to hold down interest expenses and the risks of debt while still using debt to increase the rate of return on equity.

SOURCES OF COMPARATIVE RATIOS

comparative ratio analysis

The analysis based on a comparison of a firm's ratios with those of other firms in the same industry.

The preceding analysis of Carter Chemical Company pointed out the usefulness of **comparative ratio analysis** among firms in the same industry. Comparative ratios are available from a number of sources. One useful set of comparative data is compiled by Dun & Bradstreet, Inc. (D&B), which provides 14 ratios calculated for a large number of industries. Useful ratios can also be found in the *Annual Statement Studies* published by Robert Morris Associates, the national association of bank loan officers. The Federal Trade Commission's *Quarterly Financial Report,* which is found in most libraries, gives a set of

Financial managers interested in comparing their company ratios with those of other industry firms can find this information in several sources, such as the *Key Business Ratios* compiled by Dun & Bradstreet. This excerpt from the D&B data provides 14 ratios for several manufacturing industries.

MANUFACTURING

Line of Business (and number of concerns reporting)	Quick Ratio	Current Ratio	Current liabilities to net worth	Current liabilities to inventory	Total liabilities to net worth	Fixed assets to net worth	Collection period	Net sales to inventory	Total assets to net sales	Net sales to net working capital	Accounts payable to net sales	Return on net sales	Return on total assets	Return on net worth
	Times	Times	Percent	Percent	Percent	Percent	Days	Times	Percent	Times	Percent	Percent	Percent	Percent
2011-2017 Meat Products (113)	2.1 1.3 0.8	4.2 2.2 1.6	20.4 47.0 118.0	89.2 144.8 221.5	33.3 71.8 177.2	31.9 57.9 82.6	12.7 17.8 24.8	44.2 29.0 16.3	14.0 19.2 28.9	31.0 15.3 11.0	0.9 1.8 3.2	2.9 1.5 0.6	11.6 6.5 2.4	25.7 13.9 4.8
2021-2026 Dairy Products (125)	1.2 1.0 0.7	2.0 1.4 1.2	52.0 84.6 149.4	133.7 228.8 434.2	64.3 114.7 205.0	43.7 68.2 92.4	18.9 26.4 32.8	55.0 26.9 13.9	18.6 23.1 33.2	41.3 19.1 12.5	3.7 5.6 7.7	2.8 1.2 0.5	9.5 5.2 1.1	23.1 11.1 3.1
2051-2052 Bakery Products (113)	2.0 1.1 0.8	3.3 1.9 1.3	16.9 36.2 66.1	116.4 216.8 362.6	24.1 49.1 112.0	58.9 85.6 133.5	17.0 24.4 31.7	41.5 29.8 17.4	27.3 37.0 48.2	32.5 15.0 7.1	2.5 4.3 6.2	5.5 2.4 1.2	12.7 6.9 2.7	21.8 13.8 6.7
2082-2087 Beverages (140)	1.5 0.9 0.5	3.3 2.0 1.3	20.3 38.7 70.4	61.8 118.1 188.1	34.0 68.2 136.7	41.4 72.1 100.7	16.7 24.9 37.2	20.1 13.2 5.1	33.4 44.8 68.1	17.6 9.6 5.2	2.9 4.8 7.4	7.3 4.1 1.8	14.6 8.3 3.6	27.3 15.6 8.5
2321-2329 Men's & Boy's Apparel (114)	1.6 1.0 0.6	3.5 2.4 1.7	39.9 80.9 146.2	63.5 99.8 144.5	43.4 97.2 180.9	5.5 11.8 35.6	23.3 43.8 66.0	10.8 6.3 4.2	27.8 42.1 56.1	8.3 5.2 3.7	3.3 6.4 10.1	5.5 3.0 1.6	10.2 5.1 2.4	23.3 11.4 6.2
2331-2339 Women's, Misses' & Juniors' Outerwear (107)	1.5 1.0 0.7	2.7 1.7 1.4	35.4 104.3 207.3	112.0 159.0 237.6	59.7 131.6 235.9	3.3 7.7 18.6	23.7 43.0 62.6	16.4 10.7 7.3	25.1 32.5 43.5	14.8 9.4 5.6	4.3 7.4 10.5	3.2 2.0 0.5	10.4 6.2 1.2	31.4 16.3 3.8
2421 Sawmills & Planing Mills, General (128)	2.1 0.9 0.3	4.7 2.4 1.3	11.9 30.2 84.6	58.3 94.9 173.2	22.9 63.2 150.0	31.7 67.9 108.9	14.2 20.4 29.5	13.2 8.0 5.0	40.3 57.9 84.2	12.8 6.4 3.4	1.6 2.6 4.8	6.4 4.3 1.6	10.6 7.1 3.3	17.9 10.7 6.2
2511-2519 Household Furniture (116)	2.0 1.1 0.7	3.9 2.5 1.8	27.6 46.9 97.2	55.6 83.6 130.2	31.3 71.3 148.4	19.7 35.9 70.3	18.2 34.1 47.4	13.2 9.4 5.2	29.0 42.2 51.8	10.9 6.9 4.2	2.5 3.6 6.5	6.1 3.0 0.9	13.5 7.0 2.6	25.9 13.2 4.2
2651-2655 Paperboard Containers & Boxes (115)	2.1 1.3 0.9	3.3 2.1 1.5	28.1 56.3 110.0	81.1 146.8 248.0	39.6 99.6 197.4	32.6 58.3 107.7	30.2 41.5 46.3	21.9 13.1 7.6	31.5 43.8 55.8	14.0 8.8 4.8	3.1 4.8 7.6	5.0 3.4 0.9	9.7 7.0 2.6	18.7 12.5 4.6
2731-2732 Books (101)	1.9 1.2 0.7	4.2 2.7 1.8	20.4 42.2 90.0	57.1 98.0 167.8	30.0 69.4 150.5	5.6 20.1 45.4	32.1 48.5 81.3	14.1 7.3 3.6	45.0 62.7 97.7	6.8 3.7 2.4	2.6 6.0 10.6	12.6 6.7 2.8	14.8 9.3 5.4	20.7 13.5 7.6

Source: Reprinted by permission of Dun & Bradstreet Credit Services, a company of The Dun & Bradstreet Corporation.

ratios for manufacturing firms by industry group and size of firm. Trade associations and individual firms' credit departments also compile industry average financial ratios. Finally, financial statement data are available on magnetic tapes for thousands of corporations, and because most of the larger brokerage houses, banks, and other financial institutions have access to these data, security analysts can and do generate comparative ratios tailored to their own individual needs.

Each of these organizations uses a somewhat different set of ratios, designed for the organization's own purposes. For example, D&B deals mainly with small firms, many of which are proprietorships, and they are concerned largely with the creditors' viewpoint. Accordingly, their ratios emphasize current assets and liabilities, and D&B is completely unconcerned with market value ratios. Therefore, when you select a comparative data source, you should either be sure that your emphasis is similar to that of the agency or recognize the limitations of its ratios for your purposes. In addition, there are often minor definitional differences in the ratios presented by different sources. Before using any source, be sure to verify the exact definitions of their ratios.

LIMITATIONS OF RATIO ANALYSIS

Ratio analysis can provide useful information about a company's operations and financial condition. However, it does have some inherent problems and limitations that necessitate care and judgment.

1. Many large firms operate a number of different divisions in quite different industries, making it difficult to develop a meaningful set of industry averages for comparative purposes. This tends to make ratio analysis more useful for small than for large firms.

2. Most firms want to be better than average (although about half will be above and half below), so merely attaining average performance is not necessarily good. As a target for high-level performance, it is preferable to look at industry leaders' ratios.

3. Inflation has badly distorted firms' balance sheets. Further, because inflation affects both depreciation charges and inventory costs, profits are also affected. Thus a ratio analysis for one firm over time, or a comparative analysis of firms of different ages, must be interpreted with care and judgment.

4. The ratios can be distorted. For example, the inventory utilization ratio for a food processor will be radically different if the balance sheet figure used for inventory is the one just before versus just after the close of the canning season. This problem can be minimized by using average inventory figures.

window dressing
Techniques used by a firm to make a financial statement look better to credit analysts.

5. Firms can employ **window dressing** techniques to make their financial statements look better to credit analysts. To illustrate, a Dallas manufacturer borrowed on a two-year basis on December 29, 1987, held the proceeds of the loan as cash for a few days, and then paid off the loan ahead of time on January 4, 1988. This action improved the firm's current and quick ratios and made the year-end 1987 balance sheet look good. This improvement was strictly temporary, however; a week later the balance sheet was back to its old level.

6. Different operating and accounting practices can distort comparisons. As noted earlier, inventory valuation and depreciation methods can affect the financial statements and thus distort interfirm comparisons. Also, if one firm leases a substantial amount of its productive equipment, its assets may seem to be low relative to sales because leased assets may not appear on the balance sheet; at the same time, the lease liability will not be shown as a debt. Thus leasing can artificially improve the debt and turnover ratios. The accounting profession has recently taken steps that reduce but do not eliminate this problem, which we will discuss in Chapter 23.

7. It is difficult to generalize about whether a particular ratio is good or bad. For example, a high current ratio may show a strong liquidity position, which is good, or excessive cash, which is bad because excess cash in the bank is a nonearning asset. Similarly, high asset utilization ratios may denote either a firm that uses assets efficiently or an undercapitalized firm that simply cannot afford to buy enough assets.

8. A firm may have some ratios which look good and others which look bad, making it difficult to tell whether the firm is, on balance, in a strong or a weak position. However, statistical procedures can be used to analyze the *net effects* of a set of ratios. Many banks and other lending organizations use these procedures to analyze firms' financial ratios and, on the basis of their analyses, classify companies according to their probability of getting into financial distress.[6]

Ratio analysis is useful in spite of these problems, but analysts should be aware of them and make adjustments as necessary. Ratio analysis conducted in a mechanical, unthinking manner is dangerous, but used intelligently and with good judgment, ratios can provide useful insights into a firm's operations. Your judgment in interpreting a set of ratios is probably weak at this point, but it will be greatly enhanced as we go through the remainder of the book.

---

[6]For a discussion of the use of discriminant analysis to predict bankruptcy, see Edward I. Altman, "Financial Ratios, Discriminate Analysis, and the Prediction of Corporate Bankruptcy," *Journal of Finance,* September 1968, 589–602, or Eugene F. Brigham and Louis C. Gapenski, *Intermediate Financial Management,* Second Edition, Chapter 20.

RESOLUTION TO DECISION IN FINANCE

Cooking the Books

When important income and asset figures are misreported, as they were at PepsiCo, the results can be far reaching. Because such numbers are key components of many liquidity, asset management, debt management, profitability, and market value ratios, a financial analysis based on them can become badly distorted. As a result, managers, creditors, shareholdes, stock analysts, and the general public may draw false conclusions and make wrong decisions.

In a highly publicized case like that of PepsiCo, the company itself pays dearly because its reputation is publicly tarnished. Such negative publicity raises questions about managerial competence and the effectiveness of corporate financial controls. Top management, whether it is a victim or an accomplice, usually gets blamed for middle-management fraud. Particularly when a number of employees are involved and when the situation continues undiscovered for several years, suspicions mount that management is either negligent or responsible.

Management is victimized in other ways, too. It may set goals based on false information, allocate investments or take out loans based on phony numbers, and pay bonuses to dishonest employees. Honest managers may actually get

punished; they may lose bonuses and promotions while their dishonest counterparts move quickly ahead.

Fraud affects shareholders as well, because they may buy or sell stock in response to erroneous information. For example, people may have bought PepsiCo's stock because they liked its healthy earnings per share and strong growth overseas. Shareholders' wealth may be further affected when the fraud comes to light. Stock prices can be expected to fall in response to such bad news, and their recovery depends on the size of the misstatement, the way that management handles the situation, and the company's overall reputation. It can take a long time for the market to regain confidence in a company that has suffered financial fraud.

In response to the falsified reports from its Mexican and Philippine operations, PepsiCo fired at least four employees, including a vice president at its corporate headquarters. At least eight other employees were replaced, although not all were fired.

In December 1982, two separate shareholder suits were filed, charging PepsiCo and its directors with filing false financial statements. But the law on middle-management fraud is fuzzy. Some attorneys believe that it is hard to prove damages and management responsibility. Without proof, they contend, shareholders cannot determine either the amount of their losses or who should pay for them.

Source: Adapted from "Cooking the Books" by Arlene Hershman with Henriette Sender. Reprinted with the permission of *Dun's Business Month* (formerly *Dun's Review*), January 1983. Copyright 1983, Dun & Bradstreet Publications Corporation.

SUMMARY

The primary purpose of this chapter has been to discuss the techniques used by investors, creditors, and managers to analyze businesses' financial statements. Financial analysis is designed to determine the relative strengths and weaknesses of a company — whether the firm is financially sound and profitable relative to other firms in its industry and whether its position is improving or deteriorating over time. Investors need such information in order to estimate both future cash flows from the firm and the riskiness of these flows. Managers need to be aware of their firms' financial positions in order to detect and strengthen weaknesses in a continuous quest for improvement.

Our study of financial analysis concentrated on a set of ratios designed to highlight the key aspects of a firm's operations. These ratios were broken down into five categories: (1) liquidity ratios, (2) asset management ratios, (3) debt management ratios, (4) profitability ratios, and (5) market value ratios. The ratios for a given firm are calculated, then compared with those of other firms in the same industry to judge the relative strength of the firm in question. Trends in the ratios are also analyzed, and the Du Pont system is used to pinpoint the cause of any weakness that is uncovered. Ratio analysis has limitations, but used with care and judgment, it can be most helpful.

QUESTIONS

7-1 How does inflation distort ratio analysis comparisons, both for one company over time (trend analysis) and when different companies are compared? Are only balance sheet items, or both balance sheet and income statement items, affected?

7-2 If a firm's ROE is low and management wants to improve it, explain how using more debt might provide a solution.

7-3 Suppose a firm used debt to leverage up its ROE, and in the process EPS was also boosted. Would this necessarily lead to an increase in the price of the firm's stock?

7-4 How might **(a)** seasonal factors and **(b)** different growth rates over time or across companies distort a comparative ratio analysis? Give some examples. How might these problems be alleviated?

7-5 Seasonal factors and differing growth rates are two problems that distort ratio analysis comparisons. What are some of the other factors that limit the effectiveness of ratio analysis?

7-6 Indicate the effects of the transactions listed on pages 171 and 172 on each of the following: total current assets, net working capital, current ratio, and net profit. Use (+) to indicate an increase, (−) to indicate a decrease, and (0) to indicate no effect or indeterminate effect. State necessary assumptions and assume an initial current ratio of more than 1 to 1. (Note: As an introductory finance student, you are not expected to be familiar with all of the transactions listed. The purpose of this question is to stimulate thought about the effects of these transactions.)

	Total Current Assets	Net Working Capital[a]	Current Ratio	Effect on Net Profit
1. Cash is acquired through issuance of additional common stock.				
2. Merchandise is sold for cash.				
3. Federal income tax due for the previous year is paid.				
4. A fixed asset is sold for less than book value.				
5. A fixed asset is sold for more than book value.				

[a]*Net working capital* is defined as current assets minus current liabilities.

	Total Current Assets	Net Working Capital[a]	Current Ratio	Effect on Net Profit
6. Merchandise is sold on credit.	___	___	___	___
7. Payment is made to trade creditors for previous purchases.	___	___	___	___
8. A cash dividend is declared and paid.	___	___	___	___
9. Cash is obtained through short-term bank loans.	___	___	___	___
10. Short-term notes receivable are sold at a discount.	___	___	___	___
11. Short-term marketable securities are sold below cost.	___	___	___	___
12. Advances are made to employees.	___	___	___	___
13. Short-term promissory notes are issued to trade creditors for prior purchases.	___	___	___	___
14. Ten-year notes are issued to pay off accounts payable.	___	___	___	___
15. A fully depreciated asset is retired.	___	___	___	___
16. Accounts receivable are collected.	___	___	___	___
17. Equipment is purchased with short-term notes.	___	___	___	___
18. Merchandise is purchased on credit.	___	___	___	___
19. The estimated taxes payable are increased.	___	___	___	___

[a]*Net working capital* is defined as current assets minus current liabilities.

SELF-TEST PROBLEMS

ST-1 H. B. Jones & Co. had earnings per share of $3 last year, and it paid a $1.50 dividend. Book value per share at year end was $30, whereas total retained earnings increased by $9 million during the year. Jones has no preferred stock, and no new common stock was issued during the year. If Jones's year-end debt (which equals its total liabilities) was $90 million, what was the company's year-end debt/assets ratio?

ST-2 The following data apply to Cavendish & Company (dollar amounts in millions):

Cash and marketable securities	$100.00
Fixed assets	$283.50
Sales	$1,000.00
Net income	$50.00
Quick ratio	2.0 ×
Current ratio	3.0 ×
Average collection period (ACP)	40 days
ROE	0.12 or 12%

Cavendish has no preferred stock — only common equity, current liabilites, and long-term debt. Find Cavendish's **(a)** accounts receivable (A/R), **(b)** current liabilities, **(c)** current assets, **(d)** total assets, **(e)** ROA, **(f)** common equity, and **(g)** long-term debt.

ST-3   In the preceding problem you should have found that Cavendish's accounts receivable (A/R) = $111.1 million. If Cavendish could reduce its ACP from 40 days to 30 days while holding other things constant, how much cash would it generate? If this cash were used to buy back common stock (at book value) and thus to reduce the amount of common equity, how would this affect **(a)** the ROE, **(b)** the ROA, and **(c)** the total debt/total assets ratio?

PROBLEMS

7-1   **Du Pont analysis.** Northwest Equipment's net profit margin is 5 percent, its total asset utilization (turnover) ratio is 2.0 times, and its equity multiplier (assets/equity ratio) is 1.49 times. What is its rate of return on equity?

7-2   **Rate of return.** Massachusetts Manufacturing is 100 percent equity financed. Given the following information, calculate the firm's return on equity:

$$
\begin{aligned}
\text{Earnings before taxes} &= \$8 \text{ million} \\
\text{Sales} &= \$40 \text{ million} \\
\text{Dividend payout ratio} &= 60 \text{ percent} \\
\text{Total asset utilization (turnover)} &= 2.0 \text{ times} \\
\text{Combined federal and state tax rate} &= 40 \text{ percent}
\end{aligned}
$$

7-3   **Leverage ratio.** Air Nevada, an emerging regional airline, earns 8 percent on total assets but has a return on equity of 20 percent. What percentage of the airline's assets are financed with debt?

7-4   **Du Pont analysis.** Laura Stark, president of Quality Products, has been reviewing her firm's financial statements. She knows that the firm's return on equity is 18 percent, the debt/total assets ratio is 0.32, and the total asset turnover is 5 times. She is sure the firm's accountant told her the net profit margin before he went home, but she can't remember. Would you determine the firm's net profit margin for her?

7-5   **Average collection period.** Leonard's Department Store had sales of $4,500,000 this year. Of those sales, 25 percent were for cash. If the firm maintains an accounts receivable balance of $375,000, what is the firm's average collection period?

7-6   **Inventory utilization.** Main Street Appliance Stores, Inc. had sales of $5,400,000 last year. If the firm maintains $1,800,000 in inventory, what is its inventory utilization (turnover)? What is its inventory utilization (turnover) period?

7-7   **Average collection period.** Plumber's Supply House has sales of $14,400,000. Its accounts receivable balance is $1,720,000.
a. If all sales are on credit, what is the company's average collection period?
b. What is the firm's average collection period if 10 percent of the firm's sales are for cash?

7-8   **Liquidity ratios.** Craftsman Products has $3,500,000 in current assets and $1,400,000 in current liabilities. Its initial inventory level is $1,000,000, and it will raise funds as additional notes payable and use them to increase inventory. How much can its short-term debt (notes payable) increase without exceeding a current ratio of 2 to 1? What will the firm's quick ratio be after the company has raised the maximum amount of short-term funds?

7-9   **Ratio calculations.** Boulder Software Emporium finds itself with more debt than it would like to have. Currently, the firm has $27 million in sales, an average collection period of 40 days, and an inventory turnover of 6 times. Doc Kolb, the firm's financial manager, is certain he can lower the average collection period to 30 days and increase the inventory utilization (turnover) to 8 times without lowering sales. How much would be available to reduce debt if Doc succeeds in his proposed reduction of current assets?

7-10   **Ratio calculations.** Quan Distribution Company has a quick ratio of 1.0, a current ratio of 3.0 times, an inventory turnover of 6 times, and current assets of $500,000. What are the firm's annual sales and, if cash and marketable securities are negligible, its average collection period?

7-11   **Pro forma statement.** Complete the balance sheet below by using the following financial information:

$$\text{Total assets utilization (turnover)} = 2.0 \text{ times}$$
$$\text{Current ratio} = 2.0 \text{ times}$$
$$\text{Average collection period} = 36 \text{ days}$$
$$\text{Inventory utilization (turnover)} = 4.5 \text{ times}$$
$$\text{Debt/total assets} = 40\%$$
$$\text{Fixed assets turnover} = 6 \text{ times}$$
$$\text{Sales} = \$2,700,000$$

Cash	$ 30,000	Current liabilities	$
Accounts receivable		Long-term debt	_____
Inventory	_____	Total debt	
Current assets		Common stock	100,000
Fixed assets	_____	Retained earnings	_____
Total assets	$ _____	Total claims	$ _____

7-12   **Ratio analysis.** Data for Saratoga Computer Company and its industry averages follow.
a. Calculate the indicated ratios for Saratoga.
b. Construct the Du Pont equation for both Saratoga and the industry.
c. Outline Saratoga's strengths and weaknesses as revealed by your analysis.

Saratoga Computer Company
Balance Sheet as of December 31, 1987

Cash	$ 310,000	Accounts payable	$ 516,000
Receivables	1,344,000	Notes payable	336,000
Inventory	966,000	Other current liabilities	468,000
Total current assets	$2,620,000	Total current liabilities	$1,320,000
Net fixed assets	1,170,000	Long-term debt	1,026,000
		Common equity	1,444,000
Total assets	$3,790,000	Total claims	$3,790,000

Saratoga Computer Company
Income Statement for Year Ended December 31, 1987

Sales		$6,430,000
Cost of goods sold:		
Materials	$2,868,000	
Labor	1,812,000	
Heat, light, and power	272,000	
Indirect labor	452,000	
Depreciation	166,000	5,570,000
Gross profit		860,000
Selling expenses		460,000
General and administrative expenses		120,000
Earnings before interest and taxes		$ 280,000
Interest expense		98,000
Net income before taxes		182,000
Federal income taxes (40%)		72,800
Net income		$ 109,200

Ratio	Saratoga	Industry Average
Current assets/current liabilities	_____	2.0×
Average collection period	_____	35 days
Sales/inventories	_____	6.7×
Sales/total assets	_____	2.9×
Net income/sales	_____	1.2%
Net income/total assets	_____	3.4%
Net income/equity	_____	8.3%
Total debt/total assets	_____	60.0%

d. Suppose that Saratoga's sales as well as its inventories, accounts receivable, and common equity had doubled during 1987. How would the information about this rapid growth affect the validity of your ratio analysis? (*Hint:* Think about averages and the effects of rapid growth on ratios if averages are not used. No calculations are needed.)

7-13 **Du Pont analysis.** The High Point Furniture Company, a manufacturer and wholesaler of high-quality home furnishings, has been experiencing low profitability in recent years. As a result, the board of directors has replaced the president of the firm with a new president, Greg Underwood, who has asked you to make an analysis of the firm's financial position using the Du Pont system. The most recent industry-average ratios and High Point's financial statements follow.

a. Calculate ratios to compare High Point Furniture Company with the industry-average ratios.

b. Construct a Du Pont equation for the firm and the industry and compare the resulting composite ratios.

c. Do the balance sheet accounts or the income statement figures seem to be primarily responsible for the low profits?

Industry Average Ratios

Current ratio	2×	Sales/fixed assets	6×
Total debt/total assets	30%	Sales/total assets	3×
Times interest earned	7×	Net profit on sales	3%
Sales/inventory	10×	Return on total assets	9%
Average collection period	24 days	Return on common equity	12.8%

High Point Furniture Company:
Balance Sheet as of December 31, 1987 (Millions of Dollars)

	1987		1987
Cash	$ 33	Accounts payable	$ 42
Marketable securities	26	Notes payable	30
Accounts receivable	40	Other current liabilities	18
Inventories	125	Total current liabilities	$ 90
Total current assets	$224	Long-term debt	22
Gross fixed assets	$185	Total liabilities	$112
Less: Depreciation	61	Common stock	$ 76
Net fixed assets	$124	Retained earnings	160
		Total stockholders' equity	$236
Total assets	$348	Total claims on assets	$348

High Point Furniture Company:
Income Statement for Year Ended December 31, 1987
(Millions of Dollars)

	1987
Net sales	$560
Cost of goods sold	465
Gross profit	$ 95
Operating expenses	51
Depreciation expense	13
Interest expense	5
Total expenses	$ 69
Net income before tax	$ 26
Taxes (50%)	13
Net income	$ 13

d. Which specific accounts seem to be most out of line in relation to other firms in the industry?

e. If High Point had a pronounced seasonal sales pattern, or if it had grown rapidly during the year, how might this affect the validity of your ratio analysis? How might you correct for such potential problems?

7-14   **Ratio analysis.** The following data pertain to Brennan Products, Inc. (BPI):

1. BPI has outstanding debt in the form of accounts payable, 6-month notes payable, and long-term bonds. The notes carry a 14 percent interest rate, and the bonds carry a 12 percent rate. Both the notes and bonds were outstanding for the entire year.

2. Retained earnings at the beginning of the year are $14,000.

3. The dividend payout ratio is 33.3 percent.

4. The debt to assets ratio is 60 percent.

5. The profit margin is 6 percent.

6. The return on equity (ROE) is 5 percent.

7. The inventory utilization ratio is 5 times.

8. The average collection period (ACP) is 122.4 days.

a. Given this information, complete BPI's balance sheet and income statement that follow.

b. The industry average inventory utilization ratio is 6 times, and the industry average ACP is 72 days. Assume that at the beginning of the year BPI had been able to adjust its inventory utilization and ACP to the industry averages and that this (1) freed up capital and (2) reduced storage costs and bad debt losses. Assume that the reduction of storage costs and bad debts raised the profit margin to 10 percent. Assume further that the freed-up capital was used at the start of the year to pay an extra, one-time dividend which reduced the beginning retained earnings figure. What would have been the effect on BPI's ROE for 1987? (*Hint:* Construct a new balance sheet which will show lower inventories and accounts receivable and a different value for December 31, 1987, retained earnings. The balance sheet will not balance; force it into balance by reducing accounts payable. Then calculate the new ROE. You can get the new net profit figures directly.)

Brennan Products, Inc.:
Balance Sheet at December 31, 1987

Cash	$ 7,500	Accounts payable	
Inventories		Notes payable	$10,000
Accounts receivable	_____		
Total current assets		Total current liabilities	
Net fixed assets	54,000	Bonds payable	30,000
		Total debt	
		Common stock	
		Retained earnings	_____
		Total common equity	_____
Total assets	_____	Total claims	_____

Brennan Products, Inc.:
Income Statement for Year Ended December 31, 1987

Sales	$25,000
Cost of goods sold	_____
Gross profit	
Selling expenses	2,700
General and administrative expenses	1,900
EBIT	
Interest expense	_____
Net profit before taxes	
Taxes	1,200
Net profit	_____

7-15 **Du Pont analysis.** The Ameritronic Corporation's balance sheets for 1987 and 1986 are as follows (millions of dollars):

	1987	1986
Cash	$ 21	$ 45
Marketable securities	0	33
Receivables	90	66
Inventories	225	159
Total current assets	$336	$303
Gross fixed assets	450	225
Less: Accumulated depreciation	(123)	(78)
Net fixed assets	$327	$147
Total assets	$663	$450
Accounts payable	$ 54	$ 45
Notes payable	9	45
Accruals	45	21
Total current liabilities	$108	$111
Long-term debt	78	24
Common stock	192	114
Retained earnings	285	201
Total long-term capital	$555	$339
Total claims	$663	$450

Additionally, Ameritronic's 1987 income statement is as follows (millions of dollars):

Sales	$1,365
Cost of goods sold	888
General expenses	282
EBIT	$ 195
Interest	10
EBT	$ 185
Taxes (46%)	85
Net income	$ 100

a. What was Ameritronic's dividend payout ratio in 1987?

b. The following extended Du Pont equation is the industry average for 1987:

Profit margin × Asset turnover × Equity multiplier = ROE			
6.52% ×	1.82 ×	1.77	= 21.00%

Construct Ameritronic's 1987 extended Du Pont equation. What does the Du Pont analysis indicate about Ameritronic's expense control, asset utilization, and debt utilization? What is the industry's debt to assets ratio?

c. Construct Ameritronic's 1987 statement of cash flows. What does it suggest about the company's operations?

7-16 **Ratio trend analysis.** The Kellor Corporation's forecasted 1988 financial statements follow, along with some industry average ratios.

a. Calculate Kellor's 1988 forecasted ratios, compare them with the industry average data, and comment briefly on Kellor's projected strengths and weaknesses.

(Do Part b only if you are using the computerized problem diskette.)

b. Suppose Kellor is considering installing a new computer system, which would provide tighter control of inventory, accounts receivable, and accounts payable. If the new system is installed, the following data are projected rather than the data now given in certain balance sheet and income statement categories:

Cash	$ 81,000
Accounts receivable	400,000
Inventory	750,000
Other fixed assets	91,000
Accounts payable	300,000
Accruals	133,000
Retained earnings	279,710
Cost of goods sold	3,510,000
Administrative and selling expense	228,320
P/E ratio	6 ×

(1) How does this affect the projected ratios and the comparison to the industry averages?

(2) If the new computer system is either more efficient or less efficient and causes the cost of goods sold to decrease or increase by $200,000 from the new projections, what effect does that have on the company's position?

Kellor Corporation:
Pro Forma Balance Sheet as of December 31, 1988

	1988
Cash	$ 72,000
Accounts receivable	439,000
Inventory	894,000
Total current assets	$1,405,000
Land and building	238,000
Machinery	132,000
Other fixed assets	61,000
Total assets	$1,836,000
Accounts and notes payable	$ 432,000
Accruals	170,000
Total current liabilities	$ 602,000
Long-term debt	404,290
Common stock	575,000
Retained earnings	254,710
Total liabilities and equity	$1,836,000

Kellor Corporation:
Pro Forma Income Statement for 1988

	1988
Sales	$4,290,000
Cost of goods sold	3,580,000
Gross operating profit	$ 710,000
General administrative and selling expenses	236,320
Depreciation	159,000
Miscellaneous	134,000
Taxable income	$ 180,680
Taxes (40%)	72,272
Net income	$ 108,408
Number of shares outstanding	23,000

Per-Share Data:

EPS	$4.71
Cash dividends	$0.95
P/E ratio	5×
Market price (average)	$23.57

Industry Financial Ratios (1988)[a]

Quick ratio	1.0×
Current ratio	2.7×
Inventory turnover[b]	7×
Average collection period	32 days
Fixed assets turnover[b]	13.0×
Total assets turnover[b]	2.6×
Return on total assets	9.1%
Return on equity	18.2%
Debt ratio	50%
Profit margin on sales	3.5%
P/E ratio	6×

[a]Industry average ratios have been constant for the past four years.
[b]Based on year-end balance sheet figures.

ANSWERS TO SELF-TEST PROBLEMS

ST-1   Jones paid $1.50 in dividends and retained $1.50 per share. Since total retained earnings increased by $9 million, there must be 6 million shares outstanding. With a book value of $30 per share, total common stock equity must be $30(6 million) = $180 million. Thus the debt ratio must be 33.3 percent:

$$\frac{\text{Debt}}{\text{Total assets}} = \frac{\text{Debt}}{\text{Debt} + \text{Equity}} = \frac{\$90}{\$90 + \$180} = 33.3\%$$

ST-2 **a.**

$$\text{ACP} = \frac{\text{Accounts receivable}}{\text{Sales}/360}$$

$$40 = \frac{\text{A/R}}{\$1{,}000/360}$$

$$\text{A/R} = 40(\$2.778) = \$111.1 \text{ million.}$$

b.
$$\text{Quick ratio} = \frac{\text{Current assets} - \text{Inventories}}{\text{Current liabilities}} = 2.0$$

$$= \frac{\text{Cash and marketable securities} + \text{A/R}}{\text{Current liabilities}} = 2.0.$$

Current liabilities = ($100 + $111.1)/2 = $105.5 million.

c.
$$\text{Current ratio} = \frac{\text{Current assets}}{\text{Current liabilities}} = 3.0.$$

Current assets = 3.0($105.5) = $316.5 million.

d.
$$\text{Total assets} = \text{Current assets} + \text{Fixed assets}$$
$$= \$316.5 + \$283.5 = \$600 \text{ million.}$$

e.
$$\text{ROA} = \text{Profit margin} \times \text{Total assets utilization}$$

$$= \frac{\text{Net income}}{\text{Sales}} \times \frac{\text{Sales}}{\text{Total assets}}$$

$$= \frac{\$50}{\$1,000} \times \frac{\$1,000}{\$600}$$

$$= 0.05 \times 1.667 = 0.0833 = 8.33\%.$$

f.
$$\text{ROE} = \text{ROA} \times \frac{\text{Assets}}{\text{Equity}}$$

$$12.0\% = 8.33\% \times \frac{\$600}{\text{Equity}}$$

$$\text{Equity} = \frac{(8.33\%)(\$600)}{12.0\%}$$

$$= \$416.5 \text{ million.}$$

g.
$$\text{Total assets} = \text{Total claims} = \$600$$

$$\text{Current liabilities} + \text{Long-term debt} + \text{Equity} = \$600$$

$$\$105.5 + \text{Long-term debt} + \$416.5 = \$600$$

$$\text{Long-term debt} = \$600 - \$105.5 - \$416.5 = \$78 \text{ million.}$$

Note: We could have found equity as follows:

$$\text{ROE} = \frac{\text{Net income}}{\text{Equity}}$$

$$0.12 = \frac{\$50}{\text{Equity}}$$

$$\text{Equity} = \$50/0.12$$

$$= \$416.67 \text{ million (rounding error difference).}$$

Then we could have gone on to find current liabilities and long-term debt.

ST-3   Cavendish's average sales per day were $1,000/360 = \$2.777777$ million. Its ACP was 40, so A/R $= 40(\$2,777,777) = \$111,111,111$. Its new ACP of 30 would cause A/R $= 30(\$2,777,777) = \$83,333,333$. The reduction in A/R $= \$111,111,111 - \$83,333,333 = \$27,777,777$, which would equal the amount of new cash generated.

a.
$$\text{New equity} = \text{Old equity} - \text{Stock bought back}$$
$$= \$416,500,000 - \$27,777,777$$
$$= \$388,722,223.$$

Thus

$$\text{New ROE} = \frac{\text{Net income}}{\text{New equity}}$$
$$= \frac{\$50,000,000}{\$388,722,223}$$
$$= 12.86\% \text{ (versus old ROE of } 12.00\%).$$

b.
$$\text{New ROA} = \frac{\text{Net income}}{\text{Total assets} - \text{Reduction in A/R}}$$
$$= \frac{\$50,000,000}{\$600,000,000 - \$27,777,777}$$
$$= 8.74\% \text{ (versus old ROA of } 8.33\%).$$

c. The old debt is the same as the new debt:

$$\text{New debt} = \text{Total claims} - \text{Equity}$$
$$= \$600 - \$416.5 = \$183.5 \text{ million.}$$

$$\text{Old total assets} = \$600 \text{ million.}$$

$$\text{New total assets} = \text{Old total assets} - \text{Reduction in A/R}$$
$$= \$600 - \$27.78$$
$$= \$572.22 \text{ million.}$$

Therefore

$$\frac{\text{Od debt}}{\text{Old total assets}} = \frac{\$183.5}{\$600} = 30.6\%,$$

whereas

$$\frac{\text{New debt}}{\text{New total assets}} = \frac{\$183.5}{\$572.22} = 32.1\%.$$

Chapter 8

Determining Future Financial Needs

Their Crystal Ball Was Off . . . by $1.2 Billion!

Myron Picoult of Oppenhenheimer & Co., like many other insurance analysts, must have thought he was seeing things when he got the flash about Cigna Corp. from the Dow Jones news wire: "Cigna said it is strengthening its property and casualty reserves, which will result in a charge of $1.2 billion against . . . earnings." After blinking a couple of times, Picoult fell to muttering about those "fools" at Dow Jones: "They put the decimal in the wrong place. No could be off $1.2 billion."

But Dow Jones hadn't misplaced a decimal. Instead, it was Cigna that had made a miscalculation of its future financial needs. Now the insurance giant was owning up, with shocking suddenness, to a $1.2 billion misestimate of costs.

Forecasting errors are common in the insurance business. The accounting practices in the insurance industry give an indistinct picture of even a company's present financial status. The premiums earned on a policy and all costs associated with that policy must be reflected in the same accounting period. But some claims are not made, or are not paid, until months or years into the future. Thus insurance firms must estimate the costs of these future claims and charge them, right now, to earnings. These future payouts, commonly called reserves and representing claims costs charged against earnings but not yet paid out, then move to the liability side of the balance sheet. Projecting the optimal amount of reserves to hold is a decidedly iffy proposition.

Precision is an impossible goal in the game of projecting reserves. One insurance company or another is always announcing that it is strengthening reserves — that is, making a new estimate to correct a past one that is now judged to have been too low. Still, no company has ever strengthened reserves by anything close to $1.2 billion in a single year. How could Cigna's estimates have been off by that much?

As you read this chapter, consider how Cigna may have misjudged its future financial needs? How could it have protected itself against such a large misestimate? How would such a large adjustment in reserves affect the value of the company?

See end of chapter for resolution.

pro forma statement
A financial statement that shows how an actual statement will look if certain specified assumptions are realized; used to forecast financial requirements.

As noted in Chapter 7, both managers and investors are vitally concerned with *future* financial statements. Also, managers regularly construct **pro forma,** or projected, **statements** and consider alternative courses of action in terms of the actions' effects on these projections. In this chapter we discuss how pro forma statements are constructed and how they are used to help estimate the need for capital.

SALES FORECASTS

sales (demand) forecast
Forecast of unit and dollar sales for some future period. Generally, sales forecasts are based on recent trends in sales plus forecasts of the economic prospects for the nation, region, industry, and so forth.

The most important element in financial planning is a **sales** (or **demand**) **forecast.** Because such forecasts are critical for production scheduling, for plant design, for financial planning, and so on, the entire management team participates in their preparation. In fact, most of the larger firms have a *planning group* or *planning committee,* with its own staff of economists, which coordinates the corporation's sales forecast. A great deal of work lies behind all good sales forecasts. Companies must project the state of the national economy, economic conditions within their own geographic areas, and conditions in the product markets they serve. Further, they must consider their own pricing strategies, credit policies, advertising programs, capacity limitations, and the like. Companies also must consider the strategies and policies of their competitors, such as the introduction of new products or changes in competitive pricing of key products.

If the sales forecast is off, the consequences can be serious. First, if the market expands *more* than the firm has expected and geared up for, the firm will not be able to meet its customers' needs. Orders will back up, delivery times will lengthen, repair and installations will be harder to schedule, and customer dissatisfaction will increase. Customers will end up going elsewhere, and the firm will lose market share. On the other hand, if its projections are overly optimistic, the firm could end up with too much plant, equipment, and inventory. This would mean low turnover ratios, high costs for depreciation and storage, and, possibly, high write-offs of obsolete inventory and equipment. All of this would result in a low rate of return on equity, which in turn would depress the company's stock price. If the firm financed the expansion with debt, its problems would, of course, be compounded. Thus an accurate sales forecast is critical to the well-being of the firm. Because sales forecasting is a rather specialized subject, we do not consider the mechanics of the forecasting process in this chapter. Rather, we simply take the sales forecast as given and use it to illustrate various types of financial decisions.

FORECASTING FINANCIAL REQUIREMENTS: THE PERCENTAGE OF SALES METHOD

Several methods are used to forecast financial statements. In this chapter we focus on the percentage of sales method and explain when this method can and cannot be used. We also discuss the growing use of computerized models for forecasting financial statements.

Table 8-1 **Addison Products Company: 1987 Financial Statements**

I. Balance Sheet, December 31, 1987 (Thousands of Dollars)

Cash	$ 10	Accounts payable	$ 40
Accounts receivable	90	Notes payable	10
Inventories	200	Accrued wages and taxes	50
Total current assets	$300	Total current liabilities	$100
Net fixed assets	300	Mortgage bonds	150
		Common stock	50
		Retained earnings	300
Total assets	$600	Total claims	$600

II. Summary Income Statement, 1987

Sales	$400,000
Net income	40,000
Dividends paid	24,000

The **percentage of sales method** is a simple but often practical method of forecasting financial statement variables. The procedure is based on two assumptions: (1) that most balance sheet accounts are tied directly to sales and (2) that the current levels of all assets are optimal for the current sales level. We illustrate the process by examining the Addison Products Company, whose December 31, 1987, balance sheet and summary income statement are given in Table 8-1. Addison operated its fixed assets at full capacity to support its 1987 sales of $400,000, and it had no unnecessary stocks of current assets. Its profit margin was 10 percent, and it distributed 60 percent of its net income to stockholders as dividends. If Addison's sales increase to $600,000 in 1988, what will be the condition of its pro forma December 31, 1988, balance sheet, and how much additional financing will the company require during 1988?

Our first step is to isolate those balance sheet items that vary directly with sales. Because Addison is operating at full capacity, each asset item must increase if the higher level of sales is to be attained. More cash will be needed for transactions; receivables will be higher; additional inventory must be stocked; and new plant must be added.[1]

If assets are to increase, liabilities and net worth must likewise rise; the balance sheet must balance, and increases in assets must be financed in some manner. Some of these funds will result spontaneously from routine business transactions, whereas other funds must be raised through formal means. **Spontaneously generated funds** come from sources such as accounts payable

percentage of sales method
A method of forecasting financial requirements by expressing various balance sheet items as a percentage of sales and then multiplying these percentages by expected future sales to construct pro forma balance sheets.

spontaneously generated funds
Funds that arise automatically from routine business transactions.

---

[1]Some assets, such as marketable securities, are not tied directly to operations and hence do not vary directly with sales. Also, as we shall see later in this chapter, if some assets (such as fixed assets) are not being full utilized, sales can increase without increasing those assets.

and accruals, which will increase spontaneously with sales. As sales increase, so will purchases, and larger purchases will result in higher levels of accounts payable. Thus, if sales double, accounts payable also will double. Similarly, because a higher level of operations will require more labor, accrued wages will increase, and assuming profit margins are maintained, an increase in profits will pull up accrued taxes. Retained earnings also will increase, but not in direct proportion to the increase in sales. Other sources of financing require formal action by the firm's financial manager. For example, neither notes payable, mortgage bonds, nor common stock increase automatically with sales. Management must obtain these funds from financial intermediaries or from investors.

We can use this information to construct a pro forma balance sheet for December 31, 1988, proceeding as follows:

- **Step 1** In Table 8-2, Column 1 shows those balance sheet items that vary directly with sales as a percentage of 1987 sales. An item that does not vary directly with sales, such as notes payable, is designated n.a., or "not applicable."

- **Step 2** Next these percentages are multiplied by the $600,000 projected 1988 sales to obtain the projected amounts as of December 31, 1988; these are shown in Column 2 of the table.

- **Step 3** We simply insert figures for notes payable, mortgage bonds, and common stock from the December 31, 1987, balance sheet. At least one of these accounts may have to be changed later in the analysis.

dividend payout ratio
The percentage of earnings paid out in dividends.

- **Step 4** Next we add the addition to retained earnings estimated for 1988 to the figure shown on the December 31, 1987, balance sheet to obtain the December 31, 1988, projected retained earnings. Recall that Addison expects to earn 10 percent on sales of $600,000, or $60,000, and it expects to pay 60 percent of this out in dividends to stockholders, making the **dividend payout ratio** 60 percent. Therefore, retained earnings for the year are projected to be $60,000 − 0.6($60,000) = $24,000. Adding the $24,000 addition to retained earnings to the $300,000 beginning balance gives the $324,000 projected retained earnings shown in Column 2.

- **Step 5** Next we sum the asset accounts, obtaining a total projected assets figure of $900,000, and also add the projected liabilities and net worth items to obtain $669,000, the estimate of available funds. Because liabilities and net worth must total $900,000, but only $669,000 is projected, we have a shortfall of $231,000 "additional funds needed," which presumably will be raised by bank borrowing or issuing securities or both. For simplicity, we disregard depreciation by assuming that cash flows from depreciation are reinvested to replace worn-out fixed assets.

Table 8-2 **Addison Products Company: December 31, 1987, Balance Sheet Expressed as a Percentage of Sales and December 31, 1988, Pro Forma Balance Sheet (Thousands of Dollars)**

	Balance Sheet Items on Dec. 31, 1987 (as a % of the $400 1987 Sales) (1)	Pro Forma Balance Sheet on Dec. 31, 1988 (= Projected Sales of $600 Times Column 1) (2)
Cash	2.5%	$ 15
Accounts receivable	22.5	135
Inventories	50.0	300
Total current assets	75.0%	$450
Net fixed assets	75.0	450
Total assets	150.0%	$900
Accounts payable	10.0%	$ 60
Notes payable	n.a.[a]	10[b]
Accrued wages and taxes	12.5	75
Total current liabilities	22.5%	$145
Mortgage bonds	n.a.	150[b]
Common stock	n.a.	50[b]
Retained earnings	n.a.	324[c]
Funds available		$669
Additional funds needed[d]		231
Total claims	22.5%	$900

[a]n.a. = not applicable. (Item does not vary spontaneously with sales.)
[b]Initially projected at the 1987 level. Later financing decisions might change this level.
[c]December 31, 1987, balance in retained earnings plus 1988 addition to retained earnings, as explained in Step 4.
[d]"Additional funds needed" is a balancing figure: $900 − $669 = $231.

- **Step 6** Addison could use short-term bank loans (notes payable), mortgage bonds, common stock, or a combination of these securities to make up the shortfall. Ordinarily it would make this choice on the basis of the relative costs of these different types of securities. In this case, however, the company has a contractual agreement with its bondholders to keep total debt at or below 50 percent of total assets, as well as to keep the current ratio at a level of 3.0 or greater. These provisions restrict the financing choices as follows:

1. Restriction on additional debt
Maximum debt permitted = 0.5 × Total assets
                       = 0.5 × $900,000 = $450,000
Less: Debt already projected for December 31, 1985:
              Current liabilities $145,000
              Mortgage bonds   150,000 = 295,000
Maximum additional debt $155,000

INDUSTRY PRACTICE

Why Industry Forecasts Go Wrong: The Case of the Computer Industry

Item: In June 1982, a respected computer industry guru projected that by 1990 Storage Technology Corp. would be the third-largest computer company, behind IBM and Digital Equipment Corp.

Item: In 1981, a major market research firm predicted that one in every three large corporations would have its own teleconferencing system by 1986.

Item: In the early 1980s, forecasters heralded IBM's new microcomputer, the 8100, as a sure winner — one of the most important products to come out of the computer giant in years.

As it developed, these projections proved wildly off the mark. Storage Tech not only didn't make it to the uppermost echelons of the computer industry, it filed for bankruptcy. Teleconferencing, also known as videoconferencing, proved too expensive and technologically cumbersome. And the sales of IBM's 8100 turned out to be far below expectations.

These projections are examples of the rosy scenario forecasting that characterized the salad days of the computer business. "According to the reports many forecasters turned out, we'd reached Nirvana," says John J. Connell, president of the Office Technology Research Group, an organization of some of the largest users in the country. "These electronic Pied Pipers were telling people — the vendors, users, and the venture capitalists — exactly what they wanted to hear," the former head of a now defunct computer service adds bitterly. "If a CPA provided a corporate client with the kind of num-

bers some of these people were putting out, they'd be indicted," he says.

To be sure, some wild-eyed forecasts are not forgotten. Take, for example, Future Computing Inc., a Dallas-based forecaster of personal computer sales. Carol Bunevich, a marketing director for Scholastic Software in New York, recalls Future's projections of educational software sales were "off by hundreds of millions of dollars." Future Computing is no more: a victim of the industry shakeout, it folded in 1986.

But the users who bought products based on overly optimistic reports also paid a steep price. For example, Atlantic Richfield spent an estimated $20 million upgrading its terrestrial intracorporate network to a satellite system with teleconferencing capabilities. Today, that teleconferencing system is in limited use. "Companies were stuck with products from vendors that had gone out of business or technologies that simply didn't perform as promised," says consultant Philip H. Dorn.

The euphoria was brought up short in 1983. "Senior people began to question the return on investments in PCs and other new technologies," says Connell. "When users admitted they didn't have the foggiest idea about return on investment, top management said, 'no more.'"

As a result, today's users discount projections. "There's a healthy skepticism now," says Connell. "The buying decision is more under the control of the information systems people. They've been burned often enough so they're not likely to be sold a bill of goods again."

But will they? If another lusty computer market emerges, the circumstances that fashioned the pie-in-the-sky projections could reappear. And many market research firms as well as users are worried that executives will fail to spot phony projections. Estimating the size of a market is always a dicey business. But the projections of some firms were not research, but busi-

Source: Adapted from "Why Industry Forecasts Go Wrong," Laton McCartney, *Dun's Business Month,* August 1986, pages 79 and 81. Reprinted with permission, *Business Month* magazine. Copyright © 1985 by *Business Month* Corporation, 38 Commercial Wharf, Boston, MA 02110.

ness-getting tools. The research firms sold an entrepreneur on a new business opportunity by making projections of a lucrative potential market. "They hoped he'd buy their research," recalls Howard Anderson, president of the Yankee Group. In effect, the researchers became paid cheerleaders of the vendor's offerings. "They were putting out press releases, not valid reports," he says.

These projections turned out to be great publicity. Soon the entrepreneurs sought out the researchers to make projections. With these "objective" reports, they went around to financial backers, customers, and the press to drum up support.

Not surprisingly, much of the research methodology was unprofessional. "Instead of asking users what they were going to buy, they asked vendors and dealers how much they planned to sell," says the ex-service company chief. "Naturally, sales were going to be astronomical."

How does a corporate client evaluate the quality of projections? Industry experts say users must investigate the financial strength of market research firms to see that no individual client accounts for a big part of its business. They must also scrutinize the report for signs that the researchers polled users in sufficient number and of comparable size. And finally, any user or vendor, before making a major commitment, ought to do primary research; that is, poll users themselves.

These extreme cautions are necessary, argues the Yankee Group's Anderson, because the pressure to make bullish predictions can be excruciating. "For example, there's nobody more down on the future of videotext than we are," he notes. "We said five years ago it had the stench of death. As a result, people in the business sent shock troops around with horse heads under their arms like the guys in *The Godfather.* They wanted to know who was this jerk raining on their parade."

Today's tough-mindedness is likely to fade when new dazzling technologies re-emerge. And hunger for business will probably lead a new generation of researchers into playing fast and loose with projections. Then, those who buy them despite the lessons of the past will have themselves to blame.

2. Restriction on additional current liabilities

Maximum current liabilities = ⅓ of current assets

$$= \$450{,}000 \div 3 = \$150{,}000$$

Current liabilities already projected	145,000
Maximum additional current liabilities	$ 5,000

3. Common equity requirements

Total external funds required (from Table 8-2)	$231,000
Maximum additional debt permitted	155,000
Common equity funds required	$ 76,000

We see, then, that Addison needs a total of $231,000 from external sources. Its existing debt contract limits new debt to $155,000, and of that amount, only $5,000 can be short-term debt. Thus Addison must plan to sell common stock in the amount of $76,000, in addition to its debt financing, to cover its financial requirements.

Projected Financial Statements and Ratios

Addison's financial manager can now construct a set of projected, or pro forma, financial statements and then analyze the ratios that are implied by these statements. Table 8-3 gives abbreviated versions of the final projected balance sheet, income statement, statement of cash flows, and a few key ratios. These statements, in turn, can be used by the financial manager to show the other executives the implications of the planned sales increase. For example, the projected rate of return on equity is 13.3 percent. Is this a reasonable target, or can it be improved? Also, the preliminary forecast calls for the sale of some common stock—but does top management really want to sell any new stock? Suppose Addison Products Company is owned entirely by Maddie Addison, who does not want to sell any stock and thereby lose her exclusive control of the company. How then can the needed funds be raised, or what adjustments should be made? In the remainder of the chapter, we consider approaches to answering questions such as these.

The Relationship between Growth in Sales and Capital Requirements

Although the forecast of capital requirements can be made by constructing pro forma balance sheets, as described previously, it often is easier to use a simple forecasting formula. In addition, the following formula can be used to clarify the relationship between sales growth and financial requirements.

$$
\begin{bmatrix} \text{Additional} \\ \text{funds} \\ \text{needed} \end{bmatrix} = \begin{bmatrix} \text{Required} \\ \text{increase} \\ \text{in assets} \end{bmatrix} - \begin{bmatrix} \text{Spontaneous} \\ \text{increase in} \\ \text{liabilities} \end{bmatrix} - \begin{bmatrix} \text{Increase in} \\ \text{retained} \\ \text{earnings} \end{bmatrix} \quad \textbf{(8-1)}
$$

$$
\text{AFN} = \frac{A}{S}(\Delta S) \quad - \frac{L}{S}(\Delta S) \quad - MS_1(1 - d).
$$

Here,

AFN = additional funds needed.

$\dfrac{A}{S}$ = assets that increase spontaneously with sales as a percent of sales, or required dollar increase in assets per $1 increase in sales. A/S = 600/400 = 150%, or 1.5, for Addison.

$\dfrac{L}{S}$ = liabilities that increase spontaneously with sales as a percent of sales, or spontaneously generated financing per $1 increase in sales. L/S = 90/400 = 22.5% for Addison.

S_1 = total sales projected for next year. Note that S_0 = last year's sales. S_1 = $600,000 for Addison.

ΔS = change in sales = $S_1 - S_0$ = $600,000 - $400,000 = $200,000 for Addison.

**Table 8-3 Addison Products Company:
Projected Financial Statements for 1988
(Thousands of Dollars)**

I. Projected Balance Sheet, Dec. 31, 1988

Cash	$ 15	Accounts payable	$ 60
Accounts receivable	135	Notes payable[a]	15
Inventories	300	Accruals	75
Total current assets	$450	Total current liabilities	$150
Net fixed assets	$450	Long-term debt[b]	$300
		Common stock[c]	126
		Retained earnings	324
		Total equity	$450
Total assets	$900	Total claims	$900

II. Projected Income Statement, 1988

Sales	$600
Total costs	500
Taxable income	$100
Taxes (40%)	40
Net income after taxes	$ 60
Dividends	36
Addition to retained earnings	$ 24

III. Projected Statement of Cash Flows, 1988

Funds Provided by (Used in) Operations

Sources:		Financing Activities:	
Net income	$ 60	Increase in notes payble	$ 5
Increase in accounts payable	20	Sale of bonds	150
Increase in accruals	25	Sale of common stock	76
Total sources from operations	$ 105[d]	Net funds from financing	$231
Uses:		Total funds from operations	
Increase in accounts receivable	$ 45	and financing	$ 41
Increase in inventories	100	Less: Dividends	36
Increase in fixed assets	150	Increase (decrease) in cash	
Total uses in operations	$ 295	and equivalents	$ 5
Net funds from operations	$(190)		

IV. Key Ratios Projected for December 31, 1988

1. Current ratio   3.0×
2. Total debt/total assets   50%
3. Rate of return on equity   13.3%
(Other ratios could be calculated and analyzed by the Du Pont system.)

[a]Assumes additional $5,000 is borrowed from bank. This is the maximum permissible increase in short-term debt.
[b]Assumes $150,000 additional long-term debt is sold. This is the maximum permissible increase in long-term debt, given the $5,000 increase in notes payable.
[c]Assumes $76,000 additional common stock is sold.
[d]*Funds from operations* normally includes depreciation. Here we have assumed that depreciation is reinvested in fixed assets; that is, depreciation is netted out against fixed asset additions.

M = profit margin, or rate of profit per \$1 of sales. M = 10%, or 0.10, for Addison.

d = percentage of earnings paid out in dividends, or the dividend payout ratio; d = 60%. Notice that $1 - d = 1.0 - 0.6 = 0.4$, or 40%. This is the percentage of earnings that Addison retains, often called the **retention rate** or *retention ratio*.

retention rate

The percentage of earnings retained after payment of dividends.

Inserting values for Addison into Equation 8-1, we find the additional funds needed as follows:

$$AFN = 1.5 (\Delta S) - 0.225(\Delta S) - 0.1(S_1)(1 - 0.6)$$

$$= 1.5(\$200,000) - 0.225(\$200,000) - 0.1(\$600,000)(0.4)$$

$$= \$300,000 - \$45,000 - \$24,000$$

$$= \$231,000.$$

additional funds needed

Funds that must be acquired by a firm through borrowing or by selling new stock.

To increase sales by \$200,000, Addison must increase assets by \$300,000. The \$300,000 of new assets must be financed in some manner. Of the total, \$45,000 will come from a spontaneous increase in liabilities, whereas another \$24,000 will be raised from retained earnings. The **additional funds needed** to finance this projected growth amount to \$231,000, which must be raised over and above the internally and spontaneously generated funds. This value must, of course, agree with the figure developed in Table 8-2.

Graph of the Relationship between Growth and Funds Requirements

The faster Addison's growth rate in sales, the greater its need for external financing. We can use Equation 8-1, which is plotted in Figure 8-1, to indicate this relationship. The lower section shows Addison's external financial requirements at various growth rates, and these data are plotted in the graph. Several points that can be seen from the figure are discussed in the following sections.

Financial Planning. At low growth rates Addison needs no external financing. However, if the company grows faster than 3.239 percent, it must raise capital from outside sources. If for any reason management foresees difficulties in raising this capital — perhaps because Addison's owner does not want to sell additional stock — the company might need to reconsider the feasibility of its expansion plans.

The Effect of Dividend Policy on Financing Needs. Dividend policy also affects external capital requirements, so if Addison foresees difficulties in raising capital, it might want to consider a reduction in the dividend payout ratio. This would lower, or shift to the right, the line in Figure 8-1, indicating lower external capital requirements at all growth rates. Before making this decision,

Figure 8-1 **Relationship between Growth in Sales and Financial Requirements, Assuming S_0 = \$400,000**

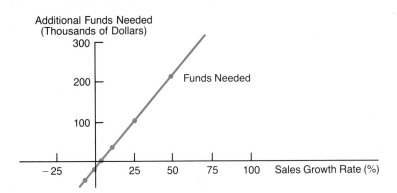

Growth Rate in Sales (1)	Increase (Decrease) in Sales, ΔS (2)	Forecasted Sales, S_1 (3)	Additional Funds Needed[a] (4)
50%	\$200	\$600	\$231.0
10	40	440	33.4
3.239	12.956	412.956	0.0
0	0	400	(16.0)
−10	(40)	360	(65.4)

Explanation of Columns:
Col. 1: Growth rate in sales, g.
Col. 2: Increase (decrease) in sales, $\Delta S = g(S_0)$.
Col. 3: Forecasted sales, $S_1 = S_0 + g(S_0) = S_0(1 + g)$.
Col. 4: Additional funds needed = $1.5(\Delta S) - 0.225(\Delta S) - 0.04(S_1)$.
[a]Negative additional funds required = surplus funds available.

however, management should consider the effects of changes in dividends on stock prices. These effects are described in Chapter 21.

Notice that the line in Figure 8-1 does *not* pass through the origin. Thus, at low growth rates (for Addison below a growth rate of 3.239 percent), surplus funds (therefore negative additional funds needed) will be produced, because new retained earnings plus spontaneous funds will exceed the required asset increases. Only if the dividend payout ratio is 100 percent, meaning that the firm does not retain any of its earnings, will the "funds required" line pass through the origin.

Capital Intensity. The amount of assets required per dollar of sales, A/S in Equation 8-1, is often called the **capital intensity ratio.** This factor has a major effect on capital requirements per unit of sales growth. If the capital intensity ratio is low, sales can grow rapidly without much outside capital. However, if the firm is capital intensive, even a small amount of growth in output will require a great deal of outside capital. Note that the capital intensity

capital intensity ratio
The amount of assets required per dollar of sales (A/S).

Unaudited Pro Forma Condensed Balance Sheet
American Telephone and Telegraph Company

The following Unaudited Consolidated Historical Balance Sheet as of June 30, 1983, is derived from the unaudited financial statements of the Company and its consolidated subsidiaries included in its Quarterly Report filed with the Securities and Exchange Commission on Form 10-Q.

The following Unaudited Pro Forma Condensed Balance Sheet gives effect to the divestiture of the telephone subsidiaries by the Company as if it had occurred on June 30, 1983, in accordance with the Plan and reflects concurrent divestiture-related extraordinary charge for the discontinued application of accounting principles appropriate only for a rate-regulated enterprise. The pro forma balance sheet is presented as of June 30, 1983 as a result of agreements reached with the Securities and Exchange Commission for the November 16, 1983 Form 8-K filing. Even though divestiture occurred on January 1, 1984, final data is not readily available for all of the divested companies and actual balances and adjustments will vary from those presented in the pro forma balance sheet below. The Unaudited Pro Forma Condensed Balance Sheet should be read in conjunction with the audited consolidated financial statements and notes for the years ended December 31, 1983, 1982 and 1981.

DOLLARS IN MILLIONS	Consolidated Historical June 30, 1983	Divestiture Pro Forma Adjustments	Divestiture-Related Extraordinary Charge	Pro Forma Consolidated June 30, 1983
		See Note (1)	See Note (2)	
ASSETS				
TELEPHONE PLANT–Net of Accumulated Depreciation	$130,056.5	$(121,087.1)(a) 15,431.3 (b) 377.0 (d) 3,993.3 (e)	$(8,857.0)	$19,914.0
INVESTMENTS	5,960.0	57,692.2 (a) (9,213.7)(b) (46,668.0)(c) (5,017.1)(e) (2,128.4)(f)	—	625.0
CURRENT ASSETS	14,887.3	(9,030.9)(a) 374.4 (b) 5,234.8 (e) 90.4 (f)	—	11,556.0
OTHER ASSETS AND DEFERRED CHARGES	2,614.6	(2,099.3)(a) 44.3 (b) 7.0 (e) 57.9 (f)	—	624.5
TOTAL ASSETS	$153,518.4	$(111,941.9)	$(8,857.0)	$32,719.5

See accompanying Notes to Unaudited Pro Forma Condensed Balance Sheet.

DOLLARS IN MILLIONS	Consolidated Historical June 30, 1983	Divestiture Pro Forma Adjustments	Divestiture-Related Extraordinary Charge	Pro Forma Consolidated June 30, 1983
		See Note (1)	See Note (2)	
INVESTED CAPITAL, LIABILITIES, AND DEFERRED CREDITS				
COMMON SHAREOWNERS' EQUITY:				
Common Shares–par value $1 per share	$ 936.7	$ —	$ —	$ 936.7
Proceeds in Excess of Par Value	34,629.6	(25,233.7)(c)	—	9,395.9
Reinvested Earnings	29,580.7	(21,495.4)(c)	(5,497.9)	2,587.4
CONVERTIBLE PREFERRED SHARES SUBJECT TO REDEMPTION	277.9	—	—	277.9
PREFERRED SHARES SUBJECT TO MANDATORY REDEMPTION	1,537.2	—	—	1,537.2
OWNERSHIP INTEREST OF OTHERS IN CONSOLIDATED SUBSIDIARIES	535.8	(535.8)(a)	—	—
LONG AND INTERMEDIATE TERM DEBT	45,319.5	(37,554.3)(a) 845.9 (b) 1,085.8 (e) (228.0)(f)	—	9,468.9
DEBT MATURING WITHIN ONE YEAR	1,617.4	(1,719.6)(a) 1,252.8 (b) 333.6 (e) (1,117.8)(f)	—	366.4
OTHER CURRENT LIABILITIES	11,277.0	(8,852.7)(a) 218.7 (b) 1,642.6 (e) (634.3)(f)	400.1	4,051.4
DEFERRED TAXES AND OTHER DEFERRED CREDITS	27,806.6	(25,862.7)(a) 4,318.9 (b) 61.1 (e) 377.0 (d) 1,156.0 (e)	(3,759.2)	4,097.7
TOTAL INVESTED CAPITAL, LIABILITIES, AND DEFERRED CREDITS	$153,518.4	$(111,941.9)	$(8,857.0)	$32,719.5

Notes to Unaudited Pro Forma Condensed Balance Sheet
Dollars in Millions (except per share amounts)

(1) Divestiture Pro Forma Adjustments

(A) This adjustment reflects the deconsolidation of the BOCs and the reversal of consolidating intercompany eliminations.

(B) This adjustment transfers assets and liabilities to and from the BOCs at net book value. The transfers are tax-free under the Internal Revenue Code. Accumulated deferred income tax reserves and unamortized investment credits are transferred along with the associated assets.

This adjustment also reflects the removal of debt by the Company from the BOCs as required by the provisions of the Plan. The amount expected to be removed at divestiture under terms of Reorganization and Divestiture Agreements between the Company and each RHC is approximately $2.6 billion. The Company's debt ratio (debt as a percent of total debt and equity) at the time of divestiture was approximately 40%.

(C) This adjustment reflects the divestiture of the investment in the BOCs.

(D) Under this adjustment, pursuant to a 1967 closing agreement with the IRS, telephone plant transferred to AT&T Information Systems is increased to original cost and the depreciation reserve is increased to what it would have been had the telephone plant been depreciated on the basis of the original cost. The closing agreement requires that when property ceases to be public utility property, the liability for deferred taxes associated with Western Electric profits reverts back to Western Electric. See Accounting Policies section of Historical Financial Statements, "Purchases From Western Electric," and "Telephone Plant."

(E) This adjustment effects the consolidation of Western Electric and Bell Laboratories.

(F) This adjustment eliminates significant intercompany accounts receivable and payable.

See Note (A) to Historical Financial Statements. These amounts differ from the amounts announced initially because of regulatory events and other adjustments.

See Note (Q) to Historical Financial Statements.

(2) Divestiture-Related Extraordinary Charge

(3) Contingent Liabilities

This unaudited Pro Forma Consolidated Balance Sheet, published by AT&T in its 1983 Annual Report, is one of the few instances of a major corporation making its financial forecasts public. Most firms are reluctant to publish their financial predictions, but AT&T, which was poised on the verge of divestiture, decided to publish this forecast of future company profits and dividends to reassure stockholders that divestiture would not adversely affect shareholder value. Following divestiture, AT&T no longer included this information in its annual reports, and a company spokesperson remarked that the publication of financial forecasts in 1983 was "unique to the special circumstances of that year."

26

27

28

ratio is the reciprocal of the total asset utilization ratio only when *all* assets grow proportionally with sales.

The Profit Margin and the Need for External Funds. The profit margin, M, is also an important determinant of the funds-required equation; the higher the margin, the lower the funds requirements, other things held constant. Addison's profit margin was 10 percent. Now suppose M increased to 15 percent. This new value could be inserted into the funds-required formula, and the effect would be to reduce the additional funds needed at all positive growth rates. In terms of the graph, an increase in the profit margin would cause the line to shift down, and its slope would also become less steep. Because of the relationship between profit margins and external capital requirements, some very rapidly growing firms do not need much external capital. For example, Xerox grew very rapidly with very little borrowing or stock sales. However, as the company lost patent protection and as competition intensified in the copier industry, Xerox's profit margin declined, its needs for external capital rose, and it began to borrow heavily from banks and other sources. IBM has had a similar experience.

FORECASTING FINANCIAL REQUIREMENTS WHEN THE BALANCE SHEET RATIOS ARE SUBJECT TO CHANGE

To this point we have been assuming that the balance sheet ratios of assets and liabilities to sales (A/S and L/S) will remain constant over time. For this to happen, each asset and liability item must increase at the same rate as sales. In graph form, this assumes the type of relationship indicated in Panel a of Figure 8-2, a relationship that is linear and passes through the origin. Under these conditions, if the company grows and sales expand from $200 million to $400 million, inventories will increase proportionately from $100 million to $200 million.

The assumption of constant ratios is appropriate at times, but there are times when it is incorrect. Three such conditions are described in the following sections.

Economies of Scale

There are economies of scale in the use of many kinds of assets, and where economies occur, the ratios are likely to change over time as the size of the firm increases. For example, firms often need to maintain base stocks of different inventory items, even if sales levels are quite low. Then, as sales expand, inventories grow less rapidly than sales, so the ratio of inventory to sales (I/S) declines. This situation is depicted in Panel b of Figure 8-2. Here we see that the inventory/sales ratio is 1.5, or 150 percent, when sales are $200 million, but it declines to 1.0 when sales climb to $400 million.

Figure 8-2 **Three Possible Ratio Relationships (Millions of Dollars)**

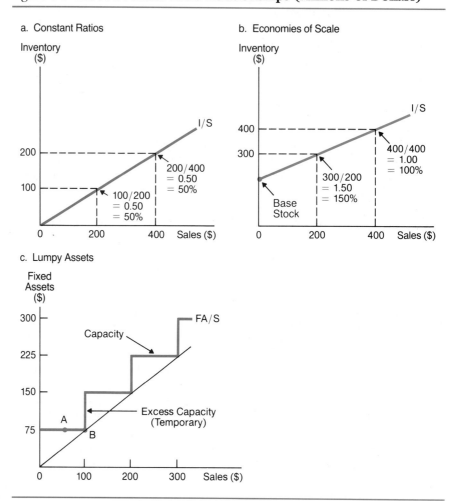

Although the relationship shown here for economies of scale is linear, this is not necessarily the case. Indeed, as we shall see in Chapters 11 and 12, if the firm uses the most popular model for establishing inventory and cash levels, the EOQ model, then the levels of these items will rise with the square root of sales. This means that the graph in Figure 8-2 would tend to be a curved line whose slope decreases at higher sales levels.

"Lumpy" Assets

"lumpy" assets
Assets that cannot be acquired in small increments but must be obtained in large, discrete amounts.

In many industries, technological considerations dictate that if a firm is to be competitive, it must add fixed assets in large, discrete units; such assets are often referred to as **"lumpy" assets.** In the paper industry, for example, there are strong economies of scale in basic paper mill equipment, so when paper companies expand capacity, they must do so in large, or lumpy, increments. This type of situation is depicted in Panel c of Figure 8-2. Here we assume that the minimum-size feasible plant has a cost of $75 million and that such a plant can produce enough output to attain a sales level of $100 million. If the firm is to be competitive, it simply must have at least $75 million of fixed assets.

This situation has a major effect on the fixed assets/sales (FA/S) ratios at different sales levels and, consequently, on financial requirements. At Point A in Figure 8-2c, which represents a sales level of $50 million, the fixed assets are $75 million, so the ratio FA/S = $75/$50 = 1.5. However, sales can expand by $50 million, out to $100 million, with no required increase in fixed assets. At that point, represented by Point B, the ratio FA/S = $75/$100 = 0.75. If the firm is operating at capacity, even a small increase in sales would require a doubling of plant capacity, so a small projected sales increase would bring with it very large financial requirements.

Cyclical Changes

Panels a, b, and c of Figure 8-2 all focus on target, or projected, relationships between sales and assets. Actual sales, however, are often different from projected sales, and the actual asset/sales ratio for a given period may thus be quite different from the planned ratio. To illustrate, the firm depicted in Panel b of Figure 8-2 might, when its sales are at $200 million and its inventories at $300 million, project a sales expansion to $400 million and then increase its inventories to $400 million in anticipation of the sales expansion. Yet suppose an unforeseen economic downturn holds sales to only $300 million. In this case, actual inventories will be $400 million, but only about $350 million will be needed to support sales of $300 million. If the firm was making its forecast for the following year, it would have to recognize that sales could expand by $100 million with no increase in inventories, but that any sales expansion beyond $100 million would require additional financing to build inventories.

Modifying the Forecast of Additional Funds Needed

If any of the asset/sales ratios in Table 8-2 are subject to any of the conditions noted above, then the simple percentage of sales forecasting method should not be used. Rather, it is necessary (1) to make separate forecasts of the requirements for each type of asset given the projected sales level, (2) to forecast spontaneously generated funds, and (3) to subtract the spontaneously generated funds from the forecasted asset requirements to determine the external funds needed.

To illustrate, consider again the Addison example set forth in Tables 8-1 and 8-2. Now suppose that a ratio analysis along the lines described in Chapter 7 suggests that the cash, receivables, and inventory ratios indicated in Table 8-2 are appropriate, as are the liability ratios and the retained earnings calculations, but that **excess capacity** exists in fixed assets. Specifically, assume that in 1987 fixed assets were being utilized at only 80 percent of capacity. To use

excess capacity
Capacity that exists when an asset is not being fully utilized; in the context of this chapter, excess capacity exists when the firm's fixed assets are operated at less than full capacity.

the existing fixed assets at full capacity, 1987 sales could have been as high as $500,000:

$$\text{Full capacity sales} = \frac{\text{Current sales}}{\text{Percentage at which fixed assets were operated}} = \frac{\$400,000}{0.80} = \$500,000 \text{ sales at full capacity.}$$

This suggests that Addison's target fixed assets/sales ratio should be

$$\frac{\text{Fixed assets}}{\text{Full capacity sales}} = \frac{\$300,000}{\$500,000} = 0.6,$$

not the 0.75 that actually exists. Therefore, at the projected sales level of $600,000, Addison would need fixed assets of only 0.6($600,000) = $360,000, up only $60,000 from the $300,000 currently on hand, rather than up $150,000.

We estimated earlier that Addison would need an additional $231,000 of capital and that at least $76,000 of this amount would have to be raised by selling common stock. However, those estimates were based on the assumption that $450,000 − $300,000 = $150,000 of additional fixed assets would be required. If Addison could attain a sales level of $600,000 with only $360,000 of fixed assets, the external funds needed would decline by $450,000 − $360,000 = $90,000, to $141,000.

COMPUTERIZED FINANCIAL PLANNING MODELS

Although the type of financial forecasting described in this chapter can be done by hand, most well-managed firms with sales greater than a few million dollars employ some type of computerized financial planning model. Such models can be programmed to show the effects of different sales levels, different ratios of sales to operating assets, and even different assumptions about sales prices and input costs (labor, materials, and so forth). Plans are then made regarding how financial requirements are to be met — through bank loans, thus increasing short-term notes payable; by selling long-term bonds; or by selling new common stock. Pro forma balance sheets and income statements are generated under the different financing plans, and earnings per share are projected, along with such risk measures as the current ratio, the debt/assets ratio, and the times-interest-earned ratio.

Depending on how these projections look, management may modify its initial plans. For example, the firm may conclude that its sales forecast must be cut because the requirements for external capital exceed the firm's ability to raise money. Or management may decide to reduce dividends and thus generate more funds internally. Alternatively, the company may decide to investigate production processes that require fewer fixed assets, or to consider the possibility of buying rather than manufacturing certain components, thus eliminating raw materials and work-in process inventories, as well as certain manufacturing facilities.

In subsequent chapters we examine in detail ways of analyzing policy changes such as those mentioned previously. In all such considerations, the basic issue is the effect that a specific action will have on future earnings, on the riskiness of these earnings, and hence on the price of the firm's stock. Because computerized models help management assess these effects, such planning models are playing an ever-increasing role in corporate management.[2]

SUMMARY

This chapter has described in broad outline how firms go about projecting their financial statements and determining their overall financial requirements. In brief, management establishes a target balance sheet based on the type of ratio analysis discussed in Chapter 7. Assuming that each balance sheet ratio is at the desired level and that the optimal levels for these ratios are stable, the *percentage of sales method* can be used to forecast the external financial requirements associated with any given increase in sales. If the balance sheet ratios are subject to change, as they will be if excess capacity exists, each item in the projected balance sheet must be forecast separately.

The type of forecasting described here is important for several reasons. First, if the projected operating results look poor, management can "go back to the drawing board" and reformulate its plans for the coming year. Second, it is possible that the funds required to meet the sales forecast simply cannot be obtained. If so, it is obviously better to know this in advance and to scale back the projected level of operations. And third, even if the required funds can be raised, it is desirable to plan for the acquisition of these funds well in advance. As we see in later chapters, raising capital takes time and is expensive, and both time and money can be saved by careful forward planning.

---

[2]It is becoming increasingly easy for companies to develop planning models as a result of the dramatic improvements that have been made in computer hardware and software in recent years. *Lotus 1-2-3* is one system that can be used, and a more elaborate system is the *Interactive Financial Planning System (IFPS)*. Both systems are used by literally thousands of companies, including 3M Corporation, Shell Oil, and Florida Power & Light. Increasingly, a knowledge of these or similar planning systems is becoming a requirement for getting even an entry-level job in the finance department of many corporations.

Note that in this chapter we have concentrated on long-run, or strategic, financial planning. Within the framework of the long-run strategic plan, firms also develop short-run financial plans. For example, in Table 8-2 we saw that Addison Products expects to need $231,000 by the end of 1988, and that it plans to raise this capital by using short-term debt, long-term debt, and common stock. However, we do not know when during the year the need for funds will occur or when Addison will obtain each of its different types of capital. To address these issues, the firm must develop a short-run financial plan, the centerpiece of which is the *cash budget,* which is a projection of cash inflows and outflows on a daily, weekly, or monthly basis during the coming year (or other budget period). Although considering the cash budget here would complete our examination of the basic types of analysis done in connection with financial planning, we nevertheless defer this discussion to Chapter 10, "Managing Cash and Marketable Securities," because cash budgets can best be understood after we have discussed the firm's target cash balance.

SMALL BUSINESS

Franchising to Lever a Good Idea

As was mentioned in Chapter 1, the small business often has limited access to capital markets and, especially, lacks human resources. What can a small business owner with a great idea and limited resources do to fully capitalize on this idea? In some instances, the owner can attract venture capital if capital is the real bottleneck to developing the business. However, if developing the idea requires both substantial capital and human resources that the owner can't provide, there is another avenue to follow — franchising.

Franchising uses other people's money, energy, and desire to build a business to lever the concept that the franchiser has developed. In an ideal franchise setting, the franchiser is better off by being able to sell franchises, and the franchisee is provided with a relatively simple way of getting started in a successful business.

Nearly everyone is familiar with McDonald's, Taco Bell, and other large fast-food franchise operations. Yet products or services offered by franchise businesses range across the full spectrum, including automotive services, video outlets, personnel services, and even medical care.

The franchiser may provide many benefits to franchisees, including some of the following:

- an idea
- a proprietary product
- a recognized trade name
- a volume buying service
- advertising
- training in a method of providing a service
- plans and designs for facilities and operations
- profit planning

Typically the franchiser will have already expended the costs of product development and will have built one or more prototypes of the business. Those prototypes give the franchiser a testing ground for working out many of the "bugs" in the business. Thus the franchisee saves the expense of unanticipated problems with the business. Once the prototypes are successful, the franchiser is ready to begin marketing franchises.

An Example

To illustrate, suppose you and a friend develop a recipe that allows you to make amazingly tasty cookies that bake very quickly. Also, you come up with an oven that is easy to load and unload and that pushes the aroma of the cookies into the surrounding air. You open a shop. Soon, you learn which varieties of cookies sell well and which don't. You also begin to develop relationships with suppliers that are reliable, and you learn (through trial and error) which ones will provide consistently high-quality ingredients. As you operate your first cookie shop, you begin to learn what hours have the highest traffic and may require more than one employee. Although your store's first location is a disaster, the second is highly successful.

As you operate the shop, you learn a good deal about cash flow from your mother, a financial vice president with a larger firm. She helps you develop a solid, realistic cash-flow plan for timing cash inflows and outflows.

Finally, you experiment with a number of color schemes and names until you create an image for the shop that is most effective. You register the name as a trade name.

By the time you have opened your second successful shop, many of the pitfalls that could hinder such a business have been overcome. So, as you think about opening new shops, you know that these problems will not again cost you the time and money that you have already expended. The second shop is easier than the first one, and the third one is a breeze.

Why sell franchises? Perhaps the strongest motivation is that you have neither the time nor the money to get the maximum benefit from your idea on your own. You have already had to sell your 300ZX and buy a Yugo to get cash, and the bank has gone about as far as it wants to go with your business. There's only one of you now (your partner tired of the long hours and was unwilling to sell her 325e). Time is limited. The shops you've opened are profitable, but they generate only enough cash to let you open a new outlet about every six months.

Further, you realize that although selling franchises will let others profit from your idea, there will be more than enough profit for the two of you to share. The franchisee benefits from your ideas and methods, your research and product development, your plans and designs, your quality control and connections with suppliers and manufacturers, and your understanding of the business. You benefit from someone paying you a franchise fee, paying you royalties on their sales, opening shops that help increase your name recognition, and, finally, buying supplies through you so that you can take advantage of larger volume purchasing.

Successful Franchises

Venture magazine* recently published a survey of 50 successful franchise operations. *Venture* defined success in terms of the number of franchise outlets rather than in terms of profit or market value. The survey is interesting both because of the wide range of products and services that proved successful and because of the different strategies the franchisers used.

The most successful new franchiser, by *Venture's* standards, was a company named Novus Franchising, Inc., which sells franchises for a windshield repair and scratch removal service. The company, which sold its first franchise in October 1985, had sold 525 franchises by the end of 1986 — an average of 35 franchises per month. (These numbers are a bit misleading, because the owner had been licensing the service for several years and created a large proportion of his franchises by converting licensees into franchisees.)

A second success story was T. J. Cinnamons. The parent company, Signature Foods, Inc., was founded in 1983 and began selling franchises for shops selling its high-quality cinnamon rolls in September 1985. By the end of 1986, the firm owned seven units of its own and had sold franchises on another seventy units (in a separate article on T. J. Cinnamons, *Venture* said the company had sold 140 franchises in six months). The success of T. J. Cinnamons came only after the owners had spent several years perfecting their product and ideas. In fact, they had been asked to sell franchises long before they decided they were ready to do so — getting the details right was important to the couple that started the business.

Controlled Growth

As this chapter emphasized, a rapidly growing firm quickly exhausts its ability to finance its growth internally. Thus, financial pressures created by growth may lead a profitable but fast-growing business to get out of control financially. Although a franchise strategy can help a business sustain faster growth than it could otherwise achieve financially, there are still limits on growth. *Venture* reports that many of the successful franchisers in its sample are "intentionally keeping a tight rein on growth, recognizing that an unbridled system cannot be supervised. . ."† Even with the benefits of franchising, the franchiser will have to devote time, energy, and money to the development of the business. Quality is especially difficult to control if the number of franchises grows too rapidly.

Conclusion

Small businesses suffer from resource poverty. Franchising can offer an alternative to help the business overcome some of its capital and human resource constraints. In a well-conceived franchise operation, both the franchiser and the franchisees benefit by their agreement to work together.

---

*"Franchising: The Art of Reproduction," *Venture*, February 1987, 38–51.

†Ibid., 49.

RESOLUTION TO DECISION IN FINANCE

Their Crystal Ball Was Off . . . by $1.2 Billion!

Robert D. Kilpatrick, Cigna's chairman, is remarkably unembarrassed by Cigna's public admission of its mistakes. Startlingly, he rejects the notion that anything went wrong, instead asserting that the company identified its problem expeditiously and "stepped up to the problem with forthrightness."

Kilpatrick says that Cigna felt comfortable with its reserves at the end of 1983. The company had just come to the end of a ten-year period of very stable claims patterns. In 1984, however, the incidence and severity of claims suddenly worsened. Figuratively, Cigna had had forty quarters of shiny red apples and four quarters of wormy ones.

The company was inclined to view the "worms" as an aberration. This rosy outlook was reinforced by a 1984 study done by an actuarial consulting firm retained by Cigna that assessed the company's reserves relative to those held by its chief competitors. Its verdict: Cigna looked conservative and ranked second or third best, depending on the measures used.

In light of this evidence, Cigna decided to assume that the 1984 data were anomalous. Still, it boosted its reserves for 1983 and earlier years by $224 million, leaving the company with a slim profit of $103 million for 1983. At the time Chairman Kilpatrick thought the move to strengthen reserves was "way on the conservative side."

Source: Carol J. Loomis, "How Cigna Took a $1.2-Billion Bath," *Fortune,* March 17, 1986, 46–47.

In 1985 Cigna probably missed its opportunity to see what the future held. Despite the warnings signalled by the 1984 data, Cigna conducted only its normal, rather cursory monthly and quarterly reviews of reserves. After all, says the company, the claims experience appeared to be taking a distinct turn for the better.

Then it was time for the company's regular, intensive year-end review, and with it came the startling revelation that the favorable claims data applied only to policies covering occurrences in 1985. The negative claims data for 1984 had continued for policies written for that year and earlier. For those years, the company now had eight quarters of wormy apples and all indicators pointing to the worms taking over the farm. So Cigna owned up to past miscalculations and stepped up its reserves by $1.2 billion.

How did the stock market treat a company that suddenly announced it was $1.2 billion poorer? With surprising leniency. The day the $1.2 billion write-down was announced Cigna's stock fell sharply, but it quickly snapped back, in part because of a market that was hot for property and casualty stocks.

That's especially good news for Cigna, which might have been vulnerable to lawsuits from shareholders pressing claims that they had bought Cigna stock (before the write-down) on the basis of misleading financial information. Luckily for Cigna, it's hard for shareholders to prove they have been injured when the stock price goes up.

QUESTIONS

8-1 Certain liability and net worth items generally increase spontaneously with increases in sales. Put a check ($\sqrt{}$) by those items that typically increase spontaneously:

Accounts payable   _____
Notes payable to banks   _____
Accrued wages   _____
Accrued taxes   _____
Mortgage bonds   _____
Common stock   _____
Retained earnings   _____
Marketable securities   _____

8-2 The following equation can, under certain assumptions, be used to forecast financial requirements:

$$\text{Additional funds needed} = \frac{A}{S}(\Delta S) - \frac{L}{S}(\Delta S) - MS_1(1 - d).$$

Under what conditions does the equation give satisfactory predictions, and when should it not be used?

8-3 Assume that an average firm in the office supply business has a 6 percent after-tax profit margin, a 40 percent debt/assets ratio, a turnover of 2 times, and a dividend payout ratio of 40 percent. Is it true that if such a firm is to have *any* sales growth ($g > 0$), it will be forced to sell either bonds or common stock (that is, will it need some nonspontaneous external capital, even if g is very small)?

8-4 Is it true that computerized corporate planning models were a fad during the 1970s, but, because of a need for flexibility in corporate planning, they have been dropped by most firms?

8-5 Suppose a firm makes the following policy changes. If the change means that external, nonspontaneous financial requirements for any rate of growth will increase, indicate this by a (+); indicate decreases by a (−); and indicate indeterminant or no effect by a (0). Think in terms of the immediate, short-run effect on funds requirements.
  a. The dividend payout ratio is increased.   _____
  b. The firm contracts to buy rather than make certain components used in its products.   _____
  c. The firm decides to pay all suppliers on delivery, rather than after a 30-day delay, in order to take advantage of discounts for rapid payment.   _____
  d. The firm begins to sell on credit; previously all sales had been on a cash basis.   _____
  e. The firm's profit margin is eroded by increased competition.   _____
  f. Advertising expenditures are stepped up.   _____
  g. A decision is made to substitute long-term mortgage bonds for short-term bank loans.   _____
  h. The firm begins to pay employees on a weekly basis; previously it paid them at the end of each month.   _____

SELF-TEST PROBLEMS

ST-1   J. Sarwark Productions, Inc. has the following ratios: $A/S = 1.6$; $L/S = 0.4$; profit margin $= 0.10$; and dividend payout ratio $= 0.45$, or 45 percent. Sales last year were $100 million. Assuming that these ratios will remain constant and that all liabilities increase spontaneously with increases in sales, what is the maximum growth rate Sarwark can achieve without having to employ nonspontaneous external funds?

ST-2   Suppose Sarwark's financial consultants report (1) that the inventory utilization ratio is sales/inventory $= 3$ times versus an industry average of 4 times, and (2) that Sarwark could raise its utilization ratio to 4 times without affecting sales, the profit margin, or the other asset utilization ratios. Under these conditions, what amount of additional funds would Sarwark expect to require during each of the next 2 years if sales grow at a rate of 20 percent per year?

PROBLEMS

8-1   **Pro forma balance sheet.** A group of investors is planning to set up a new company, The Adios Running Shoe, Ltd., to manufacture and distribute a novel type of running shoe. To help plan the new operation's financial requirements, you have been asked to construct a pro forma balance sheet for December 31, 1988, the end of the first year of operations. Sales for 1988 are projected at $30 million, and the following are industry average ratios for athletic shoe companies:

Sales to common equity	$5\times$
Current debt to equity	50%
Total debt to equity	80%
Current ratio	$2.2\times$
Net sales to inventory	$8\times$
Accounts receivable to sales	9%
Fixed assets to equity	70%
Profit margin	3%
Dividend payout ratio	30%

The Adios Running Shoe, Ltd.
Pro Forma Balance Sheet, December 31, 1988 (Millions of Dollars)

Cash	$_____	Current debt	$_____
Accounts receivable	_____	Long-term debt	_____
Inventories	_____	Total debt	_____
Total current assets	_____	Equity	_____
Fixed assets	_____		
Total assets	$_____	Total claims	$_____

a. Complete the preceding pro forma balance sheet, assuming that 1988 sales are $30 million.

b. If the group supplies all of the new firm's equity, how much external capital will it be required to put up by December 31, 1988?

8-2 **Long-term financing needed.** At year-end 1987, FSA, Inc.'s total assets were $2.4 million. Sales, which were $5 million, will increase by 25 percent in 1988. The 1987 ratio of assets to sales will be maintained in 1988. Common stock amounted to $850,000 in 1987, and retained earnings were $590,000. Accounts payable will continue to be 15 percent of sales in 1988, and the company plans to sell new common stock in the amount of $150,000. Net income after taxes is expected to be 6 percent of sales, and 50 percent of earnings will be paid out as dividends.
a. What was FSA's total debt in 1987?
b. How much new, long-term debt financing will be needed in 1988? (*Hint:* AFN − New stock = New long-term debt.)

8-3 **Ratios and short-term financing needed.** Pettit Restaurant Supply has been growing at a rapid rate lately. As a result Mr. Pettit has been unable to devote proper attention to the management of the firm's assets. Expected sales for next year are $2.7 million with a net profit margin of 3 percent. At the beginning of the year retained earnings were $390,000 and current liabilities were $200,000. Long-term debt and common stock have remained constant for some time. Pettit computed the following financial ratios:

Average collection period = 40 days,

Inventory utilization = 6 times,

Fixed asset utilization = 4 times.

Pettit anticipates no dividend payout this year. Complete the following pro forma balance sheet. Short-term debt is the appropriate balancing item. According to your projections:
a. How much will Pettit have to raise to support the expected level of sales?
b. How much of the total will be raised internally (equity); externally (debt)?
c. What is Pettit's debt ratio?
d. What is Pettit's current ratio?
e. What is the firm's return on assets?

Pettit Restaurant Supply: Pro Forma Balance Sheet

Cash	$ 60,000	Short-term debt	$ 489 00
Accounts receivable	300 000	Long-term debt	375,000
Inventory	450 000	Total debt	864 000
Current assets	810000	Common stock	150,000
Fixed assets	675 000	Retained earnings	471000
Total assets	$ 1485 000	Total claims	$ 1485000

8-4 **Ratios and short-term financing needed.** After making the projections in Problem 8-3, Mr. Pettit is determined to streamline his company's balance sheet. He is certain that the average collection period can be reduced to 30 days and that the inventory utilization can be increased to 8 times. He believes that cash and fixed assets will remain at their current level, however. Make another projection regarding Pettit's financial needs. Specifically:

DEBT UP 289
RETAINED EARNINGS UP 81000

a. How much will Pettit have to raise to support sales under these new conditions?

b. How much of the total will be raised internally (equity)? externally (debt)?

c. What is Pettit's debt ratio?

d. What is Pettit's current ratio?

e. What is the firm's return on assets?

8-5   **Sales growth.** Aunt Kay's, Inc. has these ratios:

$$A/S = 1.8$$

$$L/S = 0.5$$

Net profit margin, $M = 8\%$

Dividend payout ratio, $d = 35\%$

Sales last year were $200 million. Assuming that these ratios remain constant and that all liabilities increase spontaneously with increases in sales, what is the maximum growth rate Aunt Kay's can achieve without having to employ nonspontaneous external funds?

8-6   **Additional funds needed.** The 1987 balance sheet for Janice Zima and Associates is shown below (in millions of dollars):

Cash	$12	Accounts payable	$ 8
Accounts receivable	12	Notes payable	6
Inventory	20	Long-term debt	12
Current assets	$44	Total debt	$26
Fixed assets	12	Common equity	30
Total assets	$56	Total claims	$56

Management believes that sales will increase in the next year by 20 percent over the current level of $240 million. The profit margin is expected to be 5 percent, and the dividend payout will remain at 40 percent. If the firm has no excess capacity, what additional funding is required for 1988?

8-7   **Additional funds needed — excess capacity.** Refer to Problem 8-6. Assume that all relationships hold *except* for the capacity constraint. *Now* assume that the firm has excess capacity and that no increase in fixed assets will be required to support the sales increase. Under this new condition, how much additional funding will be required for 1988?

8-8   **Pro forma statements and ratios.** Coast Computers makes bulk purchases of small computers, stocks them in conveniently located warehouses, and then ships them to its chain of retail stores. Coast's balance sheet as of December 31, 1987, is shown here (in millions of dollars):

Cash	$ 3.0	Accounts payable	$ 7.0
Accounts receivable	22.5	Notes payable	15.0
Inventories	49.5	Accruals	8.0
Total current assets	$75.0	Total current liabilities	$ 30.0
Net fixed assets	30.3	Mortgage loan	5.1
		Common stock	12.6
		Retained earnings	57.6
Total assets	$105.3	Total liabilities and net worth	$105.3

Sales for 1987 were $300 million, while net income after taxes for the year was $9 million. Coast paid dividends of $4 million to common stockholders. The firm is operating at full capacity.

a. If sales are projected to increase by $75 million, or by 25 percent, during 1988, what are Coast's projected external capital requirements?

b. Construct Coast's pro forma balance sheet for December 31, 1988. Assume that all external capital requirements are met by bank loans and are reflected in notes payable.

c. Now calculate the following ratios, based on your projected December 31, 1988, balance sheet. Coast's 1987 ratios and industry average ratios are shown here for comparison.

	Coast Computers Dec. 31, 1988	**Coast Computers Dec. 31, 1987**	**Industry Average Dec. 31, 1987**
Current ratio	_____	2.5×	3×
Debt/total assets	_____	33.9%	30%
Rate of return on net worth	_____	13.0%	12%

d. Now assume that Coast grows by the same $75 million but that the growth is spread over 5 years; that is, sales grow by $15 million each year.

1. Calculate total external financial requirements over the 5-year period.

2. Construct a pro forma balance sheet as of December 31, 1992, using notes payable as the balancing item.

3. Calculate the current ratio, debt/assets ratio, and rate of return on net worth as of December 31, 1992. [*Hint:* Be sure to use *total sales,* which amount to $1,725 million, to calculate retained earnings, but use 1992 profits to calculate the rate of return on net worth — that is, (1992 profits)/(December 31, 1992, net worth).]

e. Do the plans outlined in Parts c and d seem feasible to you? In other words, do you think Coast could borrow the required capital, and would the company be raising the odds on its bankruptcy to an excessive level in the event of some temporary misfortune?

8-9   Additional funds needed. The Doenges-Tavis Company's 1987 sales were $36 million. The percentage of sales of each balance sheet item that varies directly with sales is as follows:

Cash	3%
Accounts receivable	20
Inventories	25
Net fixed assets	40
Accounts payable	15
Accruals	10
Profit rate (after taxes) on sales	5

The dividend payout ratio is 40 percent; the December 31, 1986, balance sheet account for retained earnings was $12.3 million; and both common stock and mortgage bonds are constant and equal to the amounts shown on the balance sheet below.

a. Complete the following balance sheet.

Doenges-Tavis Company:
Balance Sheet, December 31, 1987
(Thousands of Dollars)

Cash	$____	Accounts payable	$____
Accounts receivable	____	Notes payable	3,300
Inventories	____	Accruals	____
Total current assets	____	Total current liabilities	____
Net fixed assets	____	Mortgage bonds	3,000
		Common stock	3,000
		Retained earnings	____
Total assets	$====	Total liabilities and net worth	$====

    b. Now suppose that 1988 sales increase by 10 percent over 1987 sales. How much additional external capital will be required? The company was operating at full capacity in 1987. Use Equation 8-1 to answer this question.

    c. Develop a pro forma balance sheet for December 31, 1988. Assume that any required financing is borrowed as notes payable.

    d. What would happen to external funds requirements under each of the following conditions? Answer in words, without calculations.

        1. The profit margin went (i) from 5 to 7 percent, (ii) from 5 to 3 percent.

        2. The dividend payout ratio (i) was raised from 40 to 90 percent, (ii) was lowered from 40 to 20 percent.

        3. Credit terms on sales were relaxed substantially, giving customers longer to pay.

        4. The company had excess manufacturing capacity at December 31, 1987.

8-10   **Excess capacity.** American Business Machines' (ABM) 1987 sales were $100 million. The percentage of sales of each balance sheet item except notes payable, mortgage bonds, and common stock is as follows:

Cash	4%
Accounts receivable	25
Inventories	30
Net fixed assets	50
Accounts payable	15
Accruals	5
Profit margin (after taxes) on sales	5

The dividend payout ratio is 60 percent; the December 31, 1986, balance sheet account for retained earnings was $58 million; and both common stock and mortgage bonds are constant and equal to the amounts shown on the balance sheet below.

    a. Complete the balance sheet on the following page.

American Business Machines
Balance Sheet, December 31, 1987
(Millions of Dollars)

Cash	$_____	Accounts payable	$_____
Accounts receivable	_____	Notes payable	9.5
Inventories	_____	Accruals	_____
Total current assets	_____	Total current liabilities	_____
Net fixed assets	_____	Mortgage bonds	13.5
		Common stock	6.0
		Retained earnings	_____
Total assets	$_____	Total liabilities and net worth	$_____

b. Assume that the company was operating at full capacity in 1987 with regard to all items *except* fixed assets; had the fixed assets been used to full capacity, the fixed assets/sales ratio would have been 40 percent in 1987. By what percentage could 1988 sales increase over 1987 sales without the need for an increase in fixed assets?

c. Now suppose that 1988 sales increase by 20 percent over 1987 sales. How much additional external capital will be required? Assume that ABM cannot sell any fixed assets. Assume that any required financing is borrowed as notes payable.

d. Suppose the industry averages for receivables and inventories are 20 percent and 25 percent, respectively, and that ABM matches these figures in 1988 and then uses the funds released to reduce equity. (It could pay a special dividend out of retained earnings.) What would this do to the rate of return on year-end 1988 equity?

8-11 **Additional funds needed.** The 1987 sales of Koehlman Technologies, Inc., were $3 million. Common stock and notes payable are constant. The dividend payout ratio is 50 percent. Retained earnings as shown on the December 31, 1986, balance sheet were $105,000. The percentage of sales in each balance sheet item that varies directly with sales is expected to be as follows:

Cash	4%
Receivables	10
Inventories	20
Net fixed assets	35
Accounts payable	12
Accruals	6
Profit margin (after taxes) on sales	3

a. Complete the balance sheet that follows.

b. Suppose that in 1988 sales will increase by 10 percent over 1987 sales levels. How much additional capital will be required? Assume that the firm operated at full capacity in 1987.

c. Construct the year-end 1988 balance sheet. Assume that 50 percent of the additional capital required will be financed by selling common stock and the remainder by borrowing as notes payable.

d. If the profit margin after taxes remains at 3 percent and the dividend payout rate remains at 50 percent, at what growth rate in sales will the additional financing requirements be exactly zero?

Koehlman Technologies, Inc.
Balance Sheet, December 31, 1987

Cash	$	Accounts payable	$
Receivables		Notes payable	130,000
Inventories	_____	Accruals	_____
Total current assets		Total current liabilities	
Fixed assets	_____	Common stock	1,250,000
		Retained earnings	_____
Total assets	$_____	Total claims	$_____

8-12 **External financing requirements.** The 1987 balance sheet for the Duncan Company is shown below. Sales in 1987 totaled $7 million. The ratio of net profits to sales was 3 percent, and the dividend payout ratio was 60 percent of net income.

   a. The firm operated at full capacity in 1987. It expects sales to increase by 20 percent during 1988. Use the percent-of-sales method to determine how much outside financing is required, then develop the firm's pro forma balance sheet using AFN as the balancing item.

   b. If the firm must maintain a current ratio of 2.5 and a debt ratio of 40 percent, how much financing will be obtained using notes payable, long-term debt, and common stock.

   (Do Part c only if you are using the computerized problem diskette.)

   c. Suppose that the firm expects sales to increase by 30 percent during 1988 and that its current ratio must be at least 2.5 but its debt ratio can be as high as 50 percent. Under this situation, how much external financing would the firm require, and how would those funds be obtained?

Duncan Company
Balance Sheet as of December 31, 1987
(Thousands of Dollars)

Assets		*Liabilities*	
Cash	$ 105	Accounts payable	$ 70
Accounts receivable	245	Accruals	35
Inventory	525	Notes payable	245
Total current assets	$ 875	Total current liabilities	$ 350
Fixed assets	2,625	Long-term debt	1,050
		Total debt	$1,400
		Common stock	1,225
		Retained earnings	875
Total assets	$3,500	Total liabilities and equity	$3,500

ANSWERS TO SELF-TEST PROBLEMS

ST-1   To solve this problem, we will use the three following equations:

$$\Delta S = S_0(g).$$

$$S_1 = S_0(1 + g).$$

$$AFN = (A/S)\Delta S - (L/S)\Delta S - M(1 - d)S_1.$$

Set AFN $= 0$, substitute in known values for A/S, L/S, M, d, and S_0, and then solve for g:

$$0 = 1.6(\$100g) - 0.4(\$100g) - 0.1(0.55)[\$100(1 + g)]$$
$$= \$160g - \$40g - 0.055(\$100 + \$100g)$$
$$= \$160g - \$40g - \$5.5 - \$5.5g$$
$$\$114.5g = \$5.5$$

$$g = \$5.5/\$114.5 = 0.048 = 4.8\% = \begin{array}{l}\text{Maximum growth rate} \\ \text{without external financing.}\end{array}$$

ST-2   Note that assets consist of cash, marketable securities, receivables, inventories, and fixed assets. Therefore, we can break the A/S ratio into its components — cash/sales, inventories/sales, and so forth. Then

$$\frac{A}{S} = \frac{A - \text{Inventories}}{S} + \frac{\text{Inventories}}{S} = 1.6.$$

We know that the inventory utilization ratio is sales/inventories $= 3$ times, so inventories/sales $= \frac{1}{3} = 0.3333$. Furthermore, if the inventory utilization ratio could be increased to 4 times, then the inventory/sales ratio would fall to $\frac{1}{4} = 0.25$, a difference of $0.3333 - 0.2500 = 0.0833$. This, in turn, would cause the A/S ratio to fall from A/S $= 1.6$ to A/S $= 1.6 - 0.0833 = 1.5167$.

This change would have two effects: (1) it would change the AFN equation, and (2) it would mean that Sarwark currently has excessive inventories, so there could be some sales growth without any additional inventories. Therefore, we could set up the revised AFN equation, estimate the funds needed next year, and then subtract out the excess inventories currently on hand:

Present conditions:

$$\frac{\text{Sales}}{\text{Inventories}} = \frac{\$100}{\text{Inventories}} = 3,$$

so

$$\text{Current level of inventories} = \$100/3 = \$33.3 \text{ million.}$$

New conditions:

$$\frac{\text{Sales}}{\text{Inventories}} = \frac{\$100}{\text{Inventories}} = 4,$$

so

$$\text{New level of inventories} = \$100/4 = \$25 \text{ million.}$$

Therefore,

$$\text{Excess inventories} = \$33.3 - \$25 = \$8.3 \text{ million.}$$

Forecast of funds needed, first year:

$$\Delta S \text{ in first year} = 0.2(\$100 \text{ million}) = \$20 \text{ million.}$$

$$AFN = 1.5167(\$20) - 0.4(\$20) - 0.1(0.55)(\$120) - \$8.3$$
$$= \$30.3 - \$8 - \$6.6 - \$8.3$$
$$= \$7.4 \text{ million.}$$

Forecast of funds needed, second year:

$$\Delta S \text{ in second year} = 0.2(\$120 \text{ million}) = \$24 \text{ million.}$$

$$AFN = 1.5167(\$24) - 0.4(\$24) - 0.1(0.55)(\$144)$$
$$= \$36.4 - \$9.6 - \$7.9$$
$$= \$18.9 \text{ million.}$$

Part IV

Working Capital

If a poll were taken, financial managers would reveal that the greater part of their workday is taken up with managing and financing the firm's short-term assets. Thus this section devotes four chapters to the important topic of working capital management and policy.

Chapter 9 demonstrates that the level of current assets and how those assets are financed contribute significantly to the firm's profitability and risk exposure. In the next two chapters we turn to the management of four current asset accounts. Chapter 10 considers cash and marketable securities, whereas Chapter 11 analyzes the management of accounts receivable and inventories. Chapter 12 discusses the various types of short-term credit that can be used to finance current assets. This chapter also evaluates the cost of these sources of short-term funds.

Chapter 9

Working Capital Policy and Management

Getting Tough in the Cookie Business

In 1983, the cookie business was not a pretty sight. There they were, all the giant cookie manufacturers, engaged in an all-out, hair pulling, eye-gouging battle for dominance in the "just like mom's" soft cookie market. Millions of dollars were being pumped into product development, marketing, and sales of the new "homemade" cookies. The advertising hoopla sent waves of consumers into stores looking for new kinds of cookies.

And where was Pepperidge Farm during this battle for the cookie buck? Bringing out a line of cookies licensed from the spectacularly successful *Star Wars* movies—just as the *Star Wars* phenomenon was fading from collective memory. The cookie, aimed at children, garnered no interest from Pepperidge Farm's traditional target market: upscale adults. The ill-fated cookie cost the company $2 million in losses.

Richard Shea took over as president of Pepperidge Farm in the wake of the Star Wars disaster. He took the helm of the company with a

strong brand name, extensive assets in the form of plant and personnel, an inventory of products that nobody wanted, and a less than profitable balance sheet. A good example of the company's state of affairs was the frozen food division in Richmond, Utah. The plant was operating at a pathetic 14% of capacity cranking out a variety of unpopular pastry-wrapped fruits, vegetables, and meats.

Shea's work was clearly cut out for him — Pepperidge needed to reduce its costly assets while increasing its sales to stem the tide of the company's losses. When Margaret Rudkin founded the company to market the whole wheat bread she baked for her children, she only had her family to answer to. But Pepperidge Farm was now a subsidiary of Campbell Soup Company and Shea's superiors expected him to cut costs and increase sales — and fast.

As you read this chapter, think about what your strategy might be if you were Richard Shea. How would you handle the company's capital investments in plant and equipment? What would you do about the performance of the Utah plant? How would you manage inventory?

See end of chapter for resolution.

In Part III we saw (1) that a firm's investment in assets is closely related to actual and projected sales, (2) that the various liability and equity accounts must be analyzed in terms of their relationships to assets, and (3) that risk, profitability, and consequently stock prices are all dependent on decisions relating to the acquisition and financing of assets. This discussion was very general, however, and we looked more at industry averages than at specific economic determinants of the different types of assets. Now, in Part IV, we examine the effect of the levels of current assets and current liabilities. We find that the level of current assets and how they are financed contribute significantly to both the firm's profitability and its risk exposure.

DEFINING WORKING CAPITAL

Working capital policy involves decisions that relate to current assets, including decisions the financial manager must make about the financing of current assets. The term *working capital* originated in the days of the old Yankee peddler who would load up his wagon with goods and then go off on his route to sell his wares. The merchandise was defined as his "working capital" because it was actually sold or "turned over" to produce profits; the wagon and horse were his fixed assets. If he brought $4,000 of goods (working capital) and sold them for $5,000, he would make $1,000 per trip. If he made five trips per year, he would turn over his working capital five times and make a profit of $5 \times \$1,000 = \$5,000$ for the year.

The days of the Yankee peddler have long since passed, but the importance of working capital remains. About 40 percent of the typical firm's capital is invested in current assets, yet this doesn't tell the entire story about its importance. Financial managers probably spend more of their daily time and energy on working capital matters than on any other single function discussed in this text. In contrast, the choice of business projects and the associated fixed asset commitment occurs, for most firms, perhaps once or twice a year. As we shall see, whether the decision concerns fixed or current assets, it will affect the firm's level of risk and return.

Before taking up the topics of primary interest in this chapter, we will review the concepts of working capital and working capital management. We begin by defining the following terms:

working capital
A firm's investment in short-term assets — cash, marketable securities, inventory, and accounts receivable.

1. Working capital, sometimes termed *gross working capital,* simply refers to the firm's current assets (often called *short-term assets*) — commonly cash, marketable securities, inventory, and accounts receivable.

net working capital
Current assets minus current liabilities.

2. Net working capital is defined as current assets minus current liabilities. As we discuss later in this chapter, net working capital would therefore be financed by long-term sources of funds. We shall find that the financing factor is most important in determining the firm's risk and return levels.

working capital policy
Basic policy decisions regarding target levels for each category of current assets and the financing of these assets.

3. Working capital policy refers to the firm's basic policies regarding target levels for each category of current assets and the financing of these assets as reflected in the firm's target current and quick ratios.

4. Working capital management involves the administration, within policy guidelines, of current assets and current liabilities. Important elements of working capital management include cash management, credit and collections, inventory management, and short-term borrowings.

Whereas long-term financial analysis is primarily concerned with strategic planning, working capital management is primarily concerned with day-to-day operations — making sure that production lines do not stop because the firm runs out of raw materials, that inventories do not build up because production is not slowed down when sales dip, that customers pay on time, and that enough cash is on hand to make payments when they are due. Obviously, without good working capital management, no firm can be efficient and profitable.

working capital management
The administration, within policy guidelines, of current assets and current liabilities.

THE WORKING CAPITAL CASH FLOW CYCLE

The concept of the *working capital cash flow cycle* is important in working capital management. This cycle can be described for a typical manufacturing firm as follows. (1) The firm orders and then receives the raw materials that it needs to produce the goods it expects to sell; because firms usually purchase their raw materials on credit, this transaction creates an account payable. (2) Labor is used to convert the raw materials into finished goods; to the extent that wages are not fully paid at the time the work is done, accrued wages build up. (3) The finished goods are sold, usually on credit, which creates receivables; no cash has yet been received. (4) At some point during the cycle, accounts payable and accruals must be paid, usually before the receivables have been collected, so a net cash drain occurs and must be financed. (5) The working capital cash flow cycle is completed when the firm's receivables have been collected; at this point, the firm is ready to repeat the cycle and pay off the loans that were used to finance the cycle.

Verlyn Richards and Eugene Laughlin developed a useful approach to analyzing the working capital cash cycle.[1] Their approach centers on the conversion of operating events to cash flows, and thus it is called the **cash conversion cycle** model. Here are some terms used in the model:

cash conversion cycle
The length of time between the purchase of raw materials and the collection of accounts receivable generated in the sale of the final product.

1. *Inventory conversion period,* which is the average length of time required to convert raw materials into finished goods and then to sell these goods.

2. *Receivables conversion period,* which is the average length of time required to convert the firm's receivables into cash — that is, to collect cash following a sale.

3. *Payables deferral period,* which is the length of time between the purchase of raw materials and the cash payment for them.

---

[1]See Verlyn D. Richards and Eugene J. Laughlin, "A Cash Conversion Cycle Approach to Liquidity Analysis," *Financial Management,* Spring 1980, 32–38. A similar approach was set forth earlier by Lawrence J. Gitman, "Estimating Corporate Liquidity Requirements: A Simplified Approach," *The Financial Review,* 1974, 79–88.

Figure 9-1 **The Cash Conversion Cycle**

The cash conversion cycle measures the length of time it takes for cash invested in the firm's current assets to be returned. Cash invested in inventory is recaptured only when the firm collects its accounts receivable. Generally, the shorter the cash cycle, the more profitable the firm will be.

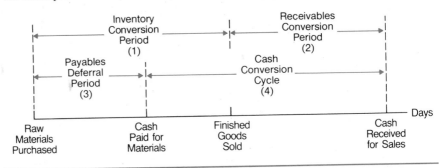

4. *Cash conversion cycle,* which is the length of time between actual cash expenditures on productive resources (raw materials and labor) and actual cash receipts from the sale of products — that is, from the day labor and suppliers are paid to the day rceivables are collected.

Now we can use these definitions to analyze the cash conversion cycle. First, the concept is diagrammed in Figure 9-1. Each component is given a number, and the cash conversion cycle can be expressed by this equation:

$$\underset{(1)}{\begin{array}{c}\text{Inventory}\\\text{conversion}\\\text{period}\end{array}} + \underset{(2)}{\begin{array}{c}\text{Receivables}\\\text{conversion}\\\text{period}\end{array}} - \underset{(3)}{\begin{array}{c}\text{Payables}\\\text{deferral}\\\text{period}\end{array}} = \underset{(4)}{\begin{array}{c}\text{Cash}\\\text{conversion}\\\text{cycle.}\end{array}}$$

To illustrate, suppose it takes an average of 50 days to convert raw materials to inventory and to sell the goods, and 40 days to collect on receivables. Also, 30 days normally elapse between purchase of materials and payment of the associated account payable. In this case, the cash conversion cycle is 60 days:

$$50 \text{ days} + 40 \text{ days} - 30 \text{ days} = 60 \text{ days.}$$

Given these data, the firm knows when it receives an order that it will have to finance the costs of processing the order for a 60-day period. The firm's goal should be to shorten the cash conversion cycle as much as possible without hurting operations. This would improve profits, because the longer the cash conversion cycle, the greater the need for external financing — and such financing has a cost.

The cash conversion cycle can be shortened (1) by reducing the inventory conversion period, that is, by processing and selling goods more quickly, (2) by reducing the receivables conversion period, that is, by speeding up collections, or (3) by lengthening the payables deferral period, that is, by slowing down its own payments. To the extent that these actions can be taken *without increasing costs or depressing sales,* they should be carried out. You should keep the cash conversion cycle in mind as we go through the remainder of this chapter and the other chapters on working capital.

WORKING CAPITAL INVESTMENT AND FINANCING POLICIES

Because it is inherently difficult to change the level of fixed assets quickly, working capital is used to make initial adjustments in operations as economic conditions change. If demand begins to rise or fall, the immediate response is in the working capital accounts, and the appropriateness of this response can spell success or failure for the firm. For example, when its sales began to decline in the late 1970s, Chrysler decided that the decline was only a temporary dip, so production levels were maintained. By the time it became clear that the "dip" was really a major recession, Chrysler had built up huge inventories of new cars. The company had borrowed heavily to finance this inventory buildup, and these loans had to be repaid. To move the cars, the only choice was to slash prices below costs. Thus the ineffective response in working capital to changes in the environment resulted in hundreds of millions of dollars in losses for Chrysler. Only after a painful period of restructuring has the company regained a healthy status in the automobile industry.

Working capital policy involves two basic questions: (1) What is the appropriate level of current assets, both in total and by specific accounts? (2) How should the required level of current assets be financed? We now turn to an examination of alternative policies regarding the level of investment in current assets and the maturities of the liabilities used to finance those assets.

Effect of Current Assets on Risk and Return

As the Chrysler experience demonstrates, unplanned changes in working capital can affect a firm in adverse ways. Therefore, financial managers must plan for levels of working capital that balance the amount of risk required to reach an acceptable level of return.

Under conditions of certainty—when sales, costs, order lead times, collection periods, and so on are known with certainty—all firms within an industry would hold the same level of current assets relative to sales. Any larger amount would increase the need for external funding without a corresponding increase in profits, whereas any smaller amount would cause late payments to suppliers, lost sales, and production inefficiencies because of inventory shortages. The picture changes when uncertainty is introduced, however. Here the firm requires some minimum amount of cash and inventories based on expected payments, sales, order lead times, and so on, plus additional amounts,

Table 9-1 **Effect of Working Capital Policies on Rates of Return (Millions of Dollars)**

	Conservative	Moderate	Aggressive
Sales	$40	$40	$40
EBIT	3	3	3
Current assets	$15	$10	$ 5
Fixed assets	10	10	10
Total assets	$25	$20	$15
Basic earning power (EBIT/TA)	12%	15%	20%

conservative working capital policy

A policy in which relatively large amounts of cash, marketable securities, and inventories are carried and in which sales are stimulated by a liberal credit policy resulting in a high level of receivables.

aggressive working capital policy

A policy in which holdings of cash, securities, inventories, and receivables are minimized.

or *safety stocks,* to help it cope if events vary from their expected values. Similarly, accounts receivable are based on credit terms, and the tougher those terms, the lower the receivables for any given level of sales.

Table 9-1 depicts three alternative policies a firm might have regarding the level of current assets that it carries. A **conservative working capital policy** means that the firm invests in larger amounts of cash or marketable securities, accounts receivable, and inventory than its level of sales seems to require. Conversely, with an **aggressive working capital policy,** the levels of cash or marketable securities, inventories, and receivables are reduced to the minimum possible amount at a given level of operations. The moderate policy is between the two extremes of working capital policy.

In general, the greater the proportion of current assets to fixed assets at any given level of output, the less risky the firm's working capital policy.[2] How does the conservative working capital policy reduce risk? In essence, all risk of shortages is removed. With high levels of working capital there will be ample inventory so that no stock outages will ever occur, sufficient cash or near-cash marketable securities will be available to prevent any conceivable liquidity problem, and accounts receivable will be expanded to prevent any loss in sales caused by a too stringent credit policy. Of course, there is a price to pay for all this safety. That price, as we illustrate in Table 9-1, comes in the form of reduced return on investment.

The lower return associated with the conservative working capital position stems from the fact that the firm has acquired more current assets than are required to support the current level of sales. Obviously, any level of sales requires the supporting assets of inventory, accounts receivable, and cash balances for business transactions. An overabundance of these assets, however, directs resources away from more productive investments. Therefore, assum-

[2]It is important to distinguish between planned and unplanned increases in current assets. Unplanned increases in inventory that cannot be sold or accounts receivable that cannot be collected are *not* examples of a conservative, risk-reducing working capital policy. Of course, such a buildup in current assets is risky and even life threatening to the firm, as the Chrysler example indicates. The planned conservative policy that we are considering here concentrates on keeping more cash, inventory, or other current assets on hand to insure that no shortages occur.

ing that net income is constant, the rate of return will be lower as the level of current assets increases.[3] We can conclude, therefore, that an overly conservative working capital policy misallocates resources, which lowers the overall earning power of the firm.

From this discussion an unwary reader might conclude that the best working capital policy would be one which aggressively slashes current assets to the bare minimum. As seen in Table 9-1, the basic earning power return rises from 12 percent under the conservative policy to 20 percent under the aggressive policy. However, just as lower returns were the price for the safety of a conservative working capital policy, there is a price associated with the higher *potential*[4] returns in the aggressive policy — higher risk.

The probability that a given level of sales cannot be maintained is one of the risks associated with an aggressive working capital policy. For example, the high rate of return resulting from the aggressive policy in Table 9-1 explicitly assumes no change in sales as levels of current assets are manipulated. How could an aggressive working capital policy affect sales? First, with lower levels of inventory, sales could decline as a result of stock outages. Second, other revenues might be lost because of a stringent credit policy that is designed to reduce accounts receivable rather than support sales. Of course, a decline in sales could result in lower returns.

Reduced sales is not the only risk associated with an aggressive working capital policy, however. Since current assets provide liquidity, their reduction may lead to difficulties in paying bills or other obligations as they come due. Slow payment could lead to poor credit ratings or even a reduction in suppliers' willingness to extend trade credit.

Therefore, an overly aggressive working capital policy can lead to exactly the opposite result than intended. As is often the case in finance, the preferred working capital policy lies somewhere between the extreme levels of aggressive and conservative policies. Even though it is difficult to prescribe an optimal level of working capital for each firm, a general guideline for working capital policy decisions does exist. *The level of current assets should be reduced as long as the marginal return from such an action is greater than the potential for resulting losses.* Thus inventory should be reduced to a point where there is only an acceptably low probability of lost sales due to stock outages. Similarly, the savings resulting from lower levels of accounts receivable must be compared to the potential losses from the more stringent credit policy. Finally, the return from minimizing cash holdings, in either demand deposits or marketable securities, must be compared to the potential losses if cash was in short supply.

---

[3]The same principle holds true for fixed assets. Idle excess capacity bloats the asset side of the balance sheet, requiring financing to support it. Because idle assets are not producing revenues but are increasing the firm's financing charges, the profitability of the firm declines.

[4]If returns *always* were higher under the more risky working capital policy, there wouldn't be any risk, would there?

Figure 9-2 **Fixed and Current Assets and Their Financing**

This figure shows an idealized model of the financing of current and fixed assets. Each season, current assets rise sharply, then gradually fall to zero. Short-term loans, used to finance these current assets, are repaid and renewed with each season. Fixed assets, on the other hand, are financed with long-term debt and owners' equity.

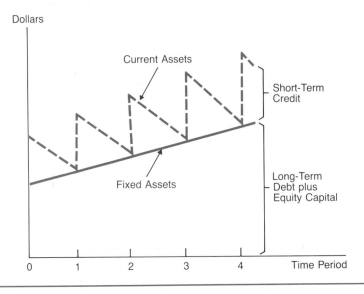

ALTERNATIVE STRATEGIES FOR FINANCING WORKING CAPITAL

The concept of financing working capital originated at a time when most industries were closely related to agriculture. Farmers would borrow to buy seed in the spring and, when the crops were harvested in the fall, repay the loan with the proceeds of the crop's sale. Similarly, processors would buy crops in the fall, process them, sell the finished product, and end up just before the next harvest with relatively low inventories. Bank loans with maximum maturities of one year were used to finance both the purchase and the processing costs, and these loans were retired with the proceeds from the sale of the finished products. Thus the loans were, in essence, self-liquidating.

This situation is depicted in Figure 9-2, in which fixed assets are shown to be growing steadily over time, whereas current assets jump at harvest season, decline during the year, and end at zero just before the next crop is harvested. Short-term credit is used to finance current assets, and long-term funds are used to finance fixed assets. Thus the top segment of the graph deals with working capital.

The figure represents an idealized situation — actually, current assets build up gradually as crops are purchased and processed; inventories are drawn down less regularly; and ending inventory balances do not decline to zero.

Figure 9-3 **Fluctuating versus Permanent Assets: Exactly Matching Maturities**

Because in the modern business world current assets rarely drop to zero, the idea of permanent current assets was developed. This figure shows these assets being financed, along with fixed assets, by long-term debt and equity capital. Those current assets that are still seasonal continue to be financed by short-term credit. Figures 9-2 and 9-3 illustrate the traditional approach of matching asset and liability maturities.

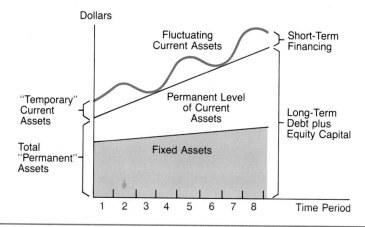

Nevertheless, the example does illustrate the general nature of the production and financing process, and working capital management consists of decisions relating to the top section of the graph — managing current assets and arranging for the short-term credit used to finance them.

Although our modern economy has become less oriented toward agriculture, seasonal or cyclical fluctuations of working capital still exist. For example, construction firms have peaks in the spring and summer, whereas retail sales often peak around Christmas. Consequently, manufacturers who supply either construction companies or retailers follow patterns similar to those of their customers, but with a lead time of several months. Similarly, virtually all businesses must build up working capital when the economy is moving up, but their inventories and receivables decline when the economy slacks off. Even when a business is at its seasonal or cyclical low, however, its current assets do not drop to zero, and this realization has led to the development of the concept of **permanent current assets.** Those current assets that rise and fall with business activity are termed **temporary current assets.** The manner in which the permanent and temporary current assets are financed constitutes the firm's *working capital financing policy.*

Maturity Matching. One commonly used financing policy is to match asset and liability maturities, as shown in Figure 9-3. Here both fixed assets and permanent current assets are financed with long-term capital — equity plus

permanent current assets

The minimum level of current assets that are required when business activity is at seasonal or cyclical lows.

temporary current assets

Current assets that fluctuate with seasonal or cyclical variations in a firm's business.

long-term debt. Temporary current assets are financed with current liabilities. This strategy reduces the risk that the firm will be unable to pay off its maturing obligations. To illustrate, suppose a firm borrowed on a one-year basis and used the funds to build and equip a plant. Because cash flows from the plant (profit plus depreciation) would almost never be sufficient to pay off the loan after only one year, the loan would have to be renewed annually. Thus the company's ability to continue operating would depend on its ability to renew the loan each year. If for some reason the lender refused to renew the loan, the firm would have serious problems. Had the plant been financed with 20-year loan, however, the required loan payments (interest plus part of the principal) would have been better matched with cash flows from profits and depreciation, and the problem of renewal would arise, if at all, only once every 20 years.[5]

At the extreme, a firm could attempt to match the maturity structure of its assets and liabilities exactly. Inventory expected to be sold in 30 days would be financed with a 30-day bank loan; a machine expected to last for 5 years would be financed with a 5-year loan; a 20-year building would be funded with a 20-year mortgage bond; and so on. Of course, uncertainty about the lives of assets prevents this exact maturity matching. For example, a firm may finance inventories with a 30-day loan, expecting to sell the inventories and use the cash generated to retire the loan. But if sales are slow, the cash will not be forthcoming, and the use of short-term credit may cause a problem.

Aggressive Approach. Figure 9-4 illustrates an aggressive working capital financing policy. Here a firm continues to finance all of its fixed assets with long-term capital but part of its permanent current assets as well as all of its temporary current assets with short-term credit. Why would a firm wish to increase the amount of assets it finances with short-term credit? Basically, short-term credit is desirable because it usually is cheaper than long-term credit. Consider the two sources of short-term debt. First, some sources of short-term financing are spontaneous; that is, they increase as the level of the firm's operations increases. Accounts payable and accruals are excellent examples of spontaneous financing. As we show in Chapter 12, when sales increase, a company obtains more raw materials from suppliers, and the increased trade credit offered by the suppliers finances the buildup in assets. Similarly, as operations increase, there is a resulting increase in accrued wages and taxes, which helps to finance the buildup in operations. Used within limits, these sources constitute "free" capital. Firms' other short-term source of funds is contractual debt, such as short-term bank loans.

The reliance on short-term credit could expand to financing all current assets (both temporary and permanent current assets) and even a portion of

---

[5]Examples of maturity matching also can be found in our personal financial lives. Few of us would even think of financing a home with only a one-year note or financing a car for 30 years. In the first case, almost no one could pay for a home in one year. In the second case, the car would have turned to rust before our payments ended. Therefore, we typically finance an asset over a period that, in some manner, reflects its expected useful life.

Figure 9-4 **Fluctuating versus Permanent Assets: Aggressive Position**

To take better advantage of cheaper, short-term credit, a firm may finance a portion of its permanent current assets from short-term sources. The remainder of its permanent current assets, along with fixed and fluctuating (seasonal) current assets, are financed in the traditional way shown in the prior two figures. A firm taking this approach sacrifices a measure of safety to lower its finance costs, in hopes of thereby increasing profits.

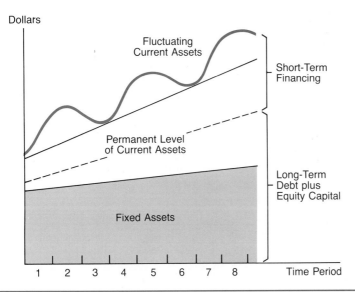

the fixed assets. This would be represented in Figure 9-4 by drawing the dashed line *below* the line designating fixed assets, which would indicate that all current and some fixed assets were being financed with short-term credit. This very aggressive financing policy would be an extremely risky, nonconservative position that would subject the firm to fluctuating interest rates and the even more critical danger of loan renewal problems. Even so, since short-term debt is often cheaper than long-term debt, some firms may be willing to sacrifice safety for possibly higher profits.

Conservative Approach. Alternatively, the firm could finance not only its fixed and permanent current assets with long-term debt and equity capital, but a portion of its temporary current assets as well. This would be represented in Figure 9-5 by drawing the dashed line *above* the line designating permanent current assets, which would indicate that permanent capital was being used to finance all permanent asset requirements as well as some or all of the seasonal demands. The humps above the dashed line in Figure 9-5 represent short-term financing; the troughs below it represent short-term security holdings. Our illustrative firm uses a small amount of short-term credit to meet its peak re-

Figure 9-5 **Fluctuating versus Permanent Assets: Conservative Position**

A very conservative approach to financing working capital is illustrated in this figure. Part of the short-term financing requirement is met by using long-term capital to "store up" marketable securities during the off season. During peak seasons these securities provide needed liquidity and are augmented by short-term borrowing.

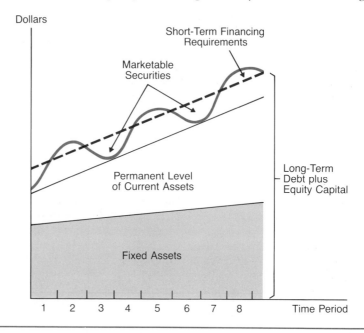

quirements, but it also meets a part of its seasonal needs by "storing liquidity" in the form of marketable securities during the off-season. This represents a very safe, conservative working capital financing policy, but one that potentially generates lower profits.

Advantages and Disadvantages of Short-Term Credit

The distinction between Figures 9-3, 9-4, and 9-5 is the relative amount of short-term debt financing employed. The aggressive policy calls for the greatest amount of short-term debt, the conservative policy uses the least amount, and the maturity matching approach falls in between. Although using short-term debt is generally more risky for the firm than using long-term debt, short-term credit does have some offsetting advantages. The pros and cons of financing with short-term debt are considered in this section.

Speed. A short-term loan can be obtained much more quickly than a long-term loan. Lenders will insist on a more thorough financial examination before

INDUSTRY PRACTICE

Turning 'Em Around

Executives are anxious, employees fearful. Everyone at the company is updating his or her resume while customers clamor for unfilled orders and suppliers call for overdue payments. Shareholders growl. The bank threatens.

Enter the turnaround specialist — a corporate hired gun whose job it is to shake things up, cut the dead wood, reorganize the business, snatch it from the jaws of bankruptcy, and generally breathe new life into the corporate corpse. The turnaround executive is a special breed. He or she must have the crisis skills of an intensive care doctor and the strategic genius of a military commander.

According to John Whitney, turnarounds are a lot like wars. By the time a turnaround specialist is called in, the situation is critical. The corporation is drowning in a sea of its own red ink. There's no time for introspection. Action is everything. The turnaround specialist must be strong, decisive, even dictatorial.

Whitney should know. A turnaround specialist himself, Whitney has orchestrated several corporate resuscitations. Now a visiting professor and executive in residence at Columbia University's Graduate School of Business, Whitney is a voice from the trenches, offering the following advice for those about to embark on the corporate turnaround trail.

Many companies assume that the only alternative for a firm battered by business downturns or the pressures of increased competition is bankruptcy; that is not necessarily the case. However, support from a bank is critical if bankruptcy is to be avoided. Anyone considering taking on a turnaround assignment should be sure to enlist the bank's support before plunging ahead. The worst news a turnaround executive can hear on arriving at a company is that the bank is going to call in its loans. It may just be a bluff and a face-to-face meeting, possibly with a bankruptcy lawyer in tow, can convince the bank that it is not going to get in as much as it thinks by calling in the loans. Still, if the bank is going to pull the plug, the situation may be terminal.

Once there is a commitment of bank support, the turnaround executive must get control of cash. No purchases over a certain amount should be made without the new leader's approval. In small companies that may mean the executive should approve all purchase orders, at least for the first month or so, just to find out what is really going on. All capital expenditures should also be cancelled until they can be reassessed by the turnaround executive.

With cash flow under control, the next task is to start making cash projections, even if they are less accurate than would be hoped. Cash projections give the executive his or her first glimpse of the future. They predict the level of sales, how much money is going to be collected, whether the business is going to get softer or weaker, and whether the company's customers are able to pay their bills.

In making the cash projections, the new leader should make every effort to sidestep established lines of communication in order to get a realistic view of the situation the company faces. The new boss should speak directly to employees on the floor, directly to key customers, and directly to vendors. He or she should also speak at length with the banker who, if the business is in really bad shape, may be the one really running the company.

Another critical task facing the turnaround specialist is finding internal sources of cash, which usually need to be wrung out of accounts receivable and inventory. Whitney suggests pur-

Source: Reprinted from the December 1986 issue of *Venture*, For Entrepreneurial Business Owners & Investors, by special permission. © 1986 Venture Magazine, Inc., 521 Fifth Ave., New York, N.Y. 10175.

suing past due accounts but avoiding going after accounts that are in dispute because collection may be too time consuming. Getting cash from inventory is a longer and more delicate process. It is important not to run out of key inventory items or rumors of corporate demise will run rampant; however, Whitney advises companies to refrain from replenishing secondary inventory items as often as under normal circumstances.

While turnaround executives must first concentrate on fixing control, cash, financial, and management information problems, a good leader will also think about marketing. Going into a new market might be too expensive and risky, but by concentrating on serving existing markets better and possibly expanding into a similar segment of the market, corporate performance can be improved.

John Whitney contends that the best turnaround leaders share many of the same characteristics as successful entrepreneurs. Both face limited resources and a sense of urgency as well as confusion. Senior managers in start-ups and turnarounds have to be adaptable and flexible. They must be able to see a promising opportunity that wasn't there a week ago and be able to shift resources in order to profit from an advantage. Turnaround specialists, according to John Whitney, like entrepreneurs, are not resource driven, they are opportunity driven.

granting long-term credit, and the loan agreement will have to be spelled out in considerably more detail, because a great number of things can happen during the life of a 10- to 20-year loan. Therefore, if funds are needed in a hurry, the firm should look to the short-term markets.

Flexibility. If its needs for funds are seasonal or cyclical, a firm may not want to commit itself to long-term debt for various reasons. First, loan initiation or flotation costs are generally higher for long-term debt. Second, although long-term debt can be repaid early, provided the loan agreement contains a prepayment provision, prepayment penalties can be expensive; accordingly, if a firm thinks its need for funds will diminish in the near future, it should choose short-term debt. Finally, long-term loan agreements always contain provisions or covenants, which constrain the firm's future actions. Short-term credit agreements are less restrictive.

Cost of Long-Term versus Short-Term Debt. In Chapter 5 we saw that the yield curve often is upward sloping, indicating that interest rates are generally lower on short-term than on long-term debt. When this situation exists, interest expense will be lower if the firm borrows on a short-term rather than a long-term basis.

Risk of Long-Term versus Short-Term Debt. Even though short-term debt is generally less expensive than long-term debt, financing with short-term debt subjects the firm to more risk for two reasons: (1) If a firm borrows on a long-

Table 9-2 **Combined Effects of Asset and
Debt Maturity Mix on Risk and Return
(Thousands of Dollars)**

	Conservative	Moderate	Aggressive
Current assets	$15,000	$10,000	$ 5,000
Fixed assets	10,000	10,000	10,000
Total assets	$25,000	$20,000	$15,000
Short-term debt (10%)	$ 3,750	$ 5,000	$ 6,000
Long-term debt (14%)	8,750	5,000	1,500
Shareholders' equity	12,500	10,000	7,500
Total liabilities and equity	$25,000	$20,000	$15,000
Sales	$40,000	$40,000	$40,000
EBIT	3,000	3,000	3,000
Less: Interest	1,600	1,200	810
EBT	$ 1,400	$ 1,800	$ 2,190
Less: Taxes (40%)	560	720	876
Net income	$ 840	$ 1,080	$ 1,314
Current ratio (assets/liabilities)	4	2	0.83
Return on equity (net income/shareholders' equity)	6.7%	10.8%	17.5%
Net working capital	$11,250	$5,000	($1,000)

term basis, its interest costs will be fixed (or if the interest rate is floating, the cost will still be relatively stable over time), but if it borrows short-term, its interest expense will fluctuate widely, at times going quite high. For example, from 1977 to 1980 the short-term rate for large corporations more than *tripled,* going from 6.25 percent to 21 percent. (2) If a firm borrows on a short-term basis, naturally there will be less time in the borrowing period to generate cash to pay the debt's principal and interest as they come due. If the firm finds itself in a weak financial position on the loan's maturity date, it is possible that the lender will not extend the loan, thereby forcing the firm into bankruptcy.

COMBINING CURRENT ASSET AND LIABILITY DECISIONS

From the preceding discussion it is obvious that a potentially profitable yet risky strategy would be to minimize investment in current assets while financing a large proportion of total assets with short-term debt. Alternatively, risk could be minimized, at the expense of profits, by increasing current assets and financing a large proportion of total assets with long-term debt.

In Table 9-2 we illustrate the results of each of these strategies along with a less extreme "moderate" plan for working capital and debt maturity policies.

For these strategies the current ratio is our measure of risk, and return on equity evaluates the profitability of each plan.

The conservative policy of building current assets and financing with more expensive long-term debt has reduced the firm's return, as expected. The firm's level of risk is quite low, however. A high current ratio indicates that the firm has sufficient liquidity to meet almost any emergency. In contrast, the aggressive policy of minimizing current asset investment and utilizing less costly short-term debt has led to a much higher return. There are dangers associated with this higher return, however. First, at this low level of current assets, it is quite possible that the firm will be unable to maintain the proposed level of sales. Second, a potentially more critical problem is indicated by the firm's low level of liquidity, as measured by the current ratio.[6] With this low current ratio, the firm may find future financing more difficult to obtain. Certainly it will be more expensive (due to the higher liquidity risk) if it can be obtained at all. The low current ratio also indicates that the firm may have substantial problems meeting bills and interest and principal payments as they come due. Thus, although an aggressive working capital policy may lead to higher profits for the firm, it may also increase the potential for bankruptcy. A more moderate approach, which represents a balancing of risk and return, may be preferred by many financial managers.

The means by which financial managers evaluate their investment in each of the current asset and liability accounts is considered in the remaining chapters on working capital.

SUMMARY

Working capital represents a firm's investment in current assets. *Net working capital* (current assets minus current liabilities) indicates the proportion of current assets that are financed from long-term sources. *Working capital policy* is concerned with the management of current assets as well as the maturity structure of the firm's debt.

The firm's expected risk and return are affected by the amount and composition of its assets and liabilities. Current assets provide the firm with the liquidity necessary for the ongoing functions of the business. Too much liquidity reduces profitability, whereas too little jeopardizes the ability of the firm to function efficiently. Short-term credit offers the advantages of lower cost and greater flexibility over long-term debt; however, an overreliance on short-term debt can lead to less predictable interest costs, refinancing problems, and even bankruptcy. Thus the financial manager must formulate a working capital policy that balances risk and return to the ultimate benefit of the shareholders.

---

[6]Note that net working capital mirrors the liquidity risk factors that are identified by the current ratio.

SMALL BUSINESS

Growth and Working Capital Needs

Working capital is one of the requirements in a new firm that is most often underestimated by the entrepreneur seeking funds to finance the business. The entrepreneur makes provisions for research and development and for the plant and equipment required to produce the products that are created. But working capital is frequently a surprise to the entrepreneur. He or she expects to come up with a product that the market will immediately accept and for which the market will pay a very substantial premium. This premium price will lead to very high profit margins, which will then "finance" all of the firm's other needs. As naive as this point of view appears to be, it nevertheless is common among less experienced founders of new businesses.

Ned was one of the founders of a new microcomputer software company that began seeking venture capital to support its products in the early part of 1988. In speaking with a venture capitalist who was concerned about the low level of funding being sought, Ned explained that the company's products had such a high profit margin that essentially the company would be self-financing.

Ned's company made and sold a computer software package. The package was shipped as three floppy disks and a set of manuals; the total cost of those materials was about $20, and the package sold for $500. With such high profit margins, Ned explained, there would be no need for financing once the marketing was well under way. In fact, he said, there would be plenty of cash to pay for new product development.

The venture capitalist — we'll call her Joanna — was a little disconcerted. She asked which firm was currently most successful in the microcomputer software business in which Ned was competing. Ned instantly answered, Microsoft. Joanna asked, "Well, if Microsoft is so successful doing what you do, why do you suppose they just raised an additional $2,500,000?" Ned fumbled around for an answer, but he got the point.

Rapid growth consumes cash; it does not generate cash. Rapid growth often does generate profits, but profits do not pay the bills — cash does. Consider what a firm must do to sustain a very high growth rate. If it is a manufacturing firm, the components of a firm's assets include raw materials inventory, work-in-process inventory, finished goods inventory, and accounts receivable, as well as fixed assets. With the exception of fixed assets, these items are all components of gross working capital. When the firm produces a product, it makes an investment in each of these working capital items before any cash is received from collection of receivables, assuming all sales are credit sales.

Imagine a small firm that chooses to finance its activities solely through the funds it generates. Recall the financial analysis in Chapter 7. Suppose the firm has an average of 120 days of sales in inventory and an average of 60 days in receivables. If the firm pays cash for all of its materials and labor, it has a cash cycle of 180 days; that is, between the payment for goods at the beginning of the cycle and the receipt of cash at the end, 180 days pass. Thus the company turns over its cash only twice per year.

If the company earns, say, 3 percent on its sales dollar (as measured by net profit margin), it has about 3 percent more money available after a cycle than before it. With two cycles per year, about 6 percent more is available for investment at the end of the year than at the beginning. Thus growth of approximately 6 percent can be supported.

If the company is growing at a rate of 20 percent and can generate only 6 percent internally, it must either obtain funds externally or face enormous pressures. How can the company improve its ability to fund growth internally?

Roughly, this concept says that the firm can grow by the product of the net margin and the number of cash cycles per year.* Thus it can support more rapid growth by either raising the profit margin or shortening the cash cycle (increasing the number of cycles).

To raise the profit margin, the company must raise prices, cut costs, or both. Raising prices may reduce growth by itself (because customers will be less eager to buy at higher prices), but it may help bring growth and financial resources more into balance.

Shortening the cash cycle requires either reducing inventory, collecting receivables more efficiently, or paying suppliers more slowly. Notice the effects of these changes. By reducing inventory by 25 percent (to 90 days) and cutting receivables to 30 days (normal credit

terms), the cycle is reduced to 120 days. If, in addition, suppliers are willing to wait 30 days for payment, the time cash is outstanding is further shortened to 90 days. Cash turnover changes to four times per year instead of two, internally fundable growth becomes 12 percent rather than 6 percent. Improving the cash cycle by increasing the rate at which the firm can support growth internally also reduces the firm's needs for outside funds to a more manageable level.

For the small business with serious constraints on obtaining outside funds, these discretionary policies can help bring the firm's rate of growth into balance with its ability to finance that growth. Furthermore, such control on the part of management may impress bankers and others with funds and may help the firm get the outside financing it would have liked to have had all along.†

---

*Several factors may mitigate the accuracy of this approximation. First, this example ignores the fact that some expenses, such as depreciation, are not *cash* expenses. Furthermore, no spontaneous sources of financing, discussed in Chapter 8, are considered. Finally, the example implicitly assumes a zero payout ratio, which may not fit every situation.

---

†Limits on growth and the concept of "sustainable growth" are explored in Chapter 6 of Robert C. Higgins, *Analysis for Financial Management* (Homewood, Ill.: Irwin, 1984).

 ## RESOLUTION TO DECISION IN FINANCE

Getting Tough in the Cookie Business

Pepperidge Farm's new president, Richard Shea, may have been a cookie novice when he took over the reins at the company, but he came to the job with a savvy instinct for the bottom line. According to Shea, in any business, "you have to have a crystal-clear product strategy and a religious appreciation for quality. Once you get

that right, you get onto production and once you get that right you get a big ad budget and you blow the product out of there."

On his first day on the job Shea made it clear to management that Pepperidge Farm would sell only top-quality products and immediately cut 300 items from the product lines. He also embarked on a large scale evaluation of every facet of production and product delivery with a keen eye to cutting costs and reducing inven-

Source: Bill Saporito, "A Smart Cookie at Pepperidge," *Fortune*, December 22, 1986, 67, 70, 74.

tory by getting the product from the ovens to the stores as fast as possible.

In an effort to cut fixed costs that were not offering good returns Shea replaced 16 top executives and sold 4 of 11 plants. At the remaining plants he replaced the company's sluggish, manual-ordering procedures in order to cut inventory costs and boost profits on units sold. By using computers to link drivers placing orders and managers on the bakery floor, the company cut down the amount of time that Pepperidge's products remained unsold. Under Shea's stewardship, operations were tightened and streamlined to the point where cookies travel from ovens to stores in close to 72 hours. By delivering not only a better cookie but a fresher one, Pepperidge Farm was better able to compete effectively with the burgeoning specialty cookie shops and in-store bakeries.

During his initial forays into corporate reorganization, Shea intended to scrap the company's frozen food operations entirely. But after visiting the plant and meeting with the workers,

Shea opted for creative use of assets instead. "We just kept telling people to come to work until we found something for them to make," recalls Shea. The answer came soon thereafter: a frozen pizza made of croissant dough that is currently selling at 30% above projections.

Shea then turned his aggressive, hands-on approach to other new products as well. In 1985, Pepperidge Farm eschewed the by now waning soft cookie battle and launched a new line of top-of-the-line cookies so loaded with chocolate, nuts, and raisins that the manufacturing engineers had a hard time getting the new cookies to hold together. The company is struggling to keep up with demand.

Shea managed to turn a sprawling company loaded with unprofitable excess plant, personnel, and inventory back into a winner. Under Shea's leadership, Pepperidge Farm has increased its operating earnings 33% to $5.1 million on sales of $455 million, making parent company, Campbell Soup, proud.

QUESTIONS

9-1 What are the differences between permanent and temporary current assets?

9-2 What is the trade-off between risk and return in the management of the firm's working capital?

9-3 Why does excess working capital reduce profits?

9-4 How would a period of rapidly increasing inflation affect the firm's working capital?

9-5 During a tight-money period, would you expect a business firm to hold higher or lower cash balances (demand deposits) than during an easy-money period? Assume the firm's volume of business remains constant over both economic periods.

9-6 How would management's ability to predict sales trends and patterns affect working capital policy?

9-7 From the standpoint of the borrower, is long-term or short-term credit riskier? Explain. Would it ever make sense to borrow on a short-term basis if short-term rates were above long-term rates?

9-8 If long-term credit exposes a borrower to less risk, why would people or firms ever borrow on a short-term basis?

PROBLEMS

9-1 **Working capital policy.** Consider the following balance sheet:

River City Industries
Balance Sheet, December 31, 1987

Assets

Cash	$ 50,000
Marketable securities	20,000
Accounts receivable	330,000
Inventory	500,000
Plant and equipment (net)	900,000
Total assets	$1,800,000

Liabilities and Shareholders' Equity

Accounts payable	$ 80,000
Notes payable	120,000
Accrued wages	20,000
Accrued taxes	70,000
Mortgage bonds	400,000
Debentures	210,000
Common stock	100,000
Paid-in-capital	200,000
Retained earnings	600,000
Total liabilities and shareholders' equity	$1,800,000

a. Determine River City Industries' investment in working capital.
b. Determine River City Industries' net working capital investment.
c. Does the firm's financing mix (long-term versus short-term) appear to be conservative or aggressive?

9-2 **Cash conversion cycle.** East Asia Import Company has an inventory conversion period of 72 days, a receivables conversion period of 38 days, and a payables deferral period of 30 days.
a. What is the length of the firm's cash conversion cycle?
b. If East Asia Import's sales are $2,700,000 and all sales are on credit, what is the firm's investment in accounts receivable?
c. How many times per year does East Asia Import turn over its inventory?

9-3 **Working capital investment.** Marshall Electric Company (MEC) is a leading manufacturer of small electric motors. MEC turns out 1,000 motors a day at a cost of $9 per motor for materials and labor. It takes the firm 20 days to convert the raw materials into a motor. The motors are shipped to dealers immediately upon completion of the manufacturing process. MEC allows its customers 30 days in which to pay for the motors, and the firm generally pays its suppliers in 20 days.
a. What is the length of MEC's cash conversion cycle?
b. In a steady state in which MEC produces 1,000 motors a day, what amount of working capital must it finance?
c. By what amount could MEC reduce its working capital financing needs if it were able to stretch its payables deferral period to 25 days?
d. MEC's management is trying to analyze the effect of a proposed new manufacturing process on the firm's working capital investment. The new production process

would allow MEC to decrease its inventory conversion period to 18 days and to increase its daily production to 1,200 motors. However, the new process would increase the cost of materials and labor to $10 per unit. Assuming the change does not affect the receivables conversion period (30 days) or the payables deferral period (20 days), what will be the length of the cash conversion cycle and the working capital financing requirement if the new production process is implemented? Assume finished goods inventory remains near zero.

9-4 **Working capital financing policies.** Ann Heath has been evaluating her firm's financing mix of short-term and long-term debt. She has projected the two following condensed balance sheets:

	Plan 1	Plan 2
Current asets	$2,500,000	$2,500,000
Fixed assets (net)	2,500,000	2,500,000
Total assets	$5,000,000	$5,000,000
Current liabilities	$ 500,000	$2,000,000
Long-term debt	2,000,000	500,000
Common stock equity	2,500,000	2,500,000
Total claims	$5,000,000	$5,000,000

Earnings before interest and taxes are $750,000 and the tax rate is 40 percent under either plan.

a. If current liabilities have a 10 percent interest rate and long-term debt has a 14 percent interest rate, what is the rate of return on equity under each plan?

b. Assume that the yield curve is inverted and that the short-term rate is 18 percent while the long-term rate is still 14 percent. What is the rate of return on equity for the two plans?

c. Which plan is riskier? Explain.

9-5 **Working capital policy.** Jim Straken, financial manager for Cleveland Cement Company, has a problem. The firm's board of directors has complained about the firm's low liquidity. Jim has been ordered to raise the current ratio to at least 2.0 within a reasonable time period. One of his plans is to sell $5,000,000 in equity and invest the proceeds in Treasury bills, which yield 8 percent before taxes. The firm has a 40 percent tax rate, and, if no Treasury bills are purchased, net income after taxes is expected to be $2,000,000. Assume 100% payout.

Cleveland Cement Company
Balance Sheet, December 31, 1987

Current assets	$10,000,000	Current liabilities	$ 6,250,000
Fixed assets	15,000,000	Long-term debt	3,750,000
		Common stock equity	15,000,000
Total assets	$25,000,000	Total claims	$25,000,000

a. Using the financial information in the accompanying balance sheet (which does not include the proposed purchase of Treasury bills), calculate the firm's current ratio, net working capital, and return on equity.

b. If Jim follows his plan and sells $5,000,000 in equity in order to purchase the 8 percent Treasury bills, what are the firm's resulting current ratio, net working capital, and return on equity?

c. What result would the plan have on the firm's liquidity?

d. Would you suggest acceptance of this plan?

9-6 **Alternate working capital financial policies.** Pinto Products' management is concerned about the way in which its new firm will be financed. The three alternative plans that have been proposed are as follows:

	Plan 1	Plan 2	Plan 3
Current assets	$4,500,000	$4,500,000	$4,500,000
Fixed assets	8,000,000	8,000,000	8,000,000
Current liabilities (8.5%)	4,500,000	1,500,000	3,000,000
Long-term debt (12%)	1,500,000	4,500,000	0
Common stock equity	6,500,000	6,500,000	9,500,000

Whichever plan is chosen, sales are expected to be $20 million and operating profits (EBIT) will be $2 million. The marginal tax rate is 40 percent.

a. For each plan, calculate the following: (1) current ratio, (2) net working capital, (3) debt/total assets ratio, and (4) return on equity.

b. Compare the risk and return associated with each plan. Which plan would you accept?

9-7 **Cash conversion cycle.** Block Printing Company's balance sheet follows.

Cash	$ 100,000	Debt	$ 448,000
Accounts receivable	350,000		
Inventory	270,000	Equity	672,000
Fixed assets (net)	400,000		
Total assets	$1,120,000	Total liabilities	$1,120,000

The company's sales are $1,800,000 annually, the payables deferral period is 35 days, and the net margin is 5 percent. Compute the firm's **(a)** inventory utilization (based on sales), **(b)** inventory conversion period, **(c)** average collection period, **(d)** cash conversion cycle, and **(e)** return on assets.

9-8 **Cash conversion cycle.** Refer to the data in Problem 9-7. The company's owner, Bob Block, is too busy in the printing shop to oversee all the financial aspects of the business. He decides to hire Sara Jefferies to reduce current assets. After some study, Jefferies concludes she can reduce the firm's inventory utilization period by 14 days and the average collection period by 20 days without reducing sales or net margin. Under these new conditions:

a. What is the new level of inventory?

b. What is the new level of accounts receivable?

c. What is the length of the firm's cash conversion cycle after these changes are implemented?

d. If all of the savings (from the reduction in inventory and accounts receivable) are used to reduce debt, what is the firm's return on assets? (Assume the net margin remains constant.)

9-9 **Working capital policy.** The Providence Corporation is attempting to determine the optimal level of current assets for the coming year. Management expects sales to increase to approximately $2 million as a result of an asset expansion presently being undertaken. Fixed assets total $1 million, and the firm wishes to maintain a 60 percent debt ratio. Providence's interest cost is currently 8 percent on both short-term and longer-term debt (which the firm uses in its permanent structure). Three alternatives regarding the projected current asset level are available to the firm: (1) an aggressive policy requiring current assets of only 45 percent of projected sales; (2) a moderate policy of 50 percent of sales in current assets; and (3) a conservative policy requiring current assets of 60 percent of sales. The firm expects to generate earnings before interest and taxes at a rate of 12 percent on total sales.

a. What is Providence's expected return on equity under each current asset level? (Assume a 40 percent federal-plus-state average tax rate.)

b. In this problem we have assumed that the level of expected sales is independent of current asset policy. Is this a valid assumption?

c. How would the overall riskiness of the firm vary under each policy?

(Do Part d only if you are using the computerized problem diskette.)

d. What would be the return on equity under each current asset level if actual sales for the year were $2.5 million? $1.6 million? If sales were $2 million under the moderate policy but $2.5 million under the conservative policy and $1.6 million under the aggressive policy? Which current asset level is the least risky over the range of probable sales from $1.6 million to $2.5 million? Which current asset level do you recommend that Providence maintain? Why?

Chapter 10

Managing Cash and Marketable Securities

To Buy Back or Not to Buy Back

There has been an old saying on Wall Street—buy on the bad news, sell on the good. But 1987 may well have been the first year that corporate America took the old adage to heart. It was definitely the year of the stock buy-back. From January through September 1987, corporations bought their own stock in record amounts. Then came Black Monday—October 19th—the day that the Dow took a sickening dive of 508 points, and companies that had never before contemplated buy-backs took advantage of the fire-sale prices of their stock. They snapped up their own shares at a rate that made the buy-backs of the previous ten months look like a trickle.

Why would a company want to spend its hard-earned money to buy its own stock? Many firms engage in share buy-back programs for restructurings, to discourage unwanted takeover attempts, to boost returns on equity, or to slow the dilution of their stock by employee stock purchase plans. Companies also buy their own stock in an attempt to bolster its price in an unfavorable market.

Allen Born, CEO of Amax, Inc., the mining giant, saw his company's ten-month rise in value from 10 points to almost 30 disappear when the market took back all those gains on Black Monday. Believing that his company's stock was fully valued at somewhere in the high 20s, Born began consulting his management team about the possibility of a stock buy-back program.

By late in the day on October 19th it became clear to everyone at Amax that the company's stock was headed well below 20. After years of courting institutional investors, 40 percent of Amax's shares were in the portfolios of pension funds, insurance companies, and mutual funds. As the market unraveled on Black Monday, these funds' automatic profit-taking and stop-loss programs impersonally dumped Amax shares along with everybody else's.

As Amax's shares plummeted below 17, Born decided that a stock buy-back was no longer an option but a necessity. As you read this chapter, imagine that you are a member of Amax's board and must vote on whether or not Allen Born should be authorized to launch a stock buy-back program. Would such a program be a wise use of Amax's assets? How could holding the company's own stock fit in with Amax's portfolio of other marketable securities?

See end of chapter for resolution.

Any business firm requires cash to pay for labor and materials, to buy fixed assets, to pay taxes, and so on. As we discussed in Chapter 9, the financial manager must consider the risk and return implications of working capital decisions. Because currency (and most commercial checking accounts) earns no interest, cash is generally considered a "nonearning" asset. Overinvestment in cash may reduce the firm's earning power, but underinvestment may cause the firm to be unable to meet some of its operating obligations. Thus the goal of the cash manager is to reduce the amount of cash held to a minimum necessary to conduct business.

CASH MANAGEMENT

cash
The total of bank demand deposits plus currency.

Approximately 1.5 percent of the average industrial firm's assets are held in the form of **cash,** which is defined as the total of bank demand deposits plus currency. In addition, sizable holdings of near-cash marketable securities such as U.S. Treasury bills (T-bills) or bank certificates of deposit (CDs) are often reported on corporate financial statements. However, cash balances vary widely both among industries and among the firms within a given industry, depending on the individual firms' specific conditions and on their owners' and managers' aversion to risk. We begin our analysis with a discussion of the factors that determine firms' cash balances. These same factors, incidentally, apply to the cash holdings of individuals and nonprofit organizations, including government agencies.

Reasons for Holding Cash

Firms hold cash for two primary reasons:

transactions balances
Cash balances associated with payments and collections; those balances necessary to conduct day-to-day business.

1. *Transactions.* Cash balances are necessary to conduct business. Payments must be made, and receipts are deposited in the cash account. Cash balances associated with routine payments and collections are known as **transactions balances.**

compensating balance
A minimum balance, usually in a checking account, that a firm must maintain with a commercial bank.

2. *Compensation to banks for providing loans and services.* A bank's revenues are generated by lending out the funds that have been deposited with it; thus depositing money in a bank helps the bank improve its profit position. If a bank is providing services to a customer, it generally requires the customer to leave a minimum balance on deposit to help offset the costs of those services. This type of balance, defined as a **compensating balance,** is discussed in detail later in this chapter.

precautionary balances
Cash balances held in reserve for random, unforeseen fluctuations in inflows and outflows.

Two other reasons for holding cash that have been noted in the finance and economics literature are (1) for precaution and (2) for speculation. Cash inflows and outflows are somewhat unpredictable, with the degree of predictability varying among firms and industries. Cash balances held in reserve for random, unforeseen fluctuations in inflows and outflows are defined as **precautionary balances.** The less predictable the firm's cash flows, the larger the necessary cash balances. However, if the firm has easy access to borrowed funds—that is, if the firm can borrow on short notice—it need not hold much, if any, cash for precautionary purposes. Also, as is noted later in this chapter, firms that do need precautionary balances tend to hold them as highly liquid marketable securities: such holdings accomplish the same purposes as cash balances while providing income in the form of interest received.

Some cash balances may be held to enable the firm to take advantage of any bargain purchases that might arise; these are defined as **speculative balances.** As with precautionary balances, firms today are more likely to rely on reserve borrowing power and on marketable securities portfolios than on actual cash holdings for speculative purposes.

Although the cash accounts of most firms can be thought of as consisting of transactions, compensating, precautionary, and speculative balances, we cannot calculate the amount needed for each type, add them together, and produce a total desired cash balance, because the same money serves all four purposes. Firms do, however, consider these four factors when establishing their target cash positions.

Although there are good reasons for holding *adequate* cash balances, there is a strong reason for not holding *excessive* balances—cash is a nonearning asset, so excessive cash balances simply lower the total asset turnover, thereby reducing both the firm's rate of return on net worth and the value of its stock. Therefore, firms are interested in establishing procedures for increasing the efficiency of their cash management; if they can make their cash work harder, they can reduce cash balances. We now turn to a discussion of the procedures business firms use to increase cash management efficiency.

The Cash Budget

The firm estimates its needs for cash as a part of its general budgeting, or forecasting, process. First it forecasts sales. Next, it forecasts the fixed assets and inventories that will be required to meet the forecast sales levels. Asset purchases and the actual payments for them are then put on a time scale, along with the actual timing of the sales and the timing of collections for sales. For example, the typical firm makes a 5-year sales forecast, which is then used to help plan fixed asset acquisitions (capital budgeting). Then the firm develops an annual forecast, in which sales and inventory purchases are projected on a monthly basis, as are the times when payments for both fixed assets and inventory purchases must be made. These forecasts are combined with projections about the timing of the collection of accounts receivable, the schedule for payment of taxes, the dates when dividend and interest payments will be made, and so on. Finally, all of this information is summarized in the **cash budget,** which shows the firm's projected cash inflows and outflows over some specified period of time.

speculative balances
Cash balances that are held to enable a firm to take advantage of any bargain purchases that might arise.

cash budget
A schedule showing cash flows (receipts, disbursements, and net cash) for a firm over a specified period.

Cash budgets can be constructed on a monthly, a weekly, or even a daily basis. Generally, firms use a monthly cash budget forecast over the next 6 to 12 months, plus a more detailed daily or weekly cash budget for the coming month. The longer-term budget is used for planning purposes, and the shorter one for actual cash control.

Constructing the Cash Budget. We shall illustrate the process with a monthly cash budget covering the last six months of 1987 for the Dayton Card Company, a leading producer of greeting cards. Dayton's birthday and get-well cards are sold year-round, but the bulk of the company's sales occur during September, when retailers are stocking up for Christmas. At the present time, Dayton offers no cash discount for early payment but it does offer a generous 60-day credit period to its customers. Small accounts, which comprise 20 percent of its total sales, are on a "cash only" basis and pay within the month of sale. However, credit customers take full advantage of Dayton's sales terms. Thus, for 70 percent of its sales, payment is made during the month after sales. A small percentage of Dayton's customers (10 percent) pay during the second month after sales. Dayton has had virtually no problem with bad debts. All bills are paid within 90 days of the original date of sale.

Rather than produce at a uniform rate throughout the year, Dayton prints cards immediately before they are required for delivery. Paper, ink, and other materials amount to 70 percent of sales and are bought the month before the company expects to sell the finished product. Its own purchase terms permit Dayton to delay payment on its purchases for one month. Accordingly, if July sales are forecast at $10 million, purchases during June will amount to $7 million, and this amount will actually be paid in July.

Other cash expenditures such as wages and rent are also built into the cash budget in Table 10-1. Dayton Printing must make tax payments of $2 million on September 15 and December 15, as well as a progress payment in October for a new plant that is under construction. Assuming that it needs to keep a **target cash balance** of $2.5 million at all times and that it will have $3 million on July 1, what are Dayton's financial requirements for the period July through December?

The monthly cash requirements are worked out in Table 10-1. The top half of the table provides a worksheet for calculating collections on sales and payments on purchases. The first line in the worksheet gives the sales forecast for the period May through January; May and June sales are necessary to determine collections for July and August. Next, cash collections are given. The first line of this section shows that 20 percent of the sales during any given month are collected that month. The first line under the heading of Collections indicates that 20 percent of sales are on a "cash only" basis, and those customers, of course, pay during month of sale. The second line shows the collections on the prior month's sales, or 70 percent of sales in the preceding month; for example, in June 70 percent of the $5,000 of May's sales, or $3,500, will be collected. The third line shows collections from sales two months earlier, or

target cash balance
The minimum cash balance that a firm must maintain in order to conduct business.

Table 10-1 Dayton Printing Company: Worksheet and Cash Budget (Thousands of Dollars)

	May	June	July	Aug.	Sept.	Oct.	Nov.	Dec.	Jan.
Worksheet									
Sales	$5,000	$5,000	$10,000	$15,000	$20,000	$10,000	$10,000	$5,000	$5,000
Collections									
During month of sale (20%)	1,000	1,000	2,000	3,000	4,000	2,000	2,000	1,000	
During first month after sale (70%)		3,500	3,500	7,000	10,500	14,000	7,000	7,000	
During second month after sale (10%)			500	500	1,000	1,500	2,000	1,000	
Total collections	$1,000	$4,500	$6,000	$10,500	$15,500	$17,500	$11,000	$9,000	
Purchases (70% of next month's sales)	$3,500	$7,000	$10,500	$14,000	$7,000	$7,000	$3,500	$3,500	
Payments (one-month lag)		$3,500	$7,000	$10,500	$14,000	$7,000	$7,000	$3,500	$3,500
Cash Budget									
(1) Collections			$6,000	$10,500	$15,500	$17,500	$11,000	$9,000	
(2) Payments									
(3) Purchases			$7,000	$10,500	$14,000	$7,000	$7,000	$3,500	
(4) Wages and salaries			750	1,000	1,250	750	750	500	
(5) Rent			250	250	250	250	250	250	
(6) Other expenses			100	150	200	100	100	50	
(7) Taxes					2,000			2,000	
(8) Payment for plant construction						5,000			
(9) Total payments			$8,100	$11,900	$17,700	$13,100	$8,100	$6,300	
(10) Net cash gain (loss) during month (Line 1 − Line 9)			($2,100)	($1,400)	($2,200)	$4,400	$2,900	$2,700	
(11) Cash at start of month if no borrowing is done			3,000	900	(500)	(2,700)	1,700	4,600	
(12) Cumulative cash (= cash at start plus gains or minus losses) (Line 10 + Line 11)			$900	($500)	($2,700)	$1,700	$4,600	$7,300	
(13) Deduct target level of cash			2,500	2,500	2,500	2,500	2,500	2,500	
(14) Total loans outstanding to maintain $2,500 cash balance			$1,600	$3,000	$5,200	$800			
(15) Surplus cash							$2,100	$4,800	

Notes

1. The amount shown on Line 11 for the first month, the $3,000 balance on July 1, is given. The values shown for each of the following months on Line 11 represent the "cumulative cash" as shown on Line 12 for the preceding month.

2. When the target cash balance of $2,500 (Line 13) is deducted from the cumulative cash balance (Line 12), if a negative figure results, it is shown on Line 14 as a required loan, whereas if a positive figure results, it is shown on Line 15 as surplus cash.

10 percent of sales in that month; for example, the July collections for May sales are $(0.10)(\$5,000) = \$500$. The collections are summed to find the total cash receipts from sales during each month covered by the cash budget; thus, the July collections represent 20 percent of July's cash sales plus 70 percent of June sales plus 10 percent of May sales.

With the worksheet completed, the cash budget itself can be constructed. Receipts from collections are given on the top line. Lines 2 through 9 summarize the cash payments made by the firm each month. Note that because we are concerned only with cash payments, depreciation does not appear in the cash budget. The difference between cash receipts and cash payments (Line 1 minus Line 9) is the net cash gain or loss during the month; for example, July had a net cash loss of $2.1 million.

Next, the cash on hand at the beginning of the month is added to the net cash gain or loss during the month to obtain the cumulative cash that would be on hand *if no financing were done;* at the end of July, Dayton would have a cumulative cash balance of $900,000.

The cumulative cash is then subtracted from the target cash balance, $2.5 million, to determine the firm's borrowing requirements or surplus cash, whichever the case may be. In July, as shown on Line 12, Dayton expects to have cumulative cash of $900,000. It has a target cash balance of $2.5 million. Thus, to maintain the target cash balance, it must borrow $1.6 million by the end of July. Assuming that this amount is indeed borrowed, loans outstanding will total $1.6 million at the end of July.

This same procedure is used in the following months. Sales will expand seasonally in August. With the increased sales will come increased payments for purchases, wages, and other items. Receipts from sales will go up, too, but the firm will still be left with $1.4 million cash outflow during the month. The total financial requirements at the end of August will be $3 million — the cumulative cash plus the target cash balance. The $3 million is also equal to the $1.6 million needed at the end of July plus the $1.4 million cash deficit for August. Thus loans outstanding will total $3 million at the end of August.

Sales peak in September, and the cash deficit during this month will hit a high of $2.2 million. The total borrowing requirements through September will increase to $5.2 million. Sales, purchases, and payments for past purchases will fall markedly in October; collections will be the highest of any month because they reflect the high September sales. As a result, Dayton will enjoy a healthy $4.4 million cash surplus during October. This surplus can be used to pay off borrowings, so loans outstanding will decline by $4.4 million, to $800,000.

Dayton will have another cash surplus in November, which will permit it to eliminate completely the need for borrowing. In fact, the company is expected to have $2.1 million in surplus cash by the month's end, and another cash surplus in December will swell the extra cash to $4.8 million. With such a large amount of unneeded funds, Dayton's treasurer will no doubt want to invest in interest-bearing securities or put the funds to use in some other way.

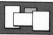

INDUSTRY PRACTICE

Controlling the Purse Strings

Everyone expects a corporate CFO to deal with banks and the investment community, to have an in-depth understanding of the larger financial environment in which the firm operates, and to balance the demands of the company's internal operations with outside market conditions. Increasingly, companies are asking their CFOs to be ace cash managers as well.

Firms used to leave their idle cash idle. They had the accountants count it. The most it did for the company was to give readers of the corporate balance sheet a warm glow knowing that there was money in the bank — or somewhere else. Well, not anymore.

In the 1970s interest rates went through the roof; credit was tight and the economy was limping through a recession. "Capital wasn't available at any cost to a lot of companies, so they had to look inwardly and see what methods they could employ to improve cash flow," notes Sy Jones, a partner in the New York office of accountants Coopers & Lybrand. What the companies discovered was that, creatively utilized, their idle cash could serve as a source of capital. Thus cash management was born.

With inflation and the prime rate in double digits, companies learned to get tough when it came to managing their cash. They swooped down on their collectibles and then cudgelled their brains to find investments that would yield a return at least as high as the rate of inflation.

In the more financially comfortable eighties, however, many corporate financial managers seem to have forgotten the lessons of the past decade. CFOs have once again loosened their hold on the company's internal purse strings. Money floats between post offices, sits fruitlessly in non-interest-bearing bank accounts, or hovers somewhere in the nether regions of the balance sheet.

But savviest financial managers haven't forgotten that one of the cheapest ways for a company to finance itself is to aggressively manage the money it already has. "People are borrowing money today at 8%," says Raymond P. Ruzek, executive director of the National Corporate Cash Management Association. "Inflation is 3%. The cost of money is still 5%. It's unfortunate that many businesses don't realize that."

Surprisingly, it's banks, themselves scrambling to be increasingly competitive, that are trying to make cash management a hot topic by offering a variety of cash management systems to their customers. The number of companies that aren't managing their cash efficiently is surprising, they contend, and banks are in a position to help corporations maximize their idle balances.

For a start, the banks are urging their larger customers to go high-tech by offering desktop computers that allow key financial managers to monitor cash balances worldwide. Says Scott E. Bates, senior vice president at First Chicago Corporation, "Their computers talk to our computers. It's getting pretty esoteric." Besides keeping an eye on cash balances, computers allow firms to transfer money electronically. Almost instantaneous electronic transactions let firms keep money in interest-bearing accounts right up until the time it's needed.

Another way that banks help their customers hold on to their cash as long as possible is by offering controlled disbursement accounts. These accounts alert the financial manager of the number and dollar amount of the company's checks that will clear on any given day at a given bank. The manager then instructs a cen-

Source: Stuart Weiss, "Making the Most of the Cash on Hand," *Business Week,* November 3, 1986, 112–113; Donna Sammons, "The Perils of Cash Management," *INC.,* June 1983; and Laurie Baum, "A Cool-Headed CFO Can Keep You Out of Hot Water," *Business Week,* November 3, 1986, 117.

tral bank to transfer the funds necessary to cover the checks just before they are presented.

A corollary system called the concentration-account system is used to collect receipts. For example, a company that has collections in a number of small towns may have a cashier make its deposits every day. The deposits are then automatically deposited in a central bank, substituting a number of relatively low-balance accounts for one larger, presumably interest-bearing one.

Another service that banks offer is a float reduction system. Essentially, this consists of a lockbox number in each local community in which the company does business. Customers send their payments to the lockbox number instead of to company headquarters. The local address cuts the amount of time that receivables wind their way unprofitably through the postal system, and it speeds up collection procedures as well. Although each lockbox transaction costs the company about 40 cents, the system pays for itself in terms of increased interest income.

What a company does with its cash balances is every bit as important as how fast it gets its hands on the money. Conservative firms hold their balances in interest-bearing accounts such as money market funds. More aggressive firms develop a corporate portfolio that may include investments in the stock market or a commodity fund. Not unexpectedly, brokerage firms are doing everything in their power to sell firms on the merits of market investments. But cash management essentially deals with the company's working capital base. Because mistakes can have grave implications, the more aggressive forms of cash management raise a host of questions. How much risk is acceptable? Should cash management play a supportive role, or should it be expected to contribute to the firm's bottom line?

Advises Coopers & Lybrands' Sy Jones: "You've got to remember what the game is. The primary game is simply the investment of temporarily idle funds. It's not to become the end game unto itself. . . You can get into trouble if you start having ideas about how you're going to take this money and outsmart the stock market. . . That's not cash management. That's making a conscious decision that you're going to do something other than your normal business."

Before concluding the discussion of the cash budget, we should make some additional points:

1. Our cash budget does not reflect interest on loans required to maintain the target level cash balance or income from the investment of surplus cash. This refinement could be added quite easily.

2. If cash inflows and outflows are not uniform during the month, Dayton could be seriously understating or overstating its financing requirements. For example, if all payments must be made on the fifth of the month, but collections come in uniformly throughout the month, Dayton would need to borrow much larger amounts than those shown in Table 10-1. In that case, the company would need to prepare cash budgets on a daily basis.

3. Because depreciation is a noncash expense, it does not appear on the cash budget.

4. Because the cash budget represents a forecast, all the values in it are *expected* values. If actual sales, purchases, and so on differ from these values, the cash deficits and surpluses that were forecast will also be incorrect. Therefore, the financial manager will wish to constantly monitor the cash budget during the period and modify it to conform to actual changes in the amount and timing of cash inflows or disbursements.

5. Computerized spreadsheet programs such as *Lotus 1-2-3* are particularly well suited for constructing and analyzing a cash budget, especially with respect to the sensitivity of cash flows to changes in sales levels, collection periods, and the like. With computerized models, one can instantly answer questions such as, "If collections slow down, what will the firm's cash needs be?"

6. Finally, the target cash balance probably would be adjusted over time, rising and falling with seasonal patterns and with longer-term changes in the scale of the firm's operations. Factors that influence the target cash balance are discussed in the following sections.

Other Factors Influencing the Target Cash Balance. Any firm's target cash balance is normally set as the larger of (1) its transactions balances plus precautionary (safety stock) balances or (2) its required compensating balances as determined by its agreements with banks. Both the transactions and the precautionary balances depend on the firm's volume of business, the degree of uncertainty inherent in its forecast of cash inflows and outflows, and its ability to borrow on short notice to cover cash shortfalls. Recalling our cash budget for Dayton Printing, the target cash balance could have been reduced if the firm had been able to predict its inflows and outflows with greater precision. Dayton, like most firms, does not know exactly when bills will come in or when payments will be received. Therefore, transactions balances must be sufficient to allow for a random increase in bills requiring payment at a time when receipts lag behind expectations. Most firms keep higher cash balances than absolutely necessary for transactions purposes to lower the probability that reduced inflows or unexpected outflows will cause the firm to run out of cash. Although we do not consider them in this book, statistical procedures are available to help improve cash flow forecasts, and the better the cash flow forecast, the lower the minimum cash balance.

Increasing the Efficiency of Cash Management

Although a carefully prepared cash budget is a necessary starting point, there are other elements of a good cash management program, some of which we describe in this section.

Cash Flow Synchronization. If you, as an individual, were to receive income on a daily basis instead of once a month, you could operate with a lower average checking account balance. If you could arrange to pay rent, tuition, and other charges on a daily basis, this would further reduce your required average cash balance. Exactly the same thing holds for business firms; by improving their forecasts and arranging things so that their cash receipts coincide

synchronized cash flows
A situation in which inflows coincide with the timing of outflows, thereby permitting a firm to hold transactions balances to a minimum.

check clearing
Process of converting a check, after it is written and mailed, into cash in the payee's account. Firms try to speed up the clearing process for checks received and to slow down the process for checks disbursed.

lockbox plan
A procedure used to speed up collections and to reduce float through the use of post office boxes in payers' local areas.

with the timing of their cash outflows, firms can hold their transactions balances to a minimum. Recognizing this point, utility companies, oil companies, and other firms arrange to bill customers and to pay their own bills on a regular schedule throughout the month. In our cash budgeting example, if Dayton Printing Company could arrange more **synchronized cash flows** and increase the certainty of its forecasts, it would be able to reduce its target cash balance and therefore its required bank loans.

Speeding Collections and Slowing Disbursements. Another important aspect of cash management deals with processing the checks a company writes and receives. It is obviously inefficient to put checks received in a drawer and deposit them every week or so; no well-run business would follow such a practice. Similarly, cash balances are drawn down unnecessarily if bills are paid earlier than required. In fact, efficient firms go to great lengths to speed up the processing of incoming checks, thus putting the funds to work faster, and they try to stretch out their own payments as long as possible.

When a customer writes and mails a check, this does *not* mean that the funds are immediately available to the receiving firm. Most of us have deposited a check in our account and then been told that we cannot write our own checks against this deposit until the **check-clearing** process is completed. Our bank must make sure that the check we deposited is good and receive funds itself before releasing funds for us to spend.

As shown on the left side of Figure 10-1, the total amount of time required for a firm to process incoming checks and obtain the use of the money can be substantial. A check first must travel through the mail and then be cleared through the banking system before the money can be put to use. Checks received from customers in distant cities are especially subject to delays. Possible mail delays can obviously cause problems, and clearing checks can also delay the effective use of funds received. Assume, for example, that you receive a check and deposit it in your bank. The bank must present the check to the bank on which it was drawn. Only when this latter bank transfers funds to your bank are they available for you to use. Checks generally are cleared through the Federal Reserve System or through a clearinghouse set up by the banks in a particular city. Of course, if the check is drawn on the bank of deposit, that bank merely transfers funds by bookkeeping entries from one of its depositors to another. The length of time required for other checks to clear is a function of the distance between the payer's and the payee's banks; in the case of private clearinghouses, it can range from one to three days. The maximum time required for checks to clear through the Federal Reserve System is two days.

The right side of Figure 10-1 shows how the process can be speeded up. First, to reduce mail and clearing delays, a **lockbox plan** can be used. Suppose a New York firm makes sales to customers all across the country. It can arrange to have its customers send payments to post office boxes (lockboxes) in their own local areas. A local bank will pick up the checks, have them cleared in the local area, and then transfer the funds by wire to the company's

Figure 10-1 **Diagram of the Check-Clearing Process**

This figure illustrates how a lockbox plan can accelerate a company's collection of receivables by three to five working days. With the regular check-clearing process, a company must wait six to eight working days for a customer's payment to pass through the mail and clear through the banks and the Federal Reserve System. When a company uses a mailing address and bank in a customer's hometown, however, the check-clearing process is expedited and the company gains quicker access to its funds. It is possible for a company to free up several million dollars in cash by using lockboxes.

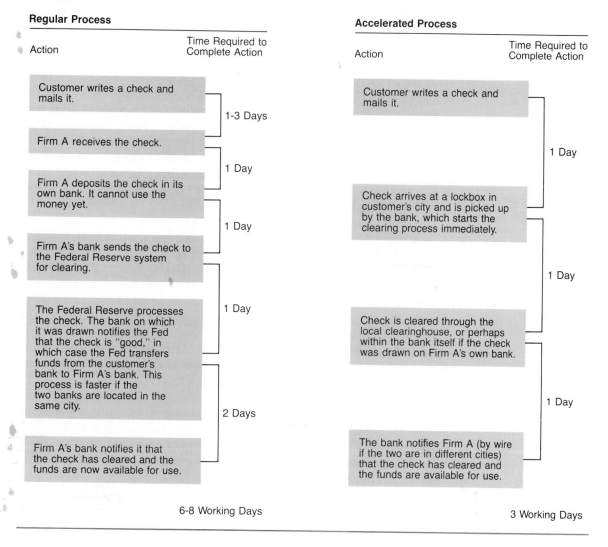

New York bank. In this way collection time can be reduced by one to five days. Examples of freeing funds in the amount of $5 million or more by this method are common. The local banks will charge the New York firm for the collection and funds-transfer services rendered. To determine whether a lockbox system is advantageous, the firm must compare the bank fees with the gains from reducing float.

Slowing Disbursements. Just as expediting the collection process conserves cash, slowing down disbursements accomplishes the same thing by keeping cash on hand for longer periods. One obviously could simply delay payments, but this involves equally obvious difficulties. Firms have, in the past, devised rather ingenious methods for "legitimately" lengthening the collection periods for their own checks. One popular method of slowing the disbursement period has been to write checks on banks located in out-of-the-way places. In the past, for example, Merrill Lynch wrote checks to its customers who lived east of the Mississippi River on a San Francisco bank, but to customers living west of the river, the checks were written on a New York bank. This delayed the check-clearing process and thus increased the length of time for which Merrill Lynch had use of the funds. Hundreds of millions of dollars were involved, and Merrill was finally forced to stop the practice as a result of a lawsuit. Other firms use banks in southeast Missouri, North Dakota, or other hard-to-get-to spots for the same purpose. Since such practices are usually recognized for what they are, there are severe limits to their use.

Another widely used procedure for delaying payouts is the use of *drafts*. Whereas a check is payable when presented to the bank on which it was drawn, a draft must be transmitted to the issuer, who approves it and deposits funds to cover it, and only then can it be collected. Insurance companies often use drafts. In handling claims, for instance, Aetna can pay a claim by draft on Friday. The recipient deposits the draft at a local bank, which must then send it to Aetna's Hartford bank. It may be Wednesday or Thursday before the draft arrives. The bank then sends it to the company's accounting department, which has until 3 P.M. that day to inspect and approve it. Not until then does Aetna have to deposit funds in the bank to pay the draft.

Using Float. The difference between the balance shown in a firm's (or an individual's) checkbook and the balance on the bank's books is known as **float.** Suppose a firm writes checks in the amount of $5,000, on the average, each day. It takes about six days for these checks to clear and to be deducted from the firm's bank account. Thus the firm's own checking account records show a balance $30,000 smaller than the bank's records. If the firm receives checks in the amount of $5,000 daily but loses only four days while these checks are being deposited and cleared, its own books have a balance that is, because of this factor, $20,000 larger than the bank's balance. Thus the firm's net float — the difference between the $30,000 and the $20,000 — is $10,000.

float

The amount of funds tied up in checks that have been written but are still in process and have not yet cleared.

If a firm's own collection and clearing process is more efficient than that of the recipients of its checks — and this is generally true of larger, more efficient firms — the firm could show a *negative* balance on its own records and a *positive* balance on the books of its bank. Some firms indicate that they *never* have true positive cash balances. One large manufacturer of construction equipment stated that, although its account according to its bank's records shows an average cash balance of about $2 million, its *actual* balance is *minus* $2 million; it has $4 million of net float. Obviously, the firm must be able to forecast its positive and negative clearings accurately to make such heavy use of float.

E. F. Hutton provides an example of pushing cash management too far. Hutton did business with banks all across the country, and it had to keep compensating balances in these banks. The sizes of the required compensating balances were known, and any excess funds in these banks were sent electronically, on a daily basis, to concentration banks, where they were immediately invested in interest-bearing securities. However, rather than waiting to see what the end-of-day balances actually were, Hutton began estimating inflows and outflows, and transferred out for investment the *estimated* end-of-day excess. Then, however, Hutton got greedy — it began to deliberately overestimate its deposits and underestimate clearings of its own checks, thereby deliberately overstating the estimated end-of-day balances. As a result, Hutton was chronically overdrawn at its local banks, and it was in effect earning interest on funds that really belonged to those local banks. It is entirely proper for a firm to forecast what the bank will have recorded as its balance and then to make decisions based on this estimate, even if that balance is different from the balance the firm's own books show. However, it is illegal to forecast an overdrawn situation but then to tell the bank that a positive balance is forecast.

Basically, a firm's net float is a function of its ability to speed up collections on checks received and to slow down collections on checks written. Efficient firms go to great lengths to speed up the processing of incoming checks, thus putting the funds to work faster, and they try to stretch their own payments out as long as possible.

Matching the Costs and Benefits Associated with Cash Management

Although a number of procedures may be used to hold down cash balance requirements, implementing these procedures is not a costless operation. How far should a firm go in making its cash operations more efficient? As a general rule, the firm should incur these expenses as long as marginal returns exceed marginal expenses.

For example, suppose that by establishing a lockbox system and increasing the accuracy of cash inflow and outflow forecasts, a firm can reduce its investment in cash by $1 million without increasing the risk of running short of

Cash management software systems for computers, such as Interplex from Manufacturers Hanover, are available to financial managers to help them increase the efficiency of cash management.

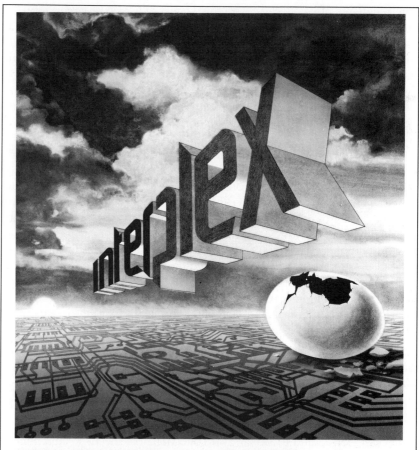

THE FINANCIAL SOURCE:

Now it's launching INTERPLEX™ to give you total control of your corporate finances automatically and earlier than ever before.

Manufacturers Hanover establishes the new standard in treasury management systems.

It's early morning as you enter your office and your financial position is waiting for you. In complete detail. Account data from all of your banks has been automatically consolidated within the integrated data base and put into a single standardized format. You're ready to perform transaction verification and account reconciliation. You know hours earlier what investment or bor-

rowing decisions to make. And you quickly realize why INTERPLEX, a fully automated treasury management system, is the industry's new standard.

INTERPLEX from Manufacturers Hanover is the microcomputer-based, multi-user, multi-task treasury management system that gives you more control. Including the ability to automatically collect data from all of your banks. Store it. Process it. Merge it. Use it. Faster.

INTERPLEX lets you conduct target balance analyses, project end of day cash posi-

tion, make cash forecasts, transfer funds, and perform many other treasury functions. Sophisticated yet simple, this system is just the beginning of a family of fully integrated financial management products from Manufacturers Hanover.

State-of-the-art leadership. Backed by a longstanding commitment to innovation. Once again, The Financial Source delivers.

Learn how you can enter the new age of INTERPLEX and gain total control. Automatically. Just contact George Chelius, Vice President, at 1-800-MHT-PLEX.

MH Financial Management Systems, Inc.

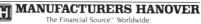

MANUFACTURERS HANOVER
The Financial Source℠ Worldwide.

Source: Courtesy of MH Financial Management Systems, Inc., New York.

cash. Furthermore, suppose the firm borrows at a cost of 12 percent. The steps taken have released $1 million, which can be used to reduce bank loans and thus save $120,000 per year. If the costs of the procedures necessary to release the $1 million are less than $120,000, the move is a good one; if the costs exceed $120,000, the greater efficiency is not worth the cost. It is clear that larger firms, with larger cash balances, can better afford to hire the personnel necessary to maintain tight control over their cash positions. Cash management is one element of business operations in which economies of scale are present.

Very clearly, the value of careful cash management depends on the costs of funds invested in cash, which in turn depend on the current rate of interest. Although interest rates have receded from their historic highs of the early 1980s, business firms continue to devote more care than ever to cash management.

Cash Management in the Multidivisional Firm. The concepts, techniques, and procedures described thus far in the chapter must be extended when applied to large, national (or multinational) firms. Such corporations have plants and sales offices all across the nation (or the world), and they deal with banks in each of their operating territories. These companies must maintain compensating balances in each of their banks, and they must be sure that no bank account becomes overdrawn. Cash inflows and outflows are subject to random fluctuations, so, in the absence of close control and coordination, there would be a tendency for some accounts to have shortages and for others to have excess balances. A sound cash management program for such multibank corporations necessarily includes provisions for keeping strict control over the level of funds in each account and for shifting funds among accounts to minimize the total corporate cash balance. Mathematical models and electronic connections between a central computer and each branch location have been developed to help with such situations; however, an in-depth discussion of these topics would go beyond the scope of this book.

Bank Relationships

Banks provide many services to firms — they clear checks, operate lockbox plans, supply credit information, and the like. Because these services cost the bank money, the bank must be compensated for rendering them.

Compensating Balances. Banks earn most of their income by lending money at interest, and most of the funds they lend are obtained in the form of deposits. If a firm maintains a deposit account with an average balance of $100,000, and if the bank can lend these funds at a net return of $8,000, the account is, in a sense, worth $8,000 to the bank. Thus it is to the bank's advantage to provide services worth up to $8,000 to attract and hold the account.

Banks determine first the costs of the services rendered to their larger customers and then the average account balances necessary to provide enough income to compensate for these costs. Firms often maintain these compensating balances to avoid paying cash service charges to the bank.[1]

Compensating balances are also required by some bank loan agreements. During periods when the supply of credit is restricted and interest rates are high, banks frequently insist that borrowers maintain accounts that average some percentage of the loan amount as a condition for granting the loan; 15 percent is a typical figure. If the balance is larger than the firm would otherwise maintain, the effective cost of the loan is increased. The excess balance presumably "compensates" the bank for making a loan at a rate below what it could earn on the funds if they were invested elsewhere.[2]

Compensating balances can be established as either (1) an *absolute minimum* (say, $100,000) below which the actual balance must never fall, or (2) a *minimum average balance* (perhaps $100,000) during some period, generally a month. The absolute minimum is a much more restrictive requirement, because the total amount of cash held during the month must be above $100,000 by the amount of the transactions balances. The $100,000 in this case is "dead money" from the firm's standpoint. The minimum average balance, however, could fall to zero one day provided it was $200,000 some other day, with the average working out to $100,000. Thus the $100,000 in this case is available for transactions.

Statistics on compensating balance requirements are not available, but average balances are typical and absolute minimums rare for business accounts. Discussions with bankers, however, indicate that absolute balance requirements are less rare during times of extremely tight money.

Overdraft Systems

overdraft systems
Systems wherein depositors may write checks in excess of their balances, with the banks automatically extending loans to cover the shortages.

Most countries other than the United States use **overdraft systems.** In such systems depositors write checks in excess of their actual balances, and the bank automatically extends loans to cover the shortages. The maximum amount of such loans must, of course, be established beforehand. Although statistics are not available on the usage of overdrafts in the United States, a number of firms have worked out informal, and in some cases formal, overdraft arrangements. Also, both banks and credit card companies regularly establish cash reserve systems for individuals. The use of overdrafts has been increasing in recent years, and if this trend continues, we can anticipate a further reduction of cash balances.

---

[1] Compensating balance arrangements apply to individuals as well as to business firms. Thus you might get "free" checking services if you maintain a minimum balance of $200, but be charged 10 cents per check if your balance falls below $200 during the month.

[2] The interest rate effect of compensating balances is discussed further in Chapter 12.

MARKETABLE SECURITIES

Sizeable holdings of such short-term **marketable securities** as U.S. Treasury bills or bank certificates of deposit are often reported on financial statements. The reasons for such holdings, as well as the factors that influence the choice of securities held, are discussed in this section.

marketable securities
Securities that can be sold on short notice for close to their quoted market prices.

Reasons for Holding Marketable Securities

Marketable securities typically provide much lower yields than firms' operating assets; for example, International Business Machines (IBM) recently held a multibillion-dollar portfolio of marketable securities that yielded about 9 percent, whereas its operating assets provided a return of about 18 percent. Why would a company like IBM have such large holdings of low-yielding assets? There are two basic reasons for these holdings: first, they serve as a substitute for cash balances, and second, they are used as a temporary investment. These points are considered next.

Marketable Securities as a Substitute for Cash. Some firms hold portfolios of marketable securities in lieu of larger cash balances, liquidating part of the portfolio to increase the cash account when cash outflows exceed inflows. In such situations the marketable securities could be a substitute for transactions balances, precautionary balances, speculative balances, or all three. In most cases the securities are held primarily for precautionary purposes. Most firms prefer to rely on bank credit to meet temporary transactions or speculative needs, but they hold some liquid assets to guard against a possible shortage of bank credit.

During the late 1970s IBM had approximately $6 billion in marketable securities. This large liquid balance had been built up as a reserve to cover possible damage payments resulting from pending antitrust suits. When it became clear that IBM would win most of the suits, the liquidity need declined, and the company spent some of the funds on other assets, including repurchases of its own stock. This is a prime example of a firm's building up its precautionary balances to handle possible emergencies.

Marketable Securities Held as a Temporary Investment. Whenever a firm has more than 1 or 2 percent of its total assets invested in marketable securities, chances are good that these funds represent a strictly temporary investment. Such temporary investments generally occur in one of the three following situations:

1. *When the firm must finance seasonal or cyclical operations.* Firms engaged in seasonal operations frequently have surplus cash flows during one part of the year and deficit cash flows during another. Such firms may purchase marketable securities during their surplus periods and then liquidate them when cash deficits occur. Other firms, however, choose to use bank financing to cover such shortages.

2. *When the firm must meet some known financial requirements.* If a major plant construction program is planned for the near future, or if a bond issue is about to mature, a firm may build up its marketable securities portfolio to provide the required funds. Furthermore, marketable securities holdings often are large immediately before quarterly corporate tax payment dates.

3. *When the firm has just sold long-term securities.* An expanding firm has to sell long-term securities (stocks or bonds) periodically. The funds from such sales can be invested in marketable securities, which can, in turn, be sold to provide funds as they are needed for permanent investments in operating assets.

Strategies Regarding Marketable Securities Holdings

Actually, each of the needs mentioned previously can be met either by obtaining short-term loans or by holding marketable securities. Consider a firm like Dayton Printing Company, which we discussed before, whose sales are growing over time but fluctuate on a seasonal basis. As we saw from Dayton's cash budget (Table 10-1), the firm plans to borrow to meet seasonal needs. As an alternative financial strategy, Dayton could hold a portfolio of marketable securities and liquidate these securities to meet its peak cash needs.

A firm's marketable securities policy is an integral part of its overall working capital policy. If the firm has a conservative working capital financing policy, its long-term capital will exceed its permanent assets, and it will hold marketable securities when inventories and receivables are low. With an aggressive policy, it will never carry any securities and will borrow heavily to meet peak needs. With a moderate policy under which maturities are matched, the firm will match permanent assets with long-term financing and will meet most seasonal increases in inventories and receivables with short-term loans, but it will also carry marketable securities at certain times.

Figure 10-2 illustrates three alternative strategies for a firm like Dayton. Under Plan A, which represents an aggressive financing policy, Dayton would hold no marketable securities, relying completely on bank loans to meet seasonal peaks. Under the conservative Plan B, Dayton would stockpile marketable securities during slack periods and then sell those securities to raise funds for peak needs. Plan C is a compromise; under this alternative, the company would hold some securities but not enough to meet all of its peak needs. Dayton actually follows Plan C.

There are advantages and disadvantages to each of these strategies. Plan A is clearly the most risky — the firm's current ratio is always lower than under the other plans, indicating that it might encounter difficulties either in borrowing the funds needed or in repaying the loan. On the other hand, Plan A requires no holdings of low-yielding marketable securities, and this will prob-

Figure 10-2 **Alternative Strategies for Meeting Seasonal Cash Needs**

This figure shows the effects of three different approaches to the use of marketable securities to finance short-term needs for cash. Under Plan A a company holds no marketable securities and relies entirely on bank loans for its short-term cash. Although it may create problems in borrowing funds or repaying loans, Plan A should provide a higher return on total assets and net worth because no funds are locked into low-yielding marketable securities. Under Plan B a company accumulates a large amount of marketable securities that it then sells off to raise cash. This plan avoids borrowing but lowers the company's return on total assets and net worth. The disadvantages of Plans A and B are moderated under Plan C, which uses a combination of marketable securities and short-term loans to finance seasonal cash needs.

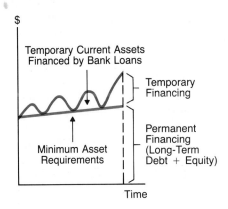

Plan A: Hold Zero Marketable Securities

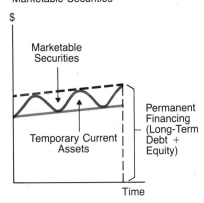

Plan B: Meet All Seasonal Needs by Sale of Marketable Securities

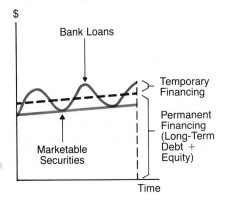

Plan C: Compromise— Hold Some Marketable Securities

ably lead to a relatively high expected rate of return on both total assets and net worth.

Factors Influencing the Choice of Securities

A wide variety of securities, differing in terms of default risk, interest rate risk, liquidity risk, and expected rate of return, are available. In this section we first consider the characteristics of different securities, and then we show how the financial manager selects the specific instruments held in the marketable securities portfolio. These same characteristics are, incidentally, as important for individuals' investment decisions as for businesses' decisions.

default risk
The risk that a borrower will not pay the interest or principal on a loan.

Default Risk. The risk that an issuer will be unable to make interest payments, or to repay the principal amount on schedule, is known as **default risk.** If the issuer is the U.S. Treasury, the default risk is negligible; thus Treasury securities are regarded as being default-free. (Treasury securities are not completely free of risk, since U.S. Government bonds are subject to risk caused by interest rate fluctuations, and they are also subject to loss of purchasing power due to inflation.) Corporate securities and bonds issued by state and local governments are subject to some degree of default risk. Several organizations (for example, Moody's Investment Service and Standard & Poor's Corporation) rate bonds. They classify them on a scale that ranges from very high quality to highly speculative with a definite chance of going into default. Ratings change from time to time. Penn Central's securities were given high ratings at one time, but the ratings were lowered as the company's financial position deteriorated.

interest rate risk
The risk to which investors are exposed due to changing interest rates.

Interest Rate Risk. We will see in Chapter 17 that bond prices vary with changes in interest rates. Furthermore, the prices of long-term bonds are much more sensitive to shifts in interest rates than are prices of short-term securities. Thus, if Dayton's treasurer purchased at par $1 million of 25-year U.S. Government bonds paying 9 percent interest, and if interest rates then rose to 14.5 percent, the market value of these bonds would fall from $1 million to just below $635,000 — a loss of almost 40 percent.[3] (This actually happened from 1980 to 1982.) If 90-day Treasury bills had been held during a period of rising interest rates, however, the loss would have been negligible.

purchasing power risk
The risk that inflation will reduce the purchasing power of a given sum of money.

Purchasing Power Risk. Another type of risk is **purchasing power risk,** or the risk that inflation will reduce the purchasing power of a given sum of money. Purchasing power risk, which is important both to firms and to indi-

---

[3]These computations are explained in detail in Chapters 13 and 17.

vidual investors during times of inflation, is generally regarded to be lower on assets whose returns can be expected to rise during inflation than on assets whose returns are fixed. Thus real estate and common stocks are thought of as being better hedges against inflation than are bonds and other fixed-income securities.[4]

Liquidity or Marketability Risk. An asset that can be sold on short notice for close to its quoted market price is defined as being highly liquid. If Dayton purchases $1 million of infrequently traded bonds of a relatively obscure company like Bigham Pork Products, it will probably have to accept a price reduction to sell the bonds on short notice. On the other hand, if Dayton buys $1 million worth of U.S. Treasury bonds, or bonds issued by AT&T, General Motors, or Exxon, it will be able to dispose of them almost instantaneously at close to the quoted market price. These latter bonds are said to have very little **liquidity or marketability risk.**

liquidity or marketability risk
The risk that securities cannot be sold at a reasonable price on short notice.

Returns on Securities. As we know from earlier chapters, the higher a security's risk, the higher the required return on the security. Thus corporate treasurers, like other investors, must make a trade-off between risk and return when choosing investments for their marketable securities portfolios. Because the liquidity portfolio is generally held for a specific known need or for use in emergencies, the firm might be financially embarrassed should the portfolio decline in value. Furthermore, most nonfinancial corporations do not have investment departments specializing in appraising securities and determining the probability of their going into default. Accordingly, the marketable securities portfolio generally is composed of highly liquid, short-term securities issued by either the U.S. Government or the very strongest corporations. Given the purpose of the securities portfolio, treasurers are unwilling to sacrifice safety for higher rates of return.

Types of Marketable Securities

Although any investor wishes to minimize needless risks, a manager investing temporary excess cash must be especially aware of liquidity risk. The manager has a wide variety of available securities to hold as near cash. These alternatives, both government and nongovernment securities, are discussed next with special emphasis given to liquidity risk. In addition, Table 10-2 provides a listing of various investment sources, an indication of their suitability as short-term investments, and an indication of their return.

---

[4]Recall from Chapter 5 that if a high rate of inflation is expected in the future, that expectation will be built into interest rates. Therefore, the real risk of inflation to bondholders is that actual inflation will exceed the expected level.

Table 10-2 **Securities Available for Investment of Surplus Cash**

Security	Typical Maturity at Time of Issue	Approximate Yields			Appropriate As a Near-Cash Reserve
		6/10/77	2/10/82	3/17/87	
Suitable to Hold as Near-Cash Reserve					
U.S. Treasury bills	91 days to 1 year	4.8%	15.1%	5.6%	Yes
Commercial paper	Up to 270 days	5.5	15.3	6.2	Yes
Negotiable certificates of deposit (CDs) of U.S. banks	Up to 1 year	6.0	15.5	6.3	Yes
Money market mutual funds	Instant liquidity	5.1	14.0	5.8	Yes
Eurodollar market time deposits	Up to 1 year	6.1	16.2	6.5	Questionable
Not Suitable to Hold as Near-Cash Reserve					
U.S. Treasury notes	3 to 10 years	6.8	14.8	6.6	Questionable
U.S. Treasury bonds	Up to 30 years	7.6	14.6	7.6	No
Corporate bonds (AAA)	Up to 40 years	8.2	16.0	8.4	No
State and local government bonds[a]	Up to 30 years	5.7	12.8	6.7	No
Common stocks of other corporations	Unlimited	Variable	Variable	Variable	No
Common stock of the firm in question	Unlimited	Variable	Variable	Variable	No

[a]Rates are lower on state/municipal government bonds because the interest they pay is exempt from federal income taxes.

Government Securities. The U.S. Treasury and other federal agencies issue a wide variety of securities with different maturities. Treasury bills are a popular outlet for excess funds, in part because Treasury bills have a large and active secondary market to insure liquidity. Also, these securities are, as a practical matter, default-free.

Treasury bills are sold at weekly auctions and have 13-week (91-day), 26-week (182-day), and 1-year maturities. Alternatively, they can be bought or sold in the secondary market with as little as one day remaining to maturity. Thus the investor has a wide choice of available maturities.

Other government securities with longer maturities are available. Treasury notes are government obligations with maturities of 3 to 5 years. Treasury bonds are issued with maturities of up to 30 years. However, because of their long maturities and potentially unstable near-term prices,[5] these longer-term securities may be poor choices as investments for **near-cash reserves.** U.S. federal agencies, such as the Federal Home Loan Bank and the Federal National Mortgage Association, also issue notes and bonds. These securities are riskier than Treasury issues, because they are not directly backed by the U.S.

near-cash reserves
Reserves that are quickly and easily converted to cash.

[5]We describe in Chapter 17 how, as interest rates rise, bond prices fall and, conversely, as interest rates fall, prices rise. Furthermore, the longer the term to maturity, the greater the price change for a given change in interest rates. These factors work against the use of bonds as a temporary store of value, since temporary excess cash should be invested in securities with stable and predictable returns.

Treasury. Therefore they yield a slightly higher return than Treasury issues. For example, on April 10, 1987, federal agency bonds yielded 8.37 percent versus 7.98 percent for 10-year Treasury bonds.

Nongovernment Securities

Commercial Paper. Short-term unsecured promissory notes issued by the largest, most financially secure corporations in America are called **commercial paper.** Dealers in commercial paper prefer to handle the paper of firms whose net worth is $50 million or more and whose annual borrowing exceeds $10 million. Regular issuers include General Motors Acceptance Corporation, Ford Motor Credit Corporation, and C.I.T. Financial Corporation. Commercial paper is sold primarily to other business firms, insurance companies, pension funds, money market mutual funds, and banks. It is traded in the secondary markets, and a firm that holds the commercial paper of another firm can sell it to raise cash in a matter of hours — it is highly liquid. The amount of commercial paper has grown rapidly in recent years. At the beginning of 1987, there was more than $337 billion of commercial paper outstanding, as compared to about $551 billion of bank loans to businesses.

Maturities of commercial paper generally vary from two to six months, with an average of about two months.[6] The rates on commercial paper fluctuate with supply and demand conditions; they are determined in the market place, varying daily as conditions change. However, the rates on commercial paper are low, relative to other securities. The low rates reflect that default risk is low, since only the most creditworthy corporations sell commercial paper. Recently, commercial paper rates have ranged from one to two percentage points below the stated prime rate but slightly above the T-bill rate. For example, in March 1987 the average rate on 3-month commercial paper was 6.2 percent, whereas the stated prime rate was 7.5 percent and the T-bill rate was 5.6 percent.

Negotiable Certificates of Deposit. Major money-center commercial banks will issue certificates of deposit (CDs) as marketable receipts for large time deposits. Usually these deposits are over $100,000 and mature within 1 to 18 months after issuance. The interest paid on these instruments is negotiated and is paid at maturity.

A secondary market for CDs exists, but it is not as well developed as that for Treasury bills. Therefore the yield on CDs is generally above Treasury bills.

These securities should not be mistaken for CDs typically purchased by individual small investors. The latter CDs are different from the marketable

commercial paper
Unsecured, short-term promissory notes of large, financially strong firms, usually issued in denominations of $100,000 or more and having an interest rate somewhat below the prime rate.

---

[6]The maximum maturity without SEC registration is 270 days. Commercial paper can be sold only to "sophisticated" investors; otherwise, SEC registration would be required even for maturities of 270 days or less.

securities in that their interest is established by the financial institution, rather than negotiated, and these smaller CDs are not marketable.

Money Market Mutual Funds. Money market funds are a popular source of liquidity for both businesses and individuals. These mutual funds hold only short-term securities such as Treasury bills, CDs, and commercial paper. Shares in these funds are easily obtained — often without commissions. Because the required initial investment is small and the liquidity is comparable to lower-yielding checking and savings accounts, the money market funds are a popular temporary investment alternative, especially for smaller firms.

Eurodollar bank time deposits
Interest-bearing time deposits, denominated in U.S. dollars, placed in banks outside the United States.

Eurodollar Bank Time Deposits. Eurodollars are interest-bearing time deposits, denominated in U.S. dollars and placed in banks outside the United States. The term **Eurodollars** may be misleading because banks in Canada, Japan, and the Caribbean are important links in the market.

In many respects the Eurodollar is an international counterpart to the negotiable certificate of deposit. Interest and maturities are negotiated; however, interest on these invested dollars is generally above the CD rate to attract investment. Like CDs, there is a secondary market for Eurodollars, but it is still in the developmental stage and is not a source of certain liquidity. Default risk is a function of the issuing bank.

SUMMARY

Firms hold cash primarily for ordinary daily business transactions and to partially compensate banks for loans and services, and to a lesser extent for precaution and speculative purposes. The key element in any cash management system is the *cash budget,* which is a forecast of cash inflows and outflows during a given planning period. The cash budget shows whether the firm can expect a cash deficit, in which case plans must be made to obtain external capital, or a cash surplus, in which case plans should be made to invest the available funds. The efficiency of cash management can be increased by speeding collections, slowing disbursements, and using *float.*

Primarily, marketable securities are held (1) as a reserve for future contingencies, (2) to meet seasonal needs, with holdings being built up during the slack season and liquidated when cash requirements are high, (3) to meet known future cash requirements such as construction progress payments or taxes, and (4) immediately after the sale of long-term securities. Given the motives for holding them, treasurers generally do not want to gamble by holding risky securities; safety is the watchword, and rarely will a treasurer sacrifice safety for the higher yields offered on risky securities.

RESOLUTION TO DECISION IN FINANCE

To Buy Back or Not to Buy Back

Allen Born used a long-dormant authorization from Amax's board to pick up something less than 1 million (1 percent) of the company's outstanding shares on Black Monday. The buying was circumscribed, however, by the Securities & Exchange Commission's "safe harbor" rule, which states that a company can buy no more than 25 percent of its average share volume of the prior 30 days. That translated to a ceiling of about 50,000 shares a day, a fraction of the more than 1 million shares the market was hemorrhaging per day. On Tuesday the market plummeted again, and Amax's shares slid to 13.

On Wednesday, Born sought approval from Amax's board for a stock buy-back of up to 4 million shares (about $60 million worth). After hurried telephone consultation, the board approved a 3 million share buy-back program. News of the buy-back program appeared on the Dow Jones ticker later that Wednesday, along with a preliminary estimate of strong earnings for the company's third quarter. The stock opened at 20 but closed the week at 17. The following Monday the stock dipped to 14.

When asked to evaluate the effects of the crash on Amax, Born responded that the Dow's

Source: James R. Norman, "Diary of a Decision: A Week in the Life of Amax," *Business Week*, November 9, 1987, 118, 123; and Kevin G. Salwen, "Share Buy-Back Plans Proliferate," *The Wall Street Journal*, January 4, 1988.

fall had "no effect on Amax's ability to show good cash flow and earnings." Amax stock ended the year trading at a little over 20 in a restabilizing market. Did the stock buy-back program buoy Amax's stock and avert a catastrophe, or would the stock have returned to a more normal value on its own as the market corrected itself? Cases like Amax's are sure to fuel the debate over whether or not stock buy-backs are good for American business.

According to Robert B. Reich, professor of political economy at Harvard's John F. Kennedy School of Government, buy-backs are poor use of a company's capital. "Companies' time horizons have been growing shorter over the past 25 years," he says. "Buy-backs pull the time horizon almost up to the front door." He argues that the increase in buy-back activity is "an unhealthy and dangerous trend because it puts corporate America on much thinner ice, should there be a major hike in interest rates or a substantial fall in demand." David Borger, director of research at Wilshire Asset Management, Los Angeles, disagrees. He argues that companies gain more from stock buy-backs than from investment in marginally productive physical assets. "The fact that they're buying back their own stocks really masks what they're doing. They're just choosing between two assets. Basically what it amounts to is making the most efficient use of your capital."

QUESTIONS

10-1 How can better methods of communication reduce the necessity for firms to hold large cash balances?

10-2 What are the two principal reasons for holding cash? Can a firm estimate its target cash balance by summing the cash held to satisfy each of the two reasons?

10-3   Explain how each of the following factors would probably affect a firm's target cash balance if all other factors were held constant.
   a. The firm institutes a new billing procedure which better synchronizes its cash inflows and outflows.
   b. The firm develops a new sales forecasting technique which improves its forecasts.
   c. The firm reduces its portfolio of U.S. Treasury bills.
   d. The firm arranges to use an overdraft system for its checking account.
   e. The firm borrows a large amount of money from its bank and also begins to pay suppliers twice as frequently as in the past; thus it must write far more checks than it did in the past even though the dollar volume of business has not changed.
   f. Interest rates on Treasury bills rise from 5 percent to 10 percent.

10-4   In the cash budget shown in Table 10-1, is the projected maximum funds requirement of $5,200,000 in September known with certainty, or should it be regarded as the expected value of a probability distribution? Consider how this peak probably would be affected by each of the following:
   a. A lengthening of the average collection period.
   b. An unanticipated decline in sales that occurred when sales were supposed to peak.
   c. A sharp drop in sales prices required to meet competition.
   d. A sharp increase in interest rates for a firm with a large amount of short-term debt outstanding.

10-5   Would a lockbox plan make more sense for a firm that makes sales all over the United States or for a firm with the same volume of business but concentrated in one city?

10-6   Would a corporate treasurer be more tempted to invest the firm's liquidity portfolio in long-term as opposed to short-term securities when the yield curve was upward sloping or downward sloping?

10-7   What does the term *liquidity* mean? Which would be more important to a firm that held a portfolio of marketable securities as precautionary balances against the possibility of losing a major lawsuit — liquidity or rate of return? Explain.

10-8   Firm A's management is very conservative, whereas Firm B's managers are more aggressive. Is it true that, other things being equal, Firm B would probably have larger holdings of short-term marketable securities? Explain.

10-9   Is it true that *interest rate risk* refers to the risk that a firm will be unable to pay the interest on its bonds? Explain.

10-10   Corporate treasurers, when selecting securities for portfolio investments, must make a trade-off between higher risk and higher returns. Is it true that most treasurers are willing to assume a fairly high exposure to risk to gain higher expected returns?

SELF-TEST PROBLEM

ST-1   David Banner, Limited, has grown from a small Houston firm, with customers concentrated in the Texas Gulf Coast area, to a large national firm serving customers throughout the United States. However, all operations, including the central billing system, have remained in Houston. On average, 5 days elapse from the time customers mail payments until the company receives and processes the checks so that it can use the money. To shorten the collection period, Banner's management is considering the installation of a lockbox system consisting of 30 local depository banks, or lockbox operations, and 8 regional concentration banks. The fixed cost of operating the system is estimated to be $14,000 per month. Under this system, customers' checks would be received by the lockbox operator 1 day after they are mailed, and daily collections would average $30,000 at each location. The collections would be transferred daily to the regional concentration banks.

One transfer mechanism involves having the local depository banks use mail depository transfer checks, or DTCs, to move the funds to the concentration banks. The alternative is to use electronic, or wire, transfers. A DTC would cost only 75 cents, but it would take 2 days for the funds to get to the concentration bank and thus be available to Banner. Therefore, float time under the DTC system would be 1 day for mail plus 2 days for transfer, or 3 days total, down from 5 days under the present system in which no concentration banking is used. Although a wire transfer would cost $11, funds would be available immediately, so float time would be only 1 day.

If Banner's opportunity cost is 11 percent, should it initate the lockbox/ concentration bank system? If so, which transfer method should be used? (Assume that there are $52 \times 5 = 260$ working days, hence 260 transfers from each lockbox, in a year.)

PROBLEMS

10-1 **Net float.** The Murchison Company is setting up a new bank account with the First National Bank. Murchison plans to issue checks in the amount of $4 million each day and to deduct them from its own records at the close of business on the day they are written. On average, the bank will receive and clear (that is, deduct from the firm's bank balance) the checks at 5 P.M. the fourth day after they are written. For example, a check written on Monday will be cleared on Friday afternoon. The firm's agreement with the bank requires it to maintain a $3 million average compensating balance. This is $1 million greater than the cash balance the firm would otherwise have on deposit; that is, without the compensating balance, it would carry an average deposit of $2 million.

    a. Assuming that the firm makes deposits at 4 P.M. each day (and the bank includes the deposit in that day's transactions), how much must the firm deposit each day to maintain a sufficient balance on the day it opens the account, during the first 4 days after it opens the account, and once it reaches a "steady state"? (Ignore weekends.)

    b. What ending daily balance should the firm try to maintain (1) on the bank's records and (2) on its own records?

    c. Explain how net float can help increase the value of the firm's common stock.

10-2 **Lockbox system.** Doc Chapman, Inc., started 5 years ago as a small medical products firm serving customers in the San Francisco Bay area. Its reputation and market area grew quickly, however, so that today Chapman has customers throughout the United States. Despite its broad customer base, Chapman has maintained its headquarters in the Bay area and keeps its central billing system there. Chapman's management is considering an alternative collection procedure to reduce its mail time and processing float. On average, it takes 5 days from the time customers mail payments until the company receives, processes, and deposits them. Chapman would like to set up a lockbox collection system, which it estimates would reduce the time lag from customer mailing to deposit by 3 days, bringing it down to 2 days. Chapman receives an average of $700,000 in payments per day.

a. How many days of collection float now exist (Chapman's customers' disbursement float) and what would it be under the lockbox system? What reduction in cash balances would Chapman achieve by initiating the lockbox system?

b. If Chapman has an opportunity cost of 9 percent, how much is the lockbox system worth on an annual basis?

c. What is the maximum monthly charge Chapman should pay for this lockbox system?

10-3   **Cash receipts.** Backroads Antique Store had sales of $60,000 in May, and it has forecast sales for its peak tourist season as follows:

Actual:	April	$ 45,000
	May	60,000
Forecast:	June	97,500
	July	135,000
	August	112,500

From experience, management estimates that 25 percent of sales are for cash, 65 percent of sales are paid after 30 days, 8 percent of sales are paid after 60 days, and 2 percent of sales are uncollectable. Prepare a schedule of cash receipts for the firm's peak season (June through August).

10-4   **Cash disbursements.** Harrison, Inc. is scheduling the production of snowmobiles to be sold next season. Orders for the next 5 months are as follows: July, 80,000 units; August, 100,000 units; September, 130,000 units; October, 80,000 units; and November, 40,000 units. Manufacturing costs for materials are $1,300 per unit, paid 1 month before manufacture. Direct labor costs equal $600 per unit, paid in the month of production. Shipping costs are $240 per unit, paid the month after manufacture. Depreciation expense is allocated on a units-of-production basis of $100 per unit in the month of production. Advertising expense is zero for July and August but will be $400,000 in September and $1,000,000 in October. Fixed overhead is $600,000 monthly. Taxes of $16 million will be paid at the end of September.

Prepare a schedule of cash disbursements for August through October.

10-5   **Cash budgeting.** Gary and Karen Burton recently leased space in the Hulen Mall and opened a new business, Art Handycrafts Gallery. Business has been good, but the Burtons have frequently run out of cash. This has necessitated late payment on certain orders, which, in turn, is beginning to cause a problem with suppliers. The Burtons plan to borrow from the bank to have cash ready as needed, but first they need to determine how much they must borrow. Accordingly, they have asked you to prepare a cash budget for a critical period around Christmas, when needs will be especially high.

Sales are made on a *cash basis only.* The Burton's purchases must be paid for the following month. The Burtons pay themselves a salary of $4,800 per month, and the rent is $2,000 per month. In addition, the Burtons must make a tax payment of $12,000 in December. The current cash on hand (on December 1) is $400, but the Burtons have agreed to maintain an average bank balance of $6,000; this is their target cash balance. (Disregard till cash, which is insignificant because the Burtons keep only a small amount on hand to lessen the chances of robbery.)

The estimated sales and purchases for December, January, and February are shown in the following table. Purchases during November amounted to $140,000.

	Sales	**Purchases**
December	$160,000	$40,000
January	40,000	40,000
February	60,000	40,000

a. Prepare a cash budget for December, January, and February.

b. Now suppose that the Burtons were to start selling on a credit basis on December 1, giving customers 30 days to pay. All customers accept these terms, and all other facts in the problem are unchanged. What would the gallery's loan requirements be at the end of December in this case? (*Hint:* The calculations required to answer this question are minimal.)

10-6 **Cash budgeting.** The Golden Empire Corporation is planning to request a line of credit from its bank. The following sales forecasts have been made for 1989 and 1990:

May 1989	$150,000
June	150,000
July	300,000
August	450,000
September	600,000
October	300,000
November	300,000
December	75,000
January 1990	150,000

Collection estimates obtained from the credit and collection department are as follows: collections within the month of sale, 5 percent; collections the month following the sale, 80 percent; collections the second month following the sale, 15 percent. Payments for labor and raw materials are typically made during the month following the one in which these costs have been incurred. Total labor and raw materials costs are estimated for each month as follows:

May 1989	$75,000
June	75,000
July	105,000
August	735,000
September	255,000
October	195,000
November	135,000
December	75,000

General and administrative salaries will amount to approximately $22,500 a month; lease payments under long-term lease contracts will be $7,500 a month; depreciation charges will be $30,000 a month; miscellaneous expenses will be $2,250 a month; income tax payments of $52,500 will be due in both September and December; and a progress payment of $150,000 on a new design studio must be paid in October. Cash on hand on July 1 will amount to $110,000, and a minimum cash balance of $75,000 will be maintained throughout the cash budget period.

a. Prepare a monthly cash budget for the last six months of 1989.

b. Prepare an estimate of the required financing (or excess funds) — that is, the amount of money that Golden Empire will need to borrow (or will have available to invest) — for each month during that period.

c. Assume that receipts from sales come in uniformly during the month (that is, cash receipts come in at the rate of 1/30 each day) but that all outflows are paid on the fifth of the month. Will this have an effect on the cash budget? In other words, would the cash budget you have prepared be valid under these assumptions? If not, what can be done to make a valid estimate of peak financing requirements? No calculations are required, although calculations can be used to illustrate the effects.

d. Golden Empire produces on a seasonal basis, just ahead of sales. Without making any calculations, discuss how the company's current ratio and debt ratio would vary during the year assuming all financial requirements were met by short-term bank loans. Could changes in these ratios affect the firm's ability to obtain bank credit?

(Do Part e only if you are using the computerized problem diskette.)

e. (1) By offering a 2 percent cash discount for paying within the month of sale, the credit manager has revised the collection percentages to 50 percent, 35 percent, and 15 percent, respectively. How will this affect the loan requirements?

(2) Return the payment percentages to their base case values and the cash discount to zero. Now suppose sales fall to only 70 percent of the forecast level. Production is maintained, so cash outflows are unchanged. How does this affect Golden Empire's financial requirements?

(3) Return sales to the forecast level (100%) and suppose collections slow down to 3%, 10%, and 87% for the three months, respectively. How does this affect financial requirements? If Golden Empire went to a cash-only sales policy, how would that affect requirements, other things held constant?

ANSWER TO SELF-TEST PROBLEM

First, determine the annual benefit to Banner from the reduction in cash balances under each of the new plans:

$$\text{Average daily collections} = (30)(\$30,000) = \$900,000.$$

DTC:

Current float: $900,000 per day × 5 days = $4,500,000
New float: $900,000 per day × 3 days = 2,700,000
Float reduction $1,800,000

Banner can reduce its cash balances by $1,800,000 by using DTCs, and it can earn 11 percent, which will provide interest income of $198,000.

$$\text{Interest earned} = \$1,800,000 \times 11\% = \$198,000.$$

Wire Transfer:

Current float: $900,000 per day × 5 days = $4,500,000
New float: $900,000 per day × 1 day   =   900,000
Float reduction   = $3,600,000

Banner can reduce its cash balances by $3,600,000 by using wire transfers, and it will earn $396,000 on the freed capital:

$$\text{Interest earned} = \$3,600,000 \times 11\% = \$396,000.$$

Next compute the annual cost of each transfer method:

$$\text{Number of transfers} = 30 \times 260 \quad = 7{,}800.$$
$$\text{Fixed costs} = \$14{,}000 \times 12 = \$168{,}000 \text{ per year.}$$

DTC:

$$\text{Total costs} = (7{,}800 \times \$0.75) + \$168{,}000 = \$173{,}850.$$

Wire Transfer:

$$\text{Total costs} = (7{,}800 \times \$11) + \$168{,}000 = \$253{,}800.$$

Finally, calculate the net annual benefit resulting from each transfer method:

DTC:

$$\text{Net benefits} = \$198{,}000 - \$173{,}850 = \$24{,}150.$$

Wire Transfer:

$$\text{Net benefits} = \$396{,}000 - \$253{,}800 = \$142{,}200.$$

Therefore, Banner should adopt the lockbox system and transfer funds from the lockbox operators to the regional concentration banks using wire transfers.

Chapter 11

Accounts Receivable and Inventories

The Price Is Wrong

When the founding partners of Contextual Design, Inc. began producing contemporary-style pine furniture, they figured that if they produced their products from scratch, they would be able to control not only the costs of materials and manufacturing but the quality and integrity of their product as well. So the foursome, all business novices in their twenties, set up their plant in the furniture capital of America, Raleigh, North Carolina. There they began to turn rough lumber into furniture components for over 70 different finished items and began selling them to more than 800 retail outlets nationwide.

Given the dozen or more steps in their production process, not to mention the space, time, and machinery involved, how did Contextual set a price? Like many companies with a good deal more experience, they chose a figure that "felt right" — in this case 50 percent of gross. How did they determine an inventory

policy? They were too busy filling orders to devote much time to analysis. Indeed, within five years, growth was so brisk that the company was number 177 on *Inc.* magazine's listing of the country's 500 fastest growing private companies. Thirteen months later the company was out of business.

Sales had been increasing exponentially, but where were the profits? Unfortunately, the company's principals had been too busy filling orders to pay much attention to the bottom line. Their approach to bookkeeping didn't help. They didn't finish the firm's June 30th end-of-the-year accounting for 1984 until practically Thanksgiving. When they finally did, they were looking at a financial statement that showed payables of $454,322 versus receivables of $189,025. What could have gone wrong?

As you read the following chapter, think of problems with inventory and pricing that could lead a rapidly growing company like Contextual Design into bankruptcy? What could Contextual have done to avert fiscal disaster?

See end of chapter for resolution.

In the previous chapter, we examined the firm's investment in cash and marketable securities. To complete the analysis of current asset management, we now turn to accounts receivable and inventories. These accounts are essential for a firm's profitability and even for its existence. Inventories are needed for sales to occur, and sales are necessary for profits. Although firms would rather sell for cash than on credit, competition forces most companies to offer credit. Accounts receivable are created when the firm sells on credit.

Firms usually have large investments in accounts receivable and inventory. For example, a typical manufacturing firm invests about 20 pecent of its total assets in accounts receivable. Inventories generally amount to another 20 percent of total assets, or more for non-manufacturers. These accounts are necessary to conduct business, but a Du Pont analysis quickly reveals that ineffective management of these accounts causes a buildup of excess accounts receivable and inventory, resulting in a lower rate of return on invested capital. Of course, too little inventory or denying credit to potential customers will lose sales and thus profit opportunities. In this chapter we present models that will help the firm optimize its investment in these current assets.

ACCOUNTS RECEIVABLE

account receivable
A balance due from a debtor on a current account.

As mentioned earlier, most firms sell on credit. When goods are shipped, inventories are reduced, and an **account receivable** is created.[1] Eventually the customer will pay the account, at which time receivables will decline and the cash account will increase. Carrying receivables results in both direct and indirect costs, but granting credit benefits the firm by increasing its sales. The financial manager tries to balance the costs and benefits of granting credit when determining the firm's credit policy. A good receivables control system is important, for without an adequate system, receivables will build up to excessive levels, cash flows will decline, and bad debts will rise to unacceptable levels. The optimal credit policy is the one at which the benefits of increased sales are exactly offset by the costs of granting credit; this is the credit policy that maximizes the value of the firm.

The optimal credit policy, and hence the optimal level of accounts receivable, depends on the firm's own unique operating conditions, however. Thus a firm with excess capacity and low variable production costs should extend credit more liberally, and therefore should carry a higher level of accounts receivable, than if it were operating at full capacity or had a slim profit margin. Although optimal credit policies can vary among firms, or even for a single

---

[1] Whenever goods are sold on credit, two accounts are created; an asset item called an *account receivable* appears on the books of the selling firm, and a liability item appears on the books of the purchaser. At this point we are analyzing the transaction from the seller's standpoint, so we concentrate on the variables under its control — in this case, receivables. The transaction will be examined from the purchaser's viewpoint in Chapter 12, where we discuss accounts payable as a source of funds and the cost of those funds relative to other sources.

firm over time, it is still useful to analyze the effectiveness of the firm's credit policy in an aggregate sense.

CREDIT POLICY

The success or failure of a business depends ultimately on the demand for its products; as a rule, the higher the demand, the greater its sales and profits and the healthier the firm. Sales, in turn, depend on a number of factors, some exogenous but others controllable by the firm. The major controllable variables that affect sales are product price and quality, advertising, and the firm's credit policy. **Credit policy** consists of the four following elements:

1. The *credit period,* which is the length of time buyers have before they must pay.

2. The *credit standards,* which refers to the minimum financial strength of acceptable credit customers.

3. The firm's *collection policy,* which is measured by its toughness or laxity in following up on slow-paying accounts.

4. *Discounts* given for early payment.

credit policy
Basic decisions that determine a firm's credit period, credit standards, collection procedures, and discounts.

Credit Period

The **credit period** is the length of time a company gives its customers to pay; for example, credit might be extended for 30, 60, or 90 days. Several factors influence the length of time over which the firm offers credit. In part this credit period is influenced heavily by the terms offered by competitors. Further, there is generally a relationship between a product's normal inventory holding period and the credit period. For example, fresh fruits and vegetables normally are sold on very short credit terms, whereas jewelry may involve a 90-day or even a 6-month credit period.

credit period
The length of time for which credit is granted.

Within these parameters there is still plenty of leeway for setting more or less generous credit terms. Lengthening the credit period may stimulate sales, but there is a cost to tying up funds in receivables. For example, if a firm changes its terms from net 30 to net 60, the average receivables for the year might rise from $100,000 to $300,000, with the increase in accounts receivable of $200,000 being caused in part by higher sales and in part by the longer credit period. Assuming that the firm's required rate of return on investment is 15 percent, the marginal return required on lengthening the credit period is $200,000 × 15% = $30,000. If the incremental profit (sales price minus all direct production, selling, and credit losses associated with the additional sales) exceeds $30,000, the change in credit policy should be made. Thus determining the optimal credit period involves many factors, but the bottom line in establishing a credit period is determining the point at which marginal profits on increased sales at least offset the costs of carrying the higher amount of accounts receivable.

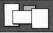

INDUSTRY PRACTICE

Formula for Disaster?

Among the important jobs a firm's chief financial officer (CFO) does is determining how much money the company has, how much it owes, and how much it is owed. This may sound fairly straightforward, but in reality it is a subtle and complex task. Legions of financial executives and accountants make their livelihood trying to keep track of the ebb and flow of corporate funds. Often the health of their enterprises depends on how well they manage to do their jobs.

One of the most problematic chores facing corporate CFOs is monitoring accounts receivable balances. Receivables comprise the money owed to a company for goods sold or services performed. They are usually tracked using the *accounts receivable collection period,* or *days sales outstanding in receivables (DSO),* method. The measure is calculated by dividing the accounts receivable balance by average daily sales over a specified period, generally monthly or quarterly. The figure derived by this method yields the average number of days between the time a firm sends an invoice and the time it receives payment.

Having a handle on accounts receivable gives the CFO an idea of how many days it is taking the company to collect on invoices. That way he or she can spot any trends in laggardly payments. Because there is currently a trend among small businesses to drag their feet in paying their bills, the CFO needs to be able to keep accounts receivable coming in on time lest his or her company should start having trouble paying *its* bills.

The problem with tracking accounts receivable using this technique, however, is that the DSO method may not be very accurate. This is because the DSO calculation is dependent on

Source: Charles W. Kyd, "Formula for Disaster?" *Inc.,* November 1986, 123, 124, 126.

two variables that have nothing to do with how quickly customers pay their accounts. One variable is recent sales trends, and the other is the time period used to calculate the daily averages.

While Charles Kyd, now a consultant for the accounting firm of Arthur Young & Co., was the controller of a high technology manufacturing firm, he ran into the problem with DSOs head-on. As controller, part of Kyd's job was to track receivables. Using the DSO method, he divided the accounts receivable balance by average daily sales over the period — in this case, one quarter (three months). His firm, which was growing at the rate of about 100 percent a year, was then purchased by a larger company whose rate of growth was much lower, close to 20 percent. After the sale, Kyd had to switch his firm's accounting practices to conform to the new parent company's, which in this case meant DSO reports every month instead of quarterly.

"As soon as we switched to the shorter period," says Kyd, "our receivables looked terrible. We were in continual trouble with headquarters over those DSO reports, and they wouldn't listen when we tried to explain that it wasn't our collections that were off, it was the formula." Changing the time period over which the DSO was calculated hadn't changed Kyd's accounts receivable situation, but it certainly changed the picture of it on the balance sheet.

The problem is that because the DSO calculations are dependent on sales averages, they can fluctuate independent of collections. Sales shifts can cause the DSO to vary widely from time period to time period, even when receivables are held steady. The DSO can also vary widely depending on which averaging period is used. When sales are rising, the longer the averaging period, the worse the days sales outstanding look. When sales are falling, the longer the averaging period, the better the receivables will look. Just when things are getting bad (sales are falling), the DSO is looking good, giving an unjustifiably rosy picture of the company's financial health.

"People often think that there must be a way to tinker with the averaging period so that the DSO numbers will be more realistic," says Kyd. "If 90 days isn't the correct period, perhaps 30 days, 60 days, or even a year. . . . The problem is that whenever you have a large blip in sales, you get unreasonable DSO figures no matter what period you use."

Kyd concludes that there is no way to accurately express the unpaid accounts receivable balance in terms of days sales outstanding. Instead, he counsels, one can generate accurate information about a company's accounts receivable performance by tracking past collection data.

Although start-up costs are high, Kyd argues that the advantages of tracking actual account collections far outweigh any inconvenience caused by having to dig up data on past receivables. Using past collection data and a spreadsheet computer program, it is possible to check at a glance on the dollar sales collected in 30-, 60-, 90-, and over-90-day periods of each month. The percentage collected in each period can then be graphed to display a clear picture of how many customers have been paying from month to month.

Credit Standards

If a firm makes credit sales only to the strongest customers, it will never have bad debt losses, nor will it incur much in the way of expenses for its credit department. On the other hand, it will probably lose sales, and the profit forgone on these lost sales could be far larger than the costs it has avoided. Determining the optimal **credit standards** involves equating the marginal costs of credit to the marginal profits on the increased sales.

Marginal costs include production and selling costs, but at this point we consider only those costs associated with the *quality* of the marginal accounts. These costs include (1) default, or bad debt losses, (2) higher investigation and collection costs, and (3) higher costs of capital tied up in receivables when selling to less creditworthy customers, who pay their accounts more slowly, causing the average collection period to lengthen.

Setting credit standards implicitly requires a measurement of *credit quality,* which is defined in terms of the probability of a customer's default. The probability estimate for a given customer is for the most part a subjective judgment; nevertheless, credit evaluation is a well-established practice, and a good credit manager can make reasonably accurate judgments of the probability of default by the different classes of customers. In this section we discuss some of the methods used by firms to measure credit quality.

credit standards
Standards that stipulate the minimum financial strength of acceptable credit customers.

The Five Cs System. The traditional method of measuring credit quality is to investigate credit customers with respect to five factors called the **five Cs of credit:**

1. *Character* refers to the probability that customers will *try* to honor their obligations. This factor is of considerable importance, because every credit

five Cs of credit
Factors used to evaluate credit risk: character, capacity, capital, collateral, and conditions.

transaction implies a *promise* to pay. Will debtors make an honest effort to pay their debts, or are they likely to try to get away with something? Experienced credit managers frequently insist that the moral factor is the most important issue in a credit evaluation. Thus credit reports provide background information on people's and firm's historical credit performance. Often credit analysts will seek this type of information from a firm's bankers, other suppliers, customers, and even competitors.

2. *Capacity* is a subjective judgment of customers' ability to pay. It is gauged in part by their past records, supplemented by physical observation of customers' plants or stores and by their business methods.

3. *Capital* is measured by the general financial position of firms as indicated by an analysis of their financial statements, with special emphasis on the risk ratios — the debt/assets ratio, the current ratio, and the times-interest-earned ratio.

4. *Collateral* is represented by assets that customers may offer as security to obtain credit.

5. *Conditions* refers to the effect of general economic trends or to special developments in certain geographic regions or sectors of the economy that may affect customers' ability to meet their obligations.

Information on these five factors comes both from the firm's previous experience with its customers and from a well-developed system of external information gatherers. Of course, once the information on the five Cs is developed, the credit manager still must make the final decision on the potential customer's overall credit quality. Because this decision is normally judgmental in nature, credit managers must rely on their experience and instincts.

Sources of Credit Information. Two major sources of external information are available. The first is *credit associations*, local groups that meet frequently and correspond with one another to exchange information on credit customers. These local groups have also banded together to create Credit Interchange, a system developed by the National Association of Credit Management for assembling and distributing information about debtors' past performances. The interchange reports show the paying records of different debtors, the industries from which they are buying, and the trading areas in which purchases are being made.

The second source of external information is *credit-reporting agencies*, which collect credit information and sell it for a fee. The best known of these agencies are Dun & Bradstreet (D&B) and TRW, Inc. D&B, TRW, and other agencies provide factual data that can be used in credit analysis; they also provide ratings similar to those available on corporate bonds.

Managing a credit department requires fast, accurate, up-to-date information, and to help make such information available, the National Association of Credit Management (a group with 43,000 member firms) persuaded TRW, Inc.,

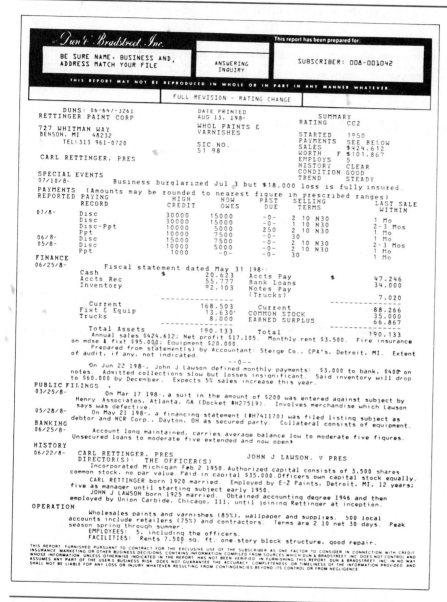

Credit reporting agencies (such as Dun & Bradstreet) compile and sell reports on specific companies; in this example, the information is on Rettinger Paint Corporation. These reports provide a credit rating (in top right corner) as well as factual information about the company's current financial status, public record of legal activities, banking, company history, and a brief description of the business.

Source: Reprinted by permission of Dun & Bradstreet Credit Services, a company of Dun & Bradstreet Corporation.

to develop a computer-based telecommunications network for the collection, storage, retrieval, and distribution of credit information. The TRW system transmits credit reports electronically, so they are available within seconds to its thousands of subscribers. Dun & Bradstreet has a similar electronic system, plus another service that provides more detailed reports through the U.S. mail.

A typical credit report would include the following information:

1. A summary balance sheet and income statement.

2. A number of key ratios, including trend information.

3. Information obtained from the firm's banks and suppliers about whether it has been paying promptly or slowly and whether it has recently failed to make any payments.

4. A description of the physical condition of the firm's operations.

5. A description of the backgrounds of the firm's owners, including any previous bankruptcies, lawsuits, fraud, and the like.

6. A summary rating, ranging from A+ for the best credit risks down to F for those judged most likely to default.

Although a great deal of credit information is available and computerized information systems can assist in making better credit decisions, in the final analysis these determinations are really exercises in informed judgment.

Management by Exception. Modern credit managers often practice *management by exception.* Under such a system, statistical procedures are used to classify customers into five or six categories according to degree of risk, and the credit manager concentrates time and attention on the weakest customers. For example, the following classes might be established:

Risk Class	Percentage of Uncollectible Credit Sales	Percentage of Customers in This Class
1	0–½%	60%
2	½–2	20
3	2–5	10
4	5–10	5
5	Over 10	5

Firms in Class 1 might be extended credit automatically and their credit status reviewed only once a year. Those in Class 2 might also receive credit (up to specified limits) automatically, but a ratio analysis of these firms' financial condition would be conducted more frequently (perhaps quarterly), and they would be moved down to Class 3 if their position deteriorated. Specific approvals might be required for credit sales to Classes 3 and 4, whereas sales to Class 5 might be on a COD (cash on delivery) basis only.

Collection Policy

collection policy
Procedures that a firm follows to collect accounts receivable.

Collection policy refers to the procedures the firm follows to collect receivables. For example, a letter may be sent to any account when the bill is 10 days past due; a more severe letter, followed by a telephone call, may be used if payment is not received within 30 days; and the account may be turned over to a collection agency after 90 days. The collection process can be expensive in terms of both out-of-pocket expenditures and lost goodwill, but some firmness is needed to prevent an undue lengthening in the collection period and to minimize outright losses. A balance must be struck between the cost and benefits of different collection policies.

Changes in collection policy influence sales, the collection period, the bad debt loss percentage, and the percentage of customers who take discounts. The effects of a change in collection policy, along with changes in the other credit policy variables, will be analyzed later in the chapter.

Cash Discounts

The last element in the credit policy decision, the use of **cash discounts** for early payment, is analyzed by balancing the costs and benefits of different discount terms. For example, Ellen Rose Fashions might decide to change its credit terms from 30 days (net 30) to allow a 2 percent discount if payment is received within 10 days (stated "2/10, net 30"). This change should produce two benefits: (1) it would attract new customers who consider discounts a type of price reduction, and (2) the discounts would cause a reduction in the average collection period, because some old customers would pay more promptly to take advantage of the discount. Offsetting these benefits is the dollar cost of the discounts taken. The optimal discount is established at the point where the costs and benefits are exactly offsetting. The methodology for analyzing changes in the discount is developed later in this chapter.

cash discount
A reduction in price given for early payment.

If sales are seasonal, a firm may use **seasonal dating** on discounts. For example, Jenson, Inc. is a swimsuit manufacturer that sells on terms of 2/10, net 30, May 1 dating. This means that the effective invoice date is May 1, so the discount may be taken until May 10, or the full amount must be paid on May 30, regardless of when the sale was made. If Jenson produces throughout the year but retail sales of bathing suits are concentrated in the spring and early summer, offering seasonal datings may induce some customers to stock up early, saving Jenson storage costs as well as "nailing down sales."

seasonal dating
Procedure which creates an invoice date during the purchaser's selling season, regardless of when the merchandise was shipped, to induce customers to buy early.

Profit Potential in Carrying Accounts Receivable

Thus far we have emphasized the costs of carrying receivables. *However, if it is possible to sell on credit and also to assess a carrying charge on the receivables that are outstanding, credit sales can actually be more profitable than cash sales.* This is especially true for consumer durables (automobiles, appliances, and so on), but it is also true for certain types of industrial equipment. Thus the General Motors Acceptance Corporation (GMAC) unit, which finances automobiles, is highly profitable, as is Sears, Roebuck's credit subsidiary. Some encyclopedia companies are even reported to lose money on cash sales but to more than make up for these losses from the carrying charges on their credit sales; obviously, such companies would rather sell on credit than for cash!

The carrying charges on outstanding credit generally run about 18 percent on an annual interest rate basis ($1\frac{1}{2}\%$ per month, so $1.5\% \times 12 = 18\%$).

Except for the early 1980s, when short-term interest rates rose to unprecedented levels, having receivables outstanding that earn 18 percent is highly profitable.

How Effective Is the Firm's Credit Policy?

As we saw in connection with the Du Pont analysis, an excessive investment in any asset account will lead to a low rate of return on net worth. For comparative purposes, we can examine the firm's average collection period (ACP) as discussed in Chapter 7. There we saw that Carter Chemical Company's average collection period was 42 days, compared to an industry average of 36 days. If Carter lowered its average collection period by 6 days to 36 days, this would mean a reduction of $8,333,333 × 6 = $49,999,998 in the amount of capital tied up in receivables. Assuming that the cost of funds tied up in receivables is 10 percent, this would mean a savings of $5 million per year, other things held constant.

The average collection period can also be compared to Carter's credit terms. Carter typically sells on terms of 1/10, net 30, so its customers, on average, are not paying their bills on time; the 42-day average collection period is greater than the 30-day credit period. Note, however, that some of the customers could be paying within 10 days to take advantage of the discount, whereas others could be taking much longer than 42 days to pay. To check against this possibility, we use an **aging schedule,** which breaks down accounts receivable according to how long they have been outstanding. Carter's aging schedule is as follows:

aging schedule

A report showing how long accounts receivable have been outstanding; it gives the percentage of receivables past due by different lengths of time.

Age of Accounts (days)	Percent of Total Value of Accounts Receivable
0–10	52%
11–30	20
31–45	13
46–60	4
Over 60	11
Total	100%

Although most of the accounts pay on schedule or after only a slight delay, a significant number are more than a month past due. This indicates that even though the majority of the firm's receivables are collected within the 30-day credit period, Carter has quite a bit of capital tied up in slow-paying accounts, some of which may eventually result in losses.

Management should constantly monitor the firm's average collection period and aging schedule to detect trends, to see how the firm's collection experience compares with its credit terms, and to see how effectively the credit department is operating in comparison with other firms in the industry. If the ACP begins to lengthen, or if the aging schedule begins to show an increasing percentage of past-due accounts, the firm's credit policy may have to be tightened.

Although a change in the ACP or the aging schedule should be a signal to the firm to investigate its credit policy, a deterioration in either of these measures does not *necessarily* indicate that the firm's credit policy has weakened.[2] In fact, if a firm experiences sharp seasonal variations, or if its sales have been growing rapidly, both the aging schedule and the ACP may be distorted. Similar problems arise with the aging schedule when sales fluctuate widely.

Investors — both stockholders and lenders — should pay close attention to accounts receivable management; otherwise they could be misled by the current financial statements and later suffer serious losses on their investments. When a sale is made, the following events occur: (1) inventories are reduced by the cost of goods sold, (2) accounts receivable are increased by the sales price, and (3) the difference is recorded as a profit. If the sale is for cash, the profit is definitely earned, but if the sale is on credit, the profit is not actually earned unless and until the account is collected. Firms have been known to encourage "sales" to very weak customers to inflate reported profits. This could boost the stock price, at least until credit losses show up and begin to lower earnings, at which time the stock price falls. An analysis along the lines suggested previously would detect any such questionable practice, as well as any unconscious deterioration in the quality of accounts receivable. Such early detection could help both investors and bankers avoid losses.

Analyzing Changes in the Credit Policy Variables

If a firm's credit policy is eased by such actions as lengthening the credit period, relaxing credit standards, following a less tough collection policy, or offering cash discounts, sales should increase; *easing the credit policy normally stimulates sales.* However, if credit policy is eased and sales *do* rise, costs will also rise because (1) more labor, materials, and so on will be required to produce the additional goods, (2) receivables outstanding will increase, which will raise carrying costs, and (3) bad debt or discount expenses will also rise. Thus the key question when deciding on a credit policy change is this: Will sales revenues rise more than costs, causing net income to increase, or will the increase in sales revenues be more than offset by higher costs?

Table 11-1 illustrates the general idea behind credit policy analysis. Column 1 shows the projected 1989 income statement for Roark Restaurant Supply Company under the assumption that the firm's current credit policy is maintained throughout the year. Because excess capacity exists, sales could be increased without adding either new plant or general overhead expense. Column 2 shows the expected effects of easing the credit policy by extending the credit period, offering larger discounts, relaxing credit standards, and easing collection efforts. Specifically, Roark is analyzing the effects of changing its credit terms from 1/10, net 30, to 2/10, net 40, relaxing its credit standards, and

---

[2]See Eugene F. Brigham and Louis C. Gapenski, *Intermediate Financial Management,* Chapter 19, for a more complete discussion of the problems with the ACP and aging schedule and how to correct for them.

Table 11-1 **Roark Restaurant Supply Company
Analysis of Credit Policy
(Millions of Dollars)**

	Projected 1989 Income Statement under Current Credit Policy (1)	Effect of Credit Policy Change (2)	Projected 1989 Income Statement under New Credit Policy (3)
Gross sales	$400.0	+ $130.0	$530.0
Less: Discounts	2.0	+ 4.0	6.0
Net sales	$398.0	+ $126.0	$524.0
Production costs, including overhead	280.0	+ 91.0	371.0
Gross profit before credit costs	$118.0	+ $ 35.0	$153.0
Credit-related costs:			
Cost of carrying receivables	3.3	+ 1.6	4.9
Credit analysis and collection expenses	5.0	− 3.0	2.0
Bad debt losses	10.0	+ 22.0	32.0
Gross profit	$ 99.7	+ $ 14.4	$114.1
Taxes (40%)	39.9	+ 5.7	45.6
Net income	$ 59.8	+ $ 8.7	$ 68.5

putting less pressure on slow-paying customers. Column 3 shows the projected 1989 income statement incorporating the expected effects of an easing in credit policy. The generally looser policy is expected to increase sales and lower collection costs, but discounts and several other types of cost will rise. The overall, bottom-line effect is an $8.7 million increase in projected profits. In the following paragraphs, we explain how the numbers in the table were calculated.

Roark's annual sales are $400 million. Under its current credit policy, 50 percent of those customers who pay do so on Day 10 and take the discount, 40 percent pay on the thirtieth day, and 10 percent pay late, on Day 40. Thus, Roark's average collection period is $(0.50)(10) + (0.40)(30) + (0.10)(40) = 21$ days.

Even though Roark spends $5 million annually to analyze accounts and to collect bad debts, 2.5 percent of sales will never be collected. Bad debt losses therefore amount to $(0.025)($400,000,000) = 10.0 million. In addition, Roark's cash collections will be reduced by the amount of discounts taken. Fifty percent of the customers who pay (97.5 percent of all customers pay) take the 1 percent discount, so discounts equal $($400,000,000)(0.975)(0.01)(0.50) = $1,950,000 \approx 2.0 million. Notice that total sales are multiplied by (1 − bad debt ratio) to obtain collected sales, and collected sales are then multiplied by the discount ratio times the percentage of customers who take the discount.

The annual cost of carrying receivables is equal to the average amount of receivables times the variable cost percentage times the cost of money used to carry receivables:

$$\begin{array}{ccccc} \text{Average} & & \text{Variable} & \text{Cost} & \text{Cost of} \\ \text{amount of} & \times & \text{cost} & \times & \text{of} & = & \text{carrying} \\ \text{receivables} & & \text{ratio} & \text{funds} & \text{receivables} \end{array} \;.$$

The average receivables balance, in turn, is equal to the average collection period times sales per day. Roark's ACP is 21 days, its variable cost ratio is 70 percent, and its cost of funds invested in receivables is 20 percent. Therefore, its cost of carrying receivables is approximately $3.3 million:

$$(\text{ACP}) \begin{pmatrix} \text{Sales} \\ \text{per} \\ \text{day} \end{pmatrix} \begin{pmatrix} \text{Variable} \\ \text{cost} \\ \text{ratio} \end{pmatrix} \begin{pmatrix} \text{Cost} \\ \text{of} \\ \text{funds} \end{pmatrix} = \begin{array}{c} \text{Cost of} \\ \text{carrying} \\ \text{receivables} \end{array}$$

$$(21) \left(\frac{\$400,000,000}{360} \right) (0.70)(0.20) = \$3,266,667 \approx \$3.3 \text{ million}.$$

Only variable costs enter into this calculation because this is the only cost element that must be financed as a result of a change in the credit policy. In other words, if a new customer buys goods worth $100, Roark will have to invest only $70 (in labor and materials), so it will have to finance only $70 even though accounts receivable rise by $100. Therefore, variable costs represent the company's investment in the goods sold.

Roark's new credit policy calls for a larger discount, a longer payment period, a relaxed collection effort, and lower credit standards. The company believes that these changes will lead to an increase in sales to $530 million per year. Under the new credit terms, management believes that 60 percent of the customers who pay will take the 2 percent discount and that bad debt losses will total 6 percent of sales, so discounts will increase to ($530,000,000)(0.94)(0.02)(0.60) = 5,978,400 ≈ $6 million. Half of the remaining paying customers will pay on the fortieth day, and the remainder on Day 50. The new ACP is thus estimated to be 24 days:

$$(0.6)(10) + (0.2)(40) + (0.2)(50) = 24 \text{ days.}$$

Also, the cost of carrying receivables will increase to $4.9 million:

$$(24) \left(\frac{\$530,000,000}{360} \right) (0.70)(0.20) = \$4,946,667 \approx \$4.9 \text{ million}.$$

Since the credit policy change will result in a longer ACP, Roark will have to wait longer to receive its profit on the goods it sells. Therefore, the firm will incur an opportunity cost due to not having the cash from these profits available for investment. The dollar amount of this opportunity cost is equal to the old sales per day times the change in ACP times the contribution margin times the cost of the funds invested in receivables, or

$$\text{Opportunity cost} = (\text{Old sales}/360)(\Delta ACP)(1 - v)(k)$$
$$= (\$400 \text{ million}/360)(3)(0.3)(0.20) = \$0.2 \text{ million.}$$

For simplicity, we have ignored this cost in our analysis.[3]

Because it will relax credit standards (hence credit checking expenses) and ease up on collections, the company expects to reduce its annual credit analysis and collection expenditures from $5 million to $2 million. However, the reduced credit standards and the relaxed collection effort are expected to raise bad debt losses from 2.5 percent to 6 percent of sales, or to $(0.06)(\$530,000,000) = \$32.0$ million.

The combined effect of all the changes in credit policy is a projected $8.7 million increase in net income. There would, of course, be corresponding changes on the projected balance sheet—the higher sales would necessitate somewhat larger cash balances, inventories, and perhaps (if the sales increase were large enough) more fixed assets. Accounts receivable would also increase. Since these asset increases would have to be financed, certain liability accounts or equity would also have to be increased.

The $8.7 million expected increase in net income is, of course, an estimate, and the actual effects of the change could be quite different. In the first place, there is uncertainty about the projected $130 million increase in sales. Conceivably, if Roark's competitors matched its changes, sales would not rise at all. Similar uncertainties must be attached to the number of customers who would take discounts, to production costs at higher or lower sales levels, to the costs of carrying additional receivables, and to the bad debt loss ratio. In view of all the uncertainties, management might deem the projected $8.7 million increase in net income insufficient to justify the change. In the final analysis, the decision to make the change will be based on judgment, but the type of quantitative analysis set forth here is essential to a good judgmental decision.

The preceding paragraphs give an overview of the way changes in credit policy are analyzed. As noted, the most important considerations have to do with changes in sales and production costs. Specific estimates of these effects are handled by the marketing and production departments within the framework set forth here. The financial manager has the responsibility for the overall analysis and also has a primary role in estimating several specific factors, including discounts taken, the cost of carrying accounts receivable, and bad debt losses. To evaluate a proposed change in credit policy, one could compare projected income statements, such as Column 1 versus Column 3 in Table 11-1. Alternatively, one could simply analyze Column 2, which shows the incremental effect (or the effect holding other things constant) of the proposed change. Of course, the two approaches are based on exactly the same data, so they must produce identical results. It is often preferable, however, to focus on the incremental approach; because firms usually change their credit poli-

---

[3]For a more complete discussion of the analysis of changes in credit policy, see Eugene F. Brigham and Louis C. Gapenski, *Intermediate Financial Management,* Chapter 19.

cies in specific divisions or on particular products and not across the board, an analysis of complete income statements might not be feasible.

INVENTORY MANAGEMENT

Inventories, which may be classified as (1) *raw materials,* (2) *work-in-process,* and (3) *finished goods,* are an essential part of most business operations. Like accounts receivable, inventory levels depend heavily on sales. However, whereas receivables build up *after* sales have been made, inventories must be acquired *before* sales are made. This is a critical difference, and the necessity of forecasting sales before establishing target inventory levels makes **inventory management** a difficult task.

The manner in which the firm's inventory is managed can have a direct effect on the value of the firm. Any procedure that allows a firm to achieve a given sales volume with a lower investment will increase the rate of return and, hence, increase the firm's value. However, actions to reduce inventory investment can also lead to lost sales because of stock-outs or costly production slowdowns. Managers must maintain inventories at levels that balance the benefits of reducing the level of investment against the costs associated with holding smaller inventories.

Inventory management focuses on three basic questions: (1) How many units of each inventory item should the firm hold in stock? (2) How many units should be ordered, or produced, at a given time? (3) At what point should inventory be ordered or produced? The remainder of this chapter is devoted to answering these questions.

inventory management
The balancing of a set of costs that increase with larger inventory holdings with a set of costs that decrease with larger order size.

Determining the Inventory Investment

In part, inventory policy is determined by the economics of the firm's industry; thus retailers have large stocks of finished goods but little, if any, raw materials or work-in-process. Moreover, the inventory policies of firms in a given industry can vary widely—inventory policy is very much subject to discretionary decisions.

No single executive establishes inventory policy. Rather, the firm's inventory policy is set by its executive committee, because production, marketing, and financial people all have a stake in inventory management. The production manager is concerned with raw materials inventory to insure continuous production; he or she has direct control over the length of the production process (which influences work-in-process inventories) and is vitally concerned with whether the firm produces on a smooth, continuous basis throughout the year, stockpiling finished goods inventories for seasonal sales, or whether it produces irregularly in response to orders. The marketing manager wants the firm to hold large stocks of inventories to insure rapid deliveries; this will make it easier to close sales. The financial manager is concerned with the level of inventories because of the effects excessive inventories have on profitability: (1) they reduce the total assets utilization ratio, and (2) there are substantial costs of carrying inventories, so excessive inventories erode the profit margin.

Table 11-2 **Costs Associated with Inventories**

	Approximate Annual Percentage Cost
Carrying Costs	
Cost of capital tied up	12.0%
Storage and handling costs	0.5
Insurance	0.5
Property taxes	1.0
Depreciation and obsolescence	12.0
Total	26.0%
Ordering, Shipping, and Receiving Costs	
Cost of placing orders, including production and set-up costs	varies
Shipping and handling costs	2.5%
Costs of Running Short	
Lost sales	varies
Loss of customer goodwill	varies
Disruption of production schedules	varies

Note: These costs vary from firm to firm, from item to item, and over time. The figures shown are U.S. Department of Commerce estimates for an average manufacturing firm. When costs vary so widely that no meaningful numbers can be assigned, we simply report "varies."

Through the accounting staff, the financial manager maintains all records relating to inventories, and in this capacity he or she is responsible for establishing information systems to monitor inventory usage and to replenish stocks as necessary. This information system is not complex in a single-product, single-plant firm, but in most modern corporations the inventory control process is as complex as it is important. Visualize an automobile or an appliance manufacturer, with thousands of dealers stocking hundreds of styles and colors of various automobiles, stoves, or refrigerators, as well as thousands of spare parts, all across the country. Production must be geared both to stocks on hand and to sales levels, and any mistake can result either in excessive stocks (which will lose value when the new models appear) or in lost sales. Grocery stores, department stores, plumbing manufacturers, textbook publishers, and most other firms are faced with similar problems.

Inventory Costs

The goal of inventory management is to provide the inventories required to sustain operations at the minimum cost. The first step is to identify all the costs involved in purchasing and maintaining inventories. Table 11-2 lists the typical costs associated with inventories, broken down into three categories: costs associated with carrying inventories, costs associated with ordering and receiving inventories, and costs associated with running short of inventory.

Figure 11-1 **Determination of the Optimal Order Quantity**

To avoid the problems that may arise from carrying too much or too little inventory, a business must determine the optimal quantity of a product to purchase each time an order is placed. As this figure shows, carrying costs rise steadily as order size increases; ordering costs, on the other hand, decline with larger order sizes. The sum of these two curves is the total cost curve, and the lowest point on that curve is the optimal order size, or economic ordering quantity (EOQ).

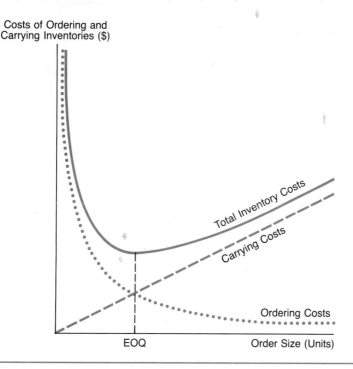

Although they may well be the most important element, we shall at this point disregard the third category of costs — the costs of running short (often called *stock-out costs*); these are dealt with by adding safety stocks, which we will discuss later. The costs that remain for consideration at this stage, then, are carrying costs and ordering, shipping, and receiving costs.

The Optimal Ordering Quantity

Inventories are obviously necessary, but it is equally obvious that a firm will suffer if it has too much or too little inventory. How can management determine the *optimal* inventory level? One commonly used approach is the *economic ordering quantity (EOQ) model,* which is described in this section.

Figure 11-1 illustrates the basic premise on which inventory theory is built, namely, that some costs rise with larger inventories while other costs decline and that there is an optimal order size that minimizes the total costs associated with inventories. The average investment in inventories depends on how frequently orders are placed; if a small order is placed every day, average inventories will be much smaller than if one large order is placed annually. Further, as Figure 11-1 shows, some inventory-associated **carrying costs** rise with larger orders; because larger orders mean larger average inventories, warehousing costs, interest on funds tied up in inventory, insurance, and obsolescence all will increase. At the same time, **ordering costs** decline with large orders, because the costs of placing orders, setting up production runs, and handling shipments all will decline if the firm orders infrequently and consequently holds larger quantities.

carrying costs
The costs associated with carrying inventories, including storage, capital, and depreciation costs; generally increase in proportion to the average amount of inventory held.

ordering costs
The costs of placing and receiving orders; these costs are fixed for each order regardless of the size of the order.

economic ordering quantity (EOQ)
The optimal (least-cost) quantity of inventory that should be ordered.

EOQ model
Formula for determining the order quantity that minimizes the total inventory cost:
$EOQ = \sqrt{2FS/CP}$.

When the carrying and ordering cost curves in Figure 11-1 are added together, the sum represents the total inventory cost. The point where the total inventory cost curve is minimized represents the **economic ordering quantity (EOQ),** and this, in turn, determines the optimal average inventory level. A graph like Figure 11-1 is useful in helping the firm determine its approximate optimal ordering quantity, but to find the exact value it would be necessary to plot every possible ordering quantity. An easier method is to use the economic ordering quantity, or **EOQ, model.** It can be shown that under certain reasonable assumptions, the order quantity that minimizes the total cost curve in Figure 11-1 can be found by using the following formula:

$$EOQ = \sqrt{\frac{2FS}{CP}}. \qquad (11\text{-}1)$$

Here

$$EOQ = \text{the economic ordering quantity, or the optimal}$$
$$\text{quantity to be ordered each time an order is placed.}$$

$$F = \text{fixed costs of placing and receiving an order.}$$

$$S = \text{annual sales in units.}$$

$$C = \text{carrying cost expressed as a percentage of inventory value.}$$

$$P = \text{purchase price per unit of inventory.}$$

The assumptions of the economic ordering quantity (EOQ) model, which will be relaxed shortly, include the following: (1) sales can be forecast perfectly, (2) sales are evenly distributed throughout the year, and (3) orders are received with no delays whatever.

To illustrate the EOQ model, consider the following data, supplied by Romantic Books, Inc., publisher of the classic novel *Madame Boudoir:*

$$S = \text{sales} = 26,000 \text{ copies per year.}$$

$$C = \text{carrying cost} = 20 \text{ percent of inventory value.}$$

P = purchase price per book to Romantic Books from a printing company = $6.1538 per copy. The sales price is $9, but this is irrelevant for our purposes.

F = fixed cost per order = $1,000. The bulk of this cost is the labor cost for setting the plates on the presses, as well as for setting up the binding equipment for the production run; the printer bills this cost separately from the $6.1538 cost per copy.

Substituting these data into Equation 11-1, we obtain

$$EOQ = \sqrt{\frac{2FS}{CP}}$$

$$= \sqrt{\frac{(2)(\$1,000)(26,000)}{(0.2)(\$6.1538)}}$$

$$= \sqrt{42,250,316}$$

$$= 6,500 \text{ copies.}$$

Average inventory holdings depend directly on the EOQ; this relationship is illustrated graphically in Figure 11-2. Immediately after an order is received, 6,500 copies are in stock. The usage rate, or sales rate, is 500 copies per week (26,000/52 weeks), so inventories are drawn down by this amount each week. Thus the actual number of units held in inventory will vary from 6,500 books just after an order is received to zero just before an order arrives. On average, the number of units held will be 6,500/2 = 3,250 books. At a cost of $6.1538 per book, the average investment in inventories will be 3,250 × $6.1538 = $19,999.85 ≈ $20,000. If inventories are financed by bank loans, the loan will vary from a high of $40,000 to a low of $0, but the average amount outstanding over the course of a year will be $20,000.

Notice that the EOQ, and hence the average inventory, rises with the square root of sales. Therefore, a given increase in sales will result in a less than proportional increase in inventories, and the inventory/sales ratio will decline as sales grow. For example, Romantic Books' EOQ is 6,500 copies at an annual sales level of 26,000, and the average inventory is 3,250 copies, worth $20,000. However, if sales increase by 100 percent, to 52,000 copies per year, the EOQ will rise to only 9,192 copies or by 41 percent, and the average inventory will rise by this same percentage. This suggests that there are economies of scale in holding individual items of inventory.

Setting the Order Point

If a 2-week lead time is required for production and shipping, what is Romantic Books' **order point,** or the inventory level at which an order should be placed? If we use a 52-week year, Romantic Books sells 26,000/52 = 500 books per week. Thus, if a 2-week lag occurs between ordering and receipt, Romantic

order point
Point at which stock on hand must be replenished.

Figure 11-2 **Inventory Position without Safety Stock**

This figure shows Romantic Books' average inventory position between orders. The EOQ of 6,500 copies represents the maximum inventory and determines the average inventory (6,500/2 = 3,250). The expected sales rate of 500 copies per week determines the order frequency (every 13 weeks). Because a 2-week lead time is required on orders, the order point is reached when inventories reach 1,000 copies. This model assumes that both the sales rate and the required lead time on orders will never change.

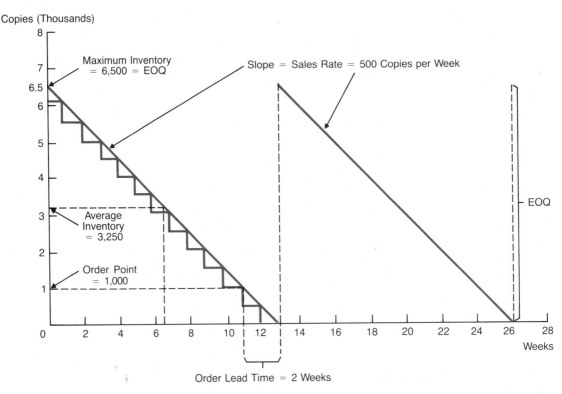

Books must place the order when there are 2(500) = 1,000 books on hand. At the end of the 2-week production and shipping period, the new inventory balance will be down to zero, but just at that time the order of new books will arrive.

Goods in Transit

If a new order must be placed before the previous order is received, the goods-in-transit inventory builds up. Goods in transit are items that have been ordered but not yet received. The goods-in-transit inventory builds up if the normal delivery lead time is longer than the time between orders. Although this complicates matters somewhat, the simplest solution to the problem is to deduct goods in transit when calculating the order point. In other words, the reorder point would be calculated as follows:

Order point = (Lead time in weeks × Weekly usage) − Goods in transit.

Goods in transit is not an issue for Romantic Books because the firm orders 26,000/6,500 = 4 times a year, or once every 13 weeks, and the delivery lead time is 2 weeks. However, suppose that Romantic Books ordered 1,000 copies of *Madame Boudoir* every 2 weeks and the delivery lead time was 3 weeks. In that case, whenever an order was placed, another order of books would be in transit. Therefore, Romantic Book's order point would be:

$$\text{Order point} = (3 \times 500) - 1,000$$
$$= 1,500 - 1,000$$
$$= 500.$$

Safety Stocks

If Romantic Books knew for certain that both the sales rate and the order lead time would never vary, it could operate exactly as shown in Figure 11-2. However, sales rates do change, and because production or shipping delays are frequently encountered, the company will carry additional inventories, or **safety stocks.**

The concept of a safety stock is illustrated in Figure 11-3. First, note that the slope of the sales line measures the expected rate of sales. The company *expects* to sell 500 copies per week, but let us assume a maximum likely sales rate of twice this amount, or 1,000 copies per week. Romantic Books initially orders 7,500, the EOQ plus a safety stock of 1,000 copies. Subsequently, it reorders the EOQ, 6,500 copies, whenever the inventory level falls to 2,000 copies (the safety stock of 1,000 copies plus the 1,000 copies expected to be used while awaiting delivery of the order). Notice that the company could, during the 2-week delivery period, sell 1,000 copies a week, doubling its normal expected sales. This maximum rate of sales is shown by the steeper dashed line in Figure 11-3. The condition that makes this higher maximum sales rate possible is the introduction of a safety stock of 1,000 copies.

The safety stock is also useful to guard against delays in receiving orders. The expected delivery time is 2 weeks; however, with a 1,000-copy safety stock, the company could maintain sales at the expected rate of 500 copies per week for an additional 2 weeks if production or shipping delays held up an order.

Safety stocks obviously are useful, but they do have a cost. For Romantic Books, the average inventory is now EOQ/2 plus a safety stock of 1,000 units, or 6,500/2 + 1,000 = 3,250 + 1,000 = 4,250 books, and the average inventory value is (4,250)($6.1538) = $26,154. The increase in average inventory resulting from the safety stock causes an increase in inventory carrying costs.

safety stocks
Additional inventories carried to guard against changes in sales rates or production/shipping delays.

Figure 11-3 **Inventory Position with Safety Stock Included**

Because sales rates and required lead times do vary, a business must carry safety
stocks. In this example 1,000 copies of safety stock are ordered in addition to the
EOQ of 6,500 copies. The order point now becomes 2,000 copies. Carrying safety
stock allows the firm to cover a sales increase to 1,000 copies per week during the
2-week reorder lead time, should that occur. If delays are encountered in receiving
orders, the company could continue its average sales rate for 2 weeks beyond the
usual 2-week delivery time.

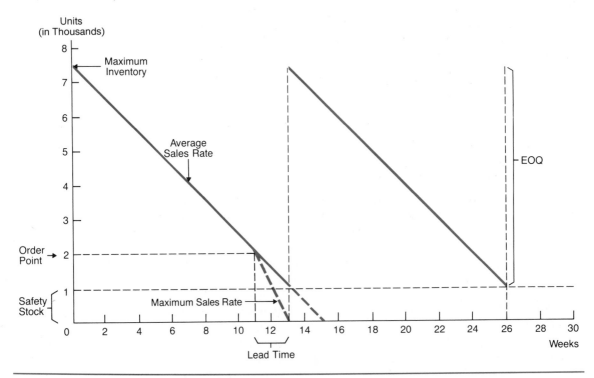

The optimal safety stock varies from situation to situation, but in general
it *increases* with (1) the uncertainty of demand forecasts, (2) the costs (in
terms of lost sales and lost goodwill) that result from inventory shortages, and
(3) the probability of delays in receiving shipments. The optimum safety stock
decreases as the cost of carrying the extra inventory increases.

Inventory Control Systems

The EOQ model, plus safety stocks, helps establish proper inventory levels,
but inventory management also involves the *inventory ordering and control
system*. There are various control systems that can be used — some simple and

some complex. One simple control procedure is the **red-line method;** here inventory items are stocked in a bin, and a red line is drawn around the inside of the bin at the level of the order point. When the red line shows, the inventory clerk places an order. The **two-bin method** has inventory items stocked in two bins. When the working bin is empty, an order is placed and inventory is drawn from the second bin.

Larger companies employ **computerized inventory control systems.** The computer starts with an inventory count in memory. As withdrawals are made, they are recorded in the computer, and the inventory balance is revised. When the order point is reached, the computer automatically places an order, and when the order is received, the recorded balance is increased. Retail stores have carried this system quite far — each merchandise item has a magnetic code and as an item is checked out, it passes over a reader that adjusts the computer's inventory balance at the same time the price is fed into the cash register. When the balance drops to the order point, an order is placed.

A good inventory control system is dynamic, not static. A company like IBM or General Motors stocks thousands of different types of items. The sales (or use) of these various items can rise or fall quite separately from rising or falling overall corporate sales. As the usage rate for an individual item begins to fall, the inventory manager must adjust its balance to avoid ending up with obsolete items — either finished goods or parts and materials for use in finished goods.

The EOQ model is useful for establishing order sizes and average inventory levels *given a correctly forecast sales or usage rate.* Usage rates change over time, however, and a good inventory management system must respond promptly to these changes in sales. One system that is used to monitor inventory usage rates and then to modify EOQs and inventory levels is the **ABC system.** Here the firm analyzes each inventory item on the basis of its cost, frequency of usage, seriousness of a stock-out, order lead time, and other criteria related to the item's importance. Items that are expensive, are frequently used, and have long order lead times are put in the A category; somewhat less important items are put in the B category; and relatively unimportant items are designated C. Management reviews the A items' recent usage rates, stock position, and delivery time situation quite frequently, say monthly, and adjusts the EOQ as necessary. Category B items are reviewed and adjusted less frequently, say every quarter, and C items are reviewed perhaps annually. Thus the inventory control group's resources are concentrated where they will do the most good.

Good inventory management will result in a relatively high inventory utilization ratio, low write-offs of obsolete or deteriorated inventories, and few instances of work stoppages or lost sales because of stockouts. All this, in turn, contributes to a high profit margin, a high total assets utilization rate, a high rate of return on investment, and a strong stock price.

red-line method
An inventory control procedure in which a red line drawn around the inside of an inventory-stocked bin indicates the order point level.

two-bin method
An inventory control procedure in which the order point is reached when one of two inventory-stocked bins is empty.

computerized inventory control system
Inventory control through the use of computers to indicate order points and to adjust inventory balances.

ABC system
A system used to categorize inventory items to ensure the most critical inventory items are reviewed most often.

Effects of Inflation on Inventory Management

Moderate inflation — say, 3 percent per year — can largely be ignored for purposes of inventory management, but the higher the rate of inflation, the more important it is to consider this factor. If the rate of inflation in the types of goods the firm stocks tends to be relatively constant, it can be dealt with quite easily — simply deduct the expected annual rate of inflation from the carrying cost percentage, C, in Equation 11-1, and use this modified version of the EOQ model to establish the working stock.

The reason for making this deduction is that inflation causes the value of the inventory to rise, thus offsetting somewhat the effects of depreciation and other carrying-cost factors. Because C will now be smaller, the calculated EOQ, and hence the average inventory, will increase. The higher the rate of inflation, however, the higher the interest rates, and this factor will increase C, thus lowering the EOQ and average inventories. On balance, there is no evidence that inflation either raises or lowers the optimal inventories of firms in the aggregate. Inflation should still be explicitly considered, though, for it will raise the individual firm's optimal holdings if the rate of inflation for its own inventories is above average (and is greater than the effects of inflation on interest rates), and vice versa.

SUMMARY

Because the typical manufacturing firm has about 40 percent of its assets invested in inventories and receivables, the management of these assets is obviously important. The investment in receivables is dependent on the firm's *credit policy,* which consists of four variables: (1) the *credit standards,* or the financial strength customers must exhibit to be granted credit; (2) the *credit period,* or length of time for which credit is extended; (3) *cash discounts* designed to encourage rapid payment; and (4) *collection policy,* which helps determine how long accounts remain outstanding. Credit policy has an important impact on the volume of sales, and the optimal credit policy involves a trade-off between the costs inherent in various credit policies and the profits generated by higher sales. From a practical standpoint, it is impossible to determine the optimal credit policy in a mathematical sense; good credit management involves a blending of quantitative analysis and business judgment.

Inventory management centers around the balancing of a set of costs that increase with larger inventory holdings (storage costs, cost of capital, physical deterioration) and a set of costs that decline with larger holdings (ordering costs, lost sales, disruptions of production schedules). Inventory management has been quantified to a greater extent than most aspects of business. The EOQ model is one important part of most inventory systems. This model can be used to determine the optimal order quantity, which, when combined with a specified safety stock, determines the average inventory level.

RESOLUTION TO DECISION IN FINANCE

The Price Is Wrong

Contextual missed the chance for profitability by inches. Although the ad hoc bookkeeping and absence of financial planning didn't help (no warning lights were in place to flash before calamity hit), the real problem was that the founders miscalculated price and mismanaged inventory. Because Contextual financed its expansion by borrowing on receivables, its miscalculations were masked by its rapid growth until it was too late to stem the tide of red ink.

The first foreshadowing of the debacle that lay ahead came when Contextual's accountants prepared a review of fiscal 1983. To estimate inventory, the accountants merely divided the total actual costs of materials by a percentage of each item's price at sale. This resulted in an estimated inventory of $246,490, which "felt high" to several of the founders but was used anyway. The plant was so busy that the figure was used again for the next six-month bookkeeping period as well. To make matters worse, in the scramble to fill orders, no one had ever analyzed what percentage of materials were wasted in the production process, which also threw inventory calculations way off. When the principals finally got worried enough to do a physical inventory, they discovered that they had overestimated the value of inventory on the plant floor by more than $100,000.

Panicked, the founding partners immediately took steps to computerize their accounting, something they had been too busy to do up until that point. When they looked at the computer screen, they didn't like what it told them. They realized that they had not only been way off on inventory, but that they must have been underestimating overhead and labor costs as well. When the four company founders had originally set out to estimate labor costs, they had performed the actual manufacturing operations themselves. When they did this, however, they managed to overlook such integral tasks as setting up the machinery and moving work in progress from one work-station to the next. In the end, the founders estimated that five parts could be completed per minute, whereas their 86 employees were actually producing a maximum of only three parts on the plant floor.

Once the numbers were revealed, the inevitability of Contextual's demise was clear. Sadly, it is easy to see how disaster could have been averted quite simply. A modest price increase as little as two years before Contextual was forced to sell its assets to a rival would have put the company in the black. Getting a handle on physical inventory as soon as there was an inkling that accounting estimates were off would have been another way to get on track. As it was, "we thought we were making money," says one of Contextual's cofounders ruefully, "almost right up to the end."

Source: Robert A. Mamis, "The Price Is Wrong," *Inc.,* May 1986, 159–160, 163, 164.

QUESTIONS

11-1 Is it true that when one firm sells to another on credit, the seller records the transaction as an account receivable while the buyer records it as an account payable and that, disregarding discounts, the receivable typically exceeds the payable by the amount of profit on the sale?

11-2   What are the four elements in a firm's credit policy? To what extent can firms set their own credit policies as opposed to having to accept credit policies dictated by "the competition"?

11-3   Suppose a firm makes a purchase and receives the shipment on February 1. The credit terms as stated on the invoice read, "20/10, net 40, May 1 dating." What is the latest date on which payment can be made and the discount still be taken? What is the date on which payment must be made if the discount is not taken?

11-4   **a.** What is the average collection period for a firm whose sales are $2,880,000 per year and whose accounts receivable are $312,000? (Use 360 days per year.)

            b. Is it true that if this firm sells on terms of 3/10, net 40, its customers probably all pay on time?

11-5   Is it true that if a firm calculates its average collection period, it has no need for an aging schedule?

11-6   Firm A had no credit losses last year, but 1 percent of Firm B's accounts receivable proved to be uncollectible and resulted in losses. Should Firm B fire its credit manager and hire A's?

11-7   Indicate by a (+), (−), or (0) whether each of the following events would probably cause accounts receivable (A/R), sales, and profits to increase, decrease, or be affected in an indeterminant manner:

	A/R	Sales	Profits
a. The firm tightens its credit standards.	___	___	___
b. The credit terms are changed from 2/10, net 30, to 3/10, net 30.	___	___	___
c. The terms are changed from 2/10, net 30, to 3/10, net 40.	___	___	___
d. The firm's major competitor changes its credit policy from 2/10, net 30 to 2/10, net 60.	___	___	___

11-8   If a firm calculates its optimal inventory of widgets to be 1,000 units when the general rate of inflation is 2 percent, is it true that the optimal inventory (in units) will almost certainly rise if the general rate of inflation climbs to 10 percent?

11-9   Indicate by a (+), (−), or (0) whether each of the following events would probably cause average annual inventories (the sum of the inventories held at the end of each month of the year divided by 12) to rise, fall, or be affected in an indeterminant manner:

            a. The firm's suppliers switch from delivering by train to air freight.   ___

            b. The firm changes from producing to meet seasonal sales to steady year-round production. Sales peak at Christmas.   ___

            c. Competition in the markets in which the firm sells increases.   ___

            d. The rate of general inflation increases.   ___

            e. Interest rates rise; other things are constant.   ___

11-10   A firm can reduce its investment in inventory by having its suppliers hold raw materials inventories and its customers hold finished goods inventories. Explain actions a firm can take that would result in larger inventories for its suppliers and customers and smaller inventories for itself. What are the limitations of such actions?

11-11   The toy business is subject to large seasonal demand fluctuations. What effect would such fluctuations have on inventory decisions of toy manufacturers and toy retailers?

SELF-TEST PROBLEMS

ST-1 The Carson Company expects to have sales of $10 million this year under its current operating policies. Its variable costs as a percentage of sales are 80 percent, and its cost of capital is 16 percent. Currently Carson's credit policy is net 25 (no discount for early payment). However, its ACP is 30 days, and its bad debt loss percentage is 2 percent. Carson spends $50,000 per year to collect bad debts, and its effective tax rate is 40 percent.

The credit manager is considering two alternative proposals (given below) for changing Carson's credit policy. Find the expected change in net income, taking into consideration anticipated changes in carrying costs for accounts receivable, the probable bad debt losses, and the discounts likely to be taken, for each proposal. Should a change in credit policy be made?

Proposal 1: Lengthen the credit period by going from net 25 to net 30. The bad debt collection expenditures will remain constant. Under this proposal, sales are expected to increase by $1 million annually, and the bad debt loss percentage on *new* sales is expected to rise to 4 percent (the loss percentage on old sales should not change). In addition, the ACP is expected to increase from 30 to 45 days on all sales.

Proposal 2: Shorten the credit period by going from net 25 to net 20. Again, collection expenses will remain constant. The anticipated effects of this change are (1) a decrease in sales of $1 million per year, (2) a decline in the ACP from 30 to 22 days, and (3) a decline in the bad debt loss percentage to 1 percent on all sales.

ST-2 The Mrs. Morris Bread Company buys and then sells (as bread) 2.6 million bushels of wheat annually. The wheat must be purchased in multiples of 2,000 bushels. Ordering costs, which include grain elevator removal charges of $3,500, are $5,000 per order. Annual carrying costs are 2 percent of the purchase price per bushel of $5. The company maintains a safety stock of 200,000 bushels. The delivery time is 6 weeks.

   a. What is the EOQ?
   b. At what inventory level should a reorder be placed to prevent having to draw on the safety stock?
   c. What are the total inventory costs?
   d. The wheat processor agrees to pay the elevator removal charges if Mrs. Morris Bread will purchase wheat in quantities of 650,000 bushels. Would it be to Mrs. Morris Bread's advantage to order under this alternative?

PROBLEMS

11-1 **Receivables investment.** Jerry Thomas, the new credit manager for Associates International, is studying the firm's credit accounts. The company sells all its products on credit terms of 2/10, net 30. Thomas's predecessor told him that the company's ACP is 36 days and that 60 percent of the customers take the discount. What is the ACP for the firm's customers that elect not to take the discount?

11-2 **Receivables investment.** Meditec, Inc., sells on terms of 2/10, net 30. Total sales for the year are $500,000. Forty-five percent of Meditec's customers pay on the tenth day and take the discount; the other 55 percent pay, on average, 45 days after their purchases.

   a. What is the average collection period?
   b. What is the average amount of receivables?

c. What would happen to the average receivables if Meditec toughened up on its collection policy with the result that all nondiscount customers paid on the thirtieth day?

11-3   **Toughening credit terms.** The Montrose Corporation with annual sales of $9 million, sells on terms of 2/10, net 30. Currently 40 percent of its customers pay on the tenth day and take discounts; the other 60 percent pay, on average, 40 days after their purchases. Montrose plans to toughen its credit policy so that all nondiscount customers will pay on the thirtieth day.

a. What is the average collection period both before and after the change?

b. What is the average collection in receivables both before and after the change?

11-4   **Easing credit terms.** Ozuna Electronics, Inc., is considering changing its credit terms from 2/15, net 30, to 3/10, net 30, to speed collections. At present, 50 percent of Ozuna's customers take the 2 percent discount. Under the new terms, discount customers are expected to rise to 60 percent. Regardless of the credit terms, half of the customers who do not take the discount are expected to pay on time, whereas the remainder will pay 10 days late. The change does not involve a relaxation of credit standards; therefore, bad debt losses are not expected to rise above their present 2 percent level. However, the more generous cash discount terms are expected to increase sales from $1 million to $1.3 million per year. Ozuna's variable cost ratio is 70 percent, its cost of capital invested in accounts receivable is 10 percent, and its average tax rate is 40 percent.

a. What is the average collection period before and after the change?

b. Calculate the discount costs before and after the change.

c. Calculate the dollar cost of carrying receivables before and after the change.

d. Calculate the bad debt losses before and after the change.

e. What is the incremental profit from the change in credit terms? Should Ozuna change its credit terms?

11-5   **Credit analysis.** University Distributors makes all sales on a credit basis, selling on terms of 2/10, net 30. Once a year it evaluates the creditworthiness of all its customers. The evaluation procedure ranks customers from 1 to 5, with 1 indicating the "best" customers. Results of the ranking are as follows:

Customer Category	Percentage of Bad Debts	Average Collection Period (Days)	Credit Decision	Annual Sales Lost Due to Credit Restrictions
1	None	10	Unlimited credit	None
2	1.0	12	Unlimited credit	None
3	3.0	20	Limited credit	$365,000
4	9.0	60	Limited credit	$182,500
5	16.0	90	Limited credit	$230,000

The variable cost ratio is 75 percent, and its average tax rate is 40 percent. The cost of capital invested in receivables is 15 percent. What would be the effect on profitability of extending unlimited credit to each of the Categories 3, 4, and 5? (*Hint:* Determine separately the effect on the income statement of changing each policy. In other words, find the change in sales, change in production costs, change in receivables and the cost of carrying receivables, change in bad debt costs, and so forth, down to the change in gross profits.)

11-6 **Tightening credit terms.** Diana Pappas, the new credit manager of the Longstreet Corporation, was alarmed to find that Longstreet sells on credit terms of net 60 days even though industrywide credit terms have recently been lowered to net 30 days. On annual credit sales of $2.5 million, Longstreet currently averages 70 days' sales in accounts receivable. Pappas estimates that tightening the credit terms to 30 days would reduce annual sales to $2.2 million, but accounts receivable would drop to 35 days of sales, and the savings on investment in receivables should more than overcome any loss in profit. Longstreet's variable cost ratio is 85 percent, and its average tax rate is 40 percent. If Longstreet's cost of funds invested in receivables is 18 percent, should the change in credit terms be made?

11-7 **Relaxing collection efforts.** The Lehigh Corporation has annual credit sales of $4 million. Current expenses for the collection department are $60,000, bad debt losses are 2 percent of sales, and the average collection period is 30 days. Lehigh is considering easing its collection efforts so that collection expenses will be reduced to $45,000 per year. The change is expected to increase bad debt losses to 3 percent as well as to increase the average collection period to 45 days. However, sales should increase to $4.3 million per year.

Lehigh's opportunity cost of funds is 13 percent, its variable cost ratio is 75 percent, and its average tax rate is 40 percent?

a. Should Lehigh relax its collection efforts?

(Do Parts b and c only if you are using the computerized problem diskette.)

b. Would the change in collection efforts be profitable if sales rose only to $4.2 million?

c. What would be Lehigh's loss if it relaxed its collection efforts and sales remained at $4 million?

11-8 **Economic ordering quantity.** Tampa Builders' Supply expects to sell 5,000 pounds of nails this year. Ordering costs are $50 per order, and carrying costs are $2 per pound.

a. What is the economic ordering quantity (EOQ)?

b. How many orders will be placed this year?

c. What is the average inventory under this plan, expressed in pounds?

11-9 **Inventory cost.** Computer Supplies, Inc., must order floppy diskettes from its supplier in lots of one dozen boxes. Given the following information, complete the table below and determine the economic ordering quantity for floppy diskettes for Computer Supplies.

Annual demand: 2,800 dozen
Cost per order placed: $5.25
Carrying cost: 20%
Price per dozen: $30

Order size (dozens)	35	56	70	140	200	2,800
Number of orders	——	——	——	——	——	——
Average inventory	——	——	——	——	——	——
Carrying cost	——	——	——	——	——	——
Order cost	——	——	——	——	——	——
Total cost	——	——	——	——	——	——

11-10 **Economic ordering quantity.** Green Thumb Garden Centers, Inc., sells 120,000 bags of lawn fertilizer annually. The optimal safety stock (which is on hand initially) is

1,000 bags. Each bag costs Green Thumb $2, inventory carrying costs are 20 percent, and the cost of placing an order with its supplier is $30.

a. What is the economic ordering quantity?

b. What is the maximum inventory of fertilizer?

c. What will Green Thumb's average inventory be?

d. How often must the company order?

11-11   **EOQ and ordering discounts.** Worthington Toys, a large manufacturer of toys and dolls, uses large quantities of flesh-colored cloth in its doll production process. Throughout the year, the firm uses 1,000,000 square yards of this cloth. The fixed costs of placing and receiving an order are $2,000, including a $1,500 set-up charge at the mill. The price of the cloth is $2.00 per square yard, and the annual cost of carrying this inventory item is 20 percent of the price. Worthington maintains a 10,000 square yard safety stock. The cloth supplier requires a two-week lead time from order to delivery.

a. What is the EOQ for this cloth?

b. What is the average inventory dollar value, including the safety stock?

c. What is the total cost of ordering and carrying the inventory, including the safety stock? (Assume that the safety stock is on hand at the beginning of the year.)

d. Using a 52-week year, at what inventory unit level should an order be placed? (Again, assume the 10,000 unit safety stock is on hand.)

11-12   **Changes in the EOQ.** The following relationships for inventory costs have been established for the Malone Corporation:

1. Annual sales are 780,000 units.

2. The purchase price per unit is $1.00.

3. The carrying cost is 15 percent of the purchase price of goods.

4. The cost per order placed is $40.

5. Desired safety stock is 15,000 units (on hand initially).

6. One week is required for delivery.

a. What is the most economical order quantity? (Round to the 100s.) What is the total cost of ordering and carrying inventories at the EOQ?

b. What is the optimal number of orders to be placed?

c. At what inventory level should Malone order?

d. If annual unit sales double, what is the percent increase in the EOQ? What is the elasticity of EOQ with respect to sales (percent change in EOQ/percent change in sales)?

e. If the cost per order doubles, what is the elasticity of EOQ with respect to cost per order?

f. If the carrying cost declines by 50 percent, what is the elasticity of EOQ with respect to that change?

g. If purchase price declines by 50 percent, what is the elasticity of EOQ with respect to that change?

ANSWERS TO SELF-TEST PROBLEMS

ST-1   Under the current credit policy, the Carson Company has no discounts, collection expenses are $50,000, bad debt losses are $(0.02)(\$10,000,000) = \$200,000$, and average accounts receivable are (ACP)(Average sales per day) $= (30)(\$10,000,000/360) =$

$833,333. The firm's cost of carrying these receivables is (Variable cost ratio) (A/R) (Cost of capital) = $(0.80)($833,333)(0.16) = $106,667$. It is necessary to multiply by the variable cost ratio because the actual *investment* in receivables is less than the dollar amount of the receivables.

Proposal 1: Lengthen the credit period so that the following occur:
1. Sales increase by $1 million.
2. Discounts = $0.
3. Bad debt losses = $(0.02)($10,000,000) + (0.04)($1,000,000)$

$$= \$200,000 + \$40,000$$

$$= \$240,000.$$

4. ACP = 45 days on all sales.
5. New average receivables = $(45)($11,000,000/360) = $1,375,000$.
6. Cost of carrying receivables = (v)(k)(Average accounts receivable)

$$= (0.80)(0.16)(\$1,375,000)$$

$$= \$176,000.$$

7. Change in cost of carrying receivables = $176,000 − $106,667

$$= \$69,333.$$

8. Collection expenses = $50,000.
   Analysis of proposed change:

	Income Statement under Current Policy	Effect of Change	Income Statement under New Policy
Gross sales	$10,000,000	+ $1,000,000	$11,000,000
Less: Discounts	0	+ 0	0
Net sales	$10,000,000	+ $1,000,000	$11,000,000
Production costs (80%)	8,000,000	+ 800,000	8,800,000
Gross profits before credit costs	$ 2,000,000	+ $ 200,000	$ 2,200,000
Credit-related costs:			
Cost of carrying receivables	106,667	+ 69,333	176,000
Collection expenses	50,000	+ 0	50,000
Bad debt losses	200,000	+ 40,000	240,000
Gross profit	$ 1,643,333	+ $ 90,667	$ 1,734,000
Taxes (40%)	657,333	+ 36,267	693,600
Net income	$ 986,000	+ 54,400	$ 1,040,400

The proposed change appears to be a good one, assuming the assumptions are correct.

Proposal 2: Shorten the credit period to net 20 so that the following occur:
1. Sales decrease by $1 million.
2. Discount = $0.
3. Bad debt losses = $(0.01)($9,000,000) = $90,000$.
4. ACP = 22 days.
5. New average receivables = $(22)($9,000,000/360) = $550,000$.

6. Cost of carrying receivables = (v)(k)(Average accounts receivable)

$$= (0.80)(0.16)(\$550,000)$$

$$= \$70,400.$$

7. Collection expenses = $50,000.

Analysis of proposed change:

	Income Statement under Current Policy	Effect of Change	Income Statement under New Policy
Gross sales	$10,000,000	− $1,000,000	$9,000,000
Less: Discounts	0	0	0
Net sales	$10,000,000	− $1,000,000	$9,000,000
Production costs (80%)	8,000,000	− 800,000	7,200,000
Gross profits before credit costs	$ 2,000,000	− $ 200,000	$1,800,000
Credit-related costs:			
Cost of carrying receivables	106,667	− 36,267	70,400
Collection expenses	50,000	0	50,000
Bad debt losses	200,000	− 110,000	90,000
Gross profit	$ 1,643,333	− $ 53,733	$1,589,600
Taxes (40%)	657,333	− 21,493	635,840
Net income	$ 986,000	− $ 32,240	$ 953,760

This change reduces net income, so it should be rejected. Carson will increase profits by accepting Proposal 1 to lengthen the credit period from 25 days to 30 days, assuming all assumptions are correct. This may or may not be the *optimal,* or profit-maximizing, credit policy, but it does appear to be a movement in the right direction.

ST-2 a.

$$EOQ = \sqrt{\frac{2(F)(S)}{(C)(P)}}$$

$$= \sqrt{\frac{(2)(\$5,000)(2,600,000)}{(0.02)(\$5.00)}}$$

$$= 509,902 \text{ bushels.}$$

Since the firm must order in multiples of 2,000 bushels, it should order in quantities of 510,000 bushels.

b. Average weekly sales = 2,600,000/52

$$= 50,000 \text{ bushels.}$$

Order point = 6 weeks' sales + Safety stock

$$= 6(50,000) + 200,000$$

$$= 300,000 + 200,000$$

$$= 500,000 \text{ bushels.}$$

c. Total inventory costs:

$$\text{TIC} = \text{CP}\left(\frac{Q}{2}\right) + \text{F}\left(\frac{S}{Q}\right) + \text{CP(Safety stock)}$$

$$= (0.02)(\$5)\left(\frac{510,000}{2}\right) + (\$5,000)\left(\frac{2,600,000}{510,000}\right) + (0.02)(\$5)(200,000)$$

$$= \$25,500 + \$25,490.20 + \$20,000$$

$$= \$70,990.20.$$

d. Ordering costs would be reduced to $1,500. By ordering 650,000 bushels at a time, Homemade Bread can lower its total inventory costs:

$$\text{TIC} = (0.02)(\$5)\left(\frac{650,000}{2}\right) + (\$1,500)\left(\frac{2,600,000}{650,000}\right) + (0.02)(\$5)(200,000)$$

$$= \$32,500 + \$6,000 + \$20,000$$

$$= \$58,500.$$

Since the firm can reduce its total inventory costs by ordering 650,000 bushels at a time, it should accept the offer and place larger orders. (Incidentally, this same type of analysis is used to consider any quantity discount offer.)

Chapter 12

Financing Current Assets: Short-Term Credit

DECISION IN FINANCE

A Bank That Looks at More than Numbers

In the mid-1970s, the Northwestern National Bank of St. Paul, Minnesota, decided on a new commercial lending policy: it would lend to promising companies early, hoping thereby to develop loyal customers. Of course, even the most conservative banks want to attract new customers with great potential. But Northwestern was determined to go most banks one better: it would aggressively pursue new business, and when it found a company it believed in, it would bend traditional banking rules to sign up the company and keep it happy.

"Once a company becomes profitable and all the financial ratios are in place, then every bank

in the country wants them," says Dennis McChesney, Northwestern's senior vice president. "We try to distinguish ourselves by being aggressive and getting them early." As a result of its willingness to work with smaller and younger companies, Northwestern has gained a reputation among financial professionals as a maverick lender, willing to take risks that other banks would find unacceptable.

As you read this chapter, look for steps that Northwestern could take to attract and hold business from promising young companies. Do you agree with the bank's decision to pursue such business? Why don't more banks follow such a policy?

See end of chapter for resolution.

As we noted in Chapter 9, working capital management involves decisions relating to current assets, including decisions about how these assets are to be financed. Any statement about the flexibility, cost, and riskiness of short-term versus long-term credit depends to a large extent on the nature of the short-term credit that actually is used. The choice of the short-term credit instrument will affect both the firm's riskiness and its expected rate of return and, hence, the market value of its stock. This chapter examines the sources and characteristics of the major types of short-term credit available to the firm. Special attention is given to the financial institution that specializes in short-term business loans — the commercial bank.

Short-term credit is defined as any liability originally scheduled for payment within one year. The four major sources of short-term credit are (1) accruals such as accrued wages and taxes, (2) trade credit among firms, (3) loans from commercial banks, and (4) commercial paper.

ACCRUED WAGES AND TAXES

Because firms generally pay employees on a weekly, biweekly, or monthly basis, the balance sheet typically will show some accrued wages. Similarly, because the firm's own estimated income taxes, sales taxes collected, and both social security and income taxes withheld from employee payrolls usually are paid on a weekly, monthly, or quarterly basis, the balance sheet will show some accrued taxes along with accrued wages.

accruals

Continually recurring short-term liabilities, such as accrued wages, accrued taxes, and accrued interest.

As we saw in Chapter 8, **accruals** increase spontaneously as a firm's operations expand. Furthermore, this type of debt is "free" in the sense that no interest must be paid on funds raised through accruals. However, a firm cannot ordinarily control its accruals; payrolls and the timing of wage payments are set by economic forces and by industry custom, whereas tax payment dates are established by law. Thus firms use all the accruals they can, but they have little control over the level of these accounts.

ACCOUNTS PAYABLE, OR TRADE CREDIT

trade credit

Interfirm debt arising through credit sales and recorded as an account receivable by the seller and as an account payable by the buyer.

Firms generally make purchases from other firms on credit, recording the debt as an *account payable*. Accounts payable, or **trade credit**, as it is commonly called, is the largest single category of short-term debt, representing about 40 percent of the current liabilities of nonfinancial corporations. This percentage is somewhat larger for smaller firms; because small companies often do not qualify for financing from other sources, they rely rather heavily on trade credit.[1]

---

[1] In a credit sale the seller records the transaction as an *account receivable,* and the buyer records it as an *account payable.* We examined accounts receivable as an asset investment in Chapter 11. Our focus in this chapter is on accounts payable, a liability item. We may also note that if a firm's accounts payable exceed its accounts receivable, it is said to be *receiving net trade credit,* whereas if its accounts receivable exceed its accounts payable, it is *extending net trade credit.* Smaller firms frequently receive net credit; larger firms extend it.

Trade credit, like accruals, is a spontaneous source of financing in that it arises from ordinary business transactions. For example, suppose a firm makes average purchases of $2,000 a day on terms of net 30. On average it will owe 30 times $2,000, or $60,000, to its suppliers. If its sales, and consequently its purchases, doubled, its accounts payable would also double, to $120,000. The firm would have spontaneously generated an additional $60,000 of financing. Similarly, if the terms of credit were extended from 30 to 40 days, accounts payable would expand from $60,000 to $80,000. Thus lengthening the credit period, as well as expanding sales and purchases, generates additional financing.

The Cost of Trade Credit

As we saw in Chapter 11 in connection with accounts receivable management, firms that sell on credit have a *credit policy* that includes setting *credit terms*. For example, Carter Chemical Company's Textile Products division sells on terms of 2/10, net 30, meaning that a 2 percent discount is given if payment is made within 10 days of the invoice date and that the full invoice amount is due and payable within 30 days if the discount is not taken.

Suppose Fall Mills, Inc. buys an average of $12 million of materials from Carter each year, minus a 2 percent discount, or net purchases of $11,760,000/360 = $32,666.67 per day. For simplicity, suppose Carter is Fall Mills's only supplier. If Fall Mills takes the discount, paying at the end of the tenth day, its payables will average (10)($32,666.67) = $326,667. Fall Mills will, on average, be receiving $326,667 of credit from its only supplier, Carter Chemical Company.

Now suppose Fall Mills decides *not* to take the discount. What will happen? First, Fall Mills will begin paying invoices after 30 days, so its accounts payable will increase to (30)($32,666.67) = $980,000.[2] Carter will now be supplying Fall Mills with an *additional* $653,333 of credit. Fall Mills could use this additional credit to pay off bank loans, to expand inventories, to add fixed assets, to build up its cash account, or even to increase its own accounts receivable.

Fall Mills's new credit from Carter Chemical Company has a cost—because Fall Mills is forgoing a 2 percent discount on its $12 million of purchases, its costs will rise by $240,000 per year. Dividing this $240,000 by the additional credit, we find the implicit percentage cost of the added trade credit as follows:

$$\text{Percentage cost} = \frac{\$240,000}{\$653,333} = 36.7\%.$$

---

[2]A question arises here: Should accounts payable reflect gross purchases or should it reflect purchases net of discounts if a company does not plan to take discounts? Although generally accepted accounting practices permit either treatment, most accountants prefer to record both inventories and payables net of discounts and then to report the higher payments that result from not taking discounts as an added expense. Thus, *we show accounts payable net of discounts even when the company does not expect to take the discount.*

Assuming that Fall Mills can borrow from its bank (or from other sources) at an interest rate of less than 36.7 percent, *it should not expand its payables by forgoing discounts.*

The following equation may be used to calculate the approximate percentage cost, on an annual basis, of not taking discounts:

$$\text{Percentage cost} = \frac{\text{Discount percent}}{100 - \left(\begin{array}{c}\text{Discount} \\ \text{percent}\end{array}\right)} \times \frac{360}{\left(\begin{array}{c}\text{Days credit} \\ \text{is} \\ \text{outstanding}\end{array}\right) - \left(\begin{array}{c}\text{Discount} \\ \text{period}\end{array}\right)}. \quad \textbf{(12-1)}$$

The numerator of the first term, discount percent, is the cost per dollar of credit, whereas the denominator in this term (100 − discount percent) represents the funds made available by not taking the discount. The second term shows how many times each year this cost is incurred. To illustrate the equation, the cost of not taking a discount when the terms are 2/10, net 30, is computed as follows:[3]

$$\text{Cost} = \frac{2}{98} \times \frac{360}{20} = 0.0204 \times 18 = 0.367 = 36.7\%.$$

Also notice that the calculated cost can be reduced by paying late. Thus, if Fall Mills pays in 60 days rather than in the specified 30, the credit period becomes 60 − 10 = 50, and the calculated cost becomes

$$\text{Cost} = \frac{2}{98} \times \frac{360}{50} = 0.0204 \times 7.2 = 0.147 = 14.7\%.$$

In periods of excess capacity, firms may be able to get away with late payments, but they may also suffer a variety of problems associated with **"stretching" accounts payable** and being labeled a "slow payer" account. These problems are discussed later in the chapter.

"stretching" accounts payable
The practice of deliberately paying accounts payable late.

---

[3]Equation 12-1 may be adequately (for most purposes) approximated as follows:

1. Divide the number of days in the year (360) by the difference in days between the end of the discount period and the date of payment.

2. Multiply this quotient by the forgone discount percentage.

Using the preceding illustration, the cost of a forgone discount of 2/10, net 30, paid on the thirtieth day, can be approximated by 360/(30 − 10) = 18, or alternatively stated, there are eighteen 20-day periods in a year. Therefore, (18)(0.02) = 36 percent is the approximate cost of forgoing the discount. However, if the payment date is delayed until the sixtieth day, 60 − 10 = 50 days, which is the difference between the discount period and the payment date. Then 360/50 = 7.2, and (7.2)(0.02) = 14.4 percent — a close approximation of the 14.7 percent determined in Equation 12-1.

Of course, both of these methods used to determine the cost of not taking advantage of a discount are approximations of the "true" or compound interest rate to be discussed in Chapter 13. As such, Equation 12-1 and its approximation, detailed in this note, may understate the cost of trade credit in a compound interest sense.

The cost of additional trade credit resulting from not taking discounts can be worked out for other purchase terms. Some illustrative costs are as follows:

Credit Terms	Cost of Additional Credit If Cash Discount Not Taken
1/10, net 20	36%
1/10, net 30	18
2/10, net 20	73
3/15, net 45	37

As these figures show, the cost of not taking discounts can be substantial. Incidentally, throughout the chapter we assume that payments are made either on the *last day* for taking discounts or on the last day of the credit period unless otherwise noted. It would be foolish to pay, say, on the fifth or twentieth day if the credit terms were 2/10, net 30.

Effects of Trade Credit on the Financial Statements

A firm's policy with regard to taking or not taking discounts can have a significant effect on its financial statements. To illustrate, let us assume that Fall Mills is just beginning its operations. On the first day, it makes net purchases of $32,666.67. This amount is recorded on the balance sheet under accounts payable.[4] The second day it buys another $32,666.67. The first day's purchases are not yet paid for, so at the end of the second day accounts payable total $65,333.34. Accounts payable increase by another $32,666.67 the third day, to a total of $98,000, and after 10 days, accounts payable are up to $326,667.

If Fall Mills takes discounts, on the eleventh day it will have to pay for the $32,666.67 of purchases made on the first day, which will reduce accounts payable. However, it will buy another $32,666.67, which will increase payables. Thus, after the tenth day of operations, Fall Mills's balance sheet will level off, showing a balance of $326,667 in accounts payable, assuming the company pays on the tenth day in order to take discounts.

Now suppose Fall Mills decides not to take discounts. In this case on the eleventh day it will add another $32,666.67 to payables, but it will not pay for the purchases made on the first day. Thus the balance sheet figure for accounts payable will rise to 11 × $32,666.67 = $359,333.37. This buildup will continue through the thirtieth day, at which point payables will total 30 × $32,666.67 = $980,000. On the thirty-first day, it will buy another $32,667 of goods, which will increase accounts payable; but it will pay for the purchases made on the first day, which will reduce payables. Thus the balance sheet item "accounts payable" will stabilize at $980,000 after 30 days, assuming Fall Mills does not take discounts.

---

[4]Of course, when the financing side of the balance sheet increases, the asset side must also increase by an equal amount for the balance sheet to balance. In this case inventories will also increase by $32,666.67 daily.

Table 12-1 Fall Mills's Balance Sheet with Different Trade Credit Policies

A. Do Not Take Discounts; Use Maximum Trade Credit

Cash	$ 500,000	Accounts payable	$ 980,000
Accounts receivable	1,000,000	Notes payable	0
Inventories	2,000,000	Accruals	500,000
Fixed assets	2,980,000	Common equity	5,000,000
	$6,480,000		$6,480,000

B. Take Discounts; Borrow from Bank

Cash	$ 500,000	Accounts payable	$ 326,667
Accounts receivable	1,000,000	Notes payable (10%)	653,333
Inventories	2,000,000	Accruals	500,000
Fixed assets	2,980,000	Common equity	5,000,000
	$6,480,000		$6,480,000

Table 12-1 shows Fall Mills's balance sheet, after it reaches a steady state, under the two trade credit policies. Total assets are unchanged by this policy decision, and we also assume that accruals and common equity are unchanged. The differences show up in accounts payable and notes payable. When Fall Mills elected to take discounts and thus gave up some of the trade credit it otherwise could have obtained, it had to raise $653,333 from some other source. It could have sold more common stock, or it could have used long-term bonds, but it chose to use bank credit, which has a 10 percent cost and is reflected in notes payable.

Table 12-2 shows Fall Mills's income statement under the two policies. If the company does not take discounts, its interest expense is zero, but it will have a $240,000 expense for "discounts lost." On the other hand, if it does take discounts, it incurs an interest expense of $65,333, but it also avoids the

Table 12-2 Fall Mills's Income Statement with Different Trade Credit Policies

	Do Not Take Discounts	Take Discounts
Sales	$15,000,000	$15,000,000
Purchases	11,760,000	11,760,000
Labor and other costs	2,000,000	2,000,000
Interest	0	65,333
Discounts lost	240,000	0
Total costs	$14,000,000	$13,825,333
Net income before tax	1,000,000	1,174,667
Tax (40%)	400,000	469,867
Net income after tax	$ 600,000	$ 704,800

cost of discounts lost. Because the cost of discounts lost exceeds the interest expense, the take-discounts policy results in the higher net income and thus in a higher stock price.

Components of Trade Credit: Free versus Costly

Based on the preceding discussion, trade credit can be divided into two components:

1. Free trade credit, which involves credit received during the discount period. For Fall Mills, this amounts to ten days of net purchases, or $326,667.[5]

2. Costly trade credit, which involves credit in excess of the free credit. This credit has an implicit cost equal to the forgone discounts. Fall Mills could obtain $653,333, or 20 days' net purchases, of such credit at a cost of approximately 37 percent.

Financial managers should always use the free component, but they should use the costly component only after analyzing the cost of this capital and determining that it is less than the cost of funds obtained from other sources. Under the terms of trade found in most industries, the costly component involves a relatively high percentage cost, so stronger firms with access to bank credit should avoid using it.

It is important to note that some firms will occasionally deviate from the stated credit terms, thus altering the percentage cost figures cited previously. To illustrate, a California manufacturing firm that buys on terms of 2/10, net 30, makes a practice of paying in 15 days (rather than 10) and still taking discounts. Its treasurer simply waits until 15 days after receipt of the goods to pay, then writes a check for the invoiced amount minus the 2 percent discount. The company's suppliers want its business, so they tolerate this practice. Similarly, a Wisconsin firm that also buys on terms of 2/10, net 30, does not take discounts, but it pays in 60 rather than in 30 days, thus "stretching" its trade credit. As we noted earlier, both practices reduce the cost of trade credit. However, neither of these firms is loved by its suppliers, and neither could continue these practices in times when suppliers were operating at full capacity and had order backlogs. These practices can and do reduce the nominal costs of trade credit during the times when suppliers have excess capacity.

SHORT-TERM BANK LOANS

Commercial banks, whose loans appear on firms' balance sheets as notes payable, are second in importance to trade credit as a source of short-term financing. The banks' influence is actually greater than appears from the dollar

free trade credit
Credit received during the discount period.

costly trade credit
Credit taken in excess of the free trade credit period, thereby forfeiting the discount offered.

---

[5]There is some question as to whether any credit is really "free," because the supplier will have a cost of carrying receivables, which must be passed on to the customer in the form of higher prices. Still, where suppliers sell on standard terms such as 2/10, net 30, and where the base price cannot be negotiated downward for early payment, for all intents and purposes the 10 days of trade credit is indeed free.

amounts they lend, because banks provide *nonspontaneous* funds. As a firm's financing needs increase, it requests its bank to provide the additional funds. If the request is denied, often the firm is forced to slow down its rate of growth. In this section we discuss factors that influence the choice of a bank, how to approach a bank for a business loan, and some features of bank loans.

Choosing a Bank

Individuals whose only contact with their bank is through the use of its checking services generally choose a bank for the convenience of its location and the competitive cost of its checking service. A business that borrows from banks must look at other criteria, however, and a potential borrower seeking banking relations should recognize that important differences exist among banks. Some of these differences include the following:

1. Banks often have different basic *policies toward risk.* Some banks follow relatively conservative lending practices; other engage in what are properly termed "creative banking practices." These policies reflect partly the personalities of the bank's officers and partly the characteristics of the bank's deposit liabilities. Thus a bank with fluctuating deposit liabilities in a static community will tend to be a conservative lender, whereas a bank whose deposits are growing with little interruption may follow liberal credit policies. A large bank with broad diversification over geographic regions or among industries served can obtain the benefit of combining and averaging risks. Thus marginal credit risks that might be unacceptable to a small bank or to a specialized unit bank can be pooled by a branch banking system to reduce the overall risks of a group of marginal accounts.

2. Some bank loan officers are active in providing *advice and counsel* and in stimulating development loans with firms in their early and formative years. Certain banks have specialized departments that make loans to firms expected to grow and thus become more important customers. The personnel of these departments can provide much counseling to customers.

3. Banks differ in the extent to which they will support the activities of the borrower in bad times. This characteristic is referred to as the banks' degree of *loyalty.* Some banks may put great pressure on a business to liquidate its loans when the firm's outlook becomes clouded, whereas others will stand by the firm and work diligently to help it get back on its feet. An especially dramatic illustration of this point was Bank of America's bailout of Memorex Corporation. The bank could have forced Memorex into bankruptcy, but instead it loaned the company additional capital and helped it survive a bad period. Memorex's stock price subsequently rose on the New York Stock Exchange from $1.50 to $68, so Bank of America's help was indeed substantial.

4. Banks differ greatly in their degrees of *loan specialization.* Larger banks have separate departments specializing in different kinds of loans — for example, real estate loans, installment loans, and commercial loans. Within these broad categories there may be a specialization by line of business, such as steel, machinery, or textiles. The strengths of banks are also likely to reflect the nature of the business and the economic environment in which they operate. For example, Texas banks have become specialists in lending to oil companies, whereas many midwestern banks are agricultural specialists. A firm can obtain more creative cooperation and more active support by going to the bank that has the greatest experience and familiarity with its particular type of business. The financial manager should therefore choose a bank with care. A bank that is excellent for one firm may be unsatisfactory for another.

5. The *maximum loan amount* a bank can lend is determined in part by its size. Because the largest loan a bank can make to any one customer is limited to 10 percent of the bank's capital accounts (capital stock plus retained earnings), it probably is not appropriate for large firms to develop borrowing relationships with small banks.

6. Banks may also supply *other services,* such as providing lockbox systems, assisting with electronic funds transfers, helping firms obtain foreign currency, and the like. Such supplementary services should be taken into account when selecting a bank. Also, if the firm is a small business whose manager owns most of its stock, the bank's willingness and ability to provide trust and estate services also should be considered.

Applying for a Bank Loan

Firms both large and small often find a temporary need for short-term funds above current resources. At those times most business firms seek interim financing from a commercial bank.

Requests for loans take many forms. A request from a major corporation may be supported by professionally prepared and audited financial statements, complete credit analysis reports from agencies such as Dun & Bradstreet, and documentation from the company's legal counsel. On the other hand, a small firm may have only an unaudited financial statement to support the loan request.

Whatever the degree of sophistication of the data presented to support the loan request, bankers use the financial statements, both historical and pro forma, to answer questions about the term and adequacy of the loan, sources of repayment, and the certainty of those sources. The borrower therefore should anticipate the banker's questions and attempt to answer them in the loan application package. A successful application package probably would contain (1) a cover letter; (2) historical financial data; (3) projected, or pro forma, financial statements; and (4) a brief history of the firm and a resumé of its major officers.

The cover letter should indicate only the most relevant factors about the loan; the purpose of the loan, the amount requested, and the loan period should be indicated here. Balance sheets, income statements, and perhaps even tax records for the past three years of operation constitute an integral part of the loan application package. These data will be used by bankers to learn more about the business, and they are especially helpful in determining management's business and financial acumen. Another important factor in a banker's evaluation is the firm's capitalization. Many small businesses are undercapitalized; that is, their long-term or permanent financing is insufficient to support a larger volume of business. A bank is not the proper source for permanent capital. Additionally, bankers demand that the owner's equity investment in the business is sufficient to give the owner a considerable stake in the success or failure of the firm.

Of course, the pro forma financial statements will receive a great deal of attention from the bank's loan officer. First, the officer will determine whether the requested loan amount is sufficient for its intended purpose. Bankers note that one of the most prevalent mistakes that novice borrowers make is to underestimate the amount needed for a loan. Second, the banker will review the projected financial statements and even the firm's purchase orders for an indication of the sources of repayment from operations and the relative certainty of those sources. If the loan is to cover only seasonal working capital requirements, a monthly or even weekly cash budget, such as the one developed in Chapter 10, is an excellent addition to the loan documentation package. Finally, if the bank's credit officers are unfamiliar with the applicants or their business, a summary of the educational and managerial backgrounds of the firm's principals and a brief history of the firm, including a review of recent company and industry trends and future prospects, should be provided.

collateral
Assets that are used to secure a loan.

Banks and bankers are in business to lend money. The loan documentation package, therefore, should provide the banker with enough data to support a positive response to the loan request. In addition, the loan request should indicate the type of security or **collateral** that is offered to support the loan. Unpleasant as the prospect is, collateral is important since it indicates a source of funds available to the bank if unforeseen events cause default. Because collateral reduces the lending risk to the bank, it may reduce the cost of the loan or may even be the determining factor in the decision to accept or reject the loan request. The topic of collateral is discussed in more detail later in this chapter.

Some Features of Bank Loans

Maturity. Although banks do make longer-term loans, *the bulk of their lending is on a short-term basis;* about two thirds of all bank loans mature in a year or less. Bank loans to businesses frequently are written as 90-day notes, so the loan must be repaid or renewed at the end of 90 days. Of course, if a borrower's financial position has deteriorated, the bank may refuse to renew the loan. This can mean serious trouble for the borrower.

Promissory Note. When a bank loan is taken out, the agreement is executed by the signing of a **promissory note.** The note specifies (1) the amount borrowed; (2) the percentage interest rate; (3) the repayment schedule, which can involve either a lump sum or a series of installments; (4) any collateral that might be put up as security for the loan; and (5) any other terms and conditions to which the bank and the borrower have agreed. When the note is signed, the bank credits the borrower's demand deposit with the amount of the loan. On the borrower's balance sheet, both cash and notes payable increase.

promissory note
A document specifying the terms and conditions of a loan such as the amount, percentage interest rate, and repayment schedule.

Compensating Balances. In Chapter 10 compensating balances were discussed in connection with a firm's cash account. A bank typically requires a regular borrower to maintain an average checking account balance of 10 to 20 percent of the face amount of the loan. This is called a **compensating balance,** and it raises the effective interest rate of the loan. For example, if a firm needs $80,000 to pay off outstanding obligations, but it must maintain a 20 percent compensating balance, it must borrow $100,000 to obtain a usable $80,000. If the stated interest rate is 8 percent, the effective cost is actually 10 percent: $8,000 divided by $80,000 equals 10 percent.[6] The effective cost of a loan with a compensating balance will be discussed in more detail later in this chapter.

compensating balance
A minimum checking account balance that a firm must maintain with a commercial bank, generally equal to 10 to 20 percent of the loan balance.

Line of Credit. A **line of credit** is a formal or informal understanding between the bank and the borrower indicating the maximum size loan the bank will allow the borrower. For example, on December 31 a bank loan officer may indicate to a financial manager that the bank considers the firm to be "good" for up to $80,000 for the forthcoming year. On January 10 the manager signs a promissory note for $15,000 for 90 days; this is called "taking down" $15,000 of the total line of credit. This amount is credited to the firm's checking account at the bank. Before repayment of the $15,000, the firm may borrow additional amounts up to a total outstanding at any one time of $80,000.

line of credit
An arrangement whereby a financial institution commits itself to lend up to a designated maximum amount of funds during a specified period.

Revolving Credit Agreement. A **revolving credit agreement** is a more formal line-of-credit arrangement often used by large firms. To illustrate, Carter Chemical Company negotiated a revolving credit agreement for $100 million with a group of banks. The banks were formally committed for 4 years to lend Carter up to $100 million if the funds were needed. Carter, in turn, paid a commitment fee of one quarter of 1 percent on the unused balance of the commitment to compensate the banks for making the funds available. Thus, if Carter did not take down any of the $100 million commitment during a year, it still would be required to pay a $250,000 fee. If it borrowed $50

revolving credit agreement
A formal line of credit extended to a firm by a bank or other financial institution.

---

[6]Note, however, that the compensating balance may be set as a minimum monthly *average;* if the firm would maintain this average anyway, the compensating balance requirement does not entail higher effective rates.

million, the unused portion of the line of credit would fall to $50 million, and the fee would fall to $125,000. Of course, interest also had to be paid on the amount of money Carter actually borrowed. As a general rule, the rate of interest on "revolvers" is pegged to the prime rate (see next section), so the cost of the loan varies over time as interest rates vary. Carter's rate was set at prime plus ½ percent.

Note that a revolving credit agreement is one type of a line of credit. However, there is an important distinguishing feature between a formal revolving credit agreement and an informal line of credit. The bank has a legal obligation to honor a revolving credit agreement, and it charges a fee for this commitment. No legal obligation exists under the informal line of credit.

The Cost of Bank Loans

prime rate
A published rate of interest that commercial banks charge very large, strong corporations.

The cost of bank loans varies for different types of borrowers at a given point in time and for all borrowers over time. Interest rates are higher for riskier borrowers. Rates also are higher on smaller loans because of the fixed costs of making and servicing loans. If a firm can qualify as a "prime risk" because of its size and financial strength, it can borrow at the **prime rate,** which has traditionally been the lowest rate banks charge. Rates on other loans are scaled up from the prime rate, which currently (June 1987) is 8.25 percent.[7]

·Bank rates vary widely over time depending on economic conditions and Federal Reserve policy. When the economy is weak, loan demand usually is slack, and the Fed also makes plenty of money available to the system. As a result, rates on all types of loans decline. Conversely, when the economy is booming, loan demand typically is strong, and the Fed generally restricts the money supply. This results in an increase in interest rates. As an indication of the kinds of fluctuations that can occur, in just five months (from August to December of 1980), the prime rate rose from 11 percent to 21 percent. Then it fell steadily until the winter of 1987, when the rate reached 7.5 percent, the lowest prime rate since 1978. Interest rates on other bank loans also vary, but generally they are kept in phase with the prime rate.

Interest rates on bank loans are calculated in three ways: as *simple* interest, as *discount* interest, and as *add-on* interest. These three methods are explained next.

Regular, or Simple, Interest. Simple interest is charged on many bank loans and is used as the basis of comparison for all other loan rates. For a loan

---

[7]Each bank sets its own prime rate, but because of competitive forces, most banks' prime rates are identical. Furthermore, most banks follow the rate set by the large New York City banks, and they, in turn, generally follow the rate set by Citibank, New York City's largest. Citibank sets the prime rate each week at 1¼ to 1½ percentage points above the average rate on large certificates of deposit (CDs) during the three weeks immediately preceding. CD rates represent the price of money in the open market, and they rise and fall with the supply of and demand for money, so CD rates are "market-clearing" rates. By tying the prime rate to CD rates, the banking system insures that the prime rate will also be a market-clearing rate.

that uses **simple interest,** the borrower receives the entire amount of the loan's face value and then repays both interest and principal at maturity. For example, on a simple interest loan of $10,000 at 10 percent for 1 year, the borrower receives the $10,000 upon approval of the loan and pays back the $10,000 principal plus $10,000(0.10) = $1,000 of interest at maturity (after 1 year). In the case of a simple interest loan, the stated or nominal rate is also the effective rate, which is 10 percent in this example:

$$\text{Effective rate of interest} = \frac{\text{Interest}}{\begin{array}{c}\text{Borrowed}\\\text{amount}\end{array}} = \frac{\$1,000}{\$10,000} = 10\%. \quad \textbf{(12-2)}$$

simple interest
Interest calculated on funds received and paid on maturity of a loan.

Discounted Interest. When a lender makes a loan with **discounted interest,** the interest is deducted from the approved loan amount before the borrower receives the proceeds of the loan. When the lender deducts the interest in advance, called *discounting* the loan, the effective rate of interest on the loan is increased. Thus, on a $10,000 loan with a nominal interest rate of 10 percent, the interest is $1,000. When the loan is discounted, the borrower has the use of only $9,000 of the loan's proceeds. Therefore, the effective rate of interest is 11.1 percent versus the stated 10 percent interest rate:

discounted interest
Interest calculated on the face amount of a loan but deducted in advance.

$$\begin{array}{c}\text{Effective rate}\\\text{of interest}\end{array} = \frac{\text{Interest}}{\text{Amount borrowed} - \text{Interest}}$$

$$= \frac{\$1,000}{\$9,000} = 11.1\%. \quad \textbf{(12-3)}$$

Installment Loans: Add-On Interest. Banks (and other lenders) typically charge **add-on interest** on automobile and other types of installment loans of under about $10,000. The term *add-on* means that interest is calculated and added on to the funds received to determine the face amount of the note. To illustrate, suppose the $10,000 loan is to be repaid in 12 monthly installments. At a 10 percent add-on rate, the borrower pays a total interest charge of $1,000. Thus the note signed is for $11,000. However, because the loan is paid off in installments, the borrower has the full $10,000 only during the first month, and by the last month eleven twelfths of the loan will have been repaid. The borrower must pay $1,000 for the use of only about half the amount received, as the *average* amount of the original loan outstanding during the year is only about $5,000. Therefore, the effective rate on the loan is *approximately* 20 percent, calculated as follows:

add-on interest
Interest calculated and added to funds received to determine the face amount of an installment loan.

$$\begin{array}{c}\text{Approximate interest rate}\\\text{on installment loan}\end{array} = \frac{\text{Interest paid}}{\text{Loan amount} \div 2}$$

$$= \frac{\$1,000}{\$5,000} = 20\%. \quad \textbf{(12-4)}$$

The main point to note here is that interest is paid on the *original* amount of the loan, not on the amount actually outstanding (the declining balance), which causes the effective interest rate to be almost double the stated rate.[8]

Effective Interest Rates When Compensating Balances Apply. Compensating balances tend to raise the effective interest rate on bank loans. To illustrate, suppose a firm needs $10,000 to pay for some equipment that it recently purchased. A bank offers to lend the company money at a 10 percent simple interest rate, but the company must maintain a compensating balance equal to 20 percent of the amount of the loan. If it did not take the loan, the firm would keep no deposits with the bank. What is the effective interest rate on the loan?

First, note that although the firm needs only $10,000, it must borrow $12,500, calculated as follows:

$$\text{Amount of loan} = \frac{\text{Funds needed}}{1.0 \ - \ \text{Compensating balance percentage}}.$$

$$= \frac{\$10,000}{0.8} = \$12,500. \tag{12-5}$$

Even though the interest paid will be $(0.10)(\$12,500) = \$1,250$, the firm will get to use only $10,000. Therefore the effective interest rate is

$$\frac{\text{Effective}}{\text{interest rate}} = \frac{\text{Interest paid}}{\text{Funds actually used}} = \frac{\$1,250}{\$10,000} = 0.125 = 12.5\%.$$

In general, we can use this formula to find the effective interest rate when compensating balances apply:

$$\frac{\text{Effective}}{\text{interest rate}} = \frac{\text{Stated interest rate}}{1.0 \ - \ \text{Compensating balance percentage}}. \tag{12-6}$$

In this example,

$$\frac{\text{Effective}}{\text{interest rate}} = \frac{10\%}{1 \ - \ 0.2} = \frac{10\%}{0.8} = 12.5\%.$$

The analysis can be extended to the case for which compensating balances are required and the loan is based on discounted interest:

$$\frac{\text{Effective}}{\text{interest rate}} = \frac{\text{Stated interest rate}}{(1.0) - \left(\begin{matrix}\text{Compensating balance} \\ \text{percentage}\end{matrix}\right) - \left(\begin{matrix}\text{Stated interest} \\ \text{rate}\end{matrix}\right)}.$$

---

[8]Equation 12-4 is an approximation of the true interest rate, which is determined by utilizing the compound interest techniques described in Chapter 13.

For example, if a firm needed $10,000 and was offered a loan with a stated interest rate of 10 percent, discounted interest, with a 20 percent compensating balance, the effective interest rate would be

$$\text{Effective interest rate} = \frac{10\%}{1.0 - 0.2 - 0.10} = \frac{10\%}{0.70} = 14.29\%.$$

The amount that the firm would need to borrow would be

$$\text{Amount borrowed} = \frac{\$10,000}{1.0 - 0.2 - 0.10} = \$14,285.71.$$

It would use this $14,285.71 as follows:

To make required payment	$10,000.00
Compensating balance (20% of $14,285.71)	2,857.14
Prepaid interest (10% of $14,285.71)	1,428.57
	$14,285.71

In this example, compensating balances and discounted interest combined to push the effective rate of interest up from 10 percent to 14.29 percent. Note, however, that our analysis assumed that the compensating balance requirements forced the firm to increase its bank deposits. Had the company had transactions balances that could supply all or part of the compensating balances, the effective interest rate would have been less than 14.29 percent. Also, if the firm earned interest on its bank deposits, including the compensating balance, the effective interest rate would decrease.

COMMERCIAL PAPER

In Chapter 10 we discussed the use of commercial paper as an investment medium for temporary excess cash. The present chapter would be incomplete if we did not include a discussion of commercial paper as a source of short-term financing available to the most financially secure firms. Commercial paper consists of unsecured promissory notes of large, strong firms and is sold primarily to other business firms, insurance companies, pension funds, money market funds, and banks in denominations of $100,000 or more. Although the amount of commercial paper outstanding is smaller than bank loans outstanding, this form of financing has grown rapidly in recent years — from $83 billion in December 1978 to an impressive $337 billion in January 1987.

Maturity and Cost

Maturities of commercial paper generally vary from two to six months from the original date of issue. The rates on commercial paper fluctuate with supply and demand conditions; they are determined in the marketplace and vary daily as conditions change. Recently, commercial paper rates have ranged from 1¼

An increasingly popular form of short-term financing among large, secure firms, *commercial paper* looks very much like a bank check, except that it is issued by a large corporation instead of a bank. Commercial paper is really just a promise to pay the bearer. It is used primarily by firms that are excellent credit risks.

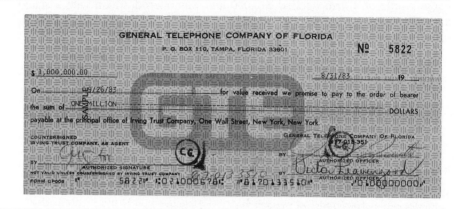

Source: Courtesy of General Telephone Company of Florida.

to 1½ percentage points below rates on prime business loans. Also, because compensating balances are not required for commercial paper, the *effective* cost differential is still wider.

Use of Commercial Paper

The use of commercial paper is restricted to a comparatively small number of large firms that are exceptionally good credit risks. As we discussed in Chapter 10, purchasers of commercial paper hold it in their temporary marketable securities portfolios as liquidity reserves, and for these purposes safety is a paramount concern. Dealers prefer to handle the paper of firms whose net worth is $50 million or more and whose annual borrowing exceeds $10 million. One potential problem with commercial paper is that a debtor who is in temporary financial difficulty may receive little help, because commercial paper dealings are generally less personal than are bank relationships. Thus a bank generally is more able and willing to help a good customer weather a temporary storm than is a commercial paper dealer. On the other hand, using commercial paper permits a corporation to tap a wide range of credit sources, including banks outside its own area and industrial corporations across the country.

USE OF SECURITY IN SHORT-TERM FINANCING

secured loan
A loan backed by collateral.

Given a choice, it is ordinarily better to borrow on an unsecured basis, as the bookkeeping costs of **secured loans** are often high. However, small or weak firms may find that they can borrow only if they put up some type of security to protect the lender or that by using some security they can borrow at a much lower rate.

Several different kinds of collateral can be employed — marketable stocks or bonds, land or buildings, equipment, inventory, and accounts receivable.

Marketable securities make excellent collateral, but few firms hold portfolios of stocks and bonds. Similarly, real property (land and buildings) and equipment are good forms of collateral, but they are generally used as security for long-term loans. However, a great deal of secured short-term business borrowing involves the use of accounts receivable and inventories.

To understand the use of security, consider the case of a Gainesville hardware dealer who wanted to modernize and expand his store. He requested a $200,000 bank loan. After examining his business's financial statements, the bank indicated that it would lend him a maximum of $100,000 and that the interest rate would be 20 percent discount, or an effective rate of 25 percent. The owner had a substantial personal portfolio of stocks, and he offered to put up $300,000 of high-quality stocks to support the $200,000 loan. The bank then granted the full $200,000 loan and at a rate of 18 percent simple interest. The store owner also might have used his inventories or receivables as security for the loan.

In the past, state laws varied greatly with regard to the use of security in financing. Today, however, all states except Louisiana operate under the **Uniform Commercial Code,** which standardizes and simplifies the procedure for establishing loan security. The heart of the Uniform Commercial Code is the **Security Agreement,** a standardized document or form on which the specific assets that are pledged are stated. The assets can be items of equipment, accounts receivable, or inventories. Procedures for financing under the Uniform Commercial Code are described in Appendix 12A.

Uniform Commercial Code
A system of standards that simplifies the procedure for establishing loan security.

Security Agreement
A standardized document that includes a description of the specific assets pledged for the purpose of securing a loan.

SUMMARY

This chapter examined the four major types of short-term credit available to a firm: (1) *accruals,* (2) *accounts payable,* or *trade credit,* (3) *bank loans,* and (4) *commercial paper.* Companies use accruals on a regular basis, but this usage is not subject to discretionary actions. The other types of credit are controllable, at least within limits.

Accounts payable may be divided into two components, *free trade credit* and *costly trade credit.* The cost of the latter is based on discounts lost, and it can be quite high. The financial manager should use all the free trade credit that is available, but costly trade credit should be used only if other credit is not available on better terms.

A third major source of short-term credit is the *commercial banking system.* Bank loans may be obtained as the need arises, or they may be obtained on a regular basis under a *line of credit.* There are three types of interest rates that may be quoted on bank loans: (1) *simple interest,* (2) *discounted interest,* and (3) *add-on interest* for installment loans. Banks often require borrowers to maintain *compensating balances;* if the required balance exceeds the balance the firm would otherwise maintain, compensating balances raise the effective cost of bank loans. *(Continues on page 324.)*

SMALL BUSINESS

Financing Receivables Directly

The growing small firm that offers its customers credit will often find that its accounts receivable grow rapidly. As discussed in Chapter 10, growth usually entails a growing need to finance the firm's working capital, and accounts receivable are a major portion of working capital. Even though growth in accounts receivable places a strain on the firm's financing ability, it may also offer the firm special opportunities to obtain financing.

Accounts receivable constitute important asset accounts within the firm, assets that may be particularly liquid and thus attractive to a lender as collateral. Two common strategies for financing receivables that make use of these desirable features are (1) pledging of receivables as collateral for debt and (2) factoring of receivables.

In the case of pledged receivables, the firm needing capital merely borrows funds and offers its receivables as collateral for the loan. For example, suppose that Main Street Builders' Supply sells materials wholesale to builders. To increase its sales, Main Street offers trade credit terms of 2/10, net 60. Most of its customers elect to delay payment. As Main Street grows, it realizes that its cash reserves are being badly strained, making it difficult to finance inventory requirements. The firm arranges to pledge its receivables to the Last Gasp National Bank. The bank, in turn, agrees to review Main Street's major receivable accounts and select the acceptable risks to serve as collateral. The bank lends Main Street about 70 percent of the face value of the acceptable accounts, reducing some of the financial pressure the firm had experienced.

Pledging of receivables makes sense when the customers of the small firm have better credit histories than the firm itself. However, the small business still bears the credit risk if its customers do not pay, and it receives only a relatively small fraction of the funds due from its accounts. Factoring receivables may be a better alternative.

Factoring involves the sale of receivables to a third party, called a factor, usually without recourse. The factor performs all of the credit services the firm might otherwise have to provide itself. It bears credit risk, it checks the creditworthiness of the customers, and it collects the receivable accounts themselves. Of course, there is a price for all these services.

Thus the small firm employing a factor gets more than just credit. If Main Street Builders' Supply employed a factor, the factor would take over Main Street's collection function almost entirely. It would be up to the factor to decide which of Main Street's customers merited credit. Also, if one of Main Street's customers, such as Reliable Homes, became unable to pay its debts, the factor would absorb the loss rather than Main Street. Of course, if Main Street wanted to sell to a customer that the factor found unacceptable, Main Street would have to bear the credit risk itself.

Main Street must decide if it is worthwhile to use a comparatively high-cost factor or to maintain its own credit and collection services. The cost of funds through the factor must be compared to the direct cost of replacing all of the factor's services internally.

There is a good reason many small firms find that using a factor's services is indeed an economical alternative; this is that the small firm has its own special expertise (in Main Street's case, buying and selling building materials), whereas the factor has its own (credit services). Because managerial talent is often especially limited in small firms, it may turn out that the factor's services are a bargain in comparison to the cost of the firm's maintaining its own credit services and exposing itself to credit risks.

The fees charged by the factor normally include an interest charge for lending the funds in advance of payment, a credit fee for evaluating customers' credit, and sometimes a charge that reflects the credit risk of the customers. Also, the factor usually does not advance all of the net proceeds, making an allowance for possible returns because of disputes between the buyer and seller.

To illustrate, suppose Main Street agrees to deliver $25,000 in building supplies to Reliable Homes on terms of net 30. Main Street approaches Factor, Inc., a wholly owned subsidiary of the major local bank holding company, and Factor accepts the account. Factor charges Main Street interest at the rate of 12 percent, 3 points over prime, resulting in an interest charge of $\frac{1}{12} \times 12\% \times \$25,000 = \$250$ on the $25,000 invoice amount. Factor charges an additional 2 percent as a credit fee, for another $500. Finally, Factor advances only $21,750 rather than $24,250, holding a 10 percent (or $2,500) allowance in case Reliable disputes the order or

finds some problem with the merchandise.

At the end of the month, Reliable pays $24,000 directly to Factor after deducting $1,000 for defective sinks it had to return to Main Street. At that point Factor pays Main Street the remaining $1,500 due the firm on its net $24,000 sale of materials to Reliable Homes.

Considering the $750 total fee paid by Main Street to Factor for 30 days' use of $24,000, the factor seems to be an expensive source of financing. Main Street must consider, however, the cost of duplicating the additional services provided by the factor.

The firm's comparative advantage is delivering a product; the factor's advantage is in providing financial and credit services. In small firms with limited managerial resources and perhaps limited experience in monitoring and collecting credit accounts, factors may be economical sources of financing and credit services.

 RESOLUTION TO DECISION IN FINANCE

A Bank That Looks at More than Numbers

The Northwestern National Bank of St. Paul uses a number of tactics to attract and hold business from promising young companies. The basis of its approach is its willingness to lend money to companies that other, more conservative banks would turn down. In fact, rather than putting the burden of proof on the customer, Northwestern often works hard on its own to justify making a loan. Even when a conventional credit analysis indicates that a company could be a

poor risk, the bank might still lend it money if the company shows compensating strengths, such as strong management talent or solid production performance.

In support of its commitment to young businesses, in 1981 Northwestern established a special division to help identify and analyze unusual lending opportunities. The division's three lending officers concentrate primarily on companies involved in high technology and

Source: Adapted from "A Bank That Looks at More than Numbers," *Inc.,* March 1983, 117–118.

other specialized areas, such as plastics and chemicals, but Northwestern's interests aren't limited to those areas alone. And its readiness to override traditional financial criteria with good judgment dates back further than the founding of the special lending division.

In fact, the bank approved its most extraordinary loan application in early 1976. At the time, the applying company had yet to generate its first dollar of revenue. Its product, a highly sophisticated supercomputer, was still in development. Based on the company's financial statements, Northwestern couldn't justify giving it a loan, so the bank decided to look instead at the product and the people. After talking to some of the company's competitors and potential customers, the bank was convinced that it could make the company a sizable loan without great risk. Thus, even though a much larger bank turned the company down, Northwestern agreed to give it a $1 million line of credit.

Ironically, the company, Cray Research, Inc., never used its new credit line. Shortly after the loan approval, the company went public, and today it is a proven performer, with annual sales in excess of $100 million.

Northwestern also believes in helping its customers survive tough financial times. For example, Detector Electronics Corporation ran into a cash crunch that threatened its ability to maintain its rapid growth. Northwestern had already given the company a fairly standard asset-based line of credit: it could borrow as needed up to 80 percent against its accounts receivable and 25 percent of the value of its inventory. But this formula wouldn't make cash available fast enough for Detector to fill all of its incoming orders.

Based on his company's assets and heavily leveraged balance sheet, Ted Larsen, Detector's president and chief executive officer, assumed that any bank would turn down his request for a larger credit line. But he hadn't taken into account Northwestern's willingness to turn aside conventional lending criteria. Because the bank believed in Detector's ability to turn its orders into sales and its sales into profits, it agreed to provide more financing for working capital by advancing cash based on a share of confirmed orders as well as on receivables and inventory. As a result, Detector was able to avert the impending financial crisis.

Of course, like any other bank, Northwestern usually charges higher rates for its riskier loans. Yet higher rates alone do not explain the bank's willingness to break with traditional lending policies. The real motivator, according to senior vice president Dennis McChesney, is the opportunity to establish ground-level relationships with newer businesses that will stay with the bank as they grow. "We think the best payoff is a loyal customer," McChesney says.

Commercial paper constitutes another important source of short-term credit, but it is available only to large, financially strong firms. Interest rates on commercial paper are generally below the prime bank rate, and the relative cost of paper is even lower when compensating balances on bank loans are considered. However, commercial paper does have disadvantages; if a firm that depends heavily on commercial paper experiences problems, its source of funds will immediately dry up. Commercial bankers are much more likely to help their customers ride out bad times.

QUESTIONS

12-1 "Firms can control their accruals within fairly wide limits; depending on the cost of accruals, financing from this source will be increased or decreased." Discuss.

12-2 Is it true that both trade credit and accruals represent a spontaneous source of capital to finance growth? Explain.

12-3 Is it true that most firms are able to obtain some "free" trade credit and that additional trade credit is often available but at a cost? Explain.

12-4 What is meant by the term *"stretching" accounts payable?*

12-5 The chapter indicated that required compensating balances usually increase the cost of a bank loan. What would be a situation in which a compensating balance does not increase the cost of a bank loan?

12-6 The availability of bank credit is often more important to a small firm than to a large one. Why?

12-7 From the standpoint of the borrower, is long-term or short-term credit riskier? Explain.

12-8 If long-term credit exposes a borrower to less risk, why would people or firms borrow on a short-term basis?

12-9 What kinds of firms use commercial paper? Could Mamma and Pappa Gus's Corner Grocery borrow using this form of credit?

12-10 Suppose that a firm can obtain funds by borrowing at the prime rate or by selling commercial paper. If the prime rate is 12 percent, what is a reasonable estimate for the cost of commercial paper?

12-11 Given that commercial paper interest rates are always lower than bank loan rates to a given borrower, why might firms that are capable of selling commercial paper also use bank credit?

SELF-TEST PROBLEM

ST-1 Kitty Burton, owner of MovieTime Rentals, is negotiating with Mechanics and Merchants Bank for a $30,000, 1-year loan. The bank has offered Burton the following alternatives. Rank the alternatives from the one with the lowest effective interest rate to the one with the highest rate. The firm will hold no balances in the bank if it does not obtain a loan from the bank.
1. A 15 percent annual rate on a simple interest loan, with no compensating balance required, interest and principal due at the end of the year.
2. A 10 percent annual rate on a simple interest loan, with a 15 percent compensating balance required and interest due at the end of the year.
3. A 9 percent annual rate on a discounted loan with a 15 percent compensating balance.
4. Interest figured as 10 percent of the $30,000 amount, payable at the end of the year, but with the $30,000 repayable in monthly installments during the year.

PROBLEMS

12-1 **Cost of trade credit.** Calculate the implicit cost of nonfree trade credit under the following terms. Assume that the discount is not taken and that payment is made on the date due.
  a. 1/10, net 30
  b. 1/15, net 30
  c. 2/10, net 30
  d. 2/15, net 40
  e. 1/10, net 60
  f. 3/10, net 60
  g. 3/10, net 20

12-2 **Cost of credit.** Lamps, Incorporated buys under terms of 2/15, net 60, but it actually pays on the 20th day and *still* takes the discount.
  a. What is the cost of its nonfree trade credit?
  b. Does it receive more or less trade credit than it would if it paid within 15 days?

12-3 **Cash discounts.** Suppose Wilson's Warehouse makes purchases of $6 million per year under terms of 2/10, net 30. It takes discounts.
  a. What is the average amount of its accounts payable, net of discounts? (Assume the $6 million purchases are net of discounts; that is, gross purchases are $6,122,450, discounts are $122,450, and net purchases are $6 million. Also, use 360 days in a year.)
  b. Is there a cost of the trade credit it uses?
  c. If it did not take discounts, what would Wilson's average payables be, and what would be the cost of this nonfree trade credit?

12-4 **Cost of bank loan.** You plan to borrow $100,000 from the bank. The bank offers to lend you the money at a 10 percent interest rate on a 1-year loan. What is the true, or effective, rate of interest for **(a)** simple interest, **(b)** discounted interest, and **(c)** add-on interest, if the loan is a 12-month installment loan?

12-5 **Cost of bank loans.** Lapin's Card Company is negotiating a $500,000, 1-year working capital loan with four area banks. The banks have provided the loan opportunities listed below. What is the effective interest rate being offered by each bank? Unless otherwise required by the terms of the loan arrangement, Lapin prefers to keep cash balances as close to zero as possible.
  a. First National Bank offered a 16.5 percent loan with principal and interest due at the end of 1 year. No compensating balance is required.
  b. Second National Bank would lend at 13 percent stated interest if Mr. Lapin kept a 20 percent compensating balance. Mr. Lapin had not planned to keep any borrowed funds in the bank.
  c. Third National Bank suggested it would approve a loan at 12 percent if Mr. Lapin, kept a 10 percent compensating balance and discounted the loan.
  d. Fourth National Bank would lend to the company at 9 percent if the principal and interest were paid in 12 equal monthly installments.

12-6 **Cost of bank loan.** Bueso's Sporting Goods needs to purchase $750,000 in inventory. The local bank agrees to the loan with a stated interest rate of 11 percent and a compensating balance of 15 percent. The loan will mature in 1 year.
  a. What is the loan's effective interest rate?

b. How much interest will Mr. Bueso pay if he agrees to the loan as stated? (*Hint:* Remember that he needs the loan proceeds to be $750,000.)

12-7 **Cost of bank loan.** Purity Bottling Company wishes to borrow $125,000 for one year. Its bank agrees to loan Purity the money at 13.5 percent, on the condition that the firm keep a 20 percent compensating balance in a 5 percent savings account for the duration of the loan. If Purity usually keeps a zero account balance, what is the effective cost of this loan?

12-8 **Trade versus bank credit.** Jim Buck of Pirate's Plumbing Warehouse is worried. Cash flow problems have prevented him from taking a 3/15, net 40, discount from his trade creditors. In fact, he has stretched payment to 55 days after purchase and his suppliers are threatening a cutoff of credit. East Carolina National Bank has agreed to lend enough money to alleviate the firm's cash flow problems and to allow Jim to take all discounts offered. The loan provides a 14 percent stated interest rate and requires a 20 percent compensating balance.
a. What is the firm's effective cost of trade credit at the present time?
b. What is the effective cost of the bank loan offered?
c. What should Jim do?

12-9 **Cost of bank loan.** Chris Miller, owner and operator of Spartan Auto Parts, is borrowing $70,000 from her local bank. Terms of the loan require a 10 percent compensating balance to qualify for a 13 percent stated interest rate. If Ms. Miller always keeps her bank cash balance as close to zero as possible, what is the effective cost of the loan? Interest and principal are due at the end of the year.

12-10 **Cost of bank loan.** Refer to Problem 12-9. Assume that rather than a zero balance, Ms. Miller, as a matter of company policy, always keeps $5,000 in the company's checking account as a cushion over expected needs. These precautionary balances may be used as part of the compensating balance. What is the effective cost of the loan under these conditions?

12-11 **Trade credit versus bank credit.** Hogan Construction has a cash flow problem that is preventing Paul Hogan from taking the trade discounts he is offered. The terms of sale are 3/10, net 30, but he has been unable to pay before 70 days after purchases are made. Understandably, his suppliers are threatening to hold him to his credit terms or withhold future credit. Hogan has discussed the matter with his bank, and it will offer his firm a 16.5 percent discounted loan that requires a 15 percent compensating balance.
a. What is the effective cost of (1) paying receivables on the 30th day; (2) continuing to pay on the 70th day; and (3) taking the bank loan?
b. What should Hogan do?

12-12 **Cost of credit agreements.** Metroplex Manufacturing has entered into a revolving credit agreement with Great Southwest National Bank. Terms of the agreement allow the firm to borrow up to $50 million as the funds are needed. The firm will pay ¼ percent for the unused balance and prime plus 2 percent for the funds that are actually borrowed. The prime rate is expected to remain at 12 percent during the period covered by the loan. Determine the effective annual percentage cost of each of the following amounts borrowed under the revolving credit agreement: **(a)** no funds are used; **(b)** $15 million; **(c)** $25 million; **(d)** $40 million; **(e)** $50 million.

12-13 **Trade credit versus bank credit.** Sound Products, Incorporated (SPI) projects an increase in sales from $2.5 million to $3 million, but the company needs an additional

$500,000 of assets to support this expansion. The money can be obtained from the bank at an interest rate of 10 percent discounted interest. Alternatively, SPI can finance the expansion by no longer taking discounts, thus increasing accounts payable. SPI purchases under terms of 2/10, net 30, but it can delay payment for an additional 30 days, paying in 60 days and thus becoming 30 days past due, without penalty at this time.

a. Based strictly on an interest rate comparison, how should SPI finance its expansion? Show your work.

b. What additional qualitative factors should SPI consider in reaching a decision?

12-14   **Bank financing.** Rocco Fashions had sales of $2 million last year and earned a 3 percent return, after taxes, on sales. Although its terms of purchase are net 30 days, its accounts payable represent 60 days' purchases. The president of the company is seeking to increase the company's bank borrowings to become current (that is, have 30 days' payables outstanding) in meeting its trade obligations. The company's balance sheet follows.

a. How much bank financing is needed to eliminate past-due accounts payable?

b. Would you as a bank loan officer make the loan? Why?

Rocco Fashions: Balance Sheet

Cash	$ 25,000	Accounts payable	$ 300,000
Accounts receivable	125,000	Bank loans	250,000
Inventory	650,000	Accruals	125,000
Current assets	$ 800,000	Current liabilities	$ 675,000
Land and buildings	250,000	Mortgage on real estate	250,000
Equipment	250,000	Common stock, par 10 cents	125,000
		Retained earnings	250,000
Total assets	$1,300,000	Total liabilities and net worth	$1,300,000

12-15   **Cost of trade credit.** Solomon and Sons sells on terms of 2/10, net 40. Annual sales last year were $4.6 million. Half of Solomon's customers pay on the tenth day and take discounts.

a. If accounts receivable averaged $447,230, what is Solomon's average collection period *on nondiscount sales?*

b. What rate of return is Solomon earning on its nondiscount receivables, where this rate of return is defined as being equal to the cost of this trade credit to the nondiscount customers?

12-16   **Short-term financing analysis.** Price and Daughters, Inc., has the following balance sheet:

Price & Daughters: Balance Sheet

Cash	$ 50,000	Accounts payable[a]	$ 500,000
Accounts receivable	450,000	Notes payable	50,000
Inventories	750,000	Accruals	50,000
Total current assets	$1,250,000	Total current liabilities	$ 600,000
		Long-term debt	150,000
Fixed assets	750,000	Common equity	1,250,000
Total assets	$2,000,000	Total liabilities and equity	$2,000,000

[a]Stated net of discounts, even though discounts may not be taken.

Price buys on terms of 1/10, net 30, but it has not been taking discounts and has actually been paying in 70 days rather than 30 days. Now Price's suppliers are threatening to stop shipments unless the company begins making prompt payments (that is, pays in 30 days or less). Price can borrow on a 1-year note (call this a current liability) from its bank at a rate of 9 percent, discounted interest, with a 20 percent compensating balance required. (All of the cash now on hand is needed for transactions; it cannot be used as part of the compensating balance.)

a. Determine what action Price should take by (1) calculating the cost of nonfree trade credit and (2) calculating the cost of the bank loan.

b. Based on your decision in Part a, construct a pro forma balance sheet. (*Hint:* You will need to include an account entitled "prepaid interest" under current assets. Also, ignore discounts lost, if any, in your calculations.

ANSWER TO SELF-TEST PROBLEM

Effective rates:

1. $\dfrac{(15\%)(\$30,000)}{\$30,000} = \dfrac{\$4,500}{\$30,000} = 15\%.$

2. $\dfrac{10\%(\$30,000)}{\$30,000 - \$4,500} = \dfrac{\$3,000}{\$25,500} = 11.76\%.$

Alternative solution:

$\dfrac{10\%}{1 - 15\%} = 11.76\%.$

3. $\dfrac{(9\%)(\$30,000)}{\$30,000 - \$2,700 - \$4,500} = \dfrac{\$2,700}{\$22,800} = 11.84\%.$

Alternative solution:

$\dfrac{9\%}{1 - 9\% - 15\%} = 11.84\%.$

4. $\dfrac{(10\%)(\$30,000)}{(\$30,000/2)} = \dfrac{\$3,000}{\$15,000} = 20\%.$

Appendix 12A

The Use of Security in Short-Term Financing

Procedures under the Uniform Commercial Code for using accounts receivable and inventories as security for short-term credit are described in this appendix. As noted in this chapter, secured short-term loans involve quite a bit of paperwork and other administrative costs; hence they are relatively expensive. However, weak firms often find that they can borrow only if they put up some type of collateral to protect the lender, or they find that by using security they can borrow at a lower rate than would otherwise be possible.

Accounts Receivable Financing

Accounts receivable financing involves either the pledging of receivables or the selling of receivables (factoring). The **pledging of accounts receivable** is characterized by the fact that the lender not only has a claim against the receivables but also has recourse to the borrower (seller), meaning that if the person or firm that bought the goods does not pay, the selling firm (borrower) must take the loss. The risk of default on the pledged accounts receivable remains with the borrower. Also, the buyer of the goods is not ordinarily notified about the pledging of the receivables. The financial institution that lends on the security of accounts receivable is generally either a commercial bank or one of the large industrial finance companies.

   Factoring, or *selling accounts receivable,* involves the purchase of accounts receivable by the lender without recourse to the borrower (seller). Under a factoring arrangement, the buyer of the goods is typically notified of the transfer and asked to make payments directly to the financial institution. Because the factoring firm assumes the risk of default on bad accounts, it must make the credit check. Accordingly, factors provide not only money but also a credit department for the borrower. Incidentally, the same financial institutions that make loans against pledged receivables also serve as factors. Thus, depending on the circumstances and the wishes of the borrower, a financial institution will provide either form of receivables financing.

Procedure for Pledging Accounts Receivable

The financing of accounts receivable is initiated by a legally binding agreement between the seller of the goods and the financing institution. The agreement sets forth in detail the procedures to be followed and the legal obligations of both parties. Once the working relationship has been established, the seller periodically sends a batch of invoices to the financing institution. The lender reviews the invoices and makes credit appraisals of the buyers. Invoices of companies that do not meet the lender's credit standards are not accepted for pledging.

   The financial institution seeks to protect itself at every phase of the operation. Selection of sound invoices is the essential first step by which the financial institution protects itself. If the buyer of the goods does not pay the invoice, the lender still has recourse against the seller of the goods. Additional protection is afforded the lender in that the loan generally will be for less than 100 percent of the pledged receivables; for example, the lender may advance the selling firm only 75 percent of the amount of the pledged receivables.

Procedure for Factoring Accounts Receivable

The procedure for factoring is somewhat different from that used for pledging. Again, an agreement between the seller and the factor is made to specify legal obligations and procedural arrangements. When the seller receives an order from a buyer, a credit approval slip is written and is immediately sent to the factoring company for a credit check. If the factor approves the credit, shipment is made and the invoice is stamped to notify the buyer to make payment directly to the factoring company. If the factor does not approve the sale, the seller generally refuses to fill the order; if the sale is made anyway, the factor will not buy the account.

   The factor performs three functions in carrying out the normal procedure outlined here: (1) credit checking, (2) lending, and (3) risk bearing. The seller can select various combinations of these functions by changing provisions in the factoring agreement. For example, a small or medium-sized firm can avoid establishing a credit department by factoring receivables. The factor's service may well be less costly than maintaining a credit department that may have excess capacity for the firm's credit volume. At the same time, if the firm uses an unqualified person to act as a credit analyst, then that person's lack of education, training, and experience may result in excessive losses.

The seller may use the factor to perform the credit-checking and risk-taking functions but not the lending function. The following procedure is carried out on receipt of a $10,000 order. The factor checks and approves the invoices. The goods are shipped on terms of net 30. Payment is made to the factor, who remits to the seller. If the buyer defaults, the $10,000 must still be remitted to the seller, and if the $10,000 is never paid, the factor will sustain a $10,000 loss. Note, however, that in this situation the factor does not remit funds to the seller until either they are received from the buyer of the goods or the credit period has expired. Thus the factor does not supply any credit.

Now consider the more typical situation in which the factor performs the lending, risk-bearing, and credit-checking functions. The goods are shipped and, even though payment is not due for 30 days, the factor immediately makes funds available to the seller. Suppose $10,000 of goods is shipped. The factoring commission sometimes called a credit fee, for credit checking is 2.5 percent of the invoice price, or $250, and the interest expense is computed at a 9 percent annual rate on the invoice balance, or $75.[1] The seller's accounting entry is as follows:

Cash	$ 9,175
Interest expense	75
Factoring commission	250
Reserve due from factor on collection of account	500
Accounts receivable	$10,000

The $500 due from the factor on collection of account is a reserve established by the factor to cover disputes between sellers and buyers on damaged goods, goods returned by the buyers to the seller, and failure to make outright sale of goods. The reserve is paid to the selling firm when the factor collects on the account.

Factoring is normally a continuous process instead of the single cycle described here. The firm selling the goods receives orders; it transmits the purchase orders to the factor for approval; on approval, the goods are shipped; the factor advances the money to the seller; the buyers pay the factor when payment is due; and the factor periodically remits any excess reserve to the seller of the goods. Once a routine is established, a continuous circular flow of goods and funds takes place between the seller, and buyers of the goods, and the factor. Thus, once the factoring agreement is in force, funds from this source are *spontaneous,* in that an increase in sales will automatically generate additional credit.

---

[1] Because the interest is for only 1 month, we take one twelfth of the stated rate, 9 percent, and multiply this by the $10,000 invoice price:

$$(1/12)(0.09)($10,000) = $75.$$

Note that the effective rate of interest is really above 9 percent, because (1) the term is for less than one year and (2) since a discounting procedure is used, the borrower does not get the full $10,000. In many instances, however, the factoring contract calls for interest to be computed on the invoice price minus the factoring commission and the reserve account.

Cost of Receivables Financing

Accounts receivable pledging and factoring services are both convenient and advantageous, but they can be costly. The credit-checking commission is 1 to 3 percent of the dollar amount of invoices accepted by the factor. The cost of money is reflected in the interest rate (usually two to three percentage points over the prime rate) charged on the unpaid balance of the funds advanced by the factor. When risk to the factoring firm is excessive, it purchases the invoices (with or without recourse) at discounts from their face value.

Evaluation of Receivables Financing

It cannot be said categorically that accounts receivable financing is always either a good or a poor method of raising funds for an individual business. Among the advantages is, first, the flexibility of this source of financing. As the firm's sales expand and more financing is needed, a larger volume of invoices is generated automatically. Because the dollar amounts of invoices vary directly with sales, the amount of readily available financing increases. Second, receivables provide security for a loan that a firm might otherwise be unable to obtain. Third, factoring can provide the services of a credit department that might otherwise be available to the firm only under much more expensive conditions.

Accounts receivable financing also has disadvantages. First is the cost; as discussed previously, financing charges are higher than those on unsecured credit. Second, the firm itself will incur additional administrative expenses to handle the paperwork, and if the invoices are numerous and relatively small in dollar amount, these administrative costs may be excessive. Third, some of a firm's trade creditors may refuse to sell to it on credit if it factors or pledges its receivables. This refusal is due in part to the fact that for a long time accounts receivable financing was frowned upon by most trade creditors as a sign of a firm's unsound financial position. It is no longer regarded in this light by most firms, because many financially sound firms engage in receivables factoring or pledging. Another reason is that since accounts receivables represents a firm's most liquid noncash assets, factoring removes these liquid assets and accordingly weakens the position of other creditors.

Future Use of Receivables Financing

We will make a prediction at this point: in the future, accounts receivable financing will increase in relative importance. Computer technology is rapidly advancing toward the point where credit records of individuals and firms can be kept on disks and magnetic tapes. Systems are in use that allow a retailer to insert a customer's magnetic credit card into a scanner linking the store to the bank. A positive signal indicates that the credit is good and that the bank is willing to "buy" the receivable created when the store completes the sale. The cost of handling invoices is greatly reduced over older procedures because the newer systems are highly automated. This makes it possible to use accounts receivable financing for very small sales, and it reduces the cost of all receivables financing. The net result will be a marked expansion of accounts receivable financing. In fact, when consumers use credit cards like MasterCard or Visa, the seller is in effect factoring receivables. The seller normally receives the amount of the purchase, minus a percentage fee, the next working day. The buyer receives about 30 days' credit, at which time she or he remits payment to the credit card company or sponsoring bank.

Inventory Financing

A substantial amount of credit is secured by business inventories. If a firm is a relatively good credit risk, the mere existence of the inventory may be a sufficient basis for receiving an unsecured loan. If the firm is a relatively poor risk, however, the lending institution may insist on security, which often takes the form of a *blanket lien* against the inventory. Alternatively, *trust receipts* or *warehouse receipts* can be used to secure the loan. These methods of using inventories as security are discussed in the following sections.

Blanket Inventory Lien. The **blanket inventory lien** gives the lending institution a lien against all inventories of the borrower. However, the borrower is free to sell inventories; thus the value of the collateral can be reduced.

> **blanket inventory lien**
> A claim on all of the borrower's inventories as security for a loan.

Trust Receipts. Because of the inherent weakness of the blanket lien for inventory financing, another kind of security is used — the **trust receipt.** A trust receipt is an instrument acknowledging that the borrower holds the goods in trust for the lender. When trust receipts are used, the borrowing firm, as a condition for receiving funds from the lender, signs and delivers a trust receipt for the goods. The goods can be stored in a public warehouse or held on the borrower's premises. The trust receipt states that the goods are held in trust for the lender or are segregated on the borrower's premises on behalf of the lender, and proceeds from the sale of goods held under trust receipts are transmitted to the lender at the end of each day. Automobile dealer financing is the most common example of trust receipt financing.

> **trust receipt**
> An instrument acknowledging that the borrower holds certain goods in trust for the lender.

One defect of trust receipt financing is the requirement that a trust receipt must be issued for specific goods. For example, if the security is bags of coffee beans, the trust receipts must indicate the bags by number. To validate its trust receipts, the lending institution has to send someone to the borrower's premises to see that the bag numbers are correctly listed. Such care is necessary because borrowers who are in financial difficulty have been known to sell the assets backing the trust receipts and then to use the funds obtained for other operations rather than for repaying the bank. Obviously administrative problems are compounded if borrowers are widely separated geographically from the lender. To offset these inconveniences, *warehousing* has come into wide use as a method of securing loans with inventory.

Warehouse Receipt Financing. Like trust receipts, **warehouse receipt financing** uses inventory as security. A *public warehouse* is an independent third-party operation engaged in the business of storing goods. Under a warehouse receipt financing arrangement, the lending institution employs the warehousing company to exercise control over the inventory and to act as its agent. Items that must age, such as tobacco and liquor, are often financed and stored in public warehouses. The value of the inventory increases as it ages, so the lender's position improves with the passage of time. However, at times a public warehouse is not practical because of the bulkiness of goods, the expense of transporting them to and from the borrower's premises, or the need for the borrower to process them on a continuous basis. In such cases, a *field warehouse* may be established on the borrower's grounds. The field warehouse arrangement is overseen by an independent third party, the field warehouse company, just as a public warehouse is run by a warehousing firm.

> **warehouse receipt financing**
> An arrangement under which the lending institution employs a third party to exercise control over the borrower's inventory and to act as the lender's agent.

Field warehousing is illustrated by a simple example. Suppose a potential borrower firm has iron stacked in an open yard on its premises. A field warehouse can be established if a field warehousing concern places a temporary fence around the iron and erects a sign stating: "This is a field warehouse supervised and conducted by the Smith Field Warehousing Corporation." These are minimal conditions, of course.

The example illustrates the three elements in the establishment of a warehouse: (1) public notification, (2) physical control of the inventory, and (3) supervision of the field warehouse by a custodian of the field warehousing concern. When the field warehousing operation is relatively small, the third condition is sometimes violated by hiring one of the borrower's employees to supervise the inventory. This practice is viewed as undesirable by the lending institution, because there is no control over the collateral by a person independent of the borrowing concern.[2]

The field warehouse financing operation is best described by an actual case. A Florida vegetable cannery was interested in financing its operations by bank borrowing. The cannery had sufficient funds to finance 15 to 20 percent of its operations during the canning season. These funds were adequate to purchase and process only an initial batch of vegetables. As the cans were put into boxes and rolled into the storerooms, the cannery needed additional funds for both raw materials and labor. Because of the cannery's poor credit rating, the bank decided that a field warehousing operation would be necessary to secure its loans.

The field warehouse was established, and the custodian notified the bank of the description, by number, of the boxes of canned vegetables in storage and under warehouse control. With this inventory as collateral, the bank established a demand deposit for the cannery on which it could draw. From this point on, the bank financed the operations. The cannery needed only enough cash to initiate the cycle. Farmers brought more vegetables; the cannery processed them; the cans were boxed and the boxes were put into the field warehouse; field warehouse receipts were drawn up and sent to the bank; the bank established further deposits for the cannery on the basis of the receipts; and the cannery could draw on the deposits to continue the cycle.

Of course, the cannery's ultimate objective was to sell the canned vegetables. As the cannery received purchase orders, it transmitted them to the bank, and the bank directed the custodian to release the inventories. It was agreed that, as remittances were received by the cannery, they would be turned over to the bank. These remittances by the cannery paid off the loans made by the bank.

Typically, a seasonal pattern exists. In this example, at the beginning of the harvesting and canning season, the cannery's cash needs and loan requirements began to rise and reached a maximum at the end of the canning season. It was hoped that well before the new canning season begins, the cannery would have sold a sufficient volume to have paid off the loan completely. If for some reason the cannery had a bad year, the bank might carry it over another year to enable it to work off its inventory.

Acceptable Products. In addition to canned food, which accounts for about 17 percent of all field warehousing loans, many other product inventories provide a basis for field warehouse financing. Some of these are miscellaneous groceries, which represent

---

[2]This absence of independent control was the main cause of the breakdown that resulted in the huge losses connected with the loans to the Allied Crude Vegetable Oil Company. American Express Field Warehousing Company hired men from Allied's staff as custodians. Their dishonesty was not discovered because of another breakdown — the fact that the American Express touring inspector did not actually take a physical inventory of the warehouses. As a consequence, the swindle was not discovered until losses running into the hundreds of millions of dollars had been suffered. See N. C. Miller, *The Great Salad Oil Swindle* (Baltimore, Md.: Penguin Books, 1965), 72–77.

about 13 percent; lumber products, about 10 percent; and coal and coke, about 6 percent. These products are relatively nonperishable and are sold in well-developed, organized markets. Nonperishability protects the lender if it should have to take over the security. For this reason a bank would not make a field warehousing loan on perishables such as fresh fish. However, frozen fish, which can be stored for a long time, can be field warehoused. An organized market aids the lender in disposing of an inventory that it takes over. Banks are not interested in going into the canning or the fish business. They want to be able to dispose of an inventory with the expenditure of a minimum of time.

Cost of Financing. The fixed costs of a field warehousing arrangement are relatively high; such financing is therefore not suitable for a very small firm. If a field warehousing company sets up the field warehouse itself, it will typically set a minimum charge of about $5,000 a year, plus about 1 to 2 percent of the amount of credit extended to the borrower. Furthermore, the financing institution will charge an interest rate of two to three percentage points over the prime rate. An efficient field warehousing operation requires a minimum inventory of about $1 million.

Appraisal. The use of field warehouse financing as a source of funds for business firms has many advantages. First, the amount of funds available is flexible because the financing is tied to the growth of inventories, which in turn is related directly to financing needs. Second, the field warehousing arrangement increases the acceptability of inventories as loan collateral. Some inventories would not be accepted by a bank as security without a field warehousing arrangement. Third, the necessity for inventory control, safekeeping, and the use of specialists in warehousing results in improved warehousing practices, which in turn save handling costs, insurance charges, theft losses, and so on. Thus field warehousing companies often have saved money for firms in spite of the financing charges. The major disadvantages of a field warehousing operation are the paperwork, physical separation requirements, and, for small firms, the fixed-cost element.

PROBLEMS

12A-1   The Lathrop Corporation is considering two methods of raising working capital: (1) a commercial bank loan secured by accounts receivable and (2) factoring accounts receivable. Lathrop's bank has agreed to lend the firm 75 percent of its average monthly accounts receivable balance of $250,000 at an annual interest rate of 9 percent. The loan would be discounted, and a 20 percent compensating balance would also be required.

A factor has agreed to purchase Lathrop's accounts receivable and to advance 85 percent of the balance to the firm. The factor would charge a 3.5 percent factoring commission and annual interest of 9 percent on the invoice price, minus both the factoring commission and the reserve account. The monthly interest payment would be deducted from the advance. If Lathrop chooses the factoring arrangement, it can eliminate its credit department and reduce operating expenses by $4,000 per month. In addition, bad debt losses of 2 percent of the monthly receivables will be avoided.

a. What is the annual cost associated with each financial arrangement?

b. Discuss some considerations other than cost that might influence management's decision between factoring and a commercial bank loan.

12A-2   **Inventory financing.** Because of crop failures last year, the Big Valley Packing Company has no funds available to finance its canning operations during the next six months. It estimates that it will require $1,200,000 for inventory financing during the period. One alternative is to establish a six-month, $1,500,000 line of credit with terms of 9 percent annual interest on the used portion, a 1 percent commitment fee on the unused portion, and a $300,000 compensating balance at all times.

Expected inventory levels to be financed are as follows:

Month	Amount
July 1989	$ 250,000
August	1,000,000
September	1,200,000
October	950,000
November	600,000
December	0

Calculate the cost of funds from this source, including interest charges and commitment fees. (*Hint:* Each month's borrowings will be $300,000 greater than the inventory level to be financed because of the compensating balance requirement.)

12A-3   **Field warehouse financing.** Because canned vegetables have a relatively long shelf life, field warehouse financing would also be appropriate for the Big Valley Packing Company in Problem 12A-2. The costs of the field warehousing alternative in this case would be a flat fee of $2,000, plus 8 percent annual interest on all outstanding credit, plus 1 percent of the maximum amount of credit extended.

   a. Calculate the total cost of the field warehousing operation.

   b. Compare the cost of the field warehousing arrangement to the line of credit cost in Problem 12A-2.

Which alternative should Big Valley choose?

12A-4   **Factoring receivables.** Muriel Industries needs an additional $250,000, which it plans to obtain through a factoring arrangement. The factor would purchase Muriel's accounts receivable and advance the invoice amount, minus a 2 percent commission, on the invoices purchased each month. Muriel sells on terms of net 30 days. In addition, the factor charges a 16 percent annual interest rate on the total invoice amount, to be deducted in advance.

   a. What amount of accounts receivable must be factored to net $250,000?

   b. If Muriel can reduce credit expenses by $1,500 per month and avoid bad debt losses of 3 percent on the factored amount, what is the total dollar cost of the factoring arrangement?

   (Do Parts c and d only if you are using the computerized problem diskette.)

   c. Would it be to Muriel's advantage to offer to pay the factor a commission of 2.5 percent if it would lower the interest rate to 14 percent annually?

   d. Assume a commission of 2 percent and an interest rate of 16 percent. What would be the total cost of the factoring arrangement if the amount of funds Muriel needed rose to $500,000? Would the factoring arrangement be profitable under these circumstances?

Part V

CAPITAL BUDGETING: INVESTMENT IN FIXED ASSETS

The previous section dealt with investment decisions that concerned assets with short-term lives. In this section we present techniques for evaluating investment opportunities in long-term assets.

Because financial management often deals with future cash returns for present cash expenditures, techniques that correctly evaluate cash flows from different time periods must be developed. This important concept, the time value of money, is presented in Chapter 13. This concept's first application is in Chapter 14, in which cash flows are first discussed and the basic methods of capital budgeting analysis are introduced. Chapter 15 formally introduces the risk dimension, discussing ways of measuring risk and emphasizing the effect of risk on the capital budgeting decision. Chapter 16 extends and refines basic capital budgeting analysis and emphasizes how risk is handled in capital budgeting analysis.

Chapter 13

Time Value of Money

 DECISION IN FINANCE

Reenlisting with the Generals

When the troubled U.S. Football League was trying to lure players into its fledgling organization with multi-million dollar deals, quarterback Steve Young signed a contract with the Los Angeles Express. The terms: approximately $40 million over 43 years, an impressive deal even in the big-money world of professional sports. Yet running back Herschel Walker, who renegotiated his own contract with another USFL team, the New Jersey Generals, for an estimated $6 million over four years, didn't think that Young got the better deal.

Because no deferred payments were involved, Walker thought that his contract extension with the Generals would win the money race with Young in the long run. All involved with Walker's contract agree that the running back probably got the better deal.

"It's better now," said Walker once his contract was signed. "Eventually it will be a whole lot better," he remarked, referring to his faith in the International Management Group, who invests his money for him. "If you have good people around you, you don't have to defer money," Walker said.

As you read this chapter, consider the pros and cons of Herschel Walker's contract. How is it possible that Walker's $6 million deal could be worth more than Young's $40 million contract? If you could choose, which contract would you accept—Walker's or Young's? Why?

See end of chapter for resolution.

In the first chapter of this text we said that the goal of the firm is to maximize the shareholders' wealth by maximizing the market value of the firm's common stock. One of the variables critical to meeting that goal is the timing of the cash flows investors expect to receive. In this chapter we learn why earlier cash flows are better than later ones. This concept is quantified in this chapter and extended in later chapters.

We hesitate to claim that one chapter in this text is more important than another. Such a claim tends to start arguments, but, more importantly, a reader might be encouraged to think that the other chapters are not important. Even so, because the principles of the time value of money, as developed in this chapter, have many applications, ranging from determining the value of stocks and bonds to making decisions about the acquisition of new equipment, we must emphasize that *of all the techniques used in finance, none is more important than the time value of money.* A thorough understanding of the material in this chapter is vital, because this concept will be used throughout the remainder of the text to evaluate a wide array of financial topics.[1]

FUTURE VALUE (OR COMPOUND VALUE)

The first law of finance, simply stated, is: *A dollar today is worth more than a dollar tomorrow.* Why? Because today's dollar can be invested today so that tomorrow the dollar will have earned interest.[2] Before we begin, let us define terms that will be used throughout this chapter:

PV = the *present value* of an amount of money.

rate of return (k)
The rate of interest offered by or required of an investment.

k = the **rate of return** offered by or required of an investment opportunity.

future value (FV)
The amount to which a payment or series of payments will grow by a given future date when compounded by a given interest rate.

FV = the **future value** of an investment some number of periods, n, from now; sometimes referred to as *terminal value.*

n = the *number of periods* covered by an investment.

---

[1]This chapter (indeed the entire book) is written assuming that the reader does not have a financial calculator. However, since the cost of these calculators is falling rapidly, this assumption is increasingly questionable.

Although a financial calculator is a valuable tool, it can present a danger. People sometimes learn how to use it in a "cookbook" fashion without understanding the logical processes that underlie financial mathematics; then, when confronted with a new type of problem, they do not understand the underlying process well enough to set it up. We urge you, therefore, to work through the illustrative problems without the financial application keys on your calculator. Doing so will ensure that you understand the financial concepts involved, so that your financial calculator will be a more useful tool in the future.

[2]What about inflation? Doesn't that lower the value of tomorrow's dollar? Although we address this question in detail in later chapters, it is important to at least mention the answer now. The simple answer is that the rate of return must indemnify the investor for all the risks faced in the investment. Therefore, since the loss of purchasing power is one of today's largest risks, the investor must believe an investment will provide a rate of return that will be larger than the inflation rate. Otherwise the investor would not make the investment.

To illustrate, suppose you have $100 that you wish to invest for 1 year at a rate of 8 percent compounded annually. How much would you have at the end of 1 year? Using our general terminology, we have

$$FV = PV(1 + k)^n. \qquad \textbf{(13-1)}$$

Substituting numbers for the general terms, we have

$$FV = \$100(1 + 0.08)^1$$
$$= \$100(1) + \$100(0.08)^1$$
$$= \$100 + \$8$$
$$= \$108.$$

If you decided to invest both the principal and interest for another year, you would have

$$FV = \$100(1.08)^1 + \$8(1.08)^1$$
$$= \$108 + \$8.64$$
$$= \$116.64.$$

Note that the increase in the value of the investment at the end of 2 years is larger than the value of the interest in the first year ($8) paid twice. This is because the second year's interest was computed on the principal plus the accumulated interest from the first year. Thus interest was paid on interest; in other words, the interest was **compounded.** Another way to express this relationship is

compounding
The arithmetic process of determining the final value of a payment or series of payments when compound interest is applied.

$$FV = \$100(1 + 0.08)^2$$
$$= \$116.64.$$

Now suppose you wish to leave your funds invested for 5 years; how much will you have at the end of the fifth year? The answer is $146.93, which is computed in Table 13-1. Notice the following points: (1) You start with $100 earning $8 in interest during the first year and end the year with $108 in your account. (2) You start the second year with $108, earn $8.64 on this now larger account, and end the second year with a total of $116.64; your second year's interest, $8.64 is larger because you earned interest on the first year's interest. (3) This process continues, and since in each year the beginning balance is higher, your interest earned increases. (4) The total interest earned, $46.93, is reflected in the ending balance of $146.93. Notice that we can arrive at the same conclusion with a great savings in effort by utilizing Equation 13-1:

$$FV = PV(1 + k)^n$$
$$= \$100 (1 + 0.08)^5$$
$$= \$146.93.$$

Table 13-1 **Compound Interest Calculations**

Year	Beginning Amount, PV	×	(1 + k)	=	Ending Amount, FV	Interest Earned, PV(R)
1	$100.00		(1 + 0.08)		$108.00	$ 8.00
2	108.00		(1 + 0.08)		116.64	8.64
3	116.64		(1 + 0.08)		125.97	9.33
4	125.97		(1 + 0.08)		136.05	10.08
5	136.05		(1 + 0.08)		146.93	10.88
						$46.93

This is, of course, the same value that was found (after a great deal more work) in Table 13-1.

If an electronic calculator is available, it is easy enough to calculate the interest factor, $(1 + k)^n$, directly. But as the number of periods, n, becomes large, the calculations of the interest factor, even with a calculator, become cumbersome. Therefore, tables have been constructed for values of $(1 + k)^n$ for wide ranges of k and n. Table 13-2 is illustrative; a much more detailed table (Appendix A) is included at the end of this text.

Notice that we have used the word *period* rather than *year* in Table 13-2. Although annual compounding will be assumed in most of the text material, compounding can occur over periods of time other than one year. Appendix 13A demonstrates how the time value of money is affected by multiperiod (semiannual, quarterly, monthly, and the like) compounding.

We set the term *future value interest factor,* IF, equal to $(1 + k)^n$. Thus Equation 13-1, $FV = PV(1 + k)^n$, can be further rewritten to

$$FV = PV(IF). \qquad \textbf{(13-1a)}$$

It is only necessary to go to the appropriate table to find the proper interest factor. In the previous example the correct interest factor for the 5-year, 8 percent illustration can be found in Table 13-2. Look down the Period column to 5, then across this row to the 8 percent column to find the interest factor, 1.4693. Then, using this interest factor, find the value of $100 after 5 years:

$$FV = PV(IF)$$

$$= \$100(1.4693)$$

$$= \$146.93.$$

This is identical to the values obtained by the long method in Table 13-1 and the direct utilization of Equation 13-1.

Graphic View of the Compounding Process: Growth

Figure 13-1 shows how $1 (or any other sum) grows over time at various rates of interest. The points plotted on the 5 percent and 10 percent curves are taken from the appropriate columns of Table 13-2. Notice that the higher the

Table 13-2 **Future Value of \$1 at the End of n Periods: IF $= (1 + k)^n$**

Period (n)	1%	2%	3%	4%	5%	6%	7%	8%	9%	10%
0	1.0000	1.0000	1.0000	1.0000	1.0000	1.0000	1.0000	1.0000	1.0000	1.0000
1	1.0100	1.0200	1.0300	1.0400	1.0500	1.0600	1.0700	1.0800	1.0900	1.1000
2	1.0201	1.0404	1.0609	1.0816	1.1025	1.1236	1.1449	1.1664	1.1881	1.2100
3	1.0303	1.0612	1.0927	1.1249	1.1576	1.1910	1.2250	1.2597	1.2950	1.3310
4	1.0406	1.0824	1.1255	1.1699	1.2155	1.2625	1.3108	1.3605	1.4116	1.4641
5	1.0510	1.1041	1.1593	1.2167	1.2763	1.3382	1.4026	1.4693	1.5386	1.6105
6	1.0615	1.1262	1.1941	1.2653	1.3401	1.4185	1.5007	1.5869	1.6771	1.7716
7	1.0721	1.1487	1.2299	1.3159	1.4071	1.5036	1.6058	1.7138	1.8280	1.9487
8	1.0829	1.1717	1.2668	1.3686	1.4775	1.5938	1.7182	1.8509	1.9926	2.1436
9	1.0937	1.1951	1.3048	1.4233	1.5513	1.6895	1.8385	1.9990	2.1719	2.3579
10	1.1046	1.2190	1.3439	1.4802	1.6289	1.7908	1.9672	2.1589	2.3674	2.5937
11	1.1157	1.2434	1.3842	1.5395	1.7103	1.8983	2.1049	2.3316	2.5804	2.8531
12	1.1268	1.2682	1.4258	1.6010	1.7959	2.0122	2.2522	2.5182	2.8127	3.1384
13	1.1381	1.2936	1.4685	1.6651	1.8856	2.1329	2.4098	2.7196	3.0658	3.4523
14	1.1495	1.3195	1.5126	1.7317	1.9799	2.2609	2.5785	2.9372	3.3417	3.7975
15	1.1610	1.3459	1.5580	1.8009	2.0789	2.3966	2.7590	3.1722	3.6425	4.1772

rate of interest, the faster the rate of growth.[3] The interest rate is, in fact, a growth rate. Thus, if a sum is invested at a rate of 5 percent, the investment fund will grow at a rate of 5 percent per period. Further, it should be clear that the concepts in this chapter can be applied to anything that is growing — sales, population, earnings per share, inflation, and so on.

PRESENT VALUE

Suppose you are offered the alternatives of receiving \$146.93 in 5 years or some amount today. Let's assume that there is no question that the \$146.93 will be paid exactly 5 years from today. Further assume that you have no current need for the money (a highly theoretical yet necessary assumption) and will therefore invest it at 8 percent. (Eight percent is defined as your opportunity cost, which is the rate you could earn on alternative investments of equal risk.) What amount of money today would make you indifferent to receiving \$146.93 in 5 years or that X amount today?

Table 13-1 shows that an initial investment of \$100 growing at 8 percent a year yields \$146.93 at the end of 5 years. Therefore, in a strictly financial sense,

---

[3]We should emphasize that this relationship is curvilinear and not linear, which means that the value of funds invested at 10 percent will grow at a rate that is *more* than twice as fast as the value of funds invested at 5 percent. This is, of course, due to compounding one fund at a faster rate than the other. The difference between the funds will grow as either time or the rate of interest increases.

Figure 13-1 **Relationships among Future Value Interest Factors, Interest Rates, and Time**

This figure shows the future value of $1.00 for several interest rates over various periods of time. Because of compounding, the higher the interest rate, the faster the growth in future value. Thus $1.00 invested at 10 percent will grow *more than* twice as fast as $1.00 invested at 5 percent. Note, for example, that for a 10-year period, the future value of $1.00 at 5 percent is only $1.63, but its future value at 10 percent is $2.59.

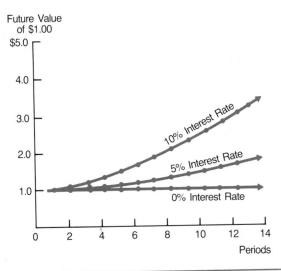

present value (PV)
The value today of a future payment or series of payments, discounted at the appropriate discount rate.

you would be indifferent in your choice between $100 today and $146.93 at the end of 5 years. The $100 is defined as the **present value, PV,** of the future $146.93, due in 5 years, when the applicable return rate (opportunity cost) is 8 percent. Therefore, if the unknown present amount is any sum less than $100, you would prefer the future promised amount, $146.93. Conversely, if the amount X is greater than $100, you would accept that present offering because, when invested at 8 percent, its value 5 years hence would be greater than $146.93.

The present value of any future sum is the amount that must be invested today to provide that future amount. Because $100 would grow to $146.93 in 5 years at an 8 percent rate, the $100 amount is the *present value* of $146.93 due in 5 years when the appropriate interest rate is 8 percent.

discounting
The process of finding the present value of a payment or a series of future cash flows; discounting is the reverse of compounding.

Finding the present value of some future amount (or **discounting** that future value, as the process is often called) is simply the reverse of compounding. We can use Equation 13-1 to illustrate this point.

$$FV = PV(1 + k)^n. \qquad \textbf{(13-1)}$$

Table 13-3 **Present Value of $1 Due at the End of n Periods: DF $= 1/(1 + k)^n = [1/(1 + k)]^n$**

Period (n)	1%	2%	3%	4%	5%	6%	7%	8%	9%	10%	12%	14%	15%
1	.9901	.9804	.9709	.9615	.9524	.9434	.9346	.9259	.9174	.9091	.8929	.8772	.8696
2	.9803	.9612	.9426	.9246	.9070	.8900	.8734	.8573	.8417	.8264	.7972	.7695	.7561
3	.9706	.9423	.9151	.8890	.8638	.8396	.8163	.7938	.7722	.7513	.7118	.6750	.6575
4	.9610	.9238	.8885	.8548	.8227	.7921	.7629	.7350	.7084	.6830	.6355	.5921	.5718
5	.9515	.9057	.8626	.8219	.7835	.7473	.7130	.6806	.6499	.6209	.5674	.5194	.4972
6	.9420	.8880	.8375	.7903	.7462	.7050	.6663	.6302	.5963	.5645	.5066	.4556	.4323
7	.9327	.8706	.8131	.7599	.7107	.6651	.6227	.5835	.5470	.5132	.4523	.3996	.3759
8	.9235	.8535	.7894	.7307	.6768	.6274	.5820	.5403	.5019	.4665	.4039	.3506	.3269
9	.9143	.8368	.7664	.7026	.6446	.5919	.5439	.5002	.4604	.4241	.3606	.3075	.2843
10	.9053	.8203	.7441	.6756	.6139	.5584	.5083	.4632	.4224	.3855	.3220	.2697	.2472

To solve for the present value, PV, divide both sides of the equation by the interest factor, $(1 + k)^n$.

$$PV = \frac{FV}{(1 + k)^n}.$$

Since dividing by a number and multiplying by its reciprocal give equivalent results,[4] we can rewrite our equation to be

$$PV = FV \left[\frac{1}{(1 + k)^n} \right]. \qquad (13\text{-}2)$$

The term in the brackets is called a **discount factor (DF),** and it is equal to the reciprocal of the interest factor, 1/IF. Just as with the interest factor, a table has been constructed for the discount factor, DF, corresponding to various values of k and n as illustrated by Table 13-3. (For a more complete table of discount factors, see Appendix B at the end of this text.) Therefore, rather than directly utilizing Equation 13-2, we can use a modified version of that equation that utilizes the discount factors in Table 13-3:

$$PV = FV(DF). \qquad (13\text{-}2a)$$

discount factor (DF)
The factor used to determine the present value of a lump sum due in n periods in the future discounted at k percent per period.

Using the table values of k and n makes direct computation of these variables in Equation 13-2 unnecessary.

Reverting to the original problem and using Equation 13-2a, we can find the discount factor, DF, by looking down the 8 percent column in Table 13-3 to the row for the fifth period, n. The number shown there, .6806, is the dis-

---

[4]For example, dividing by 2 is the same as multiplying by ½, or dividing by 4 is equivalent to multiplying by ¼.

count factor, DF, used to determine the present value of $146.93 to be received in 5 years, discounted at 8 percent:

$$PV = FV(DF)$$
$$= \$146.93(.6806)$$
$$= \$100.00.$$

Graphic View of the Discounting Process

Figure 13-2 graphically depicts how the discount factors decrease as the discounting period increases. These curves, plotted with the data presented in Table 13-3, show that the present value of a sum to be received at some future time decreases either as the payment date is extended further into the future or as the discount rate increases. To illustrate, the present value of $1 due in 10 years is about 61 cents if the discount rate is 5 percent, but it is worth only 25 cents today if the discount rate is 15 percent. Thus, since you are investing in a project with a higher rate of return, a smaller initial payment is required to earn $1 in the future. The length of time until money is paid or received is also important. For example, $1 due in 5 years at 10 percent is worth 62 cents today, but at the same discount rate $1 due in 10 years is worth only about 39 cents today.

Thus present values are dependent on two factors, the discount rate and time. If relatively high discount rates apply, funds due in the future are worth comparatively little today. Even at relatively low discount rates, the present values of funds due in the distant future are quite small. Notice that when no investment opportunity exists or no investment is made, the discount rate (interest rate) is zero, which means the present and future values of a dollar are the same.

PRESENT VALUE VERSUS FUTURE VALUE

By now you have noticed that Equations 13-1 and 13-2 (and their equivalent versions, Equations 13-1a and 13-2a, which have the table values computed for them) are really two ways of looking at the same process. People in everyday life must decide, just as financial managers do, how much to invest in order to receive future returns. The problem is that present and future amounts cannot be directly compared. We must either compound present amounts into the future or discount future dollars back to the present by using the appropriate formulas.

To illustrate this point, let's use the following farfetched example. Conrad Dunn is a college student who is going to sell his car for $5,000 and invest the money in a project that promises a 12 percent return. An uncle suggests that he would like to have the car, but he cannot pay cash for it. He does, however, have several government bonds that mature in 15 years. Although their current value is below $5,000, they will mature in 15 years at $20,000, which is four

Figure 13-2 **Relationships among Present Value Interest Factors, Interest Rates, and Time**

This graph shows the discounting process at various interest rates. The longer the time until payment or the higher the interest rate, the less invested funds will be worth in today's dollars. For example, if the interest rate is 10 percent, the present value of $1.00 due in 4 years is $0.68, but the value drops to about $0.39 if due in 10 years. If we vary the interest rate, we see that $1.00 invested at 5 percent for 10 years has a present value of about $.61, whereas if it is invested at 15 percent for 10 years, its present value is about $0.25.

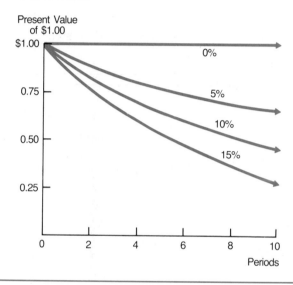

times the car's value, Conrad's uncle notes. Should Conrad give his uncle the car in anticipation of the future $20,000 or sell it for $5,000 cash today?

Even though the value of the future sum is four times the value of the car, we cannot compare the amounts because one is a future value and the other is a present sum. To make the values comparable, we must discount the future payment back to the present *or* we must compound the present amount into the future. Even though we will arrive at the same decision (to accept or reject the uncle's offer), we will use both methods.

If we wish to discount the future amount back to the present, we can use Equation 13-2a, employing a discount factor from Appendix B for 12 percent, 15 years:

$$PV = FV(DF)$$

$$= \$20,000(.1827)$$

$$= \$3,654.$$

Figure 13-3 **Discounting and Compounding Compared**

To compare a present value to a future value, we must either compound the present sum into the future or discount the future amount back to the present. Whichever method is used, the result gives the only firm basis on which to compare the two values. In this figure the future values are shown on the right ($27,368 was arrived at by compounding $5,000 over 15 periods), and the present values are shown on the left ($3,654 was reached by discounting $20,000 over 15 periods).

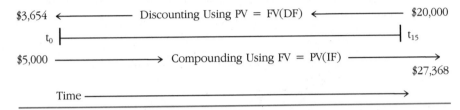

Obviously, the offer made by Conrad's uncle is not financially attractive to him, because the present value of $20,000 discounted at 12 percent for 15 years is less than the amount Conrad could receive if he sold the car today.

We come to the same conclusion if the cash value of the car if sold, $5,000, is compounded 15 years into the future. We use the interest factors from Appendix A for 12 percent, 15 years, in Equation 13-1a:

$$FV = PV(IF)$$

$$= \$5,000(5.4736)$$

$$= \$27,368.$$

As we expected, the value of $5,000 invested at a 12 percent rate of interest for 15 years exceeds the $20,000 Conrad's uncle promised for the car.

Figure 13-3 serves to illustrate the point that present and future values cannot be directly compared. A present amount can be compounded into the future and thus compared with a promised future amount. Conversely, a future sum can be discounted back to the present and compared with the present value of the uncle's offer. Thus we can compare $5,000 with $3,654 or $27,368 with $20,000, but we cannot compare $5,000 with $20,000. Conrad may wish to give his uncle the car for the promise of $20,000 in the future, but it will not be for financial reasons.

FUTURE VALUE OF AN ANNUITY

annuity
A series of equal payments or receipts for a specified number of periods.

So far we have been dealing with situations characterized by a single payment or receipt in the present and a single amount in the future. We now turn to a discussion of a special case of equal annual payments or receipts, called *annuities*. An **annuity** is defined as *a series of equal payments or receipts for a*

Figure 13-4 **Time Line for an Annuity: Future Value with k = 7%**

This figure shows how the future value of an annuity is calculated. In this case there is a promise to pay $1,000 per year for 3 years, so a $1,000 payment is received at the end of each of three periods. Upon receipt, each payment is invested at 7 percent interest. The first payment is compounded for 2 years, the second for 1 year, and the third is not compounded at all. The sum of the three future values is the total value of the annuity.

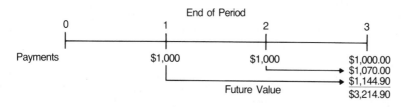

specified number of periods. If the payments are made or received at the beginning of each period, it is called an **annuity due.** However, because **regular annuities** are far more common in finance, when the word *annuity* is used in this book, you may assume that payments are received at the end of each period, unless otherwise indicated.

annuity due
A series of payments of a fixed amount for a specified number of periods, with the payments occurring at the beginning of the period.

regular annuity
A series of payments of a fixed amount for a specified number of periods, with the payments occurring at the end of the period.

Regular Annuity

A promise to pay $1,000 annually for 3 years is a 3-year annuity. If you were to receive such an annuity and deposited each annual payment in a savings account paying 7 percent interest, how much would you have at the end of 3 years? The process is shown graphically as a *time line* in Figure 13-4. The first payment is made at the end of Year 1, the second at the end of Year 2, and the third at the end of Year 3. The last payment is not compounded at all, the second year's payment is compounded for 1 year, and the first is compounded for 2 years. When the future values of each of the $1,000 payments are added, their total is the sum of an annuity, which in this case is equal to $3,214.90.

Of course, you could go through the effort of calculating the interest factors yourself,[5] but the interest factor for an annuity (IFa) has already been

---

[5]Expressed algebraically, the future value of an annuity, FVa, can be computed by multiplying the annuity, PMT, by the interest factor for an annuity, IFa:

$$\mathrm{FVa} = \mathrm{PMT}(1 + k)^{n-1} + \mathrm{PMT}(1 + k)^{n-2} + \cdots + \mathrm{PMT}(1 + k)^{1} + \mathrm{PMT}(1 + k)^{0}$$

$$= \mathrm{PMT}[(1 + k)^{n-1} + (1 + k)^{n-2} + \cdots + (1 + k)^{1} + (1 + k)^{0}]$$

$$= \mathrm{PMT} \sum_{t=1}^{n}(1 + k)^{n-t}$$

$$= \mathrm{PMT}(\mathrm{IFa}).$$

Table 13-4 **Sum of an Annuity of $1 per Period for n Periods:**

$$IFa = \sum_{t=1}^{n} (1 + k)^{n-t} = \frac{(1 + k)^n - 1}{k}.$$

Period (n)	1%	2%	3%	4%	5%	6%	7%	8%
1	1.0000	1.0000	1.0000	1.0000	1.0000	1.0000	1.0000	1.0000
2	2.0100	2.0200	2.0300	2.0400	2.0500	2.0600	2.0700	2.0800
3	3.0301	3.0604	3.0909	3.1216	3.1525	3.1836	3.2149	3.2464
4	4.0604	4.1216	4.1836	4.2465	4.3101	4.3746	4.4399	4.5061
5	5.1010	5.2040	5.3091	5.4163	5.5256	5.6371	5.7507	5.8666
6	6.1520	6.3081	6.4684	6.6330	6.8019	6.9753	7.1533	7.3359
7	7.2135	7.4343	7.6625	7.8983	8.1420	8.3938	8.6540	8.9228
8	8.2857	8.5830	8.8923	9.2142	9.5491	9.8975	10.2598	10.6366
9	9.3685	9.7546	10.1591	10.5828	11.0266	11.4913	11.9780	12.4876
10	10.4622	10.9497	11.4639	12.0061	12.5779	13.1808	13.8164	14.4866

calculated for various combinations of interest rates, k, and time periods, n, in Appendix C. An illustrative set of these annuity factors is given in Table 13-4. To answer the preceding question, you would utilize Equation 13-3:

$$FVa = PMT(IFa),$$ (13-3)

where

FVa = the future compound value of an annuity.

PMT = the annuity payment or receipt.

IFa = the future value interest factor for an annuity.

To find the future value of the 3-year, $1,000 annuity problem posed earlier, first find the interest factor for an annuity, IFa, by simply referring to Table 13-4. Look down the 7 percent column to the third-period row, and multiply the factor 3.2149 by the $1,000:

$$FVa = PMT(IFa)$$

$$= \$1,000(3.2149)$$

$$= \$3,214.90.$$

Thus the future value of an annuity of $1,000 a year, received at the end of each year and invested at 7 pecent annually, is $3,214.90.

Annuity Due

Had the annuity in the previous example been an *annuity due,* each of the three payments would have occurred at the beginning rather than the end of the period, or at t = 0, t = 1, t = 2. In terms of Figure 13-4, each payment would have been shifted to the left, so there would have been $1,000 under Period 0 and a zero under Period 3, meaning that each payment would be compounded for one more period.

We can modify Equation 13-3 to handle annuities due in the following manner:

$$\text{FVa(Annuity due)} = \text{PMT(IFa)}(1 + k). \qquad \textbf{(13-3a)}$$

Because each payment is compounded for one extra year, multiplying PMT (IFa) by (1 + k) takes care of this extra compounding. Applying Equation 13-3a to the previous example, we obtain

$$\text{FVa(Annuity due)} = \$1,000(3.2149)(1.07) = \$3,439.90$$

versus the $3,214.90 for the regular annuity.[6] Since payments on an annuity due come earlier, it will always provide a higher future value than a regular annuity.

PRESENT VALUE OF AN ANNUITY

The preceding section presented techniques that allow you to determine the value in some future period of a stream of equal annual payments or receipts. You may also wish to determine the present value of an annuity. Suppose you were offered the alternatives of a 4-year annuity of $1,000 at the end of each year or a single (lump sum) payment today. Let's assume that you have no immediate need for the money during the next 4 years (remember that we said finance was sometimes a theoretical subject), so if you accept the annuity, you would simply deposit the annual payments in an investment venture that pays 9 percent interest. How large must today's lump-sum payment be to make it equivalent to the annuity? The time line in Figure 13-5 will help explain the problem.

Rather than multiplying each year's receipt by factors from Table 13-3 and summing the results, as suggested by Figure 13-5, a table has been constructed to facilitate the computation of the present value of an annuity. Table 13-5 is

---

[6]A more mechanical technique can also be used to solve for the future value of an annuity due. First look up the IFa for n + 1 years in the table. Then subtract 1.0 from that amount to get the IFa for the annuity due. Using the previous example, the fourth period interest factor is 4.4399. This factor assumes 4 payments and 3 compounding periods, so by subtracting one payment, we will have the desired 3 payments and 3 compounding periods. Thus:

$$\text{IFa(Annuity due)} = \$1,000(4.4399 - 1.0) = \$3,439.90.$$

Figure 13-5 **Time Line for an Annuity: Present Value with k = 9%**

This figure shows how to derive the present value of a 4-year annuity of $1,000 per year at an interest rate of 9 percent. The present value is calculated by multiplying each year's receipt by the appropriate discount factor from Table 13-3 and adding the resulting amounts. One can then compare this present value with any other present value to determine the wisdom of accepting this annuity.

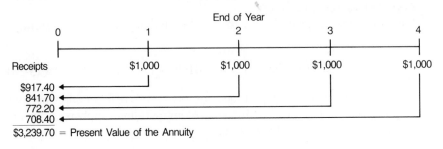

illustrative of the more complete set of discount factors for an annuity, DFa[7], that is presented in Appendix D. Utilizing Equation 13-4 and the appropriate DFa contained in Table 13-5, we can solve the problem in a direct fashion:

$$PVa = PMT(DFa) \qquad\qquad (13\text{-}4)$$

$$= \$1,000(3.2397)$$

$$= \$3,239.70.$$

Thus the present value of an annuity, PVa, equals the annuity multiplied by the appropriate discount factor for an annuity, DFa. In the present problem the DFa for a 4-year, 9 percent annuity is found from Table 13-5 to be 3.2397. Multiplying this factor by the $1,000 annual receipt gives $3,239.70, the present value of the annuity. This figure is, of course, identical to the long method suggested by Figure 13-5.

Notice that the entry for each period n in Table 13-5 is equal to the sum of the entries in Table 13-3 up to and including Period n. For example, the

---

[7]The discount factor for an annuity, DFa, is computed by summing the discount factors for each year's receipt. The present value of the first receipt is a $[1/(1 + k)]$, the second is a $[1/(1 + k)^2]$, and so on. Thus:

$$PVa = PMT \left(\frac{1}{1 + k}\right)^1 + PMT \left(\frac{1}{1 + k}\right)^2 + \cdots + PMT\left(\frac{1}{1 + k}\right)^n$$

$$= PMT \left(\frac{1}{(1 + k)^1} + \frac{1}{(1 + k)^2} + \cdots + \frac{1}{(1 + k)^n}\right]$$

$$= PMT \sum_{t=1}^{n} \left(\frac{1}{1 + k}\right)^t$$

$$= PMT(DFa). \qquad\qquad (13\text{-}4)$$

Table 13-5 **Present Value of an Annuity of $1 per Period for n Periods:**

$$DFa = \sum_{t=1}^{n} \frac{1}{(1 + k)^t} = \frac{1 - [1/(1 + k)^n]}{k}$$

Number of Periods (n)	1%	2%	3%	4%	5%	6%	7%	8%	9%	10%
1	0.9901	0.9804	0.9709	0.9615	0.9524	0.9434	0.9346	0.9259	0.9174	0.9091
2	1.9704	1.9416	1.9135	1.8861	1.8594	1.8334	1.8080	1.7833	1.7591	1.7355
3	2.9410	2.8839	2.8286	2.7751	2.7232	2.6730	2.6243	2.5771	2.5313	2.4869
4	3.9020	3.8077	3.7171	3.6299	3.5460	3.4651	3.3872	3.3121	3.2397	3.1699
5	4.8534	4.7135	4.5797	4.4518	4.3295	4.2124	4.1002	3.9927	3.8897	3.7908
6	5.7955	5.6014	5.4172	5.2421	5.0757	4.9173	4.7665	4.6229	4.4859	4.3553
7	6.7282	6.4720	6.2303	6.0021	5.7864	5.5824	5.3893	5.2064	5.0330	4.8684
8	7.6517	7.3255	7.0197	6.7327	6.4632	6.2098	5.9713	5.7466	5.5348	5.3349
9	8.5660	8.1622	7.7861	7.4353	7.1078	6.8017	6.5152	6.2469	5.9952	5.7590
10	9.4713	8.9826	8.5302	8.1109	7.7217	7.3601	7.0236	6.7101	6.4177	6.1446

DFa for 9 percent, 4 periods in Table 13-5 could have been calculated by summing the DF for Periods 1 through 4 from Table 13-3:

$$0.9174 + 0.8417 + 0.7722 + 0.7084 = 3.2397.$$

PERPETUITIES

Most annuities call for payments to be made over a definite time period — for example, $1,000 per year for 4 years. However, some annuities go on indefinitely; here the payments constitute an *infinite series* and the series is called a **perpetuity.** The present value of a perpetuity is found by applying Equation 13-5:

perpetuity
A stream of equal payments expected to last forever.

$$PV(perpetuity) = \frac{Payment}{Discount\ rate} = \frac{PMT}{k}. \qquad (13\text{-}5)$$

To illustrate, in 1815 after the Napoleonic Wars, the British government sold a huge bond issue and used the proceeds to pay off many smaller issues that had been floated in prior years to finance the wars. Because the purpose of the new bonds was to *consolidate* past debts, the bonds were called **consols.** Suppose each consol promised to pay $90 interest per year in perpetuity. (Actually, the interest was stated in pounds.) What would each bond be worth if the going rate of interest, or the discount rate, was 8 percent? The answer is $1,125:

consol
A perpetual bond, such as that issued by the British government to consolidate past debts; in general, any perpetual bond.

$$Value = \$90/0.08 = \$1,125.$$

Table 13-6 **Present Value of an Uneven Stream of Receipts**

Year	Stream of Receipts	×	DF (6%)	=	PV of Individual Receipts
1	$ 100		0.9434		$ 94.34
2	200		0.8900		178.00
3	200		0.8396		167.92
4	200		0.7921		158.42
5	200		0.7473		149.46
6	0		0.7050		0
7	1,000		0.6651		665.10
				PV = Sum =	$1,413.24

Perpetuities are discussed further in later chapters where procedures for finding the values of various types of securities (stocks and bonds) are analyzed.

PRESENT VALUE OF AN UNEVEN SERIES OF RECEIPTS

uneven payment stream
A series of payments in which the amount varies from one period to the next.

The definition of an annuity includes the concept of a fixed amount; in other words, annuities involve situations in which cash flows are *identical* every period. Although many financial decisions do involve constant cash flows, some important decisions concern uneven flows of cash. In particular, common stock investments ordinarily involve uneven, hopefully increasing, dividend payments over time. Consequently, it is necessary to expand the analysis to deal with **uneven payment streams.**

The present value of an uneven stream of future income payments is equal to the sum of the PVs of the individual components of the stream. For example, suppose we are trying to find the PV of the stream of receipts shown in Table 13-6, discounted at 6 percent. As shown in the table, we multiply each receipt by the appropriate DF, then sum these products to obtain the PV of the stream, $1,413.24. Figure 13-6 gives a graphic view of the cash flow stream.

The PV of the receipts shown in Table 13-6 and Figure 13-6 can also be found by using the annuity equation; the steps in this alternative solution process are as follows:

Step 1 Find the PV of $100 due in Year 1:

$$\$100(0.9434) = \$94.34.$$

Step 2 Recognize that a $200 annuity will be received during Years 2 through 5. Thus we can determine the value of a 5-year annuity, subtract from it the value of a 1-year annuity, and have remaining the value of a 4-year annuity whose first payment is due in 2 years. This result is achieved by

Figure 13-6 **Time Line for an Uneven Cash Flow Stream with k = 6%**

The method used to calculate the present value of an uneven stream of future payments is illustrated in this figure. Each amount to be received is multiplied by the appropriate discount factor from Table 13-3 to arrive at its individual present value. The resulting amounts are then totaled to arrive at the present value of the stream of receipts.

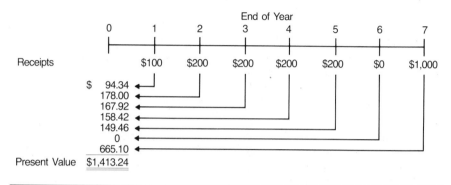

subtracting the DFa for a 1-year, 6 percent annuity from the DFa for a 5-year annuity and then multiplying the difference by $200:

$$\text{PV of the annuity} = \$200(\text{DFa}_{6\%,5 \text{ years}})$$
$$- \$200(\text{DFa}_{6\%,1 \text{ year}})$$
$$= \$200[(\text{DFa}_{6\%,5 \text{ years}})$$
$$- (\text{DFa}_{6\%,1 \text{ year}})]$$
$$= \$200(4.2124 - 0.9434)$$
$$= \$653.80.$$

Thus the present value of the annuity component of the uneven stream is $653.80.

Step 3 Find the PV of the $1,000 due in Year 7:

$$\$1,000(0.6651) = \$665.10.$$

Step 4 Sum the components:

$$\$94.34 + \$653.80 + \$665.10 = \$1,413.24.$$

Either of the methods can be used to solve problems of this type. However, the alternative (annuity) solution is easier if the annuity component runs for many years. For example, the alternative solution would be clearly superior for finding the PV of a stream consisting of $100 in Year 1, $200 in Years 2 through 29, and $1,000 in Year 30.

DETERMINING INTEREST RATES

We can use the basic equations developed previously to determine the interest rates implicit in financial contracts.

Example 1. A bank offers to lend you $1,000 if you sign a note agreeing to repay $1,610.50 at the end of 5 years. What rate of interest are you paying?

1. Recognize that $1,000 is the PV of $1,610.50 due in 5 years:

$$PV = \$1,000 = \$1,610.50(DF).$$

2. Solve for DF:

$$DF = \frac{\$1,000}{\$1,610.50} = 0.6209.$$

3. Now turn to Table 13-3 or Appendix B. Look across the row for Period 5 until you find the value 0.6209. It is in the 10 percent column, so you would be paying a 10 percent rate of interest if you took out the loan.

Example 2. A bank offers to lend you $75,000 to buy a home. You must sign a mortgage calling for a payment of $7,635.48 at the end of each of the next 25 years. What interest rate is the bank charging you?

1. Recognize that $75,000 is the PV of a 25-year, $7,635.48 annuity:

$$PVa = \$75,000 = \sum_{t=1}^{25} \$7,635.48 \left[\frac{1}{(1 + k)^t} \right] = \$7,635.48\ (DFa).$$

2. Solve for DFa:

$$DFa = \$75,000/\$7,635.48 = 9.8226.$$

3. Turn to Appendix D. Looking across the row for 25 periods, you will find 9.8226 under the column for 9 percent. Therefore the rate of interest on this mortgage loan is 9 percent.

Although the tables can be used to find the interest rate implicit in single payments and annuities, it is more difficult to find the interest rate implicit in an uneven series of payments. One can use a trial-and-error procedure, use more efficient but more complicated analytic procedures, or use a computer. We defer further discussion of this problem for now but will take it up later in the capital budgeting chapters and again in our discussion of bond values.

AMORTIZED LOANS

One of the most important applications of compound interest concepts involves loans that are to be paid off in installments, which include both principal and interest, over time. Examples include automobile loans, home mortgage loans, and most business debt other than very short-term debt. If a loan

Table 13-7 **Loan Amortization Schedule**

Year	Payment (1)	Interest[a] (2)	Repayment of Principal[b] (3)	Remaining Balance (4)
1	$ 374.11	$ 60.00	$ 314.11	$685.89
2	374.11	41.15	332.96	352.93
3	374.11	21.18	352.93	0
	$1,122.33	$122.33	$1,000.00	

[a]Interest is calculated by multiplying the loan balance at the beginning of the year by the interest rate. Therefore, interest in Year 1 is $1,000(0.06) = $60; in Year 2 interest is $685.89(0.06) = $41.15; and in Year 3 interest is $352.93(0.06) = $21.18.
[b]Repayment of principal is equal to the payment of $374.11 minus the interest charge in the first year, and so on.

is to be repaid in equal periodic amounts (monthly, quarterly, or annually), it is said to be an **amortized loan.**

To illustrate, suppose a firm borrows $1,000 to be repaid in 3 equal payments at the end of each of the next 3 years. The lender is to receive 6 percent interest on funds outstanding. The first task is to determine the amount the firm must repay each year, or the annual payment. To find this amount, recognize that the $1,000 represents the present value of an annuity of PMT dollars per year for 3 years, discounted at 6 percent:

$$\$1,000 = \text{PV of annuity} = \text{PMT(DFa)}.$$

The DFa is 2.6730, so

$$\$1,000 = \text{PMT}(2.6730).$$

Solving for PMT, we obtain

$$\text{PMT} = \$1,000/2.6730 = \$374.11.$$

If the firm pays the lender $374.11 at the end of each of the next 3 years, the percentage cost to the borrower, and the return to the lender, will be 6 percent.

Each payment consists partly of interest and partly of a repayment of principal. This breakdown is given in the **amortization schedule** shown in Table 13-7. The interest component is largest in the first year, and it declines as the outstanding balance of the loan decreases. For tax purposes the borrower reports the interest payments in Column 2 as a deductible cost each year, whereas the lender reports these same amounts as taxable income.

REVIEW OF CHAPTER CONCEPTS

In light of the seemingly large number of formulas and the importance of this chapter, we believe a review of the concepts presented in this chapter is warranted.

amortized loan
A loan in which the principal and interest is repaid in installments during the life of the loan.

amortization schedule
A schedule that shows precisely how a loan will be repaid. It gives the payment required on each specified date as well as a breakdown of each payment, showing how much of it constitutes interest and how much constitutes repayment of principal.

Table 13-8 **Applications of the Time Value of Money**

Formula	Equation Number	Interest or Discount Factor Table	Appendix
FV = PV(IF)	13-1a	13-2	A
PV = FV(DF)	13-2a	13-3	B
FVa = PMT(IFa)	13-3	13-4	C
PVa = PMT(DFa)	13-4	13-5	D

   Actually, all problems dealing with the time value of money (compounding or discounting) can be solved by utilizing one or a combination of the four formulas listed in Table 13-8.

Sample Problems

Problem: Compounding a Lump Sum to a Future Period. Your aunt has given you a $3,000 tax-free gift. If you invest it in a 5-year, 8 percent certificate of deposit, how much will you have when the certificate matures?

Discussion. The elements of this problem are a present amount, PV, of $3,000; a length of time for the investment, n, of 5 years; and an investment (interest) rate, k, of 8 percent. A future amount, FV — the value of $3,000 compounded at 8 percent for 5 years — is to be found. Because a single, present amount is being compounded, we use the IF found in either Table 13-2 or Appendix A.

Solution.

$$FV = PV(IF) \qquad\qquad \textbf{(13-1a)}$$

$$= \$3,000(1.4693)$$

$$= \$4,407.90.$$

Problem: Present Value of a Future Lump Sum. Your friend Howard has suggested that you invest, along with him, in a real estate deal. He predicts your portion of the property in question will be worth $40,000 in 8 years. If you can make an investment with equal risk at 10 percent, what is the maximum that you would wish to invest today in the venture?

Discussion. Here we are concerned with finding the present value, PV, of a future amount, FV, of $40,000 to be received in 8 years, n, with a discount rate, k, of 10 percent. With a lump-sum amount to be discounted back to the present, we use a discount factor, DF, found in Table 13-3 or in Appendix B.

Solution.

$$PV = FV(DF) \tag{13-2a}$$
$$= \$40,000(.4665)$$
$$= \$18,660.$$

Problem: Future Value of a Regular Annuity. You are planning a great vacation trip to Europe in 15 years. You plan to save $500 annually, beginning next year, after you graduate. How much will you have in your vacation fund in 15 years if you invest at 9 percent?

Discussion. In this situation you need to determine the future value, FVa, of an annuity of $500, PMT, deposited annually for 15 years, n, at 9 percent, k. To do so you would use the interest factor for an annuity, IFa, where n = 15 and k = 9%, from Appendix C.

Solution.

$$FVa = PMT(IFa) \tag{13-3}$$
$$= \$500(29.360)$$
$$= \$14,680.$$

Alternative Problem. Let's keep the scenario that you are saving for your vacation trip to Europe but change some of the elements of the problem. Now let's assume that you still want to save $500 each year for 15 years, but this time let's assume that you know the trip will cost $14,680. What is the rate of return you must earn to reach your goal?

Discussion. In this situation you use the same formula, Equation 13-3, but this time you solve for the interest factor for an annuity, IFa. Once you have the IFa, you can determine the rate of return required to meet the goal.

Solution.

$$FVa = PMT(IFa) \tag{13-3}$$
$$\$14,680 = \$500(IFa)$$
$$IFa = \$14,680/\$500$$
$$IFa = 29.360.$$

Now go to Appendix C and find the 15-year row. Moving to the right along the 15-year row, find the interest factor 29.360 in the 9 percent column. Thus 9 percent is the rate at which you must invest the annuity of $500 annually for 15 years to have a terminal value of $14,680.

Problem: Present Value of an Annuity. Lefty Holland, star center for Central State College, has been approached by the Buffalo Bouncers of the Professional Basketball League. The Bouncers have offered Lefty a generous contract that offers him a choice in the payment of his bonus. He may choose between receiving a payment of $25,000 annually for 15 years or receiving an equivalent amount today. If Lefty can invest at 8 percent, what would be the equivalent amount if the bonus were paid today? (Ignore tax consequences for the time being.)

Discussion. Under the conditions outlined, we want to find the present value of an annuity, PVa, of $25,000 annually, PMT, for 15 years, n, which could be invested at 8 percent, k. The discount factor for an annuity, DFa, is found in Appendix D.

Solution.

$$PVa \ = \ PMT(DFa) \hspace{4cm} \textbf{(13-4)}$$

$$= \ \$25,000(8.5595)$$

$$= \ \$213,987.50.$$

Alternative Problem. To demonstrate how a single formula (Equation 13-4) can be used to determine unknowns other than PVa, let's change the basketball scenario. Now assume that Lefty is given the choice of taking an immediate bonus of $213,987.50 or taking an annuity for 15 years that he could invest at 8 percent annually. What is the annuity?

Discussion. We still utilize Equation 13-4, but now we solve for the annuity, PMT. The discount factor for the annuity, 8.5595, comes from Appendix D.

Solution.

$$PVa \ = \ PMT(DFa) \hspace{4cm} \textbf{(13-4)}$$

$$\$213,987.50 \ = \ PMT(8.5595)$$

$$PMT \ = \ \$213,987.50/8.5595$$

$$PMT \ = \ \$25,000.$$

Conclusions

With a bit of practice, perhaps gained by working the end-of-chapter problems, you will find that the problems associated with the time value of money are not as difficult as they may first appear. One trick to remember is that if you wish to know a future value, you use the formulas associated with Appendix A or C. Use Appendix A if there is only a single, present investment; if the investment is an annuity, use Appendix C. On the other hand, if you wish to learn the present value of some future amount, use Appendix B or D. Use Appendix B if the future amount to be discounted is a single, lump-sum amount. If the future receipt (or payment) is an annuity, use Appendix D.

SUMMARY

Financial decisions often involve situations in which someone pays money at one point in time and receives money at another time. Dollars paid or received at different points in time cannot be evaluated directly. Rather, when analyzing financial decisions and transactions, the timing differences in cash flows must be recognized through the techniques introduced in this chapter.

The key procedures covered in the chapter include the following:

Future Value. $FV = PV(1 + k)^n$, where FV is the future value of an initial amount, PV, compounded at the percentage rate, k, for n periods. The term $(1 + k)^n$ is called IF, the *future value interest factor*.

Present Value. $PV = FV[1/(1 + k)]^n$. This equation is simply a transformation of the future value equation. The term $[1/(1+k)]^n$ is called DF, the *discount factor*. The term k, when used to find present values, is often called the *discount rate*.

Future Value of an Annuity. An annuity is defined as a series of constant or equal payments of PMT dollars per period. The sum, or future value of an annuity, is given the symbol FVa, and it is found as follows:

$$FVa = PMT \sum_{t=1}^{n} (1 + k)^{n-t}.$$

The term

$$\sum_{t=1}^{n} (1 + k)^{n-t}$$

is called IFa, the *future value interest factor for an annuity*.

Present Value of an Annuity. The present value of an annuity is given the symbol PVa, and it is found as follows:

$$PVa = PMT \sum_{t=1}^{n} \left(\frac{1}{1 + k}\right)^t.$$

The term

$$\sum_{t=1}^{n} \left(\frac{1}{1 + k}\right)^t = DFa$$

is called the *discount factor for an annuity*.

These four basic equations can be used to find the present or the future value of any lump sum or series of cash flows as well as the interest rate built into any financial contract. These concepts will be used throughout the remainder of the book. In the next chapter the same basic concepts learned in this chapter are applied to business decisions involving expenditures on capital assets. In subsequent chapters present value concepts are applied to the process of valuing bonds and stocks; there we will see that the market prices of these securities are established by determining the present values of the cash flows they are expected to provide. Present value concepts also are used in determining both the types of financing that should be used to fund the firm's assets and the cost of these funds.

RESOLUTION TO DECISION IN FINANCE

Reenlisting with the Generals

Because of the time value of money, it is not surprising that Herschel Walker's $6 million contract may well turn out to be the more lucrative in the long run. Under the terms of Walker's contract, he received all of his money within four years of signing, and he was therefore free to invest it as he wished, thus increasing its value. On the other hand, Young must wait for most of his money, with the last payment due in 2027. Because the payments extend so far into the future, their present value is greatly reduced.

Sources say that Generals owner Donald Trump laid out more money for Walker's contract than Express owner J. William Oldenburg put up for former Brigham Young quarterback Young. Young actually received only $1 million between 1984 and 1988, whereas Walker received his full $6 million from the Generals. The bulk of Young's money is reportedly in an annuity-like arrangement that will bring him about $30 million from 1990 to 2027. That's $810,810 a year, or $67,567 a month, if payments are made in equal amounts.

The Express won't say, of course, but several insurance firms used their annuity formulas—minus fees to financiers—to determine how much money the Express should have set aside

in 1984 to provide Young with $30 million. Assuming a guaranteed interest rate of 9 percent, the Express would have needed slightly less than $5.4 million. By 1990, when the payments to Young are scheduled to begin, that will have grown to more than $9 million. Still earning 9 percent, that $9 million would generate enough interest to pay the entire $30 million to Young through 2027 without ever having to make another payment to the original fund of $5.4 million.

From the players' point of view, Walker probably did get the better financial deal. On paper, Young's contract appears to offer more security than Walker's does. Young is assured payments for the next 43 years, whereas Walker's financial future carries a degree of risk. Depending on the investment decisions of his advisers, Walker's income would appear to have greater potential, both upside and downside. But Young's financial security is tied to the solvency of the U.S. Football League, which is now using its resources not to put on football games but to untangle its financial troubles in the courts.

Fortunately for Young and Walker, when the USFL folded, they were quickly scooped up by the Dallas Cowboys and the San Fransisco Forty-Niners, respectively. One can only wonder how the decisions they made regarding their USFL contracts affected the way they negotiated their contracts with the NFL.

Source: "Walker Prefers $6 Million Pact to Young's Deal," *San Jose Mercury News*, March 9, 1984, 2E.

QUESTIONS

13-1 Is it true that for all positive interest rates the following conditions hold: $IF_{k,n} \geq 1.0$; $DF_{k,n} \leq 1.0$; $FVa_{k,n} \geq$ number of periods the annuity lasts; $DFa_{k,n} \leq$ number of periods the annuity lasts?

13-2 An annuity is defined as a series of payments of a fixed amount for a specific number of periods. Thus $100 a year for 10 years is an annuity, but $100 in Year 1, $200 in Year 2, and $400 a year in Years 3 through 10 is *not* an annuity. However, the second series *contains* an annuity. Is this last statement true or false?

13-3 If a firm's earnings per share grew from $1 to $2 over a 10-year period, the *total growth* was 100 percent, but the *annual growth rate* was *less than* 10 percent. Why is this so?

13-4 To find the present value of an uneven series of payments, you must use the DF tables; the DFa tables can never be of use, even if some of the payments constitute an annuity (for example, $100 each year for Years 3, 4, 5, and 6), because the entire series is not an annuity. Is this statement true or false?

SELF-TEST PROBLEMS

ST-1 Assume it is now January 2, 1988. If you put $1,000 into a savings account on January 2, 1989, at an 8 percent interest rate, compounded annually:
  a. How much would you have in your account on January 2, 1992?
  b. Suppose that you deposited the $1,000 in 4 payments of $250 each on January 2 of 1989, 1990, 1991, and 1992. How much would you have in your account on January 2, 1992, based on 8 percent annual compounding?
  c. Suppose that you made 4 equal payments into your account as suggested in Part b. How large would each of your payments have to be for you to obtain the same ending balance you calculated in Part a?

ST-2 Assume that it is now January 2, 1988, and you will need $1,000 on January 2, 1992. Your bank compounds interest at an 8 percent rate annually.
  a. If only one deposit is made, how much must you place in your account today to have a balance of $1,000 on January 2, 1992?
  b. If you want to make equal payments on each January 2 from 1989 through 1992 to accumulate the $1,000 you need, how large must each of the 4 payments be?
  c. If your father offered either to make the payments calculated in Part b ($221.92) or to give you a lump sum of $750 on January 2, 1989, which would you choose?
  d. If you have only $750 on January 2, 1989, what interest rate, compounded annually, would you have to earn to have the necessary $1,000 on January 2, 1992?
  e. Suppose that you can deposit only $186.29 each January 2 from 1989 through 1992 but you still need $1,000 on January 2, 1992. What interest rate, with annual compounding, must you seek out to achieve your goal?

ST-3 Due to unfortunate circumstances, your sister must borrow $5,000 from you. She wants to repay the loan in 3 equal annual installments that include 9 percent interest. How much should she pay for each of the next 3 years? (*Note:* The first payment is due one year from today.)

ST-4 Your Uncle Henry promises that if you invest $7,500 today in his latest "get rich quick" scheme, he will pay you $2,651.50 each year for the next 3 years. What rate of return is his project offering?

PROBLEMS

13-1   **Present and future values for different periods.** Find the following values *without* using the tables, then work the problems *with* the tables to check your answers. Disregard rounding errors.
   a. An initial $1,000 compounded for 1 year at 8 percent.
   b. An initial $1,000 compounded for 2 years at 8 percent.
   c. The present value of $1,000 due in 1 year at a discount rate of 8 percent.
   d. The present value of $1,000 due in 2 years at a discount rate of 8 percent.

13-2   **Present and future values for different interest rates.** Use the tables to find the following values:
   a. An initial $1,000 compounded for 10 years at 6 percent.
   b. An initial $1,000 compounded for 10 years at 12 percent.
   c. The present value of $1,000 due in 10 years at a 6 percent discount rate.
   d. The present value of $3,105.80 due in 10 years at a 12 percent discount rate.

13-3   **Time for a lump sum to double.** To the closest year, how long will it take $1,000 to double if it is deposited and earns the following rates?
   a. 6 percent.
   b. 12 percent
   c. 16 percent
   d. 100 percent

13-4   **Future value of an annuity.** Find the *future value* of the following annuity if the first payment in this annuity is made at the end of the year; that is, it is a regular annuity.
   a. $1,000 per year for 10 years at 10 percent.
   b. $2,000 per year for 5 years at 5 percent.
   c. $1,000 per year for 5 years at zero percent.

13-5   **Future value of an annuity due.** Find the *future value* of the following annuity if the first payment is made today; that is, it is an annuity due.
   a. $1,000 per year for 10 years at 10 percent.
   b. $2,000 per year for 5 years at 5 percent.
   c. $1,000 per year for 5 years at zero percent.

13-6   **Present value of an annuity.** Find the *present value* of the following regular annuity:
   a. $1,000 per year for 10 years at 10 percent.
   b. $2,000 per year for 5 years at 5 percent.
   c. $1,000 per year for 5 years at zero percent.

13-7   **Present value of an annuity due.** Find the *present value* of the following annuity if the first payment is made today; that is, it is an annuity due.
   a. $1,000 per year for 10 years at 10 percent.
   b. $2,000 per year for 5 years at 5 percent.
   c. $1,000 per year for 5 years at zero percent.

13-8   **Uneven cash flows.**
   a. Find the present value of the following cash flow streams when the discount rate is 10 percent:

Year	Cash Flow Stream A	Cash Flow Stream B
1	$1,000	$5,000
2	3,000	3,000
3	3,000	3,000
4	3,000	3,000
5	5,000	1,000

b. What is the value of each cash flow stream at a zero percent discount rate?

13-9 **Uneven cash flows.** Find the present value of the following cash flow stream, discounted at 8 percent: Year 1, $10,000; Year 2, $5,000; Years 3 to 20, $1,000.

13-10 **Growth rates.** Last year Houston Chemical's sales were $5 million. Sales were $2.5 million 5 years earlier.

a. To the nearest percentage point, at what rate have sales been growing?

b. Suppose someone calculated the sales growth in Part a as follows: "Sales doubled in 5 years. This represents a growth of 100 percent in 5 years; so dividing 100 percent by 5, we find the growth rate to be 20 percent per year." Explain what is wrong with this calculation.

13-11 **Regulary annuity versus annuity due.**

a. You have decided to turn over a new leaf and begin to save money for a change. If you save $3,000 annually for the next 5 years in a 7 percent money market account, what will be the total at the end of the period? Assume that your investment will occur at the end of each year.

b. Since the savings look so good in Part a, you want to get your savings started today. What is the value of the $3,000 annual investment if your first payment is made today and continues as before with 5 annual payments at an assumed rate of 7 percent?

13-12 **Effective rate of interest.** Find the interest rates, or rates of return, on each of the following:

a. You borrow $2,000 and promise to pay back $2,200 at the end of 1 year.

b. You lend $2,000 and receive a promise of $2,200 at the end of 1 year.

c. You borrow $20,000 and promise to pay back $62,112 at the end of 10 years.

d. You borrow $20,000 and promise to make payments of $5,141.78 per year for 5 years.

13-13 **Expected rate of return.** The Dickenson Company buys a machine for $500,000 and expects a return of $119,260.50 per year for the next 10 years. What is the expected rate of return on the machine?

13-14 **Expected rate of return.** New York Orchards invests $3 million to clear a tract of land and set out some young apple trees. The trees will mature in 10 years, at which time the firm plans to sell the orchard at an expected price of $12,136,800. What is New York Orchard's expected rate of return?

13-15 **Effective rate of interest.** Your broker offers to sell you a note for $3,992.70 that will pay $1,000 per year for 5 years. If you buy the note, what rate of interest will you be earning?

13-16 **Effective rate of interest.** Great Atlantic Mortgage Company offers to lend you $150,000; the loan calls for annual payments of $16,432.08 for 20 years. What interest rate is the company charging you?

13-17   **Required lump sum payment.** To enable you to complete your last year in college and then go through law school, you need $12,000 per year for the next 4 years, starting next year (that is, you need the first payment of $12,000 one year from today). Your rich aunt has offered to provide you with a sum of money sufficient to put you through school. She plans to deposit this sum today in a bank account that is expected to yield 8 percent interest.
     a. How large must the deposit be?
     b. How much will be in the account immediately after you make the first withdrawal? After the last withdrawal?

13-18   **Required lump sum investment.** Spartan Financial Corporation is offering a note that matures in 5 years at $1,000. If you wish a 10 percent return on your investment, how much would you be willing to pay for this note? (Assume that no other cash flows accrue from the note other than the single lump-sum maturity payment.)

13-19   **Regular annuity versus annuity due.** Thompson Business Machines has just purchased equipment costing $500,000. The firm can finance the equipment at 10 percent for 15 years.
     a. If the annual payment is computed using a *regular annuity,* what is the annual payment?
     b. If, however, the annual payment is computed as an *annuity due* (that is, the first payment is due today), what is the amount of the payment?

13-20   **Compound growth.** Entertainment Video Centers plans to increase sales at an annual rate of 10 percent for the next 5 years from its current $5,000,000 level.
     a. What is the expected level of sales each year?
     b. Graph each year's sales.

13-21   **Present value of a perpetuity.** What is the present value of a perpetuity of $100 per year if the appropriate discount rate is 5 percent? If interest rates in general doubled and the appropriate discount rate rose to 10 percent, what would happen to the present value of the perpetuity?

13-22   **Amortization schedule.**
     a. Set up an amortization schedule for a $20,000 loan to be repaid in equal installments at the end of each of the next 3 years. The interest rate is 10 percent.
     (Do Parts b through d only if you are using the computerized problem diskette.)
     b. Set up an amortization schedule for a $40,000 loan to be repaid in equal installments at the end of each of the next 3 years. The interest is 10 percent.
     c. Set up an amortization schedule for a $100,000 loan to be repaid in equal installments at the end of each of the next 3 years. The interest rate is 9 percent.
     d. Recalculate Parts b and c using a 20-year amortization schedule.

ANSWERS TO SELF-TEST PROBLEMS

ST-1   **a.**

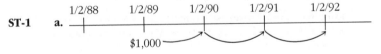

$1,000 is being compounded for 3 years, so your balance on January 2, 1992, is $1,259.71:

$$FV = PV(1 + k)^n$$

$$= \$1,000(1 + 0.08)^3$$

$$= \$1,259.71.$$

b.

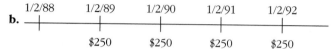

Future value of an annuity:

$$FVa = PMT(IFa) = \$250(4.5061)$$

$$= \$1,126.53.$$

c. $FVa = \$1,259.71.$

$k = 8\%.$

$n = 4.$

$$PMT(IFa) = FVa$$

$$PMT(4.5061) = \$1,259.71$$

$$PMT = \$1,259.71/4.5061$$

$$= \$279.56.$$

Therefore, you would have to make 4 payments of $279.56 at the end of each year to accumulate a balance of $1,259.71 on January 2, 1992.

ST-2 **a.** Set up a time line like those in Self-Test Problem 1 and note that your deposit will grow for 3 years at 8 percent. The deposit on January 2, 1989, is the PV, and $1,000 = FV. The solution is as follows:

$$FV = \$1,000.$$

$$n = 3.$$

$$k = 8\%.$$

$$FV(DF) = PV$$

$$\$1,000(0.7938) = \$793.80, \text{ the initial deposit}$$
$$\text{necessary to accumulate } \$1,000.$$

b. Here we are dealing with a 4-year annuity whose first payment occurs one year from today, on January 2, 1989, and whose future value must equal $1,000. The solution is as follows:

$$FVa = \$1,000.$$

$$n = 4.$$

$$k = 8\%.$$

$$PMT(IFa) = FVa$$

$$PMT = \frac{FVa}{(IFa_{8\%,4})}$$

$$= \frac{\$1,000}{4.5061}$$

$$= \$221.92.$$

c. This problem can be approached in several ways. Perhaps the simplest is to ask the question, "If I received $750 on January 2, 1989, and deposited it to earn 8 percent, would I have the required $1,000 on January 2, 1992?" The answer is no:

$$\$750(1.08)(1.08)(1.08) = \$944.78.$$

This indicates that you should let your father make the payments rather than accept the lump sum of $750.

You could also compare the $750 with the PV of the payments:

$$PMT = \$221.92.$$

$$k = 8\%.$$

$$n = 4.$$

$$PMT(DFa) = PVa$$

$$\$221.92(3.3121) = \$735.02, \text{ the present value of}$$
$$\text{the required payments.}$$

Because this is less than the $750 lump-sum offer, your initial reaction might be to accept the lump sum of $750. However, this would be a mistake. Note that if you deposited the $750 on January 2, 1989, at an 8 percent interest rate to be withdrawn on January 2, 1992, interest would be compounded for only 3 years, from January 2, 1989, to December 31, 1991 and the future value would be only

$$PV(IF) = \$750(1.2597)$$

$$= \$944.78.$$

The problem is that when you found the $735.02 present value of the annuity, you were finding the value of the annuity *today,* on January 2, 1988. You were comparing $735.02 today with the lump sum $750 one year from now. Such a comparison is, of course, invalid. What you should have done was take the $735.02, recognize that this is the present value of an annuity as of January 2, 1988, multiply $735.02 times 1.08 to get $793.82, and compare $793.82 with the lump sum of $750. You would then take your father's offer to pay off the loan rather than the lump sum on January 2, 1989.

d. $$PV = \$750.$$

$$FV = \$1,000.$$

$$n = 3.$$

$$k = ?$$

$$PV(IF) = FV$$

$$IF = \frac{FV}{PV}$$

$$= \frac{\$1,000}{\$750}$$

$$= 1.3333.$$

Use the future value of $1 (Appendix A at the end of the book) for 3 periods to find the interest rate corresponding to an IF of 1.3333. Look across the third-period row of Appendix A until you come to 1.3333. The closest value is 1.3310 in the 10 percent column. Therefore, you would require an interest rate of approximately 10 percent to achieve your $1,000 goal. The exact rate required, found with a financial calculator, is 10.0642 percent.

e.

$$FVa = \$1,000.$$

$$PMT = \$186.29.$$

$$k = ?$$

$$n = 4.$$

$$PMT(IFa) = FVa$$

$$\$186.29(IFa) = \$1,000$$

$$= \frac{\$1,000}{\$186.29}$$

$$= 5.3680.$$

Using the sum of an annuity table for 4 periods (Appendix C at the end of the book), you find that 5.3680 corresponds to a 20 percent interest rate. You might be able to find a borrower willing to offer you a 20 percent interest rate, but there would be some risk involved, and he or she might not actually pay you your $1,000!

ST-3

$$PVa = \$5,000.$$

$$PMT = ?$$

$$k = 9\%.$$

$$n = 3.$$

$$PVa = PMT(DFa)$$

$$\$5,000 = PMT(2.5313)$$

$$PMT = \$5,000/2.5313$$

$$= \$1,975.27.$$

By dividing each side of the equation by the DFa for 3 years at 9 percent, DFa = 2.5313, we can solve for the annuity required to repay the loan in 3 years with a 9 percent return to the lender, which is $1,975.27.

ST-4

$$PVa = \$7,500.$$

$$PMT = \$2,651.50.$$

$$k = ?$$

$$n = 3.$$

$$PVa = PMT(DFa)$$

$$\$7,500 = \$2,651.50(DFa)$$

$$DFa = \$7,500/\$2,651.50$$

$$= 2.8286.$$

Using the present value of an annuity table (found in Appendix D), go down to the third row (n = 3) and go across the row until you find the discount factor, DFa = 2.8286. We find that 2.8286 corresponds to only a 3 percent rate of return. Apparently this is not a very profitable investment opportunity.

Appendix 13A

Semi-Annual and Other Compounding Periods

In all of the examples thus far, it has been assumed that returns are received once a year, or annually. Suppose, however, that you put $1,000 in a bank which advertises that it pays 6 percent compounded *semiannually*. How much will you have at the end of 1 year? Semiannual compounding means that interest is actually paid every 6 months. The procedures for semiannual compounding are illustrated in the calculations in Table 13A-1. Here the annual interest rate is divided by 2, but twice as many compounding periods are used because interest is paid twice a year. Comparing the amount on hand at the end of the second 6-month period, $1,060.90, with what would have been on hand under annual compounding, $1,060, you see that semiannual compounding is better from your standpoint as a saver. This result occurs because you can earn *interest on interest* more frequently.

    Throughout the economy, different types of investments use different compounding periods. For example, bank accounts generally pay interest monthly or daily; most bonds pay interest semiannually; stocks pay dividends quarterly; and many loans pay interest annually. Thus, if securities with different compounding periods are to be compared, one needs to put them on a common basis. This need requires an understanding of the terms *nominal,* or *stated, interest rate* versus the *effective annual rate,* also called the *annual percentage rate (APR).* The **nominal, or stated, interest rate** is the quoted rate; thus, in this example, the nominal rate is 6 percent. The **effective annual rate,** or *annual percentage rate,* is the rate that would have produced the final compound value, $1,060.90, under annual rather than semiannual compounding. In this case, the effective annual rate is 6.09 percent, found by solving for k in the following equation:

nominal (stated) interest rate
The contracted, or stated, interest rate.

effective annual rate
The annual rate of interest actually being earned as opposed to the stated rate; also called the *annual percentage rate (APR).*

Table 13A-1 **Future Value Calculations with Semiannual Compounding**

Period	Beginning Amount, PV	×	(1 + k/2)	=	Ending Amount, FV
1	$1,000.00		(1.03)		$1,030.00
2	1,030.00		(1.03)		1,060.90

$$\$1{,}000(1 + k) = \$1{,}060.90$$

$$k = \frac{\$1{,}060.90}{\$1{,}000} - 1 = 0.0609 = 6.09\%.$$

Thus, if one bank offered 6 percent with semiannual compounding while another offered 6.09 percent with annual compounding, they would both be paying the same effective annual rate of interest.

In general, the effective annual percentage rate can be determined, given the nominal rate, by solving Equation 13A-1:

$$\text{Effective annual rate} = \left(1 + \frac{k_{\text{Nom}}}{m}\right)^{m} - 1.0. \qquad \textbf{(13A-1)}$$

Here k_{Nom} is the nominal, or stated, interest rate, and m is the number of compounding periods per year. For example, to find the effective annual rate if the nominal rate is 6 percent, compounded semiannually, the following calculation is made:

$$\text{Effective annual rate} = \left(1 + \frac{0.06}{2}\right)^{2} - 1.0$$

$$= (1.03)^{2} - 1.0$$

$$= 1.0609 - 1.0$$

$$= 0.0609 = 6.09\%.$$

The points made about semiannual compounding can be generalized as follows. When compounding periods are more frequent than once a year, a modified version of Equation 13A-2 is used to find the future value of a lump sum:

$$\text{Annual compounding: FV} = \text{PV}(1 + k)^{n}. \qquad \textbf{(13A-2)}$$

$$\text{More frequent compounding: FV} = \text{PV}\left(1 + \frac{k_{\text{Nom}}}{m}\right)^{mn}. \qquad \textbf{(13A-2a)}$$

Here m is the number of times per year compounding occurs, and n is the number of years. Therefore, if $1,000 is invested for 1 year at a nominal rate of 6 percent, compounded semiannually, the ending value can be computed using Equation 13A-2a:

$$\text{FV} = \$1{,}000(1 + \{0.06/2\})^{2 \times 1}$$

$$= \$1{,}000(1.0609)$$

$$= \$1{,}060.90.$$

If the investment period is 3 years rather than 1 year, then:

$$FV = \$1,000(1 + \{0.06/2\})^{2 \times 3}$$

$$= \$1,000(1.1941)$$

$$= \$1,194.10.$$

The interest tables often can be used when compounding occurs more than once a year. Simply divide the nominal, or stated, interest rate by the number of times compounding occurs during the year (m), then multiply the years (n) by the number of compounding periods per year (m). For example, to find the amount to which $1,000 will grow after 5 years if semiannual compounding is applied to a stated 8 percent interest rate, divide 8 percent by 2, the number of compounding periods in the year when semiannual compounding is used, and multiply the 5-year period by 2, also because of semiannual compounding. Then look in Appendix A under the 4 percent column and the row for Period 10. You will find an interest factor of 1.4802. Multiplying this by the initial $1,000 gives a value of $1,480.20, the amount to which $1,000 will grow in 5 years at 8 percent, compounded semiannually. This compares to $1,469.30 for annual compounding.

The same procedure is applied in all the cases covered — compounding, discounting, single payments, and annuities. To illustrate semiannual discounting when finding the present value of an annuity, consider the case of an annuity of $1,000 a year for 3 years, discounted at 12 percent. With annual discounting, the discount factor is 2.4018 and the present value of the annual annuity is $2,401.80. For semiannual discounting, look under the 6 percent column and in the Period 6 row of Appendix D to find the discount factor of 4.9173. This discount factor is now multiplied by half of the $1,000, or $500 received each six months, to get the present value of the annuity, PVa = $2,458.65. Because the payments come a little more rapidly, (the first $500 is paid after only six months), the annuity is a little more valuable if payments are received semiannually rather than annually.

PROBLEMS

13A-1   **Future value for various compounding periods.** Find the amount to which $200 will grow under each of the following conditions:
    a. 12 percent compounded annually for 4 years.
    b. 12 percent compounded semiannually for 4 years.
    c. 12 percent compounded quarterly for 4 years.
    d. 12 percent compounded monthly for 1 year.

13A-2   **Present value for various compounding periods.** Find the present value of $200 due in the future under each of the following conditions:
    a. 12 percent nominal rate, semiannual compounding, discounted back 4 years.
    b. 12 percent nominal rate, quarterly compounding, discounted back 4 years.
    c. 12 percent nominal rate, monthly compounding, discounted back 1 year.

13A-3   **Annuity values for various compounding periods.** Find the indicated value of the following regular annuities:
    a. FV of $200 each 6 months for 4 years at a nominal rate of 12 percent, compounded semiannually.
    b. PV of $200 each 3 months for 4 years at a nominal rate of 12 percent, compounded quarterly.

13A-4   **Effective versus nominal interest rates:** The First National Bank pays 11 percent interest, compounded annually, on time deposits. The Second National Bank pays 10 percent interest, compounded quarterly.

   a. In which bank would you prefer to deposit your money?

   b. Is your choice of banks influenced by the fact that you might want to withdraw your funds during the year rather than at the end of the year? In answering the question, assume that funds must be left on deposit during the entire compounding period for you to receive any interest.

Chapter 14

The Process of Capital Budgeting

GM: A Case of Capital Budgeting Gone Awry

When General Motors, the auto giant, makes mistakes, they can be giant mistakes. As the world's largest industrial company and one-time world leader in the auto industry, General Motors is used to being on top. But as the company entered the 1980s, like Gulliver among the Lilliputians, it wakened to find itself tied to the ground by a gang of smaller, more market-savvy competitors.

Relying on its long entrenched belief that money and technology can surmount all obstacles, the corporate behemoth reached deep into its pockets and launched a six-year spending spree. GM bought robots, lasers, and computers designed to boost efficiency, increase quality, and implement engineering changes faster than

before. GM hoped to increase market share by investing $40 billion into state-of-the-art manufacturing facilities and equipment. The idea was that technology, liberally applied, would make the Japanese eat GM's dust.

GM's capital-spending spree did not pay off, however. As Chief Financial Officer F. Alan Smith glumly told 500 of GM's senior executives, with the $40 billion the company put into plant and equipment, GM could have purchased Toyota and Nissan outright. Instead, the company ended up losing market share.

Obviously, something was seriously wrong with GM's capital budgeting analysis. As you read this chapter, try to figure out where GM may have miscalculated. What assumptions did GM make that may have later turned out to be faulty? What important questions did it fail to ask itself?

See end of chapter for resolution.

375

In the previous section we analyzed decisions relating to investment of funds in current assets. Now we consider investment decisions involving long-term assets, or the process of capital budgeting. The term *capital* refers to fixed assets used in production, whereas a *budget* is a plan detailing projected inflows and outflows during some future period. Thus the *capital budget* outlines the planned expenditures on fixed assets, and **capital budgeting** is the entire process of analyzing projects, including not only the analysis of fixed assets, but also the evaluation of current assets investments such as inventory or accounts receivable which would be required to support fixed asset investment projects and the determination of whether these projects should be included in the capital budget.

capital budgeting
The process of planning and analyzing expenditures on assets whose returns extend beyond one year.

Each year businesses invest hundreds of billions of dollars in fixed assets. The process of selecting projects and the real assets associated with them not only involves large sums of capital but also determines to a large extent the firm's future productivity and cash flows. Thus, by their very nature, such investments fundamentally affect the firm's future. A good decision can boost earnings sharply and increase the price of a firm's stock dramatically; a bad decision can lead to bankruptcy. Therefore, the process of capital budgeting is of fundamental importance to the success or failure of a firm, for its asset investment decisions chart the firm's course for many years into the future — indeed, these decisions *determine* its future.

Our treatment of capital budgeting is divided into three parts. First, this chapter gives an overview of the process and explains the basic techniques used in capital budgeting analysis. Then the discussion turns to measures of the risk inherent in any investment in which the future cash flows are not known with certainty. Finally, in Chapter 16 special capital budgeting situations, including risk analysis in capital budgeting, are considered.

IMPORTANCE OF CAPITAL BUDGETING

Various factors combine to make capital budgeting decisions among the most important ones financial managers must make. Because the consequences of capital budgeting decisions continue over an extended period, the decision maker loses some flexibility. The firm is making a financial commitment into the future. For example, the purchase of an asset with an economic life of ten years requires a long waiting period before the final consequences of the decision can be known. Further, asset expansion is related to expected future sales, so a decision to buy an asset that is expected to last five years involves an implicit five-year sales forecast.

An erroneous forecast of asset requirements can have serious results. If the firm has invested too much in assets, it will incur unnecessarily heavy expenses. If it has not spent enough on long-term assets, however, two problems may arise. First, the firm's equipment may not be sufficiently modern to enable it to produce competitively. Second, if it has inadequate capacity, it may lose a portion of its share of the market to rival firms, and regaining lost customers typically requires heavy selling expenses, price reductions, product improvements, and so forth.

Effective capital budgeting will improve both the timing of asset acquisitions and the quality of assets purchased. A firm that forecasts its needs for capital assets in advance will have the opportunity to purchase and install the assets before its sales are at capacity. In practice, most firms do not order capital goods until their sales approach capacity levels. If sales increase because of an increase in general market demand, all firms in the industry will tend to order capital goods at about the same time. This often results in backlogs, long waiting times for machinery, a deterioration in the quality of the capital goods, and a rise in their prices. The firm that foresees its needs and purchases capital assets early can avoid these problems.

Finally, capital budgeting is important because asset expansion typically involves substantial expenditures, and before a firm spends a large amount of money, it must make the proper plans; large amounts of funds are not available automatically. A firm contemplating a major capital expenditure program may need to arrange for its financing several years in advance to be sure of having the funds required for the expansion.

PROJECT PROPOSALS AND CLASSIFICATION

A firm's growth, development, and even its ability to remain competitive and to survive depend on a constant flow of new investment ideas. A well-managed firm will go to great lengths to develop good capital budgeting proposals. A senior executive of a major corporation recently indicated the following:

> Our R & D department is constantly searching for new products, or for ways to improve existing products. In addition, our Executive Committee, which consists of senior executives in marketing, production, and finance, identifies the products and markets in which our company will compete, and the Committee sets long-run targets for each division. These targets, which are formalized in the Corporation's strategic plan, provide a general guide to the operating executives who must meet them. These executives then seek new products, set expansion plans for existing products, and look for ways to reduce production and distribution costs. Since bonuses and promotions are based in large part on each unit's ability to meet or exceed its targets, these economic incentives encourage our operating executives to seek out profitable investment opportunities.
>
> While our senior executives are judged and rewarded on the basis of how well their units perform, people further down the line are given bonuses for specific suggestions, including ideas that lead to profitable investments. Additionally, a percentage of our corporate profit is set aside for distribution to nonexecutive employees. Our objective is to encourage lower level workers to keep on the lookout for good ideas, including those that lead to capital investments.

Not all capital project ideas come from the research and development department however. For example, a Hewlett-Packard sales representative recently reported that customers were asking for a particular type of oscilloscope that the company was not producing at the time. The sales manager discussed the idea with the marketing research group to determine the size of the market for the proposed product. It appeared likely that a substantial market did exist, so cost accountants and engineers were asked to estimate production costs. The entire analysis suggested that the product could be produced and sold to yield a good profit, and the project was undertaken.

If the firm has capable and imaginative executives and employees, and if its incentive system is working properly, many ideas for capital investment will be advanced. Because some ideas will be good ones while others will not, procedures must be established for screening projects.

Although benefits may be gained from carefully screening and analyzing capital expenditure proposals, such investigation does have a cost. For certain types of projects, a relatively refined analysis may be warranted; for others, cost/benefit studies may suggest that a simpler procedure should be used. To aid the screening process, firms generally classify projects into the following categories:

1. **Replacement: maintenance of business.** This category includes those expenditures that are necessary to replace worn-out or damaged equipment.

2. **Replacement: cost reduction.** Expenditures to replace serviceable but obsolete equipment fall into this category. The purpose of these expenditures is to lower the cost of labor, materials, or other items such as electricity.

3. **Expansion of existing products or markets.** Included here are expenditures to increase output of existing products or to expand outlets or distribution facilities in markets now being served.

4. **Expansion into new products or markets.** These are expenditures necessary to produce a new product or to expand into a geographic area not currently being served.

5. **Safety or environmental projects.** Expenditures necessary to comply with government orders, labor agreements, or insurance policy terms are listed here. These expenditures are often called *mandatory investments,* or *non-revenue-producing projects.*

6. **Other.** This catch-all includes home office buildings, parking lots, and so on.

In general, relatively simple calculations and only a few supporting documents are required to support replacement decisions, especially maintenance-type investments in profitable plants. More detailed analysis is required for cost reduction replacements, for expansion of existing product lines, and especially for investments for expansion into new products or areas. Also, within each category, projects are broken down by their dollar costs: the larger the

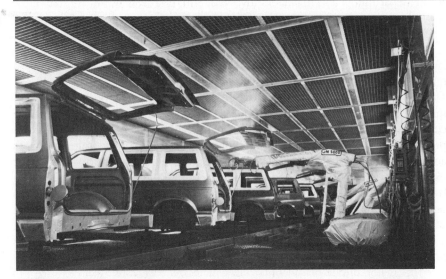

An example of a capital project in which equipment replaces human labor is robot painting in the automobile industry. This photo from Chrysler shows robots painting car interiors. The enormous capital investment in this equipment was offset by savings incurred because of the decreased cost of using equipment instead of labor.

Source: Courtesy of Chrysler Corporation.

required investment, the more detailed the analysis and the higher the level of the officer who must authorize the expenditure. A plant manager may be authorized to approve maintenance expenditures up to $25,000 on the basis of a relatively unsophisticated analysis, but the full board of directors may have to approve decisions that involve either amounts over $1 million or expansions into new products or markets.

ESTIMATING THE CASH FLOWS

The most important, but also the most difficult, step in the analysis of a capital expenditure proposal is the estimation of the **cash flows** associated with the project—the initial investment outlays that are required and the annual cash inflows that the project will produce after it goes into operation. Many variables are involved in the cash flow forecast, and many individuals and departments participate in developing them. For example, the market research group projects sales by means of industry analysis and test marketing of potential products; the marketing department determines pricing policy and anticipates competitors' actions; the production and engineering departments combine to determine the necessary capital outlays and to establish production and labor requirements, while the industrial relations department considers these labor requirements to determine wage and benefit packages. In addition, the accounting department evaluates operating costs attributable to the new project. Of course, in smaller firms these same forecasts must be accomplished with

cash flow

The actual net cash, as opposed to accounting net income, that flows into (or out of) a firm during some specified period.

fewer departments and managers involved. Still, no matter what the size of the firm, the better the forecast, the more likely it is that a poor project will be rejected and a good one accepted.

Obtaining accurate estimates of the costs and revenues associated with a large, complex project can be exceedingly difficult, and forecast errors can be quite large. For example, when several oil companies decided to build the Alaskan Pipeline, the original cost forecast was in the neighborhood of $700 million, but the final cost was closer to $7 billion. Similar miscalculations are common in product design cost estimates for items like new personal computers. As difficult as plant and equipment costs are to estimate, sales revenues and operating costs over the life of a project are even harder to forecast. For example, when AT&T developed the Picturephone, it envisaged large sales in both the residential and business markets, yet it turned out that virtually no one was willing to pay the price required to cover the project's costs. Because of its financial strength, AT&T was able to absorb losses on the project without a problem, but the Picturephone venture would surely have forced a weaker firm into bankruptcy.

The major duties of the financial staff in the forecasting process are (1) coordinating the efforts of the other departments, such as engineering and marketing, (2) ensuring that everyone involved with the forecast uses a consistent set of economic assumptions, and (3) making sure that no biases are inherent in the forecasts. This last point is extremely important, because division managers often become emotionally involved with pet projects or develop empire-building complexes, which leads to cash flow forecasting biases that make bad projects look good—on paper. The AT&T Picturephone project is reported to have been a good example of this problem.

It is not sufficient that the financial staff has unbiased point estimates of the key variables; as we shall see, data on probability distributions or other indications of the probable ranges of error are also essential. It is useful to know the relationship between each input variable and some basic economic variable, such as gross national product. If all production and sales variables can be related to such a basic variable, the financial manager can forecast how the project will do under different economic conditions.

One cannot overstate the importance of cash flow estimates—or the difficulties that are encountered in making these forecasts. However, there are certain principles that, if observed, will help to minimize errors.

Identifying the Relevant Cash Flows

An important element in cash flow estimation is the identification of *relevant cash flows,* which are defined as those cash flows within the firm that should be considered in the decision at hand. Errors are often made here, but there are two cardinal rules that can help financial analysts avoid mistakes: (1) Capital budgeting decisions must be based on cash flows, not on accounting income; and (2) only *incremental cash flows* are relevant to the accept/reject decision. These two rules are discussed in detail in the following sections.

Table 14-1 **Spartan Manufacturing Company: Project X**

	Effect of Project X on:	
	Reported Earnings	**Cash Transactions**
Sales	$90,000	$90,000
Less: COGS (except depreciation)	40,000	40,000
Less: Depreciation	20,000	
Gross margin	30,000	
Less: Selling and administrative	15,000	15,000
Operating profit	15,000	
Less: Taxes (40%)	6,000	6,000
Earnings after taxes	9,000	
Plus: Depreciation	20,000	
Cash flow	$29,000	$29,000

Cash Flow versus Accounting Income

In capital budgeting analysis, annual cash flows, not accounting profits, are used. Cash flows and accounting profits can be very different. To illustrate, consider Table 14-1, which shows how accounting profits and cash flows are related to each other. To better understand the importance of cash flow in the firm's capital investment decision, let's assume that Spartan Manufacturing Company has a new project, known around the firm as "Project X," which will require $100,000 in new equipment. This equipment will be depreciated on a straight line basis for the 5-year life of the project. The effect of the project on Spartan's *reported earnings* is seen in the first column of numbers in Table 14-1.

In the second column of numbers, the aggregate *cash transactions* associated with the project are listed. Costs of goods sold, COGS, is the total of all of the expenditures on the production, labor, and materials for Project X. The selling and administrative expenses are those allocated or directly attributable to the project. The taxes are, of course, those paid as a direct result of the revenues generated by the new project.

Note that each of the expenditures in the second column of Table 14-1 are actual *cash* receipts or payments. In the first column, however, one expense is only a bookkeeping entry — depreciation. As discussed in our review of accounting, depreciation is a noncash allocation of the expense of a fixed asset over its useful (or IRS-determined) life. This allocation permits the company to reduce its tax burden each period but *involves no actual payment of cash.* Therefore, we can add the *depreciation* back to the accounting-determined *after-tax earnings* attributable to the project, which in Table 14-1 equal the project's *cash flow* of $29,000.

Accounting profits are important for some purposes, but for determining the value of a project, we are interested only in cash flows. Therefore, in capital budgeting, focus must be on *net cash flows,* defined as shown on page 382.

$$\text{Net cash flow} = \text{Net income after taxes} + \text{Depreciation,}$$

not on accounting profits per se.

An equivalent method of determining the cash flow is presented in Equation 14-1:

$$\text{Cash flow} = (\$R - \$E)(1 - t) + (D)(t), \qquad \textbf{(14-1)}$$

where

$R =$ cash revenues generated by the project.

$E =$ cash expenses associated with the project.

$t =$ marginal tax rate.

$D =$ depreciation on the project's fixed assets.

When using this formula and the data from Project X found in Table 14-1,

$$
\begin{aligned}
\text{Cash flow} &= (\$R - \$E)(1 - t) + (D)(t) \\
&= (\$90{,}000 - 55{,}000)(1 - 0.4) + (\$20{,}000)(0.4) \\
&= (\$35{,}000)(0.6) + (\$20{,}000)(0.4) \\
&= \$21{,}000 + \$8{,}000 \\
&= \$29{,}000,
\end{aligned}
$$

we arrive at the same conclusion as we did when we found the *cash flow* by adding the accounting-determined *earnings after taxes* and *depreciation*.

Note that the cash flow *does not* contain any financing expenses, such as interest or preferred or common stock dividends. As you will learn in a subsequent chapter, the minimum acceptable rate of return for any project is the **cost of capital**, which is the weighted average of the required returns, or cost, of all sources of financing. If financing charges were included in determining the project's cash flow, and the net cash flows later were discounted by the cost of capital, double counting of the financing costs would occur. Therefore, the consensus is that interest charges should *not* be dealt with explicitly in capital budgeting. It is convenient to compute the project's cash flow *as if* it were financed entirely with common stock equity funding. In essence, this approach allows the analyst to concentrate on selecting the best project available. Once the best project has been identified, the optimal means by which it should be financed can be determined.

Another point about cash flows should be made here. In evaluating a capital budgeting project, we are concerned with only those cash flows that result directly from the project. These cash flows, called **incremental cash flows,** represent the change in the firm's total cash flows that occurs as a direct result of accepting or rejecting the project.

cost of capital
The discount rate that should be used in the capital budgeting process.

incremental cash flow
The net cash flow attributable to an investment project.

Changes in Net Working Capital

Normally, additional inventories are required to support a new operation, and expanded sales also produce additional accounts receivable; both of these increases in assets must be financed. At the same time, however, accounts payable and accruals also will increase spontaneously as a result of the expansion, and this will reduce the net cash needed to finance inventories and receivables. The difference between the required increase in current assets and the spontaneous increase in current liabilities is a required **change in net working capital.** If this change is positive, as it generally is for expansion projects, *additional financing* over and above the cost of the fixed assets is needed for the project. This additional financing is part of the required initial cost of the project and is just as necessary as the investment in the project's fixed assets.

As the end of the project's life approaches, inventories will be sold off and not replaced, and receivables will be collected and thus converted to cash. As these changes occur, the firm experiences an end-of-project positive cash inflow equal to the net working capital requirement that occurred when the project began.

change in net working capital
The increased current assets resulting from a new project minus the increased spontaneous liabilities.

METHODS USED TO EVALUATE PROPOSED PROJECTS

A number of different methods are used to rank projects and to decide whether or not they should be accepted for inclusion in the capital budget. The three ranking methods that are used by firms today are payback, net present value (NPV), and internal rate of return (IRR).[1]

1. Payback (or payback period). This is the number of years required to return the original investment.

2. Net present value (NPV). This is the present value of future cash flows, discounted at the appropriate cost of capital, minus the cost of the investment. The NPV method is called a *discounted cash flow (DCF)* method.

3. Internal rate of return (IRR). This is the discount rate that equates the present value of future cash flows to the initial cost of the project. The IRR is also a discounted cash flow (DCF) method.

Future cash flows are, in all cases, defined as the incremental net cash inflows from the investments. The nature and characteristics of these methods are illustrated and explained in the following sections, where the cash flow

---

[1]You should be aware that there are three other ranking methods that are sometimes used: (1) the accounting rate of return, (2) the profitability index, and (3) the discounted payback period. Each of these methods can lead to incorrect rankings for projects and are thus potentially misleading. For a more complete discussion of these methods and their potential to provide incorrect project evaluations, see Brigham and Gapenski, *Intermediate Financial Management,* 2nd ed., Chapter 7.

Table 14-2 **Cash Flows for Projects E and L**
(Investment Outlay for Each Project Is $25,000)

| Year | Net Cash Flow (After-Tax Profits Plus Depreciation) | |
	Project E	Project L
1	$12,000	$ 5,400
2	10,000	8,000
3	8,000	10,000
4	5,400	12,000
Total inflows	$35,400	$35,400

data shown in Table 14-2 is used for two projects that we call Project E and Project L. Note that the returns from Project E are much greater early in its life than those of Project L, whose returns are larger comparatively late in its life. As we have discussed, these cash flows consist of both after-tax profits and depreciation, not just profits alone. Furthermore, the **investment outlay** includes not only the cost of the fixed assets required for the project, but also any working capital outlays, such as increases in inventories and accounts receivable, that occur because of the project.[2]

investment outlay
Funds expended for fixed assets of a specified project plus working capital funds expended as a result of the project's adoption.

payback (or payback period)
The length of time required for the cash flows to return the cost of the investment.

Payback Method

The **payback period** is defined as the number of years it takes a firm to recover its original investment from net cash inflows. The payback method provides a measure of project liquidity or the speed with which cash invested in the project will be returned. In Table 14-2 each project costs $25,000. Assuming that the cash flows come in evenly during the year, the payback period for Project E is 2.375 years [$12,000 + $10,000 + ($3,000/$8,000)], and the payback period for Project L is 3.133 years [$5,400 + $8,000 + $10,000 + ($1,600/$12,000)]. Because Project E's largest cash flows occur early in its life, it is not surprising that it has the faster recovery of the initial investment. On the basis of payback, Project E is superior to Project L if the projects are of equal risk.

The payback method's principal strength is that it is easy and inexpensive to calculate and apply. This was an important consideration in the precomputer days. Prior to the 1960s payback was the most commonly used method for screening capital expenditure proposals. However, the payback technique has

[2]Of course, only the investment in fixed assets is depreciable. When the project ends, the investment in working capital is often recovered through reductions in inventory and collection of accounts receivable outstanding. This recovery is not taxable since it represents a conversion of assets without economic gain.

conceptual problems that make total reliance on this technique financially undesirable. Two of the major conceptual weaknesses of payback are the following:

1. It ignores returns beyond the payback period. One glaring weakness of the payback period is that it ignores any cash flow that occurs beyond the payback period. For example, if Project L had an additional return of $20,000 in Year 5, this fact would not influence the payback ranking of Projects E and L. Ignoring returns in the distant future means that the payback method is biased against long-term projects.

2. It ignores the time value of money. The timing of cash flows is obviously important (as the last chapter emphasized), yet the payback method ignores the time value of money. By this method a dollar in Year 3 is given the same weight as a dollar in Year 1.

In spite of the conceptual drawbacks to the payback technique, this project-screening device has shown remarkable vitality over the years. Managers still use payback because it tells them something they want to know. Firms that are short of cash necessarily place a higher value on projects with a higher degree of liquidity. A project that returns its investment quickly will allow these funds to be reinvested quickly in other projects. Such a project would be especially valuable to a small or growing firm that is unable to raise capital quickly or in large amounts. Also, the payback period is often used as one indicator of projects' relative risk. Because firms can usually forecast near-term events better than more distant ones, projects whose returns come in relatively rapidly are, other things held constant, generally less risky than longer-term projects. By focusing on the speed of cash inflows, the payback method provides important information to the financial manager. However, in light of payback's weaknesses, the technique should be used in conjunction with other, more technically correct project-screening methods such as net present value and internal rate of return.

Net Present Value (NPV) Method

As the flaws in the payback method were recognized, people began to search for methods of evaluating projects which would recognize that a dollar received immediately is preferable to a dollar received at some future date. This led to the development of **discounted cash flow (DCF) techniques** to take account of the time value of money. One such DCF technique is called the *net present value method*. To implement this approach, find the present value of the expected net cash flows of an investment, discounted at an appropriate percentage rate, and subtract from it the initial cost outlay of the project. If its net present value is positive, the project should be accepted; if negative, it should be rejected.

discounted cash flow (DCF) techniques
Methods of ranking investment proposals that employ time value of money concepts, two of which are the net present value method and the internal rate of return method.

Table 14–3 **Calculating the Net Present Values (NPVs) of Projects E and L**

	Project E			Project L		
Year	Cash Flow	DF (12%)	PV of Cash Flow	Cash Flow	DF (12%)	PV of Cash Flow
1	$12,000	.8929	$ 10,715	$ 5,400	.8929	$ 4,822
2	10,000	.7972	7,972	8,000	.7972	6,378
3	8,000	.7118	5,694	10,000	.7118	7,118
4	5,400	.6355	3,432	12,000	.6355	$ 7,626
		PV of inflows	$ 27,813		PV of inflows	$ 25,944
		Less: Cost	− 25,000		Less: Cost	− 25,000
		NPV	$ 2,813		NPV	$ 944

net present value (NPV)

A method of ranking investment proposals. The NPV is equal to the present value of future returns, discounted at the marginal cost of capital, minus the present value of the cost of the investment.

The equation for the **net present value (NPV)** is as follows:

$$NPV = \sum_{t=1}^{n} \frac{CF_t}{(1 + k)^t} - C$$

$$= \left[\frac{CF_1}{(1 + k)^1} + \frac{CF_2}{(1 + k)^2} + \cdots + \frac{CF_n}{(1 + k)^n} \right] - C$$

$$= CF_1(DF_1) + CF_2(DF_2) + \cdots + CF_n(DF_n) - C. \tag{14-2}$$

Here CF_t is the expected net cash flow from the project at Period t, n is the project's expected life, and k, represented by the discount factor, DF, is the appropriate discount rate, or the cost of capital. The cost of capital, k, depends on the riskiness of the project, the level of interest rates in the economy, and several other factors. In this chapter we take k as a given, but it is discussed in detail in Chapter 19.

The capital outlays, C, such as the cost of buying equipment or building factories, are *negative* cash outflows and are given a minus sign. In evaluating Projects E and L, only CF_0 is negative, but for many large projects, such as General Motors' Saturn project, an electric power plant, or IBM's new lap-top computer, outflows occur for several years before operations begin and positive cash in-flows are generated.

Under the assumption that the two projects are equally risky, the net present values of Projects E and L are calculated in Table 14-3, using the discounting procedures developed in Chapter 13 and Equation 14-2. Assuming a required rate of return of 12 percent for both projects, Project E has an NPV of $2,813 and Project L has an NPV of $944. On this basis, both projects should be accepted if possible; however, if only one can be chosen, Project E is the better choice because it has the higher NPV.

The rationale for the NPV method is straightforward. The value of a firm is the sum of the value of its parts; that is, the value of its various projects and investments. If the firm takes on a zero-NPV project, the position of the original investors is unchanged — the firm becomes larger but its value does not change. Thus, when the NPV is zero, the project has covered all required operating and financial costs but has no excess returns. However, when a firm adopts a project with a positive NPV, the project's returns exceed required financial and operating costs. Therefore, the value of the firm increases by the amount of the NPV, thereby improving the position of the original investors. In this example, the value of the firm, and hence the original shareholders' wealth, increases by $2,813 if the firm chooses Project E, but by only $944 if it chooses Project L. Of course, the firm's value will increase by $3,757 if it is possible to accept both projects. *The increase in the value of the firm from its capital budget for the year is the sum of the NPVs of all accepted projects.* Thus, if Projects E and L are mutually exclusive, it is easy to see why Project E is preferable to Project L, but if they are independent, both are acceptable since each has a positive NPV.[3]

The Internal Rate of Return (IRR) Method

In the previous section on NPV we said that if a project's NPV is positive, the project is acceptable, and if the NPV is negative, the project is unacceptable. When the NPV is neither positive nor negative, the rate used to discount future cash flows back to the present is the project's **internal rate of return (IRR).** More formally, the internal rate of return is the discount rate that equates the present value of the expected future cash flows, or receipts, to the initial cost of the project. The equation for calculating this rate is as follows:

$$\sum_{t=1}^{n} \frac{CF_t}{(1 + r)^t} - C = 0$$

$$\frac{CF_1}{(1 + r)^1} + \frac{CF_2}{(1 + r)^2} + \cdots \frac{CF_n}{(1 + r)^n} - C = 0$$

$$CF_1(DF_1) + CF_2(DF_2) + \cdots + CF_n(DF_n) - C = 0. \qquad \textbf{(14-3)}$$

Here we know the value of the investment outlay, C, and the cash flows, CF_1, $CF_2, \cdots, CF_n$ as well, but we do not know the value of the **discount rate,** r, that equates the future cash flows and the present value of the investment outlays. There is a value of r which will cause the sum of the discounted cash receipts to equal the initial cost of the project, making the equation equal to zero: this value of r is defined as the internal rate of return. In other words, the solution value for r is the IRR.

internal rate of return (IRR)
The rate of return on an asset investment, calculated by finding the discount rate that equates the present value of future cash flows to the cost of the investment.

discount rate
The interest rate used in the discounting process.

---

[3]*Mutually exclusive* projects are alternative investments; if one project is taken on, the other must be rejected. The installation of a conveyor belt system in a warehouse and the purchase of a fleet of forklift trucks to do the same job for the same warehouse is an example of mutually exclusive projects—accepting one implies rejection of the other. *Independent* projects are those whose costs and revenues are independent of one another. For example, the purchase of the company president's automobile and the purchase of a corporate jet would represent independent projects.

A simple example may make this concept easier to understand. If we invest $10,000 for 6 years at 14 percent, using Equation 13-1a we can determine the terminal value of the investment:

$$FV = PV(IF)$$

$$= \$10,000(2.1950)$$ **(13-1a)**

$$= \$21,950.$$

Now assume that we know that if we invest $10,000 today, the investment will return $21,950 in 6 years. What is the rate of return on this investment? We need to find the discount rate that equates the value of the investment today, $10,000, with the future value of $21,950 to be received 6 years hence. This is the same as finding the discount rate that causes the NPV of the investment to equal zero. Therefore, as Equation 14-3 suggests, we solve for the discount factor to determine the discount rate:

$$PV = FV(DF)$$

$$DF = \frac{PV}{FV}$$

$$= \frac{\$10,000}{\$21,950}$$

$$= .455581 = .4556.$$

We can find the discount factor .4556 in Appendix B by looking across the sixth-year row to the 14 percent column. The rate that equates the present cost and future return is the internal rate of return—14 percent.

Notice that the internal rate of return formula, Equation 14-3, is simply the NPV formula, Equation 14-2, solved for the particular discount rate that causes the NPV to equal zero. Thus the same basic equation is used for both methods; in the NPV method the discount rate, k, is specified and the NPV is found, whereas in the IRR method the NPV is specified to equal zero and the value of r that forces the NPV to equal zero is found.

The internal rate of return may be found in a number of ways. Several methods are discussed in the following sections.

Procedure 1: IRR with Constant Cash Inflows. If the cash flows from a project are constant, or equal in each year, the project's internal rate of return can be found by a relatively simple process. In essence, such a project is an annuity: the firm makes an outlay, C, and receives a stream of cash flow benefits, PMT, for a given number of years. The IRR for the project is found by applying Equation 13-4, discussed in Chapter 13.

To illustrate, suppose a project has a cost of $10,000 and is expected to produce cash flows of $1,627.45 each year for 10 years. The cost of the project,

$10,000, is the present value of an annuity of $1,627.45 a year for 10 years. Applying Equation 13-4, we obtain

$$PVa = PMT(DFa) \qquad\qquad (13\text{-}4)$$

$$Cost = PMT(DFa)$$

$$\frac{Cost}{PMT} = \frac{\$10,000}{\$1,627.45} = 6.1446 = DFa.$$

Looking up DFa in Appendix D (at the end of the text) across the row for Year 10, we find it located under the 10 percent column. Accordingly, 10 percent is the project's IRR. In other words, 10 percent is the value of r that would force Equation 14-3 to be zero when PMT is constant at $1,627.45 for 10 years and C is $10,000. This procedure works only if the project has constant annual cash flows; if it does not, the IRR must be found by one of the other methods discussed next.

Procedure 2: Trial and Error. In the trial-and-error method, the present value of cash flows from an investment is first computed using a somewhat arbitrarily selected discount rate. Because the cost of capital for most firms is in the range of 12 to 18 percent, it is hoped that projects will promise a return of at least 12 percent. Therefore, 12 percent is a good starting point for most problems. Then the present value thus obtained is compared with the investment's cost. Suppose the present value of the inflows is larger than the project's cost. What do we do now? We must *lower* the present value, and to do this we must *raise* the discount rate and go through the process again. Conversely, if the present value is lower than the cost, we lower the discount rate and repeat the process. This process is continued until the present value of the flows from the investment is approximately equal to the project's cost. The discount rate that brings about this equality is the internal rate of return. Thus, *the discount rate that forces a project's NPV to equal zero is defined as the project's internal rate of return.*

This calculation process is illustrated next for the same Projects E and L that were analyzed earlier. In Table 14-4 the steps required to find the IRR for Project L are reviewed. First, the 12 percent interest factors are obtained from Appendix B at the end of the text. These factors are then multiplied by the cash flows for the corresponding years, and the present values of the cash flows are placed in the appropriate columns. Next, the present values of the yearly cash flows are summed to obtain the investment's total present value. Subtracting the cost of the project from this figure gives the net present value of the project's cash flow. Because the NPV of Project L's cash flow is positive, we know that the internal rate of return of this investment opportunity is greater than 12 percent. However, the NPV is rather small, indicating that the IRR is close to 12 percent. Thus we increase the discount rate slightly to 14

Table 14-4 **Finding the Internal Rate of Return of Project L**

		12%		14%	
Year	**Cash Flow**	**DF**	**PV**	**DF**	**PV**
1	$ 5,400	.8929	$ 4,822	.8772	$ 4,737
2	8,000	.7972	6,378	.7695	6,156
3	10,000	.7118	7,118	.6750	6,750
4	12,000	.6355	7,626	.5921	7,105
		PV of inflows	$ 25,944		$ 24,748
		Less: Cost	− 25,000		− 25,000
		NPV	$ 944		$ (252)

percent. At 14 percent the NPV of Project L is a negative $252. Because the internal rate of return (IRR) causes the NPV to equal zero, we know that the internal rate of return for Project L is between 12 and 14 percent.

If we wish the IRR to be more accurate, we can interpolate between these results. To do so, we bracket the discount rate that causes the project's NPV to equal zero:

$$
\left.
\begin{array}{l}
PV = \$25,944 \text{ at } 12.\ 0\% \\[4pt]
PV = \$25,000 \text{ at } 12.+\% \\[4pt]
PV = \$24,748 \text{ at } \underline{14.\ 0\%} \\
\phantom{PV = \$24,748 \text{ at } } 2.\ 0\%
\end{array}
\right\}
$$

$\left.\begin{array}{l}\$944\end{array}\right\}$ $\left.\begin{array}{l}\\ \\ \end{array}\right\}\$1,196$

Thus

$$IRR = 12.00\% + (\$944/\$1,196)(2.0\%)$$

$$= 12.00\% + 0.789(2.0\%)$$

$$= 13.58\%.$$

The IRR lies 944/1196 percent of the way between 12 and 14 percent. Since there is a two-percentage-point difference between 12 and 14 percent, we multiply the fraction by 2 percent before adding the quantity to 12 percent to obtain the IRR of 13.58 percent. For all practical purposes, an IRR that is accurate to within one-half percent is usually sufficient. The calculations may be carried out to several decimal places, but for most projects, when the assumptions associated with forecasting cash flows several years into the future are considered, this is spurious accuracy.

Table 14-5 **Finding the Internal Rate of Return of Project E**

Year	Cash Flow	12%		16%		18%	
		DF	PV	DF	PV	DF	PV
1	$12,000	.8929	$ 10,715	.8621	$ 10,345	.8475	$ 10,170
2	10,000	.7972	7,972	.7432	7,432	.7182	7,182
3	8,000	.7118	5,694	.6407	5,126	.6086	4,869
4	5,400	.6355	3,432	.5523	2,982	.5158	2,785
		PV of inflows	$ 27,813		$ 25,885		$ 25,006
		Less: Cost	− 25,000		− 25,000		− 25,000
		NPV	$ 2,813		$ 885		$ 6

Just as we found the IRR of Project L, we now trace the steps in determining the IRR for Project E (see Table 14-5). Again, the 12 percent discount rate is employed as a starting point in the search for the project's internal rate of return. The firm's cost of capital, or the return on the best alternative investment opportunity, is usually the first discount rate used in the trial-and-error process. The NPV at 12 percent is positive, so we know the project's IRR is greater than 12 percent. Because the NPV is significantly greater than zero at 12 percent, we know the IRR is much greater than that rate. Multiplying the project's cash flows by a greater discount rate (the rate of 16 percent is chosen arbitrarily), we find that the NPV is still positive, though less than before. At 18 percent the NPV is barely larger than zero; thus for all practical purposes the IRR of Project E is 18 percent, because at that rate the project's NPV is essentially zero.

Procedure 3: Graphic Solution. The graphic method for finding IRRs involves plotting a curve that shows the relationship between a project's NPV and the discount rate used to calculate the NPV. Such a curve is defined as the project's **net present value profile.** NPV profiles for Projects E and L are shown in Figure 14-1. To construct them, we first note that at a zero discount rate, the NPV is simply the total of the undiscounted cash flows of the project less the project's cost; thus, at a zero discount rate, the NPV of both projects is $10,400. These values are plotted as the vertical axis intercepts in Figure 14-1. Next we calculate the projects' NPVs at three discount rates, say, 5, 10, and 15 percent, and plot these values. The data points plotted on the graph are shown at the bottom of the figure. When we connect these points, we have the net present value profiles.

Since the IRR is defined as the discount rate at which a project's NPV equals zero, *the point at which its net present value profile crosses the horizontal axis indicates the project's internal rate of return.* Figure 14-1 indicates that IRR$_E$ is 18 percent, whereas IRR$_L$ is 13.6 percent. With graph paper and a sharp pencil, the graphic method yields reasonably accurate results.

net present value profile
A curve showing the relationship between a project's NPV and the discount rate used to calculate it.

Figure 14-1 **Net Present Value Profiles**
NPVs of Projects E and L at Different Discount Rates

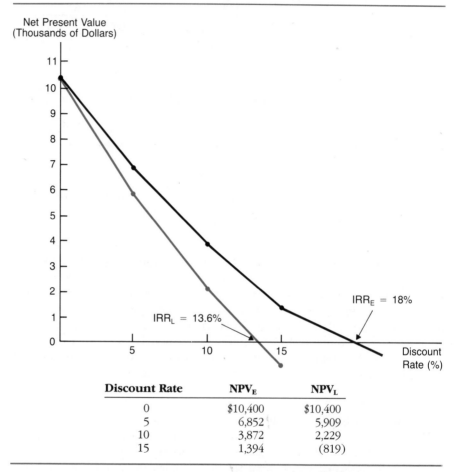

Discount Rate	NPV_E	NPV_L
0	$10,400	$10,400
5	6,852	5,909
10	3,872	2,229
15	1,394	(819)

Procedure 4: Financial Calculator and Computer Solutions. Internal rates of return can be calculated easily by computers. Most larger firms have computerized their capital budgeting processes and automatically generate IRRs, NPVs and paybacks for all projects. Also, many hand-held calculators have built-in functions for calculating IRRs. Thus business firms have no difficulty whatever with the mechanical side of capital budgeting.

Rationale and Use of the IRR Method. What is so special about the particular discount rate that equates a project's cost with the present value of its receipts (its IRR)? To answer this question, first assume that our illustrative firm obtains the $25,000 needed to take on Project E by borrowing from a bank at an interest rate of 18 percent. Since the internal rate of return of this

Table 14-6 **Analysis of Project E's IRR as a Loan Rate**

Year	Loan Amount at Beginning of Year (2)	Cash Flow (3)	Interest on the Loan at 18.0% 0.18 × (2) = (4)	Repayment of Principal (3) − (4) = (5)	Ending Loan Balance (2) − (5) = (6)
1	$25,000	$12,000	$4,500	$7,500	$17,500
2	17,500	10,000	3,150	6,850	10,650
3	10,650	8,000	1,917	6,083	4,567
4	4,567	5,400	822	4,578	11[a]

[a]The exact value of IRR$_E$ is 18.01325 percent. Had that value been used, the ending balance would have been zero. Note that the difference between this residual and that in Figure 14-5 is simply the result of rounding differences.

project was calculated to be 18 percent, the same as the cost of the bank loan, the firm can invest in the project, use the cash flows generated by the investment to pay off the principal and interest on the loan, and come out exactly even on the transaction. This point is demonstrated in Table 14-6, which shows that Project E provides cash flows that are just sufficient to pay 18 percent interest on the unpaid balance of the bank loan, retire the loan over the life of the project, and end up with a balance that differs from zero only by a rounding error of $10.94.

If the internal rate of return exceeds the cost of the funds used to finance a project, a surplus will remain after paying for the capital. This surplus will accrue to the firm's stockholders, so taking on the project will increase the value of the firm's stock. If the internal rate of return is less than the cost of capital, taking on the project will impose a cost on existing stockholders, so accepting the project will result in a reduction of value. It is this "breakeven" characteristic that makes us interested in the internal rate of return.[4]

Continuing with the example of Projects E and L, if both projects have a cost of capital of 12 percent, the internal rate of return rule indicates that if the projects are independent, both should be accepted — they both do better than break even. If they are mutually exclusive, E ranks higher and should be accepted whereas L should be rejected. If the cost of capital is above 18.0 percent, both projects should be rejected.

EVALUATION OF THE DECISION RULES

We have presented three possible capital budgeting rules, all of which are used to a greater or lesser extent in practice. However, because the methods can lead to quite different accept/reject decisions, we need to answer this question: Which method is best? Obviously, the best method is the one that selects

---

[4]This example illustrates the logic of the IRR method, but for technical correctness, the capital used to finance the project should be assumed to be a mix of debt and equity, not debt alone.

that set of projects which will maximize shareholder wealth. If more than one method does this, the best method would be the one that is easiest to use in practice.

Here are three properties that must be exhibited by a capital budgeting method if it is to lead to consistently correct decisions:

1. The method must consider all cash flows throughout the entire life of a project.

2. The method must consider the time value of money—that is, it must reflect the fact that dollars which come in sooner are more valuable than those expected in the distant future.

3. When the method is used to select from a set of mutually exclusive projects, it must choose that project which will maximize the firm's value.

How do the three decision methods stand in regard to the required properties? The payback method violates Properties 1 and 2; it does not consider all cash flows, and it ignores the time value of money. Both the NPV and IRR methods satisfy Properties 1 and 2, and both lead to identical (and correct) accept/reject decisions for independent projects. However, only the NPV method satisfies Property 3 under all conditions. As we shall see in Appendix 14A, there are certain conditions under which the IRR method fails to correctly identify that project in a set of mutually exclusive projects which will maximize the firm's stock price.

A CASE OF CAPITAL BUDGETING

expansion project
A project that is intended to increase sales.

An **expansion project** is one that calls for the firm to invest in new facilities in order to increase sales. For example, suppose Houston Trucking Company buys a new delivery van at a cost of $10,000. The van has a 5-year ACRS life (see Chapter 6 for a review of ACRS depreciation); additional sales attributable to the new van will amount to $28,000 per year for five years; and Houston expects to be able to sell the van for $500 at the end of its 5-year service life. Operating costs (fuel, labor, and so forth) will amount to $20,000 per year. Houston's marginal federal-plus-state income tax rate is 40 percent, and its cost of capital is 10 percent. Table 14-7 works out the cash flows over the van's 5-year life.

Now we need to determine the company's initial investment, or CF_0. Houston must write a check for $10,000 to pay for the van. Also, Houston's net working capital (inventories plus accounts receivable, minus accounts payable) will rise by $3,000 if it purchases the van; this net working capital will be recovered when the van is sold. Thus the net investment in the van at (approximately) t = 0 is as follows:

Purchase price of van	$10,000
Plus investment in working capital	3,000
Net investment at t = 0	$13,000

Table 14-7 **Analysis of an Expansion Project:**
Houston Trucking Company

	Year 1	Year 2	Year 3	Year 4	Year 5
Sales attributable to the project (S)	$28,000	$28,000	$28,000	$28,000	$28,000
Operating costs (OC)	20,000	20,000	20,000	20,000	20,000
Depreciation (Dep)	2,000	3,200	2,000	1,400	1,400
Income before tax	$ 6,000	$ 4,800	$ 6,000	$ 6,600	$ 6,600
Taxes (40%)	2,400	1,920	2,400	2,640	2,640
Net income after taxes (NI)	$ 3,600	$ 2,880	$ 3,600	3,960	3,960
Net cash flow (CF$_t$ = NI + Dep)	$ 5,600	$ 6,080	$ 5,600	$ 5,360	$ 5,360

When the van is disposed of at the end of five years, Houston expects to sell it for $500. Since the truck will be fully depreciated, yet will have a value of $500, in economic terms it has been "overdepreciated." Under the tax laws, the government gets to "recapture" this depreciation by treating any salvage value in excess of the original depreciable basis as ordinary income rather than as a capital gain. Therefore, the $500 will be taxed as ordinary income at a rate of 40 percent. The after-tax proceeds from the sale will be as follows:

Salvage value after tax = Amount before tax − Tax

$$= \text{Amount before tax} - \text{Amount before tax(Tax rate)}$$

$$= \text{Amount before tax}(1 - T)$$

$$= \$500(0.6)$$

$$= \$300 \text{ recovered at end of Year 5.}$$

The annual net cash flows attributable to the investment in the van are equal to net income after taxes plus depreciation. These cash flows are developed in Table 14-7. Note that depreciation under ACRS for a 5-year class life project such as the van is calculated as follows:

1. The *depreciable basis* is equal to the total cost of the truck, which is $10,000. Note that delivery, installation, and similar charges are included in the depreciable basis.

2. Annual depreciation:

Year	ACRS Percent[a]	Basis	Annual Depreciation
1	0.20	$10,000	$ 2,000
2	0.32	10,000	3,200
3	0.20	10,000	2,000
4	0.14	10,000	1,400
5	0.14	10,000	1,400
	1.00		$10,000

[a]We assume that these ACRS percentages apply.

Now we have all the information necessary for calculating the project's NPV at the 10 percent cost of capital:

Year	Cash Flow	$DF_{10\%,t}$	Product
1	$5,600	0.9091	$ 5,091
2	6,080	0.8264	5,025
3	5,600	0.7513	4,207
4	5,360	0.6830	3,661
5	8,660[a]	0.6209	5,377
		Total	$23,361
		Less: Net investment at t = 0	13,000
		Net present value (NPV)	$10,361

[a]$5,360 from operations + $3,000 recovery of net working capital + $300 after-tax salvage.

Alternatively, we could set up the problem as follows:

$$NPV = \sum_{t=1}^{n} \frac{CF_t}{(1 + k)^t} - Cost$$

$$= \frac{\$5,600}{(1.10)^1} + \frac{\$6,080}{(1.10)^2} + \frac{\$5,600}{(1.10)^3} + \frac{\$5,360}{(1.10)^4} + \frac{\$8,660}{(1.10)^5} - \$13,000$$

$$= \$10,361.$$

Alternatively, we could input the cash flow data and the cost of capital into a financial calculator, press the NPV button, and obtain the NPV, $10,361. If the project had a fairly long life, the calculator solution would be much more efficient.

We could also solve for r in the following equation to find the van's IRR:

$$NPV = 0 = \frac{\$5,600}{(1 + r)^1} + \frac{\$6,080}{(1 + r)^2} + \frac{\$5,600}{(1 + r)^3}$$
$$+ \frac{\$5,360}{(1 + r)^4} + \frac{\$8,660}{(1 + r)^5} - \$13,000.$$

The solution value is r = IRR = 36.25%, found with a financial calculator.

The question still remains: Should Houston Trucking invest in the delivery van? Assuming the forecasts of revenues and costs are reasonably correct, yes, the firm should invest in the van; the NPV is positive at the company's required rate of return and the IRR is greater than the required rate of return.[5] However, the financial managers's responsibility for the purchase does not end with the acceptance of the investment opportunity. The purchase must be monitored closely by means of a *post-audit* to determine if it is living up to expectations.

---

[5]As we note later, if a single project has a positive NPV, the project's IRR will always be larger than the project's required rate of return. However, complications *may* arise when comparing two or more investment opportunities. In that situation, the NPV ranking of multiple projects *may* differ from the IRR ranking.

THE POST-AUDIT

The final aspect of the capital budgeting process is the *post-completion audit,* or **post-audit,** which involves a comparison of actual results to those pre- dicted in the request for funds and an explanation of observed differences. For example, firms often require that the operating divisions send a monthly re- port for the first six months after a project goes into operation and a quarterly report thereafter until the project's results are up to expectations. From then on, reports on the operation are handled like those on other operations.

post-audit
A comparison of the actual and expected results for a given capital project.

    The post-audit has several purposes, including the following:

1. Improve forecasts. When decision makers systematically compare their projections to actual outcomes, there is a tendency for estimates to improve. Conscious or unconscious biases are observed and eliminated; new forecasting methods are sought as the need for them becomes apparent; and people simply tend to do everything better, including forecasting, if they know that their actions are being monitored.

2. Improve operations. Businesses are run by people, and people can perform at higher or lower levels of efficiency. When a divisional team has made a forecast about a new installation, its members are, in a sense, putting their reputations on the line. If costs are above predicted levels, sales below expectations, and so on, executives in production, sales, and other areas will strive to improve operations and to bring results into line with forecasts.

    The post-audit is not a simple process. First, one must recognize that each element of the cash flow forecast is subject to uncertainty, so a percentage of all projects undertaken by any reasonably venturesome firm will go awry. This fact must be considered when appraising the performances of the operating executives who submit capital expenditure requests. Second, projects some- times fail to meet expectations for reasons beyond the control of the operating executives and for reasons that no one could realistically be expected to antic- ipate. For example, the dramatic and unexpected decline in oil prices in 1986 hurt many projects. Third, it is often difficult to separate the operating results of one investment from those of a larger system. Even though projects must stand alone to permit ready identification of costs and revenues, the actual cost savings that result from a replacement project may be very hard to measure. Fourth, if the post-audit process is not used with care, executives may be re- luctant to suggest potentially profitable but risky projects. And fifth, the exec- utives who were actually responsible for a given decision may have moved on by the time the results of the decision are known.

    Because of these difficulties, some firms tend to play down the importance of the post-audit. However, observations of both businesses and government units suggest that the best-run and most successful organizations are the ones that put the greatest stress on post-audits. Accordingly, the post-audit is one of the most important elements in a good capital budgeting system.

SUMMARY

Capital budgeting requires the financial manager to estimate future cash flows, appraise risks and incorporate that evaluation into the required rate of return, and adjust the expected cash flows to a present value basis; if a project's *net present value* is positive, it is accepted.

The capital budgeting process centers around the following steps:

1. Ideas for projects are developed.

2. Projects are classified by type of investment: replacement, expansion of existing product lines, expansion into new markets, safety, and "other."

3. The expected future cash flows from a project are estimated. This involves estimating the investment outlay required for the project and estimating the cash inflows over the project's projected life.

4. The riskiness inherent in the project is appraised. This important subject is taken up in Chapters 15 and 16.

5. The projects are ranked by their NPVs or IRRs; those with NPV > 0 or IRR > the cost of capital are accepted.

6. Finally, in a good capital budgeting system, the *post-audit* is conducted. This involves comparing actual to predicted results. Post-audits help obtain the best results from every accepted project; they also lead to improvements in the forecasting process and hence to better future capital budgeting decisions.

Although this chapter has presented the basic elements of the capital budgeting process, there are many other aspects of this important topic. Some of the more technical ones are discussed in the appendix to this chapter, and others are taken up in Chapter 16.

 RESOLUTION TO DECISION IN FINANCE

GM: A Case of Capital Budgeting Gone Awry

Even GM's top executives now admit publicly that management's attempt to gain market share, increase productivity, and cut cost by infusing the corporate giant with $40 billion of technologically advanced equipment backfired. Obviously, GM was unrealistically optimistic in forecasting the cash inflows it would receive from the new plant and equipment. Worse, GM management acted as though the automaker was doing business in a vacuum. It made little attempt to understand its competitors' role in the company's budgeting process. Management

Source: Anne B. Fisher, "GM Is Tougher Than You Think," *Fortune,* November 10, 1986, 56–58, 60, 62, 64.

seemed to assume that by boosting technology there would be a concomitant increase in market share. Unfortunately for GM, while it was improving its production capacity, so were its competitors. No wonder GM's earnings, revenues, and cash flows fell way below expectations.

GM may have finally learned the valuable lesson that money can't solve all problems and that capital budgets should be well planned and meticulously scrutinized. Throwing big money into projects without taking careful aim is at best a risky enterprise. Lasers, robots, and other high-tech wizardry did not make a dent in GM's manufacturing costs, which are still the U.S. industry's highest.

What went wrong became clear when GM executives took a long hard look at the GM-Toyota joint venture that manufactures the Corolla-based Chevy Nova in Fremont, California. The facility, called New United Motor Manufacturing Inc., or Nummi for short, wasn't the recipient of any of GM's recently acquired robots or lasers, yet its productivity is double that of most GM plants and its Novas have earned the highest customer satisfaction ratings and lowest warranty costs of any GM car. The reason: worker participatory management and the labor agreement that made it possible.

After evaluating its failed capital budgeting program in light of its success at Nummi, GM is beginning to get tough where it should have

gotten tough all along—on itself. A sprawling and rigid bureaucracy glutted with middle managers and buried under memos, GM's own corporate culture has always been its biggest stumbling block to competitiveness.

But GM Chairman Roger B. Smith is adamant that he is up to the challenge of breaking through the corporate bureaucracy to get GM into fighting trim. He is striving to deemphasize capital spending and focus instead on managing workers well. There do seem to be some signs that he is succeeding.

Several plants have now copied Nummi's way of organizing workers into teams so that a dozen or so workers are responsible for a given assembly operation and make their own decisions about how to divide up the work. At stamping plants in Lansing, Michigan, and Lordstown, Ohio, that supply parts to Buick, Oldsmobile, and Cadillac, such innovative management has cut the time needed for a typical die change from 12 hours to 15 minutes.

However, other industry observers say that GM still has a long, long way to go. Wall Street analysts bemoan all those robots that can't be laid off in times of slow sales. H. Ross Perot, a former GM board member, thinks that Smith is facing an uphill battle. With its nightmare of overlapping departments and ossified standard operating procedures, Perot says teaching GM to be competitive is like teaching an elephant to tap dance.

QUESTIONS

14-1 How is a project classification scheme (for example, replacement, expansion into new markets, and so forth) used in the capital budgeting process?

14-2 Why is working capital included in a capital budgeting analysis?

14-3 Why are spontaneous liabilities such as accounts payables and accruals deducted from working capital in the analysis of capital budgeting costs?

14-4 If a firm like Carter Chemical Company used straight line rather than an accelerated depreciation method, how would this affect (a) the total amount of depreciation, net income, and net cash flows over the project's expected life; **(b)** the timing of depreciation, net income, and net cash flows; and **(c)** the project's payback and NPV?

14-5 Net cash flows rather than profits are listed in Table 14-1. What is the basis for this emphasis on cash as opposed to profits?

14-6 Is the NPV of a long-term project, defined as one with a high percentage of its cash flows expected in the distant future, more sensitive to changes in the cost of capital than the NPV of a short-term project?

14-7 Explain why, if two mutually exclusive projects are being compared, the short-term project might have the higher ranking under the NPV criterion if the cost of capital is high, but the long-term project might be deemed better if the cost of capital is low. Would changes in the cost of capital ever cause a change in the IRR ranking of two such projects?

14-8 Are there conditions under which a firm might be better off if it were to choose a project with a rapid payback rather than one with a larger NPV?

14-9 A firm has $100 million available for capital expenditures. It is considering investment in one of two projects, each costing $100 million. Project A has an IRR of 20 percent and an NPV of $9 million. It will be terminated at the end of one year at a profit of $20 million, resulting in an immediate increase in earnings per share (EPS). Project B, which cannot be postponed for one year in order to take on Project A, has an NPV of $50 million and an IRR of 30 percent. However, the firm's short-run EPS will be reduced if it accepts Project B, because no revenues will be generated by the project for several years.
a. Should the short-run effects on EPS influence the choice between the two projects?
b. How might situations like the one described here influence a firm's decision to use payback as a part of the capital budgeting process?

SELF-TEST PROBLEMS

ST-1 Paschal Products is considering the purchase of a new machine that will dramatically increase the firm's manufacturing capacity. The machine, if purchased today, would cost $40,550,000 and provide annual cash flows after taxes (net income plus depreciation) of $13,425,000 per year for 6 years.
a. Determine the project's payback.
b. Determine the project's NPV if the required return is 15 percent.
c. Determine the project's IRR.

ST-2 Bio-Technical Engineering (BTE) is considering an investment in a gene splicing project. The investment involves acquiring land, developing a new plant, operating the plant during the project, and then disposing of the salvageable assets from the project. The following is a summary of the project's characteristics (dollars in millions):
1. A total of $50 has been spent thus far to investigate the feasibility of the process used in the project. These funds were expensed.
2. BTE will purchase the land immediately at a cost of $300.
3. A BTE operations building will be put up at a cost of $400. This expenditure will occur at t = 1, that is, at the end of Year 1.
4. Equipment will be installed at a cost of $200. This outlay will occur at t = 2, the end of Year 2.

5. BTE will bring in net working capital with a cost of $100. This outlay will occur at the end of Year 3, t = 3, and the working capital will be recovered at the end of the project's life, t = 8, the end of Year 8.

6. The plant will commence operations at the beginning of Year 4. The operations will continue for 5 years, until the end of Year 8. After-tax cash flows from the project (net income plus depreciation) will equal $425 annually for the 5-year operating period.

7. Even though the operating assets will be fully depreciated, management believes the building and equipment will have a combined salvage value of $150 at the end of Year 8.

8. BTE's effective tax rate is 40 percent.

9. Assume that the project is not eligible for an investment tax credit.

If the required return for a high-risk project, such as the gene splicing project at BTE, is 20 percent, should the firm invest in this project?

PROBLEMS

14-1 **Payback, NPV, and IRR calculations.** Sound Design's Renaissance Project has a cost of $250,740, and its expected annual cash inflows are $90,000 per year for 8 years.
  a. What is the project's payback?
  b. The firm's cost of capital is 14 percent. What is the project's NPV?
  c. What is the project's IRR? (*Hint:* Recognize that the project's cash inflows are an annuity.)

14-2 **Payback, NPV, and IRR calculations.** Walter Construction Company's proposed Nino Project has a cost of $5 million, and its expected net cash inflows are $1,319,000 per year for 5 years.
  a. What is the payback for the Nino Project?
  b. The cost of capital is 8 percent. What is the project's NPV?
  c. What is the project's IRR? (*Hint:* Recognize that the project's cash flows are an annuity.)

14-3 **Payback, NPV, and IRR calculations.** Accurex Associates is investigating a project that costs $1 million and is expected to produce cash flows of $334,381 annually for 5 years.
  a. What is the project's payback?
  b. If the cost of capital is 12 percent, what is the project's NPV?
  c. What is the project's IRR?

14-4 **Payback, NPV, and IRR calculations.** The management of Graham's Inc., is evaluating the following investment opportunity, which costs $47,678.50 today but promises to return the following cash flows:

Year	Cash Flow
1	$20,000
2	15,000
3	10,000
4	20,000

  a. What is this project's payback?
  b. What is the project's NPV if Graham's cost of capital is 14 percent?
  c. What is the project's IRR?

14-5   **Payback, NPV, and IRR calculations.** RaeTel is evaluating an investment opportunity that costs $50,000 today but promises to return the following cash flows (net income plus depreciation) over the next 4 years:

Year	Cash Flow
1	$10,000
2	20,000
3	18,000
4	12,000

a. What is the investment's payback?
b. What is the NPV of the project if the required return is 10 percent?
c. Is the IRR of the investment greater or less than the required return?

14-6   **NPV and IRR calculations.** Scientific Measurement Corporation is considering an investment in a new machine that will provide dramatic cost savings over the next 5 years. The cost of the machine is $72,107.10. Annual after-tax cash flows (net income plus depreciation) are projected as follows:

Year	Cash Flow
1	$18,000
2	25,000
3	22,000
4	20,000
5	20,000

a. If the firm's required return for a project of this type is 12 percent, what is the investment's NPV?
b. What is the project's IRR?

14-7   **NPVs and IRRs for mutually exclusive projects.** Chung Engineering is considering including two pieces of equipment, a truck and an overhead pulley system, in this year's capital budget. These projects are mutually exclusive. The cash outlay for the truck is $17,350, and that for the pulley system is $24,225. The firm's cost of capital is 15 percent. After-tax cash flows, including depreciation, are as follows:

Years	Truck	Pulley
1–5	$5,300	$8,100

Calculate the IRR and the NPV for each project, and indicate the correct accept/reject decision for each.

14-8   **NPVs and IRRs for mutually exclusive projects.** Florida Industries must choose between a gas-powered and an electric-powered forklift for moving materials in its factory. Because both forklifts perform the same function, the firm will choose only one. (They are mutually exclusive investments.) The electric-powered forklift will cost more, but it will be less expensive to operate; it will cost $22,000, whereas the gas-powered one will cost $17,600. The cost of capital that applies to both investments is 10 percent. The life for both equipment types is estimated to be 6 years, during which time the net cash flows for the electric-powered forklift will be $6,600 annually and for the gas-powered forklift will be $5,300 per year. Annual net cash flows include depreciation expenses. Calculate the NPV and IRR for each type of forklift, and decide which to recommend for purchase.

14-9 **NPVs and IRRs for independent projects.** The net cash flows for Projects X and Y follow. Each project has a cost of $40,000.

Year	Project X	Project Y
1	$26,000	$14,000
2	12,000	14,000
3	12,000	14,000
4	4,000	14,000

a. Calculate each project's payback.
b. Calculate each project's NPV at a 10 percent cost of capital.
c. Calculate each project's IRR. (*Hints:* Use the graphic approach for Project X, and notice that Project Y is an annuity.)
d. Should X or Y or both be accepted if they are independent projects?
e. Which of the two projects should be accepted if they are mutually exclusive?
f. How might a change in the cost of capital produce a conflict between NPV and IRR? At what values of k would this conflict exist?

14-10 **Project evaluation.** BackPacker Manufacturing Company is considering a new production line for its rapidly expanding camping equipment division. The line will have a cost of $480,000 and will be depreciated toward a zero salvage value over the next 3 years, using straight line depreciation. Other important factors are: (1) The new camping products will be responsible for new sales of $500,000 next year, $550,000 the following year, and $600,000 in the last year. (2) Cost of goods sold (excluding depreciation) is 40 percent of sales. (3) The increase in selling and administrative expenses caused by the new line is predicted to be $40,000 annually. (4) The company's cost of capital is 15 percent, and its tax rate is 40 percent.
a. What are the project's annual cash flows?
b. What is the project's NPV?

14-11 **Project evaluation.** The director of capital budgeting for Hytec Electronics is analyzing a proposal to build a new plant in Arizona. The following data have been developed thus far:

Land acquisition, cost incurred at start of Year 1 (t = 0)	$ 300,000
Plant construction, cost incurred at start of Year 2 (t = 1)	$ 700,000
Equipment purchase, cost incurred at start of Year 3 (t = 2)	$1,000,000
Net working capital, investment made at start of Year 4 (t = 3)	$ 400,000

Operations will begin in Year 4 and will continue for 10 years, through Year 13. Sales revenues and operating costs are assumed to come at the end of each year; since the plant will be in operation for 10 years, operating costs and revenues occur at the end of Years 4 through 13 (t = 4 to 13). The following additional assumptions are made: (1) The plant and equipment will be depreciated over a 10-year life, starting in Year 4. The buildings and equipment will be worthless after 10 years' use, but Hytec expects to sell the land for $300,000 when the plant is closed down. The firm's management also expects its investment in working capital for the plant will be fully recoverable when the plant is closed. Hytec uses straight line depreciation. (2) Hytec uses a cost of capital of 14 percent to evaluate projects like this one. (3) Annual sales = 10,000 units at $140 per unit; annual sales revenue = $1,400,000. (4) Annual fixed operating costs *excluding* depreciation are $213,333. (5) Annual variable operating costs are $300,000, assuming the plant operates at full capacity. (6) Hytec's marginal income tax rate is 40 percent. (7) The project is not eligible for an investment tax credit.

a. Calculate the project's NPV. Should Hytec's management accept this project?

b. Assuming constant sales prices and constant variable costs per unit, what will happen to the NPV if unit sales fall 10 percent below the forecast level?

14-12   **Cash flow estimation.** D. Harrington and Company is considering the installation of a new production line for its rapidly expanding skate division. The line will have a cost of $100,000. The asset will be 5-year-class property for the purpose of ACRS depreciation. No salvage value is expected for the assets when the project ends in 5 years. Sales are expected to be $100,000 annually. Operating costs other than depreciation will be $70,000 annually. The company's required rate of return is 12 percent, and its tax rate is 40 percent.

Determine the project's cash flows, and then calculate the project's net present value. (Assume the following ACRS recovery allowances are in affect: Year 1, 20%; Year 2, 32%; Year 3, 20%; Years 4 and 5, 14%.)

ANSWERS TO SELF-TEST PROBLEMS

ST-1   **a.** The payback is defined as the length of time it takes to recover the investment in a project. For this proposed purchase, payback is determined in the following table:

Year	Cash Flow	Cumulative Cash Flow
1	$13,425,000	$13,425,000
2	13,425,000	26,850,000
3	13,425,000	40,275,000
4	13,425,000	

$40,550,000 − $40,275,000 = $275,000 unrecovered after 3 years.

$13,425,000/365 = $36,781 recovery per day.

$275,000/$36,781 = 7.5 days.

Therefore, the payback period is 3 years and 1 week, which would be rounded to 3 years. (Note: Since this project's cash flows are level, we could have found the payback by $40,550,000/$13,425,000 = 3.02 years, which is, of course, 3 years and 1 week.)

b. The NPV is calculated thus:

$$NPV = CF(DFa) - Cost$$

$$= \$13,425,000(3.7845) - \$40,550,000$$

$$= \$50,806,912 - \$40,550,000$$

$$= \$10,256,912.$$

c. Since the cash flows of this project take the form of an annuity, we can solve the following equation to determine the discount factor:

$$PVa = PMT(DFa)$$

$$DFa = \frac{PVa}{PMT}$$

or

$$\$40,550,000 = \$13,425,000(DFa)$$

$$DFa = \frac{\$40,550,000}{\$13,425,000}$$

$$= 3.0205.$$

For a 6-year annuity, the discount factor of 3.0205 corresponds to a 24 percent rate of return.

ST-2 The costs associated with the gene splicing project (in millions of dollars) are as follows:

Time	Cost	Purpose
$t = 0$	$300	Land
$t = 1$	$400	Building
$t = 2$	$200	Equipment
$t = 3$	$100	Working capital

$$\text{Present value of costs} = -\$300 - \$400(0.8333)$$
$$- \$200(0.6944) - \$100(0.5787)$$

$$= -\$830.07 = -\$830,070,000.$$

The cash flows associated with the project (in millions of dollars) are as follows:

Time	Cash Flow	Source
$t = 4 - 8$	$425	Cash flow from operations
$t = 8$	$100	Recapture of working capital
$t = 8$	$150	Sale of salvageable assets (taxed as ordinary income)

$$\text{Present value of cash flows} = \$425(1.7307)^* + \$100(0.2326)$$
$$+ \$150(1 - 0.4)(0.2326)$$

$$= \$779.7415 = \$779,741,500.$$

$$\text{Net present value} = \text{Discounted cash flows} - \text{Costs}$$

$$= \$779.7415 - \$830.07$$

$$= -\$50.3285 = -\$50,328,500.$$

$^*DFa_{20\%,8n} - DFa_{20\%,3n} = 3.8372 - 2.1065 = 1.7307.$

Because the project's NPV is negative, BTE should abandon the project. Of course, the same decision would have been reached if we had found the project's IRR. For single projects, a negative NPV indicates that the IRR of the project is less than the required return for the project. Whichever method is used, BTE should not invest in the gene splicing project.

Appendix 14A

Conflicts between NPV and IRR

independent project
A project whose cash flows are unaffected by the decision to accept or reject some other project.

In Chapter 14 we indicated that the two appropriate procedures for evaluating capital budgeting projects are the NPV and the IRR methods. For single projects and for two (or more) **independent projects,** the NPV and IRR methods *always* lead to the same accept/reject decisions. As noted in Table 14A-1, if the project's internal rate of return, r, is greater than the company's or project's required rate of return, k, the NPV will be positive, and the project will thus be deemed acceptable. Under normal circumstances, any project that provides a return less than the required return will be rejected. In this situation the project's NPV will always be negative. Of course, where NPV $= 0$, the project's required and internal rates of return are equal, and the firm will be indifferent between this project and other alternatives of the same risk. (Remember that k is also an opportunity cost representing the return of the best other available investment opportunity.)

mutually exclusive projects
A set of projects of which only one can be accepted.

However, when we consider *ranking* two or more investment projects, as in the following example, these decision rules may not agree. Assume that MBI Corporation has two competing, **mutually exclusive projects,** Projects A and B. Recall that with mutually exclusive projects, we can choose either Project A or Project B, or we can reject both, but we cannot accept both projects. In this example, each project requires an initial investment outlay of $1,000,000. Notice in Figure 14A-1 that if the firm's cost of capital is above 7.1 percent, both the NPV and IRR methods indicate that Project A should be selected. However, if the firm's cost of capital is below 7.1 percent, a conflict between the decision methods arises. If the firm's cost of capital is 5 percent, for example, the NPV of Project A is $180,410 whereas the NPV of Project B is $206,480, as seen in Table 14A-2. We approximate the IRRs of both projects graphically in Figure 14A-1. The IRR of Project A is 14.5 percent, but the IRR of Project B at 11.8 percent is lower. Therefore, the IRR method indicates that Project A should be selected, whereas

Table 14A-1 **Comparison of NPV and IRR Project Evaluation Rules for Single Projects**

Method	Accept	Reject	Indifferent
NPV	Positive	Negative	Zero
IRR	Greater than k	Less than k	k = r

Figure 14A-1 **Net Present Value Profiles of Projects A and B at Different Discount Rates (Thousands of Dollars)**

Conflicting results may arise when both net present value and internal rate of return are used to rank mutually exclusive capital projects. In this example, Project A has an NPV of $180,410 and an IRR of 14.5 percent, whereas Project B has an NPV of $206,480 and an IRR of 11.8 percent. Based on NPV, Project B would be preferred, but based on IRR, Project A would seem more attractive. In such cases NPV provides the least ambiguous means of ranking projects.

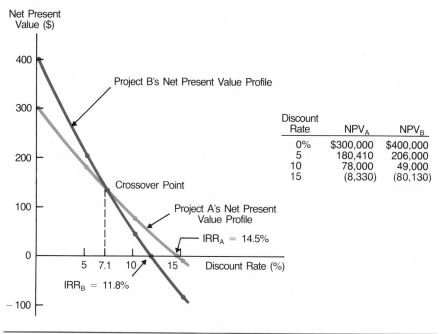

Discount Rate	NPV_A	NPV_B
0%	$300,000	$400,000
5	180,410	206,000
10	78,000	49,000
15	(8,330)	(80,130)

Note: Notice that the present value profiles are curved — they are *not* straight lines. We should also mention that under certain conditions, the NPV profiles can cross the horizontal axis several times or never cross it.

Table 14A-2 **Calculating the NPVs of Projects A and B where k = 5%**

	Project A				Project B		
Year	Cash Flow	DF = 5%	Discounted Cash Flow		Cash Flow	DF = 5%	Discounted Cash Flow
1	$500,000	.9524	$ 476,200		$100,000	.9524	$ 95,240
2	400,000	.9070	362,800		300,000	.9070	272,100
3	300,000	.8638	259,140		400,000	.8638	345,520
4	100,000	.8227	82,270		600,000	.8227	493,620
		PV of inflows	$1,180,410				$1,206,480
		Less: Cost	1,000,000				1,000,000
		NPV	$ 180,410				$ 206,480

the NPV method indicates that Project B is preferable. The critical question is, which method should we use in making capital budgeting decisions when the methods are in conflict?

Comparison of the NPV and IRR Methods

As we noted in Chapter 14, the NPV exhibits all the desired decision rule properties, and as such it provides the best method for evaluating projects. Because the NPV method is theoretically superior to the IRR, we were tempted to explain only the NPV, state that it should be used for all capital budgeting decisions, and move on to the next topic. However, the IRR method is familiar to many corporate executives, and it is widely entrenched in industry practices. Therefore, it is important that finance students thoroughly understand the IRR method and be prepared to explain why at times a project with a lower IRR may be preferable to one with a higher IRR.

Causes of Conflicting Rankings

There are two basic conditions that cause NPV profiles to cross, as in Figure 14A-1, and thus lead to potential conflicts between the NPV and IRR methods.

1. Project size or scale differences. If the cost of one project is significantly larger than that of the other, the larger project will generally have a higher NPV than the smaller one at low discount rates. If the larger project has the higher NPV at a zero discount rate, and the smaller project has the higher IRR, the NPV profiles will cross each other. For example, Project S calls for the investment of $1.00 and yields $1.50 at the end of one year. Its IRR is 50 percent and at a 10 percent cost of capital, its NPV is 36 cents. Project L costs $1 million and yields $1.25 million at the end of the year. Its IRR is only 25 percent but its NPV at 10 percent is $136,375.

2. Timing differences exist. If most of the cash flows from one project come in the early years whereas most of those from the other project come in the later years, as occurred with Projects A and B, the project with the longer-term cash flows will generally have a higher vertical axis intercept, so again the NPV profiles can cross each other. This situation is caused by the fact that high discount rates benefit projects that have early cash flows but impose a greater penalty on projects having cash flows that are slow to accrue. Therefore, long-term projects, like Project B, have NPV profiles that start high on the vertical axis but that also decline quite steeply relative to those of projects like Project A, allowing the two profiles to cross.

Resolving the NPV versus IRR Conflict

When either size or timing differences occur, the methodologies that determine the desirability of capital investment projects may be in conflict. When there is a conflict in these selection methods, it should be resolved by choosing the project that has the highest NPV. The choice of the NPV method avoids three problems where the IRR criterion can provide an incorrect capital budgeting decision: (1) the problem of absolute versus relative returns, (2) the reinvestment rate assumption, and (3) the problem of multiple rates of return.[1]

---

[1] For a much more detailed and complete discussion of these factors, see Brigham and Gapenski, *Intermediate Financial Management,* 2nd ed., Chapter 7.

Absolute versus Relative Returns

Suppose we are offered the choice between two competing one-year projects. Project Y's IRR is 10 percent, whereas Project Z's IRR is 20 percent. If we rank and select projects using the IRR criterion, we would choose the project with the larger IRR — Project Z. However, if we learned that Project Z's maximum available investment is $1,000, it would leave us with an NPV of $200; but we can invest up to $10,000 in Project Y, which gives us an NPV of $1,000. Which is the best project? The project that provides the highest true return — dollars — is the best. Thus we would opt for the project that gives the highest *absolute* return, the one with the highest NPV.

Reinvestment Assumption

When either timing or size differences occur, the firm will have different amounts of funds to invest in the intervening years of the project's life, depending on which of the mutually exclusive projects it chooses. For example, if one project costs more than the other, the firm will have more money at t = 0 to invest elsewhere if it selects the less costly project. Similarly, for projects of equal cost, the one with the larger early cash inflows will provide more funds for reinvestment in the early years. Thus the rate of return at which differential cash flows can be invested is an important consideration.

Although we do not prove it in this book, the fundamental reason behind the NPV/IRR conflict has to do with the **reinvestment rate assumptions** underlying the two methods.[2] The NPV method assumes that the firm can reinvest cash flows at the cost of capital, whereas the IRR method assumes that they can be reinvested at the IRR rate itself. The NPV method makes a much more conservative reinvestment assumption than the IRR method. The NPV assumes reinvestment at the cost of capital, which is the rate of return required by all suppliers of funds. Thus the NPV reinvestment assumption is that intervening cash inflows will be reinvested at the firm's current required rate of return. On the other hand, the IRR method assumes that the intervening cash inflows from the project will be reinvested at that project's rate of return, its IRR. Thus, if a project has a *computed* IRR of 40 percent, but the best alternative for reinvesting the intervening cash flows from the project is 8 percent, the realized rate of return from the project will definitely be less than 40 percent. This does not mean that the project may not be acceptable, only that its realized return, r, will be less than its computed IRR.

Naturally, the closer the project's IRR to the firm's opportunity cost, the less the reinvestment assumption matters. Yet there will *never* be a problem using the NPV rule in ranking competing or mutually exclusive investment opportunities.

Multiple Rates of Return

A third reason that the NPV method provides a better criterion for ranking capital budgeting projects is that, in certain situations, there can be more than one IRR. In Figure 14A-1, Projects A and B each have only one IRR, which is found where the NPV profile

reinvestment rate assumption
The assumption that cash flows from a project can be reinvested (1) at the cost of capital, if using the NPV method, or (2) at the internal rate of return, if using the IRR method.

[2]Both the NPV and the IRR methods are discounted cash flow techniques. Because both techniques utilize the time value of money, we should consider again how the present value tables are constructed. Recall that the present value of any future sum is defined as the beginning amount that, when compounded at a specified and constant rate, will grow to equal the future amount over the stated time period. From Table 13-3 we can see that the present value of $146.93 due in 5 years, when discounted at 8 percent, is $100, because $100, when reinvested and compounded at 8 percent into the future for 5 years, will grow to $146.93. Thus compounding and discounting are reciprocal relationships, and *the very construction of the discounting and compounding tables implies a reinvestment process.*

crosses the X axis — that is, where the NPV = 0. These are both normal projects in that their cash outflow (one or more cash outflows) is followed by future cash inflows. However, capital budgeting projects can have outflows followed by inflows, then by more outflows, and so on. Strip mining for coal provides an example of this nonnormal cash flow. First the land is purchased, then the coal is mined for several years, and finally the land must be returned to its natural state at the expense of the mine's owners. Oil-well drilling provides a similar example of nonnormal cash flows, as the rig must be periodically shut down and refurbished before the well can produce more cash flows.

An example of a nonnormal cash flow (in millions) is as follows:

Expected Net Cash Flow		
Year 0	Year 1	Year 2
$1.6	+ $10	− $10

If one were ranking projects based on the IRR method, this nonnormal project would create a problem, because the project's IRR is 25 percent *and* 400 percent. Both IRRs cause the NPV to equal zero, so both are correct. This situation creates confusion for firms that rely on the IRR method to select projects. However, the NPV method gives a single decision criteria, and it is thus superior to the IRR method.

PROBLEMS

14A-1   **NPV versus IRR ranking for mutually exclusive projects.** Two projects each involve an investment of $18,000. Cash flows (after-tax profits plus depreciation) are $12,000 a year for 2 years for Project S and $4,800 annually for 6 years for Project L.

   a. Compute the NPV for each project if the firm's cost of capital is zero percent and if it is 6 percent. NPVs for Project S at 10 and 20 percent, respectively, are $2,826 and $333.60, whereas NPV for Project L at 10 and 20 percent are $2,905.44 and ($2,037.60).

   b. Graph the present value profiles of the two projects, putting NPV on the Y axis and the cost of capital on the X axis, and use the graph to estimate each project's IRR.

   c. Calculate the IRR for each project, using a formula.

   d. If these projects were mutually exclusive, which one would you select, assuming a cost of capital of (1) 8 percent, (2) 10.3 percent, or (3) 12 percent? Explain. For this problem, assume that the operation will terminate at the end of the project's life, making an analysis based on equal lives unnecessary.

14A-2   **NPV and IRR analysis.** Each of two mutually exclusive projects involves an investment of $180,000. Net cash flows (after-tax profits plus depreciation) for the two projects have a different time pattern. Project M involves using some acreage for a mining operation. Because the expense of removing the ore is lower in the early years, when the ore will be closer to the surface, Project M will yield high returns in early years and lower returns in later years. Project O involves using the land for an orchard, and it will take a number of years for the trees to mature and become fully bearing. Thus Project O will yield low returns in the early years and higher returns in the later years. The cash flows from the two investments are as follows:

Year	Project M	Project O
1	$105,000	$ 15,000
2	60,000	30,000
3	45,000	45,000
4	15,000	75,000
5	15,000	120,000

a. Calculate each project's payback.

b. Compute the net present value of each project when the firm's cost of capital is 0 percent, 6 percent, and 20 percent. At 10 percent, the NPV for M is $18,410 and the NPV for O is $17,975.

c. Graph the net present value profiles of the two projects. Use the graph to estimate each project's IRR. If you have a financial calculator, use it to check your graphic estimate.

d. Which project would you select, assuming no capital rationing and a constant cost of capital of 8 percent? Of 10 percent? Of 12 percent? Explain.

e. How might a change in the cost of capital produce a conflict between NPV and IRR results? At what value of k would this conflict exist?

f. The company's capital budgeting manual states that no project with a payback greater than 4.0 should be accepted. Discuss this rule and its effects, both in general and in this specific case.

14A-3 **NPV and IRR analysis.** Southwest Construction Company (SCC) is considering two mutually exclusive investments. The projects' expected net cash flows are as follows:

	Expected Net Cash Flow	
Year	**Project A**	**Project B**
0	($300)	($405)
1	(387)	134
2	(193)	134
3	(100)	134
4	600	134
5	600	134
6	850	134
7	(180)	0

a. Construct NPV profiles for Projects A and B.

b. What is each project's IRR?

c. If you were told that each project's cost of capital was 10 percent, which project should be selected? If the cost of capital was 17 percent, what would be the proper choice?

(Do Parts e and f only if you are using the computerized problem diskette.)

d. SCC's management is confident of the projects' cash flows in Years 0 to 6 but is uncertain about what the Year 7 cash flows will be for the two projects. Under a worst case scenario, Project A's Year 7 cash flow will be − $300 and B's will be − $150, whereas under a best case scenario, the cash flows will be − $70 and + $120 for Projects A and B, respectively. Rework Parts a through c using these new cash flows. Which project should be selected under each scenario? Press the F10 function key (in the lower left corner of the keyboard) to see the NPV profiles.

e. Put the Year 7 cash flows back to − $180 for A and zero for B. Now change the cost of capital and observe what happens to NPV, IRR, and the crossover rate at k = 0%, 5%, 20%, and 400% (input as 4.0). Again, press the F10 function key to see the NPV profiles.

Chapter 15

Risk and Return

DECISION IN FINANCE

The Perilous Pursuit of Sexy Businesses

In the fiercely competitive business environment of the 1980s, more and more companies faced with stagnant or declining demand for their mainstay products have decided to buy, rather than build, businesses in such "sexy" industries as electronics, health care, biotechnology, and financial services. The idea is that it is quicker and cheaper to boost drooping revenues by buying a small but growing company that already has a hot product on the market than to enter a long-term, and potentially risky, capital investment program to develop new product lines from the ground up.

Perhaps a classic example of this type of acquisition is Schlumberger Ltd.'s purchase of Fairchild Camera & Instrument Corporation. Schlumberger (pronounced slum-ber-jay′), a manufacturer of oil-field and other heavy equip-

ment with sales in excess of $6 billion annually, was looking for a way to branch out into the fast-moving electronics industry. In 1979 it agreed to purchase Fairchild Camera & Instrument Corp., a leading-edge semiconductor company that produces microprocessors, disk drives, and a host of other products essential to the computer, aerospace, and defense industries.

Even though Fairchild's businesses were unrelated to Schlumberger's, Schlumberger's management thought that they were making a wise capital investment in acquiring Fairchild and that their expertise in managing one kind of business would apply to Fairchild's business as well.

As you read this chapter, try to think of the sorts of risks that Schlumberger was taking in entering an industry in which it was a novice. How might Schlumberger minimize these risks? Do you think buying Fairchild was a prudent capital expenditure?

_____
See end of chapter for resolution.

Up to this point in our discussion of capital budgeting project evaluations, we have assumed that future cash flows were known with virtual certainty. We now turn to a more realistic situation — the case in which future events are not known with certainty. In the following sections we define the term *risk* as it applies to financial matters, discuss procedures for measuring it, and determine how these characteristics may be incorporated into the investment decision process.[1] Then, in Chapter 16, we apply these concepts more directly to the capital budgeting decision process.

DEFINING AND MEASURING RISK

risk
The probability that actual future returns will be below expected returns.

Risk is defined in *Webster's* as "a hazard; a peril; exposure to loss or injury." Thus risk refers to the chance that some unfavorable event will occur. If you engage in skydiving, you take a chance with your life — skydiving is risky. If you bet on the horses, you risk losing your money. If you invest in speculative stocks (or, really, in *any* stock), you are taking a risk in the hope of making an appreciable return.

To illustrate the riskiness of financial assets, suppose an investor buys $100,000 of short-term government bonds with an interest rate of 8 percent. In this case the yield to maturity on the investment, 8 percent, can be estimated quite precisely, and the investment is said to be risk-free. However, if the $100,000 is invested in the stock of a company just being organized to prospect for oil in the mid-Atlantic, the investment's return cannot be estimated precisely. One might analyze the situation and conclude that the *expected* rate of return is 20 percent. However, the *actual* rate of return could range from an extremely large positive return, say +1,000 percent, to a total loss of invested capital, -100 percent. Because there is a significant danger of actually earning a return considerably lower than the expected return, the investment is described as being relatively risky.

Of course, no investment would be made unless the expected rate of return was high enough to compensate the investor for taking extra risks. In fact, we could generalize that the higher the perceived risk associated with an investment opportunity, the greater the expected return must be to persuade a manager to accept the project. In this investment example, it is clear that few, if any, investors would buy the oil company stock if its expected return were the same as that of the government bond. Naturally, the more risky investment might not realize the higher rate of return; if the highest-risk projects always provided the highest returns, there would be no risk.

Investment risk, then, is associated with the probability of earning a return less than the expected return — the greater the chance of low or negative returns, the riskier the investment. We can define risk more precisely, however, and in the following sections we will do so.

---

[1]The general approach to the investment decision process is the same whether we are investing in financial assets, such as stocks and bonds, or investing in real assets, as with capital budgeting.

Probability Distributions

An event's *probability* is defined as the chance that the event will occur. For example, a weather forecaster may state, "There is a 40 percent chance of rain today and a 60 percent chance that it will not rain." If all possible events, or outcomes, are listed, and if a probability is assigned to each event, the listing is called a **probability distribution.** For a weather forecast, we could set up the following probability distribution:

Outcome (1)	Probability (2)
Rain	0.4 = 40%
No rain	0.6 = 60%
	1.0 = 100%

probability distribution
A listing of all possible outcomes or events, with a probability (the chance of the event's occurrence) assigned to each outcome.

The possible outcomes are listed in Column 1, and the probabilities of these outcomes, expressed both as decimals and as percentages, are given in Column 2. Notice that the probabilities must sum to 1.0, or 100 percent.

Eastern Communications, Inc., a manufacturer and retailer of business and consumer telephones, is considering the expected rate of return on two of its consumer lines of telephones. The two lines consist of its Standard Phone line and its new Designer Phone line. Most of the firm's marketing managers believe that the Designer line should have a return higher than the Standard equipment in "boom" and "normal" economic periods. In recessionary periods, when consumers typically have less to spend on luxury items, the Designer line is not expected to be profitable. Before money is invested to initiate the manufacture and sale of both lines, Eastern Communications wishes to determine the risk and return of these two product lines in a more direct manner.

The state of the economy and the resulting rate of return on each product line are presented in Table 15-1. Here we see that there is a 30 percent chance of a boom, in which case both product lines will enjoy high rates of return; a 40 percent chance of a normal economy and moderate returns; and a 30 percent probability of a recession, which will mean low or even negative returns for both product lines. Of course, the profits of the luxury Designer line are more sensitive to the economic environment than the profits of the Standard line. In fact, in recessionary periods there is a fairly high probability that the return on the Designer line will drop significantly, resulting in a loss of 70 percent, whereas the Standard line has no chance for loss.

Expected Rate of Return

If we multiply each possible outcome by its probability of occurrence and then sum these products, as in Table 15-1, we have a *weighted average* of outcomes. This weighted average of outcomes can be expressed in equation form as the **expected rate of return, $\hat{k}$,** of a probability distribution:

expected rate of return, $\hat{k}$
The rate of return expected to be realized from an investment; the mean value of the probability distribution of possible returns.

$$\text{Expected rate of return} = \hat{k} = \sum_{i=1}^{n} P_i k_i. \qquad \textbf{(15-1)}$$

Table 15-1 **Projected Return on Each Phone Line Based on the State of the Economy**

Designer Phone Line

State of the Economy	Probability of This State Occurring	Rate of Return under This State
Boom	0.3	100%
Normal	0.4	15
Recession	0.3	− 70
	1.0	

Standard Phone Line

State of the Economy	Probability of This State Occurring	Rate of Return under This State
Boom	0.3	20%
Normal	0.4	15
Recession	0.3	10
	1.0	

Here the expected rate of return, $\hat{k}$, is the weighted average of each possible outcome, k_i, weighted by the probability of its occurrence, P_i. Using the data for the Designer line, we obtain its expected rate of return as follows:

$$\hat{k} = P_1(k_1) + P_2(k_2) + P_3(k_3)$$

$$= 0.3(100\%) + 0.4(15\%) + 0.3(-70\%)$$

$$= 15\%.$$

Similarly, we can use Equation 15-1 to determine the expected rate of return for the Standard line:

$$\hat{k} = 0.3(20\%) + 0.4(15\%) + 0.3(10\%)$$

$$= 15\%.$$

We can graph the rates of return to obtain a picture of the variability of the possible outcomes; this is shown in the bar charts in Figure 15-1. The height of each bar signifies the probability that a given outcome will occur. The range of probable returns for the Designer line is from 100 percent to − 70 percent, with an average or expected return of 15 percent. The expected return for the Standard line is also 15 percent, but with a much narrower range of return possibilities.

Figure 15-1 **Probability Distributions of the Rates of Return for the Designer and Standard Telephone Projects: Eastern Communications, Inc.**

The expected rate of return on a project is equal to the average of all possible outcomes, with each outcome weighted by the probability of its occurrence. These bar charts show the variability of three possible outcomes for each of two projects. An average (or expected) return of 15 percent is most probable for both, but the Designer line has a much wider range of return possibilities. Because this wider range means a greater probability that the return will differ from 15 percent, the Designer line is a riskier project.

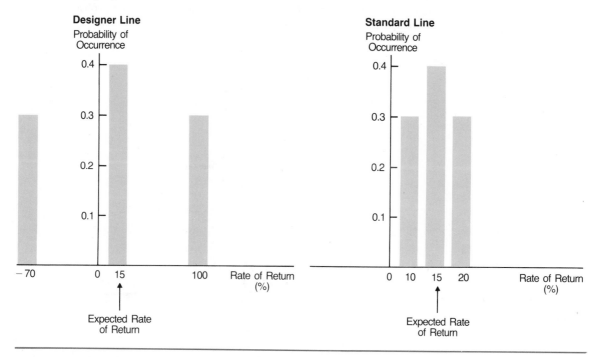

Continuous Probability Distributions

Thus far we have assumed that only three states of the economy can exist: recession, normal, and boom. Actually, of course, the state of the economy could range from a deep depression to a fantastic boom, and there are an unlimited number of possibilities in between. Suppose we had the time and patience to assign a probability to each possible state of the economy (with the sum of the probabilities still equaling 1.0) and to assign a rate of return to each project for each state of the economy. We would have an equation similar to Equation 15-1 except that it would have many more entries. This equation could be used to calculate expected rates of return as shown previously, and

Figure 15-2 **Continuous Probability Distributions of the Designer and Standard Lines' Rates of Return**

Figure 15-1 graphed the probabilities of three possible outcomes for each telephone project. In reality, both projects could have numerous rates of return, which could be illustrated best by the continuous probability curves shown here. These curves indicate that the most likely rate of return for both product lines is 15 percent. In addition, the relative flatness of the curves indicates the extent to which returns are likely to vary from 15 percent. The height of the curve for the Standard line indicates a tight probability distribution and reflects the fact that there is a very low probability that the return will be below 10 percent or above 20 percent. The curve for the Designer line is much flatter, meaning that this project has a higher probability of returning either more or less than 15 percent and is thus a higher risk.

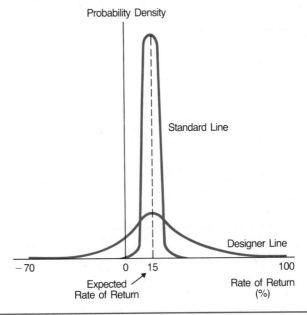

Note: The assumptions about the probabilities of various outcomes have been changed from those in Figure 15-1. There the probability of obtaining exactly 15 percent was 40 percent; here it is *much smaller,* because there are many possible outcomes instead of just three. With continuous distributions such as those in this figure, it is more appropriate to ask what the probability is of obtaining at least some specified rate of return than to ask what the probability is of obtaining exactly that rate. This cumulative probability is equal to the area under the probability distribution curve to the right of the point of interest, or 1 minus the area under the curve up to that point. This topic is covered in detail in statistic courses.

the probabilities and outcomes could be approximated by the continuous curves presented in Figure 15-2. Here we have changed the assumptions so that there is a very low probability that the Designer line's return will be less than −70 percent or more than 100 percent or that the Standard line's return will be less than 10 percent or more than 20 percent, but virtually any return within these limits is possible.

The tighter, or more peaked, the probability distribution, the more likely it is that the actual outcome will be close to the expected value and, consequently, the less likely it is that the actual return will be far below the expected return. Thus the tighter the probability distribution, the lower the risk assigned to a project. Since the Standard line has a relatively tight probability distribution, its *actual return* is likely to be closer to the 15 percent *expected return* than is that of the Designer line.

Measuring Risk: The Standard Deviation

Risk is a difficult concept to grasp, and a great deal of controversy has surrounded attempts to define and measure it. However, a common definition, and one that is satisfactory for many purposes, is stated in terms of probability distributions like those presented in Figure 15-2. *The tighter the probability distribution of expected future returns, the smaller the risk of a given investment.* According to this definition, the Standard line of telephones is less risky than the Designer line, because the chances of a large loss on the Standard line are smaller than the chances of a similar loss on the Designer line.

To be most useful, any measure of risk should have a definite value; we need a measure of the tightness of the probability distribution. One such measure is the **standard deviation**, the symbol for which is σ, pronounced "sigma." The smaller the standard deviation, the tighter the probability distribution and, accordingly, the lower the riskiness of the project. The calculation of the standard deviation is outlined as follows:

1. Calculate the expected rate of return:

$$\text{Expected rate of return} = \hat{k} = \sum_{i=1}^{n} P_i k_i. \qquad \textbf{(15-1)}$$

For both projects, we found $\hat{k} = 15\%$.[2]

2. Subtract the expected rate of return from each possible outcome to obtain a set of deviations about the expected rate of return, $\hat{k}$:

$$\text{Deviation}_i = k_i - \hat{k}.$$

3. Square each deviation, multiply the squared deviation by the probability of occurrence for its related outcome, and sum these products to obtain the *variance* of the probability distribution:

$$\text{Variance} = \sigma^2 = \sum_{i=1}^{n} (k_i - \hat{k})^2 P_i. \qquad \textbf{(15-2)}$$

measuring risk
The tighter the probability distribution of expected future returns, the smaller the risk of a given investment.

standard deviation, σ
A statistical measurement of the variability of a set of observations.

---

[2]Since we define risk in terms of the chances of returns being less than expected, it seems logical to measure risk in terms of the probability of returns being below the expected return rather than by the entire distribution. Measures of below-expected returns, known as *semivariance measures,* have been developed, but they are difficult to analyze. Additionally, if the distribution is approximately symmetric, which often happens in the case of security returns, the standard deviation is as good a risk measure as the semivariance.

4. Find the standard deviation by obtaining the square root of the variance:

$$\text{Standard deviation} = \sigma = \sqrt{\sum_{i=1}^{n} (k_i - \hat{k})^2 P_i}. \qquad \textbf{(15-3)}$$

5. We can illustrate these procedures by calculating the standard deviation for both the Designer and Standard lines:

a. Designer line:

(1) The expected rate of return, $\hat{k}$, is found, using Equation 15-1, to be 15 percent.

(2) Following the steps outlined before, we set up a table to work out the value for Equation 15-3:

(a) In Column 1, we subtract the expected return from each possible outcome to obtain Column 2, a set of deviations about $\hat{k}$.

(b) In Column 3, we square each of these deviations.

(c) In Column 4, these squared deviations are multiplied by the probability of their occurrence.

(d) In Column 5, these products are summed to obtain the variance of the probability distribution, 4,335.

(e) Below the table, we take the square root of the variance to obtain the probability distribution's standard deviation, 65.84%.

1		2	3	4	5
$k_i - \hat{k}$	=	$(k_i - \hat{k})$	$(k_i - \hat{k})^2$	$(k_i - \hat{k})^2 P_i$	
100 − 15		85	7,225	(7225) (0.3) = 2,167.5	
15 − 15		0	0	(0) (0.4) = 0.0	
−70 − 15		−85	7,225	(7225) (0.3) = 2,167.5	
				Variance = σ_k^2 = 4,335.0	

$$\text{Standard deviation} = \sigma_k = \sqrt{\sigma_k^2} = \sqrt{4335.0} = 65.84\%.$$

b. Standard line:

(1) The expected rate of return, $\hat{k}$, is 15 percent.

(2) As before, we compute the project's risk measure, the standard deviation, by utilizing the previously outlined steps to solve Equation 15-3:

1		2	3	4	5
$k_i - \hat{k}$	=	$(k_i - \hat{k})$	$(k_i - \hat{k})^2$	$(k_i - \hat{k})^2 P_i$	
20 − 15		5	25	(25) (0.3) = 7.5	
15 − 15		0	0	(0) (0.4) = 0.0	
10 − 15		−5	25	(25) (0.3) = 7.5	
				Variance = σ_k^2 = 15.0	

$$\text{Standard deviation} = \sigma_k = \sqrt{\sigma_k^2} = \sqrt{15} = 3.87\%.$$

If a probability distribution is normal, as pictured in Figure 15-3, the actual return will lie within ±1 standard deviation of the *expected* return about 68 percent (68.26 percent, to be exact) of the time. Figure 15-3 illustrates this

Figure 15-3 **Probability Ranges for a Normal Distribution**

This figure illustrates a normal probability curve. In a normal distribution the actual value will fall within ±1 standard deviation of the expected value about 68 percent of the time. Thus, in the Eastern Communications, Inc. example, 68 percent of the time the Standard line's actual return will be in the range of 15 percent ± 3.87 percent. Similarly, there is a 68 percent chance that the Designer line's return will fall in the range of 15 percent ± 65.84 percent. The normal curve again highlights the greater risk associated with the Designer line.

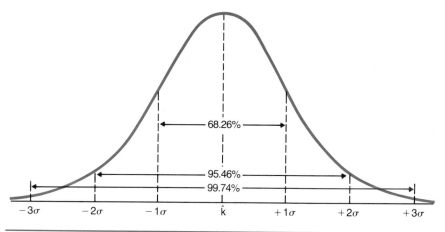

Notes:
1. The area under the normal curve equals 1.0, or 100%. *Thus the areas under any pair of normal curves drawn on the same scale, whether they are peaked or flat, must be equal.*
2. Half of the area under a normal curve is to the left of the mean, indicating that there is a 50% probability that the actual outcome will be less than the mean and a 50% probability that it will be greater than the mean, or to the right of it.
3. Of the area under the curve, 68.26% is within ±1σ of the mean, indicating that the probability is 68.26% that the actual outcome will be within the range $\hat{k} - 1\sigma$ to $\hat{k} + 1\sigma$.
4. Procedures are available for finding the probability of other earnings ranges. These procedures are covered in statistics courses.
5. For a normal distribution, the larger the value of σ, the greater the probability that the actual outcome will vary widely from, hence perhaps be far below, the expected, or most likely, outcome. *Because the probability of having the actual results turn out to be far below the expected result is our definition of risk, and because σ measures this probability, we can use σ as a measure or risk.* This definition may not be a good one, however, if we are dealing with an asset held in a diversified portfolio. This point is covered later in the chapter.

point and also shows the situation for ±2σ and ±3σ. For the Designer line, $\hat{k}$ = 15 percent and σ = 65.84 percent. Thus there is a 68.26 percent probability that the actual return will be in the range of 15 percent ± 65.84 percent, or from −50.84 percent to 80.84 percent. In a similar fashion, the expected return for the Standard line is 15 percent, but the project's standard deviation is 3.87 percent. Thus for the Standard line there is a 68.26 percent probability that the actual return will be in the range of 15 percent ± 3.87 percent, or from 11.13 to 18.87 percent. With such a small standard deviation for the Standard line, we can conclude that there will be little chance of significant loss from investing in that product line.

Measuring Risk: The Coefficient of Variation

coefficient of variation

Standardized measure of the risk per unit of return, calculated as the standard deviation divided by the expected return.

Another useful measure of risk, the **coefficient of variation,** is calculated by dividing the standard deviation by the expected value of the investment. The coefficient of variation (CV) shows the risk per unit of return, and it results in a more meaningful comparison when the expected risk and returns on two alternatives are not the same. Since the Designer line and the Standard line have the same expected return, the computation of the coefficient of variation is not particularly necessary in this case because the result is obvious; the project with the larger standard deviation, the Designer line, will have the larger coefficient of variation. In fact, the coefficient of variation for the Designer line is 65.84/15 = 4.39, whereas the CV for the Standard line is 3.87/15 = 0.26. Based on this criterion, the Designer line is riskier than the Standard line.

Now consider two other projects, A and B, which have different expected rates of return and different standard deviations. Project A has a 45 percent expected rate of return and a standard deviation of 15 percent, whereas Project B has an expected rate of return of 20 percent and a standard deviation of 10 percent. Is Project A riskier because it has the larger standard deviation? If we calculate the coefficients of variation for these two projects, we find that Project A has a coefficient of variation of 15/45 = 0.33, and Project B has a coefficient of variation of 10/20 = 0.50. Thus we see that Project B actually has more risk per unit of return than Project A, even though Project A's standard deviation is larger. Therefore, by the coefficient of variation measure, Project B is riskier. When such differences occur, the coefficient of variation is generally the better measure of risk than the standard deviation alone.

Risk Aversion and Required Returns

Suppose you have worked hard and saved $100,000, which you now plan to invest. You can buy 10 percent U.S. Treasury notes, and at the end of 1 year you will have a return of $110,000, which is your original investment plus $10,000 interest. The risk on this investment is quite low and is certainly risk-free from the standpoint of default risk. Alternatively, you can buy stock in Genetic Innovations, Inc (GII). If GII's medical research programs are successful, your stock will increase in value to $220,000; however, if the research is a failure, the value of your stock will be zero, and you will lose all of your savings. You regard GII's chances of success or failure to be 50-50, so the expected value of the stock investment is 0.5($0) + 0.5($220,000) = $110,000. Subtracting the $100,000 cost of the stock leaves an expected profit of $10,000, or an expected (but risky) 10 percent rate of return:

$$\text{Expected rate of return} = (\text{Expected investment value} - \text{Cost})/\text{Cost}$$

$$= (\$110,000 - \$100,000)/\$100,000$$

$$= \$10,000/\$100,000$$

$$= 10 \text{ percent.}$$

Thus, you have a choice between a sure $10,000 profit (representing a 10 percent rate of return) on the Treasury note or a risky expected $10,000 profit (also representing a 10 percent rate of return) on the Genetic Innovations stock. Which one would you choose? If you choose the less risky investment, you are risk averse. Most investors are indeed risk averse, and certainly the average investor is risk averse, at least with regard to his or her "serious money." Because this is a well-documented fact, we shall assume **risk aversion** throughout the remainder of this book. However, the concept of risk aversion does *not* mean that investors are afraid of taking chances; rather, risk aversion indicates that individuals or businesses will take on risks only if a stock or project's rate of return is expected to reward them for taking risks.

risk aversion
A dislike for risk. Risk-averse investors have higher required rates of return for higher-risk investments.

What are the implications of risk aversion for security prices and rates of return? The answer is that, other things held constant, the higher a security's risk, (1) the lower its price and (2) the higher its required return. To see how this works, assume two stocks are available for investment. Suppose that each stock has the same expected return and the same stock price but very different risk profiles. The first, TotWear Products, a respected manufacturer of children's clothing, has little risk, and its expected rate of return is 15 percent. TotWear's common stock sells for $75. The second firm, SilTek, is involved in new technology for superconductors. SilTek's return is also expected to be 15 percent. However, its returns have always been highly variable and thus risky, and they will remain so in the future, due to the nature of the firm's product. SilTek's stock also sells for $75. Investors are risk averse, so because of the general uncertainty about SilTek's actual return, there would be a general preference for TotWear's stock. Therefore, people with money to invest would purchase TotWear's rather than SilTek's stock. Simultaneously SilTek's stockholders would start selling it and use the money to buy TotWear's stock, and this selling pressure would cause SilTek's price to decline.

These price changes, in turn, would cause changes in the expected rates of return on the two securities. Supppose, for example, that the price of TotWear's stock was bid up from $75 to $112.50 and that the price of SilTek's stock declined from $75 to $56.25. Further, suppose this caused TotWear's expected rate of return to fall to 10 percent, while SilTek's expected return rose to 20 percent. The difference in returns, 20% − 10% = 10%, is a **risk premium, RP,** which represents the compensation investors require for assuming the additional risk of SilTek's stock.

risk premium, RP
The difference between the required rate of return on a given risky asset and the return on a less risky asset with the same expected life.

This example demonstrates a very important principle: *In a market dominated by risk-averse investors, riskier securities will have higher expected returns as estimated by the average investor than less risky securities, for if this situation does not hold, actions will occur in the market to force it to come about.* We will discuss how the market prices financial assets such as bonds and common stock in subsequent chapters. Later in this chapter, we will consider the question of *how much* higher the returns of risky assets must be, after we examine in more depth how risk should be measured.

PORTFOLIO RISK AND THE CAPITAL ASSET PRICING MODEL

In the preceding sections we considered the description and measurement of risk for an asset held in isolation. Now we analyze the effect of combining two or more investments into a portfolio of either financial or real assets. As we shall see, investing in more than one project may actually reduce the firm's overall risk. To investigate this phenomenon, we utilize a slightly different type of investment, common stock, as opposed to an investment in capital budgeting projects. We make this shift in our analysis because the risk reduction qualities of investment in multiple assets was first recognized in a stock market context. Even though the analysis in real and financial assets is quite similar on an analytical basis, we shall return to our capital budgeting framework later in Chapter 16. As we shall see, a stock held as part of a portfolio is less risky than the same stock held in isolation. This fact has been incorporated into a generalized framework for analyzing the relationship between risk and rates of return. This framework is called the **Capital Asset Pricing Model,** or **CAPM,** and it is an extremely important analytical tool in *both* financial management and investment analysis.

Capital Asset Pricing Model (CAPM)
A model based on the proposition that any stock's required rate of return is equal to the riskless rate of return plus its risk premium.

Portfolio Risk

Most financial assets are not held in isolation; rather, they are held as parts of portfolios. Banks, pension funds, insurance companies, mutual funds, and other financial institutions are required by law to hold diversified portfolios. Even individual investors — at least those individuals whose security holdings constitute a substantial part of their total wealth — generally hold stock portfolios, not just the stock of one firm. This being the case, from an investor's standpoint the fact that a particular stock goes up or down is not very important; *what is important is the value of the portfolio and the portfolio's return.* Logically, then, the risk and return of an individual security should be analyzed in terms of how that security affects the risk and return of the portfolio in which it is held.

To illustrate this point, suppose you have $100,000 to invest. You are considering two stocks. Atlas Industries and Walker Products, whose total returns (dividend yield plus capital gains or minus capital losses) over the last four years are shown in Columns 2 and 3:

Year (1)	Rate of Return		
	Atlas (2)	Walker (3)	Portfolio (4)
1985	40%	−20%	10%
1986	−10	50	20
1987	35	−9	13
1988	−5	39	17
Average return	15%	15%	15%
Standard deviation	26%	35%	4%

Figure 15-4 **Rates of Return on Atlas Industries, Walker Products, and Portfolio Consisting of 50 Percent in Each Stock**

Diversification of stock holdings reduces an investor's portfolio risk. For example, both Atlas Industries and Walker Products had widely varying rates of return from 1985 through 1988, making each a risky investment by itself. Note, however, that the two stocks' rates of return rose and fell in opposition to each other. Thus, if the two were combined into a single portfolio, their ups and downs would tend to cancel each other out. Because the fluctuations in returns would then be less pronounced, the combined investment would be less risky.

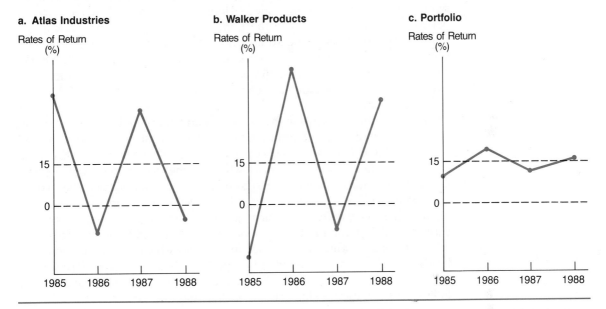

If you invested your entire $100,000 in either Atlas or Walker, and if returns in the future varied as they have in the past, your *expected return* on this one-stock portfolio would be $15,000, or 15 percent. However, your *actual return* could easily be negative. On the other hand, if you put half of your money into each stock, your expected return would still be $15,000, or 15 percent, but this return would be much less risky. Thus, although the expected return of a portfolio is simply a weighted average of the expected returns on the individual stocks in the portfolio, the same is not true for the measurement of portfolio risk. Unlike portfolio returns, the riskiness of a portfolio, σ_p, is generally *not* a weighted average of the standard deviations of the individual securities in the portfolio; the portfolio's risk will be *smaller* than the weighted average of the stock's standard deviations. These results are graphed in Figure 15-4, where we see that the ups and downs in the portfolio's returns are not nearly as pronounced as are those on the individual stocks.

What conditions are necessary for diversification to cause the riskiness of a portfolio to be less than the riskiness of the individual assets contained in the portfolio? The only condition necessary is that the returns on the stocks in the portfolio do not move together exactly. If Atlas's and Walker's returns always moved in the same direction and by the same amount, diversification into these two stocks would do no good. *In technical terms this means that for diversification to be effective, returns must not be perfectly positively correlated.* Since most stocks are not perfectly correlated, diversification generally reduces, but does not eliminate, portfolio risk.[3]

To see better how diversification affects portfolio risk, consider Figure 15-5, which shows that the riskiness of a portfolio declines as more and more randomly selected stocks are added.[4] Here risk is measured by the standard deviation of annual returns on the portfolio, σ_p. With just one stock in the portfolio, σ_p equals the standard deviation of returns on that stock, or 30 percent. Notice, however, that as more stocks are added, the portfolio's risk declines and approaches a limit, 15 percent in this example. Adding more and more stocks (diversification) can eliminate *some* of the riskiness of the portfolio, *but not all of it.*

It seems quite reasonable that stocks would tend to move together, at least to some extent, because of factors in the economy. Most stocks tend to do well when the national economy is strong and to do badly when it is weak. Certain wide ranging factors affect all stocks, whereas other factors affect only individual securities. Security returns tend to be positively (but not perfectly) correlated with one another. Therefore, risk consists of two parts: (1) *company-specific,* or *diversifiable, risk,* which can be eliminated by adding enough securities to the portfolio, and (2) *market,* or *nondiversifiable, risk,* which is related to broad swings in the stock market and which cannot be eliminated by diversification.[5] It is not especially important whether we call it *diversifiable, company-specific,* or *nonsystematic,* but the fact that part of the riskiness of any individual stock can be eliminated is vitally important.

company-specific risk
That part of a security's risk associated with random events; such risk can be eliminated by proper diversification.

Company-specific risk is caused by things like lawsuits, strikes, successful and unsuccessful marketing programs, the winning and losing of major contracts, and other events that are *unique to a particular firm.* Because these events are essentially random, their effects on a portfolio can be eliminated by

---

[3]*Correlation* is defined as the tendency of two variables to move together. The *correlation coefficient, r,* measures this tendency and can range from $+1.0$, denoting that the two variables move up and down in perfect synchronization, to -1.0, denoting that the variables always move in exactly opposite directions. A correlation coefficient of zero suggests that the two variables are not related to each other; that is, changes in one variable are independent of changes in the other. If stocks were negatively correlated, or if there were zero correlation, a properly constructed portfolio would have very little risk. However, stocks tend to be positively (but less than perfectly) correlated with one another, so all stock portfolios tend to be somewhat risky.

[4]The data used in this example are adapted from W. H. Wagner and S. C. Lau, "The Effect of Diversification on Risk," *Financial Analysts' Journal,* November–December 1971, 48–53. Wagner and Lau divided a sample of 200 New York Stock Exchange stocks into 6 subgroups based on quality ratings. Then they constructed portfolios from each of the subgroups, using from 1 to 20 randomly selected securities, and applied equal weights to each security.

[5]Market risk is sometimes called *systematic risk,* whereas company risk is called *unsystematic risk.*

Figure 15-5 **Reduction of Portfolio Risk through Diversification**

Increasing diversification decreases the risk in an investor's portfolio. When an investor owns only one stock, the risk equals the standard deviation of the returns on that stock, or, in this case, 30 percent. Risk declines as more stocks are added until the level of market risk (here, 15 percent) is reached. Market risk is related to broad swings in the stock market as a whole and cannot be eliminated through diversification.

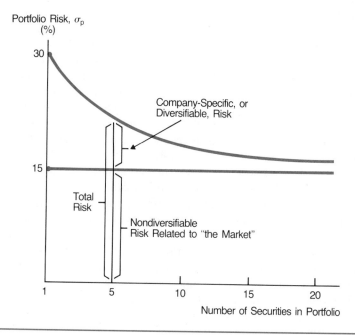

diversification; bad events in one firm will be offset by good events in another. **Market risk,** on the other hand, stems from factors that affect all firms simultaneously, like war, inflation, recessions, and high interest rates. However, not all firms are affected equally by market risk; for example, some firms are much more sensitive to changes in interest rates than others. Later in this chapter, we discuss a means by which we can measure a firm's sensitivity to market risk. Still, because all firms are affected simultaneously by these factors, market risk cannot be eliminated by diversification.

We know that investors demand a premium for bearing risk; that is, the higher the riskiness of a security, the higher its expected return must be to induce investors to buy (or to hold) it. If investors are primarily concerned with *portfolio risk* rather than the risk of the individual securities in the portfolio, how should the riskiness of the individual stocks be measured? The answer is this: *The relevant riskiness of an individual stock is its contribution to the riskiness of a well-diversified portfolio.* In other words, the riskiness of

market risk

That part of a security's risk that cannot be eliminated by diversification. It is measured by the beta coefficient.

relevant risk
The risk of a security that cannot be diversified away; that is, its market risk. This is a security's contribution to the risk of a portfolio.

Apple Computer's stock to a doctor who has a portfolio of 25 stocks or to a trust officer managing a 250-stock portfolio is the contribution that Apple's stock makes to the portfolio's riskiness. The stock may be quite risky if held by itself, but if most of its risk can be eliminated by diversification, its **relevant risk,** which is its *contribution to the portfolio's risk,* may be small.

A simple example will help make this point clear. Suppose you can flip a coin once. If a head comes up, you win $10,000, but if it comes up tails, you lose $9,500. Although this may be considered to be a good bet — the expected return is $250 — it is a highly risky proposition. Alternatively, suppose you can flip 100 coins and win $100 for each head but lose $95 for each tail. It is possible that you would hit all heads and win $10,000, and it is also possible that you would flip all tails and lose $9,500, but the chances are very high that you would actually flip about 50 heads and about 50 tails, winning a net $250. Although each individual flip is a risky bet, collectively you have a very low-risk proposition because you have diversified away most of the risk. This is the idea behind holding portfolios of stocks rather than just one stock, except that with stocks all of the risk cannot be eliminated by diversification — those risks related to broad changes in the stock market as reflected in the Dow Jones index and other stock market averages will remain.

Are all stocks equally risky in the sense that adding them to a well-diversified portfolio will have the same effect on the portfolio's riskiness? The answer is no — different stocks will affect the portfolio differently; hence different securities have different degrees of relevant risk. How can the relevant risk of a stock be measured? As we mentioned before, all risk except that related to broad market movements can, and presumably will, be diversified away. After all, why accept risk that easily can be eliminated? *The risk that remains after diversifying is market risk, or risk that is inherent in the market, and this risk can be measured by the degree to which a given stock tends to move up and down with the market.*

The Concept of Beta

beta coefficient, b
A measurement of the extent to which the returns of a given stock move with the stock market.

The tendency of a stock to move with the market is reflected in its **beta coefficient, b,** which is a measure of the stock's *volatility* relative to an average stock. Betas are discussed at an intuitive level in this section, then in more detail in Chapter 16.

An *average-risk stock* is defined as one that tends to move up and down in step with the general market as measured by some index, such as the Dow Jones Industrials, the Standard & Poor's 500, or the New York Stock Exchange Index. Such a stock will have a beta, b, of 1.0, which indicates that, in general, if the market moves up by 10 percent, the stock will also move up by 10 percent, and that if the market falls by 10 percent, the stock will likewise fall by 10 percent. A portfolio of such b = 1.0 stocks will move up and down with the broad market averages and will be just as risky as the averages. If b = 0.5, the stock is only half as volatile as the market — it will rise and fall only half

Table 15-2 **Illustrative List of Beta Coefficients**

Stock	Beta
Anheuser-Busch	1.00
Apple Computer	1.45
Campbell Soup Company	0.85
Delta Airlines	1.10
Du Pont	1.15
Exxon	0.80
General Motors	1.10
IBM	1.00
Kodak	0.85
Pillsbury Company	0.95
Polaroid	1.15
Potomac Electric Power	0.65
Procter and Gamble	0.85
Tandem Computers	1.55
Texas Air Corporation	1.35

Source: Value Line, July 24, 1987.

as much — and a portfolio of such stocks will be half as risky as a portfolio of $b = 1.0$ stocks. On the other hand, if $b = 2.0$, the stock is twice as volatile as an average stock, so a portfolio of such stocks will be twice as risky as an average portfolio.

Betas for literally thousands of companies are calculated and published by Merrill Lynch, Value Line, and numerous other organizations. The beta coefficients of some well-known companies are shown in Table 15-2. Most stocks have betas in the range of 0.50 to 1.50; the average for all stocks is 1.0, by definition.

If a high beta stock (one whose beta is greater than 1.0) is added to an average-risk ($b = 1.0$) portfolio, both the beta and the riskiness of the portfolio will increase. Conversely, if a low beta stock (one whose beta is less than 1.0) is added to an average-risk portfolio, the portfolio's beta and risk will decline. *Thus, because a stock's beta measures its contribution to the riskiness of any portfolio, beta is the appropriate measure of the stock's riskiness.*

We can summarize the analysis to this point as follows:

1. A stock's risk consists of two components, market and company-specific risk.

2. Company-specific risk can be eliminated by diversification, and most investors do indeed diversify, either directly, or indirectly by purchasing mutual funds. This leaves market risk, which is caused by general movements in the stock market and which reflects the fact that all stocks are affected by certain overall economic events like war, recession, and inflation. Market risk is the only relevant risk to a rational, diversified investor, because the investor has already eliminated company-specific risk.

3. Investors must be compensated for bearing risk; the greater the riskiness of a stock, the higher its required rate of return. However, compensation is required only for risk that cannot be eliminated by diversification. If risk premiums existed for diversifiable risk, well-diversified investors would buy these securities and bid up their prices, and their final expected returns would reflect only nondiversifiable market risk.

4. The market risk of a stock is measured by its beta coefficient, which is an index of the stock's relative volatility. Some benchmark betas are the following:

$b = 0.5$: Stock is only half as volatile, or risky, as the average stock.

$b = 1.0$: Stock is of average risk.

$b = 2.0$: Stock is twice as risky as the average stock.

5. *Because a stock's beta coefficient determines how it affects the riskiness of a diversified portfolio, beta is the most relevant measure of a stock's risk.*

THE RELATIONSHIP BETWEEN RISK AND RATE OF RETURN

Now that we have established beta as an appropriate measure of most stocks' risk, the next step in the Capital Asset Pricing Model (CAPM) framework is to specify the relationship between risk and return. This relationship is known as the **Security Market Line (SML),** and it is given by this equation:

Security Market Line (SML)
The line that shows the relationship between risk and rate of return for individual securities.

$$k = R_F + b(k_M - R_F). \tag{15-4}$$

Here:

k = the required rate of return on the stock in question. If the expected future return, $\hat{k}$, was less than k, you would not purchase this stock, or you would sell it if you owned it.

R_F = the risk-free rate of return, generally measured by the rate of return on short-term U.S. Treasury securities.

b = the beta coefficient of the stock in question.

k_M = the required rate of return on an average risk ($b = 1.0$) stock. k_M is also the required rate of return on a portfolio consisting of all stocks, which is the market portfolio.

$RP_M = (k_M - R_F)$ = the market risk premium, or the price of risk for an average stock. It is the additional return over the riskless rate required to compensate investors for assuming an average amount of risk.

$RP_i = b(k_M - R_F) =$ the risk premium on the stock in question. The stock's risk premium is less than, equal to, or greater than the premium on an average stock, depending on whether its beta is less than, equal to, or greater than 1.0

The **market risk premium, RP_M,** depends on the degree of aversion to risk that investors have in the aggregate. Let us assume that at the current time, Treasury bonds represent $R_F = 9\%$ and an average share of stock has a required return of $k_M = 13\%$. Therefore, the market risk premium is 4 percent:

$$RP_M = k_M - R_F = 13\% - 9\% = 4\%.$$

market risk premium, RP_M
The additional return over the risk-free rate needed to compensate investors for assuming an average amount of risk.

In words, the SML equation shows that the required rate of return on a given stock, k, is equal to the return required in the marketplace for securities that have no risk, R_F, plus a risk premium equal to that demanded on an average stock, $k_M - R_F$, scaled up or down by the relative riskiness of the firm as measured by its beta coefficient, b. Thus, if $R_F = 9\%$, b = 0.5, and $k_M = 13\%$, then the $RP_M = 4\%$ and the required rate of return for this lower risk stock would be

$$k = 9\% + 0.5(13\% - 9\%)$$
$$= 9\% + 0.5(4\%)$$
$$= 11\%.$$

An average-risk firm, with b = 1.0, would have the same return as an average stock:

$$k = 9\% + 1.0(4\%)$$
$$= 13\%,$$

whereas a riskier firm, with b = 2.0, would have a required rate of return of the following:

$$k = 9\% + 2.0(4\%)$$
$$= 17\%.$$

Figure 15-6 shows a graph of the SML and the required rate of return for a safe, an average, and a risky stock when $R_F = 9\%$ and $k_M = 13\%$. Several features of the graph in Figure 15-6 are worth noting:

1. Required rates of return are shown on the vertical axis, and risk as measured by beta is shown on the horizontal axis.

Figure 15-6 **The Security Market Line (SML)**

The Security Market Line reflects the relationship between a stock's riskiness and its rate of return. According to the SML equation, a stock's required rate of return equals the rate for riskless securities (U.S. Treasury bills) plus a risk premium. This premium is set according to whether a stock is considered to be of average risk (beta = 1.0), less than average risk (beta < 1.0), or greater than average risk (beta > 1.0). When the riskless rate is 9 percent, a stock with a beta of 0.5 will have a 2 percent risk premium, a stock with a beta of 1.0 will have a 4 percent risk premium, and a stock with a beta of 2.0 will have a 9 percent risk premium.

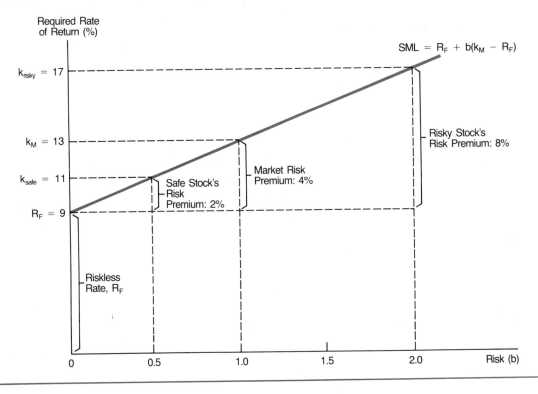

2. Riskless securities have b = 0; therefore R_F appears as the vertical axis intercept.

3. The slope of the SML reflects the degree of risk aversion in the economy; the greater the average investor's aversion to risk, (1) the steeper the slope of the line, (2) the greater the risk premium for any risky asset, and (3) the higher the required rate of return on risky assets.[6]

[6]Students sometimes confuse beta with the slope of the SML. This is a mistake. The confusion arises partly because the SML equation is generally written, in this book and throughout the finance literature, as $k_i = R_F + b_i(k_M - R_F)$, and in this form b_i looks like the slope coefficient and $(k_M - R_F)$ the variable. It would perhaps be less confusing if the second term were written $(k_M - R_F)b_i$, but this is not generally done.

4. The values for the low-risk stock with b = 0.5, the average-risk stock with b = 1.0, and the high-risk stock with b = 2.0 are shown on the graph for k_{safe}, k_M = $k_{average}$, and k_{risky}.

Both the Security Market Line and a company's position on change over time because of changes in interest rates, investors' risk aversion, and individual companies' betas. Such changes are discussed in the following sections.

The Impact of Inflation

As we discussed in Chapter 5, interest amounts to "rent" on borrowed money, or the price of money; thus R_F is the price of money to a riskless borrower. The risk-free rate as measured by the rate on U.S. Treasury securities is a *nominal rate,* and it consists of two elements: (1) a *real,* or *inflation-free, rate-of return, k*,* and (2) an *inflation premium, IP,* equal to the anticipated rate of inflation. Thus R_F = k^* + IP. The real rate on risk-free government securities has historically ranged from 2 to 4 percent, with a mean of about 3 percent. If no inflation is expected, risk-free government securities will tend to yield about 3 percent. As the expected rate of inflation increases, however, a premium must be added to the real rate of return to compensate investors for the loss of purchasing power that results from inflation. Therefore, the 9 percent R_F shown in Figure 15-6 may be thought of as consisting of a 3 percent real rate of return plus a 6 percent inflation premium: R_F = k^* + IP = 3% + 6% = 9%.

If the expected rate of inflation rises to 8 percent, this will cause R_F to rise to 11 percent. Such a change is shown in Figure 15-7. Notice that under the CAPM, the increase in R_F also causes an *equal* increase in the rate of return on all risky assets, because the inflation premium is built into the required rate of return of both riskless and risky assets. For example, in the figure the rate of return on an average stock, k_M, increases from 13 to 15 percent. Other risky securities' returns also rise by two percentage points.

Changes in Risk Aversion

The slope of the Security Market Line reflects the extent to which investors are averse to risk; the steeper the slope of the line, the greater the average investor's risk aversion. If investors were indifferent to risk and if R_F was 9 percent, risky assets would also sell to provide an expected return of 9 percent. With no risk aversion, there would be no risk premium, so the SML would be horizontal. As risk aversion increases, so does the risk premium and, thus, the slope of the SML.

Figure 15-8 illustrates an increase in risk aversion. The market risk premium rises from 4 to 6 percent, and k_M rises from 13 to 15 percent. The returns on other risky assets also rise, with the impact of this shift in risk aversion being more pronounced on riskier securities. For example, the required return on a stock with b_i = 0.5 increases by only one percentage point, from 11 to 12 percent, whereas that on a stock with b_i = 1.5 increases by three percentage points, from 15 to 18 percent.

Figure 15-7 **Shift in the SML Caused by an Increase in Inflation**

If market participants anticipate a 2 percent increase in inflation, the return on Treasury bills would rise from its original 9 percent to 11 percent to compensate purchasers for the expected inflation risk. This rise in the R_F would cause an equal rise in the rate of return for all risky assets since the inflation risk premium is part of the required return for all assets. The change in inflation expectations would therefore cause a parallel shift in the SML from SML_1 to SML_2, indicating a 2 percent greater required return for each investment risk level.

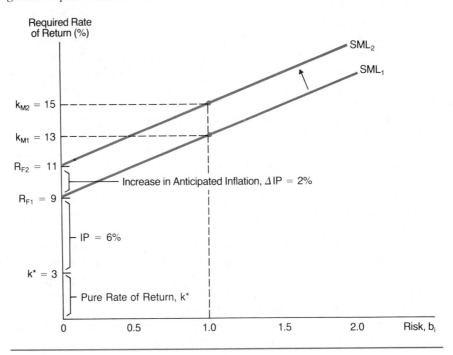

A Word of Caution

A word of caution about betas and the Capital Asset Pricing Model is in order. Although these concepts are logical, the entire theory is based on *ex ante*, or *expected*, conditions, yet we have available only *ex post*, or *past*, data. The betas we calculate show how volatile a stock has been in the *past*, but conditions may change, and the stock's *future* volatility, which is the item of real concern to investors, may be quite different from its past volatility. Thus problems may arise when one attempts to measure *future* events on the basis of *past* data. Indeed, the CAPM does have some potentially serious deficiencies when applied in practice, so estimates of k found through the SML may be subject to considerable error. In spite of the potential problems in the application of the CAPM in practice, however, it does represent an important step foreward in

Figure 15-8 **Shift in the SML Caused by Increased Risk Aversion**

If market participants grow more risk averse, they require a higher rate of return for risky investments. Therefore the difference between the return on an average risk investment and the risk-free rate, known as the market risk premium ($k_M - R_F$), will grow. In this case, the resulting SML (SML_2) will have a greater slope than before (SML_1). Note that the shift in risk aversion has no effect on the risk-free rate or on an individual investment's beta.

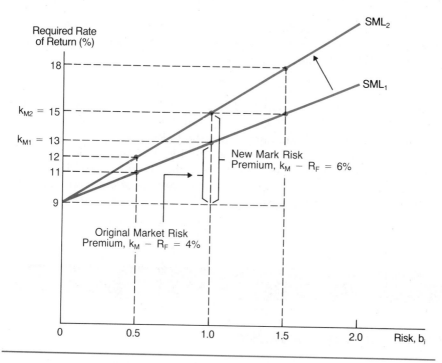

understanding how markets adjust for risk. Thus abandoning the CAPM because of these potential difficulties would be like throwing the baby out with the bath water.

SUMMARY

This chapter showed how risk is measured in financial analysis and explained how risk affects security prices and rates of return. Risk is related to the variability of expected future returns. Most rational investors hold *portfolios* of stocks, however, and such investors are more concerned with the risks of their portfolios as a whole than with the risks of individual securities.

The riskiness of a given stock can be split into two components — *market risk,* which is caused by changes in the broad stock market and which cannot be eliminated by diversification, and *company-specific risk*, which can be eliminated by holding a diversified portfolio. Because investors can and do diversify and thus eliminate company risk, the *relevant risk* inherent in stocks is their market risk, which is measured by the *beta coefficient*, b.

Betas measure the tendency of stocks to move up and down with the market; a high-beta stock is more volatile than an average stock, whereas a low-beta stock is less volatile than average. An average risk stock has a b = 1.0 by definition.

The required rate of return on a stock consists of the rate of return on risk-free securities, R_F, plus a risk premium that depends on the stock's beta coefficient and the market risk premium, RP_M:

$$k = R_F + b(k_M - R_F).$$

This formula is called the *Security Market Line (SML) equation* or, sometimes, the *Capital Asset Pricing Model (CAPM) equation,* and it is of fundamental importance in finance. Note, though, that the CAPM is based on investors' *expectations;* for example, the beta and k_M used in the SML equation should be the values that an average investor expects in the future. Because those expectations cannot be measured precisely, CAPM estimates of required returns are subject to potentially large errors.

 RESOLUTION TO DECISION IN FINANCE

The Perilous Pursuit of Sexy Businesses

Despite its lack of expertise in electronics, Schlumberger sent in its own management team to take charge of Fairchild shortly after its acquisition. Operations were decentralized in accordance with Schlumberger's management style. Salaries, bonuses, and profit-sharing plans were slashed to trim costs. As a result, Fairchild CEO Wilfred J. Corrigan and a host of key engineering personnel left the company. After this, earnings begin to plummet and new-product development ground to a near halt. In 1986, after more than six years of Schlumberger's management, Fairchild lost an estimated $150 million in operating income even though it had sales of more than $550 million. When Schlumberger ousted its own CEO, Michael Vaillaud, in the fall of 1986, analysts widely believed that the fiasco at Fairchild was the key reason for his dismissal.

What went wrong? In their rush to buy instant growth, even the biggest and savviest companies sometimes blunder. Giving cursory analysis to unfamiliar markets or technologies, they convince themselves that the potential for almost limitless growth is only an acquisition away. Instead of carefully planning the direction that they hope to take and pinpointing how a potential acquisition will fit in, they jump in and make a bid, hoping that by acting quickly and

Source: Thomas J. Murray, "The Perilous Pursuit of Sexy Businesses," *Dun's Business Month,* November 1986, 37.

covertly, they can outmaneuver competitive bidders.

"Management frequently fails to consider how it will manage the little beauty after acquisition," says David Jemison, associate professor of management at Stanford University Graduate School of Business. "You can't do it well from the back of an envelope." Corporate overconfidence is part of the explanation for this half-baked approach. Despite all evidence to the contrary, many top executives assume that if they can run their business successfully, they can run any business with the same degree of success.

Schlumberger, like many acquiring companies, believed that the best way to overcome its own lack of experience in electronics was to plunge in and take control of Fairchild as soon as possible. But often the success of entrepreneurial, high-tech firms is a product of their own unique corporate culture. When a different management style is suddenly imposed from above, the results can be disastrous.

One reason for such corporate heavy-handedness, of course, it top management's desire to generate short-term profits. This can be a mistake. According to Mark L. Feldman, mergers and acquisitions director at the May Management Consulting Group, a young company typically requires time to realize its earnings potential, especially while trying to blend its unique corporate culture with that of its new, more firmly entrenched parent company. In fact, profitability usually suffers a temporary set-back in the immediate post-acquisition period. "The short-term emphasis [on profits]," Feldman believes, "can substantially lengthen the payback period and reduce the value of the investment."

It appears that Schlumberger, in the wake of the corporate shake-up following the ouster of its CEO, may have all but written off its investment in Fairchild to experience. "I do have the feeling that Schlumberger is going to sell or spin off Fairchild," says semiconductor analyst James Crandell of Salomon Brothers.

QUESTIONS

15-1   The probability distribution of a less risky expected return is more peaked than that of a more risky return. What shape would the probability distribution have for (a) completely certain returns and (b) completely uncertain returns?

15-2   Security A has an expected return of 6 percent, a standard deviation of expected returns of 30 percent, a correlation coefficient with the market of -0.25, and a beta coefficient of -0.5. Security B has an expected return of 11 percent, a standard deviation of returns of 10 percent, a correlation with the market of 0.75, and a beta coefficient of 1.0. Which security is riskier? Why?

15-3   Suppose you owned a portfolio consisting of $500,000 worth of long-term U.S. government bonds.
   a. Would your portfolio be riskless?
   b. Now suppose you hold a portfolio consisting of $500,000 worth of 30-day Treasury bills. Every 30 days your bills mature and you reinvest the principal ($500,000) in a new batch of bills. Assume that you live on the investment income from your portfolio and that you want to maintain a constant standard of living. Is your portfolio truly riskless?
   c. You should have concluded that both long-term and short-term portfolios of government securities have some element of risk. Can you think of any asset that would be completely riskless?

15-4 A life insurance policy is a financial asset. The premiums paid represent the investment's cost.

  a. How would you calculate the expected return on a life insurance policy?

  b. Suppose the owner of the life insurance policy has no other financial assets — the person's only other asset is "human capital," or lifetime earnings capacity. What is the correlation coefficient between returns on the insurance policy and returns on the policyholder's human capital?

  c. Life insurance companies have to pay administrative costs and sales representatives' commissions; hence, the expected rate of return on insurance premiums is generally low or even negative. Use the portfolio concept to explain why people buy life insurance in spite of negative expected returns.

15-5 If investors' aversion to risk increased, would the risk premium on a high-beta stock increase more or less than that on a low-beta stock? Explain.

SELF-TEST PROBLEM

ST-1 Stocks X and Y have the following historical dividend and price data:

	Stock X		Stock Y	
Year	**Dividend**	**Year-End Price**	**Dividend**	**Year-End Price**
1983	—	$61.25	—	$110.00
1984	$5.00	48.75	$12.00	92.50
1985	5.25	55.00	13.00	97.50
1986	5.75	68.75	14.25	126.25
1987	6.50	66.25	15.25	112.50
1988	7.50	77.50	16.25	120.00

  a. Calculate the realized rate of return (or holding period return) for each stock in each year. Then assume that someone had held a portfolio consisting of 50 percent of X and 50 percent of Y. (The portfolio is rebalanced every year to maintain these percentages.) What would the realized rate of return on the portfolio have been in each year from 1984 through 1988? What would the average returns have been for each stock and for the portfolio?

  b. Now calculate the standard deviation of returns for each stock and for the portfolio.

  c. On the basis of the extent to which the portfolio has a lower risk than the stocks held individually, would you guess that the correlation coefficient between returns on the two stocks is closer to 0.95 or to −0.95?

  d. If you added more stocks at random to the portfolio, what is the most accurate statement of what would happen to σ_p?

  1. σ_p would remain constant.

  2. σ_p would decline to somewhere in the vicinity of 15 percent.

  3. σ_p would decline to zero if enough stocks were included.

PROBLEMS

15-1 **Expected risk and return.** Analysts have determined the following probability distribution of expected returns for the Reston Corporation:

Probability	Returns
0.1	− 10%
0.2	5
0.4	15
0.2	25
0.1	40

a. Calculate the expected rate of return for Reston.

b. Calculate the standard deviation of these expected returns for Reston.

15-2 **Expected returns.** Projects X and Y have the following probability distributions of expected future rates of return:

Probability	X	Y
0.1	− 40%	− 25%
0.2	0	5
0.4	20	15
0.2	40	30
0.1	70	45

a. Calculate the expected rate of return for Project Y. The expected rate of return for Project X is 19%.

b. Calculate the standard deviation of expected returns for Project X. The standard deviation of expected returns for Project Y is 17.75%.

c. Is it possible that the firm's management might regard Project X as being *less* risky than Project Y? Explain.

15-3 **Expected NPV and IRR.** Highlands Consulting has provided the following cash flow (net income + depreciation) estimates for a proposed investment project:

Annual Cash Flows	
Probability	**Amount**
0.3	$40,000
0.4	60,000
0.2	75,000
0.1	90,000

This project has a life of 10 years and is expected to have a zero salvage value. An investment of $251,550, is required to make the project operational.

a. If the firm requires a 16 percent return, what is the project's NPV?

b. What is the project's IRR?

c. Should Highlands Consulting accept or reject the proposed project?

15-4 **Risk adjusted NPVs.** Acorn Industries has a cost of capital that equals 12 percent. The company is choosing between two mutually exclusive projects. Alpha Project is of average risk and costs $1 million. Its expected cash flows are $220,000 annually for 8 years. The Omega Project is of above-average risk, and management estimates that its cost of capital should be 15 percent. Omega also costs $1 million, and it promises to provide a cash flow of $240,000 annually for 8 years. Each project will end with a zero salvage value at the end of its designated life. Calculate the risk-adjusted NPV for each project and indicate which project should be accepted and which should be rejected by Acorn Industries. What is the basis for your conclusion?

15-5   **Risk adjusted NPV.** Sierra International is considering investing in a new capital project. The project, which has an expected productive life of 10 years, would require a $500,000 investment and promises to provide a cash flow (net income + depreciation) of $100,000 annually. Sierra's cost of capital is 12 percent. However, management has determined that the project is much riskier than the firm's average projects. Sierra requires an 18 percent return on high risk-projects.
- **a.** Which rate of return, 12% or 18%, should management use in evaluating this project?
- **b.** What is the project's NPV?
- **c.** Should Sierra invest in this project?

15-6   **Required rate of return.** Olson Products is evaluating three investment opportunities. Its financial manager has forecast the risk-free rate and the expected market rate of return as being $R_F = 8\%$ and $k_M = 11\%$, respectively. What is the appropriate required rate of return for each project if:
- **a.** Project A has a beta of 0.5?
- **b.** Project B has a beta of 1.0?
- **c.** Project C has a beta of 2.0?

15-7   **Required rate of return.** Suppose that $R_F = 9\%$, $k_M = 14\%$, and the beta for Dahl Industries is 1.6.
- **a.** What is the required rate of return for Dahl's stock?
- **b.** Now suppose that R_F (1) increases to 11 percent or (2) decreases to 7 percent. The slope of the Security Market Line (SML) remains constant (that is, $[k_M - R_F]$ remains at 5 percent). How would each of these changes affect k_M and the required return on Dahl's stock?
- **c.** Now assume that the risk-free rate remains at 9 percent but that k_M (1) increases to 16 percent or (2) falls to 12 percent. The slope of the SML does not remain constant. How would each of these changes affect investors' required return for Dahl's stock?

15-8   **Risk adjusted NPVs.** Miller's Mills has an average cost of capital equaling 10 percent. The company is choosing between two mutually exclusive projects. Project B is of average risk, has a cost of $50,000, and has expected cash flows of $14,701.80 per year for 5 years. Project A is of above-average risk, and management estimates that its cost of capital would be 12 percent. Project A also costs $50,000, and it is expected to provide cash flows of $9,380.53 per year for 10 years. Each project will terminate at the end of its designated life. Calculate risk-adjusted NPVs for the two projects, and use these NPVs to choose between them.

15-9   **Expected returns.** Suppose you were offered (1) $10,000 or (2) a gamble in which you would get $20,000 if a head was flipped but zero if a tail came up.
- **a.** What is the expected value of the gamble?
- **b.** Would you take the sure $10,000 or the gamble?
- **c.** If you choose the sure $10,000, are you a risk averter or a risk seeker?
- **d.** Suppose that you actually take the sure $10,000. You can invest it in either a U.S. Treasury bond that will return $10,900 at the end of a year or a common stock that has a 50-50 chance of being either worthless or worth $23,600 at the end of the year.
  - **1.** What is the expected dollar profit on the stock investment? (The expected profit on the T-bond investment is $900.)

2. What is the expected rate of return on the stock investment? (The expected rate of return on the T-bond investment is 9 percent.)

3. Would you invest in the bond or the stock?

4. Just how large would the expected profit (or the expected rate of return) have to be on the stock investment to make *you* invest in the stock?

5. How might your decision be affected if, rather than buying one stock for $10,000, you could construct a portfolio consisting of 100 stocks with $100 in each? Each of these stocks has the same return characteristics as the one stock; that is, a 50-50 chance of being worth either zero or $236 at year-end. Would the correlation between returns on these stocks matter?

15-10   **Security Market Line.** The Wisconsin Investment Fund has a total investment of $500 million in five stocks:

Stock	Investment	Stock's Beta Coefficient
A	$150 million	0.50
B	$125 million	1.50
C	$ 75 million	2.00
D	$100 million	1.00
E	$ 50 million	1.75

The beta coefficient for a fund like Wisconsin Investment can be found as a weighted average of the fund's investments. The current risk-free rate is 9 percent. Expected market returns have the following estimated probability distribution for the next period:

Probability	Market Return
0.1	10%
0.2	12
0.4	14
0.2	16
0.1	18

a. What is the estimated equation for the Security Market Line (SML)? (*Hint:* Determine the expected market return.)

b. Compute the fund's required rate of return for the next period.

c. Suppose Wisconsin Investment Fund's management receives a proposal for a new stock. The investment needed to take a position in the stock is $50 million; it will have an expected return of 17 percent; and its estimated beta coefficient is 2.0. Should the new stock be purchased? At what expected rate of return should management be indifferent to purchasing the stock?

15-11   **Risky cash flows.** The Severn Company is faced with two mutually exclusive investment projects. Each project costs $9,000 and has an expected life of 3 years. Annual net cash flows from each project begin one year after the initial investment is made and have the following probability distributions:

Project A		Project B	
Probability	**Cash Flow**	**Probability**	**Cash Flow**
0.2	$ 8,000	0.2	$ 0
0.6	9,000	0.6	9,000
0.2	10,000	0.2	24,000

Severn has decided to evaluate the riskier project at a 12 percent rate and the less risky project at a 10 percent rate.

a. What is the expected value of the annual net cash flows from each project? The coefficient of variation (CV)? (*Hint:* Use Equation 15-3 from Chapter 15 to calculate the standard deviation of Project A. $\sigma_B = \$7,730$ and $CV_B = 0.76$)

b. What is the risk-adjusted NPV of each project?

c. If it were known that Project B was negatively correlated with other cash flows of the firm whereas Project A was positively correlated, how should this knowledge affect the decision? If Project B's cash flows were negatively correlated with gross national product (GNP), would that influence your assessment of its risk?

ANSWER TO SELF-TEST PROBLEM

ST-1 **a.** The realized return in each Period t is estimated as follows:

$$k_t = \frac{D_t + P_t - P_{t-1}}{P_t}.$$

For example, the realized return for Stock X in 1984 was -12.24 percent:

$$k_{1984} = \frac{D_{1984} + P_{1984} - P_{1983}}{P_{1983}}$$

$$= \frac{\$5.00 + \$48.75 - \$61.25}{\$61.25}$$

$$= -0.1224 = -12.24\%.$$

The table that follows shows the realized returns for each stock in each year, the averages for the five years, and the same data for the portfolio:

Year	Stock X's Return, k_X	Stock Y's Return, k_Y	Portfolio XY's Return, k_{XY}
1984	-12.24%	-5.00%	-8.62%
1985	23.59	19.46	21.52
1986	35.45	44.10	39.78
1987	5.82	1.19	3.50
1988	28.30	21.11	24.71
$k_{Avg} \approx$	16.20%	16.20%	16.20%

b. The standard deviation of returns is estimated, using Equation 15-3a, as follows[a]:

$$\text{Estimated } \sigma = S = \sqrt{\frac{\sum_{t=1}^{n} (k_t - k_{Avg})^2}{n - 1}}. \tag{15-3a}$$

---

[a]If only sample returns data over some past period are available, the standard deviation can be estimated using Equation 15-3a.

For Stock X, the estimated σ is 19.3 percent:

$$\sigma_X = \sqrt{\frac{(-12.24 - 16.2)^2 + (23.59 - 16.2)^2 + \cdots + (28.30 - 16.2)^2}{5 - 1}}$$

$$= \sqrt{\frac{1,488.15}{4}} = 19.3\%.$$

The standard deviation of returns for Stock Y and for the portfolio are similarly determined, and they are as follows:

	Stock X	**Stock Y**	**Portfolio XY**
Standard deviation	19.3	19.3	18.9

c. Because the risk reduction from diversification is small (σ_{XY} fall only from 19.3 to 18.9 percent), the more likely value of the correlation coefficient is 0.95. If the correlation coefficient were -0.95, the risk reduction would be much larger. In fact, the correlation coefficient between Stocks X and Y is 0.93.

d. If more randomly selected stocks were added to the portfolio, σ_p would decline to somewhere in the vicinity of 15 percent. σ_p would remain constant only if the correlation coefficient were $+1.0$, which is most unlikely. σ_p would decline to zero only if the correlation coefficient, r, were equal to zero and a large number of stocks were added to the portfolio, or if the proper proportions were held in a two-stock portfolio with r = -1.0.

Chapter 16

Decisions in Capital Budgeting

 DECISION IN FINANCE

Gambling on a State-of-the-Art Refinery

In the spring of 1980 Chairman William E. Greehey set an ambitious goal for Valero Energy Corp.: To diversify the $1 billion San Antonio firm into a full-fledged energy company. At the time Valero operated the nation's largest intrastate natural-gas pipeline, but that wasn't enough for Greehey. In short order he added gas storage facilities, signed up new gas sources in Texas and Mexico, and built new collection lines. If all went according to plan, Valero would soon begin production of natural gas liquids and launch its own drilling projects.

Late in 1980 Greehey took a bold step toward his goal of making Valero into an integrated energy producer: he purchased 50 percent of Saber Energy, Inc., a small gasoline marketer. What especially caught Greehey's eye was Saber's tiny refinery in Corpus Christi, Texas. The way Greehey saw it, he could turn

the refinery into a high-volume, state-of-the-art facility that would yield margins up to three times higher than the average of other refineries.

The cost of upgrading the old facility would be high — $617 million. But, according to Greehey, the economics were unbelievably promising. The new 50,000-barrel-per-day refinery would crack low-value heavy crude oil into gasoline. Because the raw material — called "resid" — could be bought from the Middle East for about $20 per barrel, Greehey projected Valero's profits at $16 per barrel. At that rate the Saber refinery could be expected to pay for itself in three years and would eventually generate more than half of Valero's profits.

As you read this chapter, look for the factors that Greehey should consider in deciding whether to replace the old refinery. Would you recommend that Valero build the new refinery? Why or why not?

See end of chapter for resolution.

RISK ANALYSIS IN CAPITAL BUDGETING

The basic principles of capital budgeting were covered in Chapter 14. However, measuring an investment's return provides only a portion of the information required when determining an investment's quality. Therefore, in Chapter 15 we introduced, in general terms, how risk is defined, the procedures managers and security analysts use to measure risk, and the relationship between risk and return. In this chapter, we continue the discussion of risk with special emphasis on how managers incorporate risk measures into their evaluation of capital budgeting projects. We then turn to several special topics in capital budgeting such as the replacement decision, the comparison of projects with unequal lives, and the effect of inflation on capital budgeting decisions.

Corporate Risk versus Beta Risk

market, or beta, risk
That part of a project's risk that cannot be eliminated by diversification; it is measured by the project's beta coefficient.

total, or corporate, risk
Risk viewed without consideration of the effects of diversification; in capital budgeting, it relates to the probability that a project will incur losses that will destabilize profits.

Two separate and distinct types of risk are relevant in capital budgeting analysis. First there is **market, or beta, risk,** which is a measure of risk from the standpoint of an investor who holds the stock of the company doing the capital budgeting analysis as just one security in a highly diversified portfolio. Second there is **total, or corporate risk,** which is the firm's risk viewed without consideration of the effects of its stockholders' personal diversification. A particular project might have highly uncertain returns, yet taking it on might not affect the firm's beta coefficient at all; in this case, the project's risk might be low from the stockholders' point of view. To understand this point more clearly, recall that the beta coefficient reflects only that part of an investor's risk which cannot be eliminated by forming a large portfolio of stocks. If an investor holds a portfolio consisting of 100 companies' stocks, and if each company is considering 20 major projects, the project in question is but one of 2,000 projects from the investor's point of view. Therefore, even if the project produces a return of minus 100 percent, this would not make much difference within the overall portfolio, and the law of large numbers suggests that the loss would be offset by gains in some of the other 1,999 remaining projects.

To illustrate the difference between corporate and beta risk, suppose 100 firms in the oil business each drill one wildcat well. Each company has $1 million of capital that it will invest in its well. If a firm strikes oil, it will get a return of $2.4 million and earn a profit of $1.4 million, whereas if it hits a dry hole, it will lose its $1 million investment and go bankrupt. The probability of striking oil is 50 percent. Each firm's expected rate of return is 20 percent, calculated as follows:

$$\frac{\text{Expected rate}}{\text{of return}} = \frac{\text{Expected profit}}{\text{Investment}} = \frac{0.5(-\$1\text{ million}) + 0.5(+\$1.4\text{ million})}{\$1\text{ million}}$$

$$= \frac{-\$500,000 + \$700,000}{\$1,000,000} = 20\%.$$

Note, however, that even though the expected return is 20 percent, there is a 50 percent probability of each firm being wiped out. From the standpoint of the individual firms, this is a very risky business.

Although the risk to each individual firm is high, if a stockholder constructs a portfolio consisting of a few shares of each of the 100 companies, the riskiness of this portfolio will not be high at all. Some of the firms will strike oil and do well, others will miss and go out of business, but the portfolio's return will be very close to the expected 20 percent. Therefore, because investors can diversify away the risks inherent in each of the individual companies, these risks are *not market-related;* that is, they do not affect the companies' beta coefficients. The firms remain quite risky from the standpoint of their managers and employees, however, who bear risks similar to those borne by undiversified stockholders.

With this background, *we may define the corporate risk of a capital budgeting project as the probability that the project will incur losses which will, at a minimum, destabilize the corporation's earnings and, at the extreme, cause it to go bankrupt.* A project with a high degree of corporate risk will not necessarily affect the firm's beta to any great extent, as our hypothetical example demonstrated. On the other hand, if a project has highly uncertain returns, and if those returns are also highly correlated with those of most other assets in the economy, the project may have a high degree of both corporate and beta risk.

For example, suppose a firm decides to undertake a major expansion to build solar-powered automobiles. Because the firm is not sure if its technology will work on a mass production basis, there are great risks in the venture. Management also estimates that the project will have a higher probability of success if the economy is strong, for then people will have the money to spend on the new automobiles. This means that the plant will tend to do well when other companies are also doing well and to do badly when others do badly; therefore, the plant's beta coefficient will be high. A project like this will have a high degree of both corporate risk and beta risk.

Beta risk is obviously important because of beta's effect on the value of a firm's stock. At the same time, corporate, or total, risk is also important for three primary reasons:

1. Undiversified stockholders, including the owners of small businesses, are more concerned about corporate risk than about beta risk.

2. Many financial theorists argue that investors, even those who are well diversified, consider factors other than market risk when setting required returns. Empirical studies of the determinants of required rates of return generally find both beta and total risk to be important.

3. A firm's stability is important to its managers, workers, customers, suppliers, and creditors, as well as to the community in which it operates. Firms that are in serious danger of bankruptcy, or even of suffering low profits and reduced output, have difficulty attracting and retaining good managers and workers. Also, both suppliers and customers will be reluctant to depend on weak firms, and such firms will have difficulty borrowing money except at high interest rates. These factors will tend to reduce risky firms' profitability and hence the price of their stock.

For all of these reasons, corporate risk can be important even to well-diversified stockholders.[1]

Beta Risk

The evaluation of total, or corporate, risk discussed thus far in the chapter provides insights into projects' risks and thus helps managers to make better accept/reject decisions. However, the measurement of total risk does not take into account the reduction of risk that is possible when projects are combined and evaluated as part of a portfolio of projects. In this section, we show how the Capital Asset Pricing Model (CAPM) can be used to evaluate projects as portfolios and thereby overcome the shortcomings of corporate risk measures. Of course, the CAPM has shortcomings of its own, but it does offer additional insights into risk analysis in capital budgeting.

The CAPM provides a framework for analyzing the relationship between risk and return. In Chapter 15 we analyzed the relationship between risk and return in portfolios of financial assets. The fundamental concept of this analysis is that the higher the risk associated with an investment, the higher the expected rate of return must be to compensate investors for assuming risk. This same principle holds for managers evaluating capital budgeting investment opportunities for a firm. The CAPM holds that there is a minimum required rate of return, even if there are no risks, plus a premium for all unavoidable risks associated with the investment. Thus

$$\text{Required return} = \text{Risk-free rate} + \text{Risk premiums},$$

which translates into the Security Market Line (SML) equation to express this risk/return relationship:

$$k = R_F + b(k_M - R_F),$$

where the required return on an investment, k, is equal to the riskless rate, R_F, plus a risk premium that is equal to the stock's beta coefficient, b, times the market risk premium, $k_M - R_F$.[2] The greater the nondiversifiable risk from a stock or project, the greater the beta and hence the larger the risk premium.

---

[1] In Chapter 15, we noted that the appropriate measure of total, or corporate, risk was the standard deviation. Other techniques for measuring corporate risk such as sensitivity analysis, scenario analysis, and simulation techniques are discussed in Brigham and Gapenski, *Intermediate Financial Management,* 2nd ed., Chapter 9.

[2] Note that both the risk-free rate, R_F, and the return on a diversified portfolio of securities, k_M, are market determined and outside the control of the firm.

For example, consider the case of Chicago Steel Company, an integrated producer operating in the Great Lakes region. Chicago Steel's beta is 1.1, so if $R_F = 8\%$ and $k_M = 12\%$, then

$$k = 8\% + 1.1(4\%) = 12.4\%.$$

This suggests that investors would be willing to give Chicago Steel money to invest in average-risk projects if the company could earn 12.4 percent or more on this money. Here again, by average risk we mean projects having risk similar to the firm's existing assets. Therefore, as a first approximation, Chicago should invest in capital projects if and only if these projects have an expected return of 12.4 percent or more.[3] In other words, Chicago should use 12.4 percent as its discount rate to determine average-risk projects' NPVs or as the "hurdle rate" if the IRR method is used.

Suppose, however, that taking on a particular project will change Chicago's beta coefficient and hence change the company's cost of equity capital. For example, the company might be considering the construction of a fleet of barges to haul iron ore, and barge operations might have betas of about 1.5. Since the corporation itself may be regarded as a portfolio of assets, and since the beta of any portfolio is a weighted average of the betas of the individual assets, taking on a barge investment will cause the overall corporate beta to rise and to end up somewhere between the original beta of 1.1 and the barge division's beta of 1.5. The exact position will depend on the relative size of the investment in barge operations versus Chicago's other assets. If 80 percent of the total corporate funds are in basic steel operations having a beta of 1.1 and 20 percent in barge operations having a beta of 1.5, the new corporate beta will be 1.18.

$$\text{New beta} = 0.8(1.1) + 0.2(1.5)$$

$$= 1.18.$$

An increase in the beta coefficient will cause the stock price to decline *unless the increased beta is offset by a higher expected rate of return*. Specifically, the overall corporate cost of capital will rise from 12.4 percent to 12.72 percent:

$$k_{(new)} = 8\% + 1.18(4\%) = 12.72\%.$$

Therefore, to keep the barge investment from lowering the value of the firm, Chicago's expected overall rate of return must rise from 12.4 percent to 12.72 percent.

If investments in basic steel earn 12.4 percent, how much must the barge investment earn for the new overall rate of return to equal 12.72 percent? We

---

[3] To simplify things somewhat, we assume at this point that the firm uses only equity capital. If debt is used, the cost of capital used must be a weighted average of the cost of debt and equity. This point is discussed at length in Chapters 19 and 20.

know that if Chicago undertakes the barge investment project, it will have 80 percent of its assets invested in basic steel earning 12.4 percent and 20 percent in barges earning X percent, and the average required rate of return will be 12.72 percent. Therefore,

$$0.8(12.4\%) + 0.2(X) = 12.72\%$$

$$X = 14.0\%.$$

In summary, if Chicago Steel makes the barge investment, its beta will rise from 1.1 to 1.18; its overall required rate of return will rise from 12.4 percent to 12.72 percent; and it will achieve this new required rate if the barge investment earns 14 percent. If the barge investment has an expected return of more than 14 percent, taking it on will increase the value of Chicago's stock. If the expected return is less than 14 percent, taking it on will decrease the stock's value. At an expected return of 14 percent, the barge project is a breakeven proposition in terms of its effect on the value of the stock.

This line of reasoning leads to the conclusion that, if the beta coefficient for each project could be determined, individual projects' costs of capital could be found as follows:

$$k_{(project)} = R_F + b_{(project)}(K_M - R_F).$$

Thus, for basic steel projects with $b = 1.1$, Chicago should use 12.4 percent as the discount rate. The barge project should be evaluated at a 14 percent discount rate:

$$k_{(barge)} = 8\% + 1.5(4\%) = 8\% + 6\% = 14\%.$$

A low-risk project such as a new steel distribution center with a beta of only 0.5 would have a cost of capital of 10 percent:

$$k_{(center)} = 8\% + 0.5(4\%) = 10\%.$$

Figure 16-1 gives a graphic summary of these concepts as applied to Chicago Steel. Note the following points:

1. The SML is the same Security Market Line that we developed in Chapter 15. It shows how investors are willing to make trade-offs between risk as measured by beta and expected returns. The higher the beta risk, the higher the rate of return needed to compensate investors for bearing this risk, and the SML specifies the nature of this relationship.

2. Chicago Steel initially had a beta of 1.1, so its required rate of return on average-risk investments is 12.4 percent.

3. High-risk investments like the fleet of barge require higher rates of return, whereas low-risk investments like the distribution center have lower required rates of return. It is not shown in Figure 16–1, but if Chicago makes relatively large investments in either high- or low-risk projects, as opposed to those

Figure 16-1 **Using the Security Market Line Concept in Capital Budgeting**

The Security Market Line can be used in the accept-reject decision for potential projects in capital budgeting decisions. A project whose expected rate of return lies above the SML should be accepted. A project whose return falls below the SML should be rejected because its return will not be high enough to overcome its higher risk. In this case Project M would be accepted, whereas Project N would be rejected.

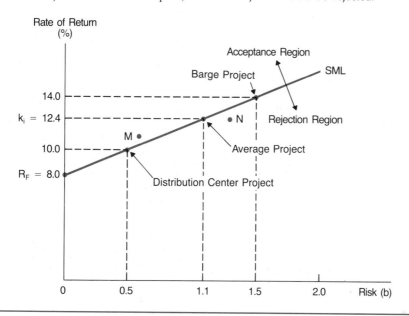

with average risks, the corporate beta and therefore the required rate of return on the common stock (k_s) will change.

4. If the expected rate of return on a given capital project lies *above* the SML, the expected rate of return on the project is more than enough to compensate for its risk, so it should be accepted. Conversely, if the project's rate of return lies *below* the SML, it should be rejected. Thus Project M in Figure 16-1 is acceptable, whereas Project N should be rejected. Even though Project N has a higher expected rate of return than Project M, the difference is not enough to offset Project N's much higher risk.

Portfolio Effects within the Firm

As we have seen, a security might be quite risky if held in isolation but not very risky if held as part of a well-diversified portfolio. The same thing is true of capital budgeting. The returns on an individual project might be highly uncertain, but if the project is small relative to the total activities of the firm, and if its returns are not highly correlated with the firm's other assets, the project may not be very risky in either the corporate or the beta sense.

Many firms do make serious efforts to diversify; often this is a specific objective of the long-run strategic plan. For example, Du Pont diversified into both coal and oil to broaden its operating base, and real estate developers have diversified geographically to lessen the effect of a slowdown in one region. The major objective of many such moves is to stabilize earnings, reduce corporate risk, and thereby raise the value of the firm's stock.

The wisdom of corporate diversification designed to reduce risk has been questioned; why should a firm diversify when stockholders can so easily diversify on their own? In other words, it may be true that if the returns on Du Pont and on Conoco are not perfectly positively correlated, merging the companies (as happened recently) will reduce their risks somewhat, but would it not be just as easy for investors to carry out this risk-reducing diversification directly without all the trouble and expense of a merger?

As you might suspect, the answer is not so simple. Although stockholders could directly obtain some of the risk-reducing benefits through personal diversification, other benefits can be gained only by diversification at the corporate level. For example, a relatively stable corporation may be able to attract a better work force, and also may be able to use more low-cost debt, than two less stable firms. Of course, there may also be spillover effects from diversification. For example, Du Pont provided Conoco with a more stable market for its oil, whereas Conoco provided Du Pont with a stable supply of raw materials. Further, the two companies' research departments are reported to have gained economies of scale from combined operations.

Project Risk Conclusions

We have discussed two types of risk in capital budgeting analyses — corporate risk and beta risk — and we have looked at ways of assessing each. However, two important questions remain: (1) Should a firm consider both corporate risk and beta risk in its capital budgeting decisions? (2) What does a firm do when its beta and corporate risk assessments lead to different conclusions?

These questions do not have easy answers. From a theoretical standpoint, well-diversified investors should be concerned primarily with beta risk and managers with stock price maximization; this leads to the conclusion that market (or beta) risk should be given the most weight in capital budgeting decisions. However, if investors are not well diversified, if market imperfections prevent the CAPM from functioning as theory says it should, or if measurement problems keep management from implementing the CAPM approach in capital budgeting, total risk may be given more weight than theory would suggest. Moreover, the CAPM does not consider bankruptcy and other costs associated with financial weakness, even though such costs are in reality often very significant, and the probability of financial distress depends on a firm's total risk, not just on its beta risk. Therefore, one could easily conclude that even well-diversified investors should want a firm's management to give at least some consideration to total risk rather than to concentrate exclusively on beta risk.

Although it would be desirable to measure project risk on some absolute scale, the best one can do in practice is to determine project risk in a somewhat nebulous, relative sense. For example, the financial manager might be able to say with a fair degree of confidence that Project A has more total risk than the firm's average project. Then, if beta risk and corporate risk are highly correlated (as most studies suggest they are), the project with more total risk is also likely to have more beta risk.

What does all this mean to the financial manager? He or she should make as good an assessment as possible of each project's relative total risk and beta risk. If both types of risk are higher than average for a given project, that project's cost of capital should be increased relative to the firm's overall cost of capital. If both types of risk are below average, the adjustment should be reversed. Unfortunately, it is impossible to specify exactly how large the adjustments should be.

OTHER TOPICS IN CAPITAL BUDGETING

Chapter 14 identified the techniques financial managers use to evaluate capital budgeting projects. Several important topics were omitted from that discussion, however. In the remainder of this chapter we will consider some of these special topics, including the replacement decision, the comparison of projects with unequal lives, and the effect of inflation on the evaluation of real assets.

Replacement Decisions

The example of Houston Trucking Company's decision to purchase a new van was used in Chapter 14 to illustrate how expansion projects are analyzed. Not all project analysis is for new projects, however. Some investment opportunities are evaluated as part of replacement decisions. Accordingly, the analysis relating to a **replacement decision** is somewhat different from that for expansion projects. These differences are illustrated here with a capital equipment (coffee roaster) replacement analysis for Gourmet Coffee International (GCI).

GCI of New Orleans roasts, blends, and packages coffee from imported beans for specialty shop owners in the Gulf Coast area. The company's management is evaluating the purchase of a new coffee bean roaster that is quicker and more efficient than GCI's old roasting machine. This old, relatively inefficient roaster was purchased five years ago at a cost of $200,000. The machine had an original expected life of 10 years and a zero estimated salvage value at the end of its expected life. It is being depreciated on a straight line basis and currently has a book value of $100,000. The production manager reports that a new, faster machine can be purchased and installed for $240,000. Over its 5-year life, the new machine will expand sales from $200,000 to $230,000 a year

replacement decision
The decision to replace an existing asset that is still productive with a new one; an example of mutually exclusive projects.

and, furthermore, will reduce labor usage sufficiently to cut annual operating costs from $140,000 to $100,000. The new machine, which will be depreciated using the ACRS method, has an estimated salvage value of $40,000 at the end of its 5-year life. The old machine's current market value is $20,000; the firm's marginal tax rate is 40 percent; and its cost of capital is 10 percent. Should GCI buy the new coffee roasting machine?

The replacement decision analysis requires five steps: (1) estimate the actual cash outlay at t = 0 attributable to the new investment; (2) determine the *incremental cash flows* over each year of the machine's operating life; (3) add the after-tax expected salvage value to the final year's cash flow; (4) find the present value of the incremental cash flows; and (5) determine whether the NPV is positive. These steps are explained further in the following sections.

Estimated Cash Outlay at t = 0. The net initial cash outlay consists of these items: (1) payment to manufacturer for the new machine and its installation, (2) proceeds from the sale of the old machine, and (3) tax effects. GCI must make a $240,000 payment to the manufacturer of the roasting machine, but it will receive a cash inflow of $20,000 from the sale of the old one. Also, its current tax bill will be reduced because of the loss it will incur when it sells the old machine:

$$\text{Tax saving} = (\text{Loss})(\text{Tax rate})$$

$$= (\$80,000)(0.4)$$

$$= \$32,000.$$

The tax reduction will occur because the old machine, which has a book value of $100,000, will produce a loss of $80,000 ($100,000 minus the $20,000 salvage value) immediately upon the purchase of the new one, and with a tax rate of 40 percent, this will reduce the tax bill by $32,000. No investment tax credit can be taken under current tax laws, but if the investment tax credit were allowed, it too would reduce the net cost of the project.

The result is that the purchase of the new machine will involve an immediate net cash outlay of $188,000, and this is its cost for capital budgeting purposes:

Invoice price of the new machine	$240,000
Less: Tax savings from loss ($80,000 × 0.4)	(32,000)
Salvage value of the old machine	(20,000)
Net cash outflow (cost)	$188,000)

If an increase in additional working capital were required as a result of the capital budgeting decision, as would generally be true for expansion investments (as opposed to cost-reducing replacement investments), this factor

Table 16-1 **Comparative Income Statement Framework for Analyzing Cash Flows, Year 1**

	Old Machine (1)	New Machine (2)	Difference (2) − (1) = (3)
Sales (S)	$200,000	$230,000	+ $30,000
Cash operating costs (OC)	140,000	100,000	− 40,000
Depreciation (D)[a]	20,000	48,000	+ 28,000
Income before taxes	$ 40,000	$ 82,000	+ $42,000
Taxes (40%)	16,000	32,800	+ 16,800
Income after taxes	$ 24,000	$ 49,200	+ $25,200
Add depreciation	20,000	48,000	+ 28,000
Net cash flow	$ 44,000	$ 97,200	+ $53,200

[a]The old machine had a cost of $200,000 and is being depreciated by the straight line method over a 10-year period; therefore, its depreciation is $20,000 annually. The new machine will be depreciated under the ACRS method, so its first-year depreciation is 20 percent of its $240,000 cost, or $(0.2)($240,000) = $48,000$. See Chapter 2 for a discussion of the ACRS method depreciation.

would have to be taken into account. The amount of net working capital (additional current assets required as a result of the expansion minus any spontaneously generated funds) would be estimated and added to the initial cash outlay. We assume that GCI will not need any additional working capital, so that factor is not relevant in this example.

Incremental Cash Flows. GCI requires a net investment of $188,000 to buy the new roaster. What will it get from this investment? Put another way, what annual cash flows can the company expect to receive from its investment? The value we seek is GCI's *incremental net cash flow,* or the *additional* cash flow the company will have if it takes on the project.

Column 1 in Table 16-1 shows GCI's estimated income from operations for Year 1 as it would be *without* the new machine, whereas Column 2 shows how the statement would look if the new investment was made. (Cash flow estimates must be made for each year, because the depreciation expense of the new machine is not a constant annual amount.) Column 3 shows the difference between the first two columns. The + $53,200 shown at the bottom of Column 3 is the *incremental net cash flow* from the project for Year 1; this is the value for CF_1 that will be used in the NPV or IRR analysis.

We could set up a series of tables like Table 16-1, one for each year of the project's life; with computer programs like *Lotus 1-2-3* this is a very simple process. If a computer is not available, however, a relatively simple equation can be used to calculate the incremental cash flows. First, note that because the project's effects on sales and operating costs were assumed to be constant in each year, the only changes in Column 3 of Table 16-1 from year to year would be those that resulted from the change in depreciation. The incremental cash flow (CF_t) can be calculated by using the following equation:

$$CF_t = (\Delta S - \Delta OC)(1 - t) + \Delta D(t) \tag{16-1}$$

$$= [(\$230,000 - \$200,000) - (\$100,000 - \$140,000)](1 - 0.4) + \$48,000(0.4) - \$20,000(0.4)$$

$$= [\$30,000 - (-\$40,000)](0.6) + \$28,000(0.4)$$

$$= (\$30,000 + \$40,000)(0.6) + \$28,000(0.4)$$

$$= \$42,000 + \$11,200$$

$$= \$53,200.$$

This value agrees with the amount shown at the bottom of Column 3 of Table 16-1.

The only numbers in Equation 16-1 that change from year to year are the values of the depreciation, specifically the change in annual depreciation that results from the purchase of the new machine. Now consider Table 16-2, which shows the annual depreciation for both the old and new machines, along with the net change in depreciation resulting from the purchase of the new machine. If we insert depreciation figures from Table 16-2, we can find the yearly incremental cash flows:

$$CF_t = (\Delta\$R - \Delta\$E)(1 - t) + D_N(t) - D_O(t)$$

$$= (\$30,000 + \$40,000)(0.6) + \Delta D(0.4)$$

$$= \$70,000(0.6) + \Delta D(0.4)$$

$$= \$42,000 + \Delta D(0.4).$$

Thus CF_1 to CF_2 can be found as follows:

$$CF_1 = \$42,000 + \$28,000(0.4) = \$53,200.$$

$$CF_2 = \$42,000 + \$56,800(0.4) = \$64,720.$$

$$CF_3 = \$42,000 + \$28,000(0.4) = \$53,200.$$

$$CF_4 = \$42,000 + \$13,600(0.4) = \$47,440.$$

$$CF_5 = \$42,000 + \$13,600(0.4) = \$47,440.$$

salvage value
The market price of a capital asset at the end of a specified period. In a capital budgeting decision, it is also the current market price of an asset being considered for replacement.

Salvage Value. The new machine has an estimated **salvage value** of $40,000; that is, GCI expects to be able to sell the machine for $40,000 after its 5 years of use. However, this salvage value will be taxable; because the machine will be fully depreciated in 5 years, income from its sale will be subject to regular corporate income taxes. Thus the after-tax cash flow from the sale of the new machine will be $24,000.

Table 16-2 **Change in Annual Depreciation Expense, ΔD**

Year (1)	Old Machine's Depreciation (2)	New Machine's Depreciation (3)	Incremental Depreciation (3) − (2)
1	$20,000	$48,000 (20%)	$28,000
2	20,000	76,800 (32%)	56,800
3	20,000	48,000 (20%)	28,000
4	20,000	33,600 (14%)	13,600
5	20,000	33,600 (14%)	13,600

The old machine had a cost of $200,000 and is being depreciated by the straight line method over a 10-year life; therefore, its depreciation is $20,000 per year. The new machine will be depreciated under the ACRS method. See Chapter 2 for a discussion of ACRS; assume the depreciation percentages in Column 3 are currently in use and are applied to a depreciable basis of $240,000.

$$\text{After-tax salvage value} = \text{Salvage value} - \text{Taxes}$$
$$= \text{Salvage value} - \text{Salvage value(T)}$$
$$= \text{Salvage value}(1 - T)$$
$$= \$40,000(0.6)$$
$$= \$24,000, \text{ which will come at the end of Year 5.}$$

Of course, when the new machine is actually retired 5 years hence, it probably will be sold for more or less than the expected $40,000, but $40,000 is the best present estimate of the new machine's salvage value. (Note also that if additional working capital had been required and included in the initial cash outlay, that amount would have been added to the final year's cash flow, because the working capital would be recovered if and when the project was completed or abandoned.)

Determining the Net Present Value. The replacement project's net cash flows, expressed in a time line, are as follows:

Year	0	1	2	3	4	5
Cost	− $188,000	—	—	—	—	—
Operating cash flow	—	$53,200	$64,720	$53,200	$47,440	$47,440
After-tax salvage value	—	—	—	—	—	$24,000
Net cash flows	− $188,000	+ $53,200	+ $64,720	+ $53,200	+ $47,440	+ $71,440

These cash flows can now be used to determine the project's NPV based on GCI's 10 percent cost of capital:

$$\text{NPV} = \sum_{t=1}^{5} \frac{CF_t}{(1 + k)^t} - \text{Cost}$$

$$= \left(\frac{\$53,200}{(1.1)^1} + \frac{\$64,720}{(1.1)^2} + \frac{\$53,200}{(1.1)^3} + \frac{\$47,440}{(1.1)^4} + \frac{\$71,440}{(1.1)^5} \right) - \$188,000$$

$$= \$53,200(.9091) + \$64,720(.8264) + \$53,200(.7513)$$
$$+ \$47,440(.6830) + \$71,440(.6209) - \$188,000$$

$$= \$218,577 - \$188,000$$

$$= \$30,577.$$

Because the NPV is positive, GCI should replace the old coffee bean roaster with the newer, more efficient machine. If the NPV had been negative, the decision would have been not to replace the old machine. Alternatively, had we set NPV equal to zero and solved for the discount rate, r, we would have found that the IRR = 16.06%. Since the required rate of return = 10%, and the IRR > 10%, this second method reaffirms the decision to replace the old machine.

In conclusion, the replacement decision is a combination of an investment decision and, to coin a phrase, a disinvestment decision. An investment decision involves an *investment outlay* of cash to purchase an asset that will produce a forecast *cash inflow* consisting of after-tax earnings and depreciation. Disinvestment is just the reverse — if the old machine is sold, the firm receives an *inflow* of cash or a cash equivalent tax credit on any book loss created by the sale. Additionally, because the company no longer owns the asset, there is an opportunity loss of the asset's cash inflow. This situation is presented in Table 16-3. Our concern is that the replacement should be considered only in terms of the net cost outlays for the asset (minus all "trade-in" allowances) and the differential increase in cash flows. To do otherwise would double-count costs or benefits associated with the asset under evaluation.

Comparing Projects with Unequal Lives

To simplify matters, our example of replacement decisions assumed that the new coffee roasting machine had a life equal to the remaining life of the existing one. Suppose, however, that we must choose between two mutually exclusive replacement alternatives that have *different* lives. For example, Machine S has an expected life of 10 years, whereas Machine L has a 15-year life. The most typical procedure for solving problems of this type is to set up a series of *replacement chains* extending out to the "common denominator" year — that is, the year in which both alternatives require replacement. For Machines S and L this would be Year 30, so it is necessary to compare a 3-chain cycle for S, the 10-year machine, with a 2-chain cycle for L, the 15-year project.

To illustrate both the replacement chain problem and its solution, suppose that a firm is considering the replacement of a fully depreciated printing press with a new one. The plant in which the press is used is profitable and is expected to continue in operation for many years. The old press could con-

Table 16-3 **Replacement Decision Framework**

New Asset Investment	Old Asset Disinvestment	Difference
− Investment outlay	+ Cash for asset	= Net cost
+ Cash flow	− Cash flow	= Incremental cash flow

tinue to be used indefinitely, but it is not as efficient as new presses. Two replacement machines are available. Press A has a cost of $36,100, will last for 5 years, and will produce after-tax incremental cash flows of $9,700 per year for 5 years. Press B has a cost of $57,500, will last for 10 years, and will produce net cash flows of $9,500 per year. Both the costs and performances of Presses A and B have been constant in recent years and are expected to remain constant in the future. The company's cost of capital is 10 percent.

Should the old press be replaced, and, if so, with A or with B? To answer these questions, we first calculate A's NPV as follows:

$$NPV_A = \$9,700(3.7908) - \$36,100 = \$36,771 - \$36,100 = \$671.$$

B's NPV is calculated as follows:

$$NPV_B = \$9,500(6.1446) - \$57,500 = \$58,374 - \$57,500 = \$874.$$

These calculations suggest that the old press should indeed be replaced and that Press B should be selected. However, the analysis is incomplete, and the decision to choose Press B is *incorrect*. If the company chooses Press A, it will have an opportunity to make another new investment after 5 years, and this second investment will *also* be profitable. However, if it chooses Press B, it will not have this second investment opportunity. Therefore, to make a proper comparison of Presses A and B, we must find the present value of Press A over a 10-year period and compare it with Press B over the same 10 years.

The NPV for Press B as calculated previously is correct as it stands. For Press A, however, we must take three additional steps: (1) determine the NPV of the second Press A 5 years hence, (2) bring this NPV back to the present, and (3) sum these two component NPVs:

1. If we assume that the cost and annual cash flows of Press A will not change if the project is repeated in 5 years and that the firm's cost of capital will remain at 10 percent, then Press A's NPV will remain the same as its first-stage NPV, $671. However, the second NPV will not accrue for five years, and hence it represents a present value at $t = 5$.

2. The present value (at $t = 0$) of the purchase of a second printing Press A is determined by discounting the second NPV (at $t = 5$) back five years at 10 percent to determine its present value at $t = 0$: $\$671(DF_{10\%, 5 \text{ years}}) = \$671(0.6209) = \$417.$

3. The true NPV of Press A is $671 + $417 = $1,088. This is the value that should be compared with the NPV of Press B, $874.

The value of the firm will increase more if the old press is replaced by Press A than if the firm goes with Press B; therefore Press A should be selected.

EFFECTS OF INFLATION ON CAPITAL BUDGETING ANALYSIS

Inflation is a fact of life in the United States and most other nations, and thus it must be considered in any sound capital budgeting analysis. Several procedures are available for dealing with inflation. The two most frequently used methods are (1) to explicitly adjust both the discount rate and the expected cash flows and (2) to make no explicit adjustment in either the discount rate or the expected cash flows to compensate for inflation. Both methods are discussed in this section.

To see how inflation enters the picture, suppose an investor lends $100 for 1 year at a rate of 5 percent. At the end of the year the investor will have $100(1.05) = $105. However, if prices rise by 6 percent during the year, the ending $105 will have a purchasing power, in terms of beginning-of-year values, of only $105/1.06 = $99. Thus the investor will have lost $1, or 1 percent of the original purchasing power, in spite of having earned 5 percent interest: $105 at the end of the year will buy only as much in goods as $99 would have bought at the beginning of the year.

Investors recognize this problem, and, as we learned in earlier chapters, they incorporate expectations about inflation into the required rate of return. For example, suppose investors seek a *real rate of return* (k_r) of 8 percent on an investment with a given degree of risk. Suppose further that they anticipate an *annual rate of inflation* (i) of 6 percent. Then, to end up with the 8 percent real rate of return, the nominal rate of return (k_n) must be a value such that

$$1 + k_n = (1 + k_r)(1 + i),$$

or

$$k_n = (1 + k_r)(1 + i) - 1$$

$$= 1 + k_r + i + k_r i - 1$$

$$= k_r + i + k_r i.$$

In words, the nominal rate (k_n) must be set equal to the real rate (k_r) plus the expected inflation (i) plus a cross-product term ($k_r i$). In this example,

$$k_n = 0.08 + 0.06 + (0.08)/(0.06)$$

$$= 0.08 + 0.06 + 0.0048$$

$$= 0.1448 = 14.48\%.$$

If the investor earns a nominal return of 14.48 percent on a $100 investment, the ending value, in real terms, will be

$$\$100(1.1448)/(1.06) = \$114.48/1.06 = \$108,$$

producing the required 8 percent real rate of return.

We can use these concepts to analyze capital budgeting under inflation. First, note that a project's NPV in the absence of inflation, where $k_r = k_n$ and RCF_t = the *real* net cash flow in Year t, is calculated as follows:

$$NPV = \sum_{t=1}^{n} \frac{RCF_t}{(1 + k_r)^t} - Cost.$$

Now suppose the situation changes. We begin to expect inflation to occur and expect both sales prices and input costs to rise at the rate i, the same inflation rate that is built into the estimated cost of capital that we find in the capital markets. In this event the *nominal* cash flow (CF_t) will increase annually at the rate of i percent, producing this situation:

$$CF_t = Actual\ cash\ flow_t = RCF_t(1 + i)^t.$$

For example, a net cash flow of $100 is expected in Year 5 in the absence of inflation, then with a 5 percent rate of inflation, $CF_t = \$100(1.05)^5 = \$127.63$.

Now if net cash flows increase at the rate of i percent per year, and if this same inflation factor is built into the cost of capital, then

$$NPV = \sum_{t=1}^{n} \frac{RCF_t(1 + i)^t}{(1 + k_r)^t(1 + i)^t} - Cost.$$

Because the $(1 + i)^t$ terms in the numerator and denominator cancel, we are left with

$$NPV = \sum_{t=1}^{n} \frac{RCF_t}{(1 + k_r)^t} - Cost = \begin{array}{l} \text{The same NPV as} \\ \text{we found earlier} \\ \text{in the absence of} \\ \text{inflation.} \end{array}$$

Thus, whenever sales prices and costs are *both* expected to rise at the rate of i percent, and if this is the same inflation rate that investors have built into the cost of capital, then (1) the inflation-adjusted NPV is identical to the inflation-free NPV, and (2) we can find a project's NPV by taking its real cash flows, RCF_t, and discounting them at the *real* risk-adjusted rate, k_r.

Sometimes the procedure just set forth is not followed. People sometimes discount cash flows that have *not* been adjusted for inflation by the *nominal* cost of capital, which *does* include an inflation premium. This is wrong! Therefore when the cost of capital, which usually includes an inflation risk premium, is used to discount constant dollar (not adjusted for expected inflation) cash flows, *the resulting NPV will be downwardly biased.* The denominator will reflect inflation, but the numerator will not, which produces the bias. If sales prices and all costs are expected to rise at exactly the same rate, the bias can be corrected by having current cash flows increase at the inflation rate, or by using the real rate as the cost of capital.

Although it is often appropriate to assume that *variable costs* will rise at the same rate as sales prices, fixed costs (especially the depreciation associated with a project) generally increase at a lower rate. In any situation where both revenues and all costs are not expected to rise at exactly the same inflation rate as is built into the cost of capital, the best procedure is to build inflation into the basic cash flow component projections for each year. If high rates of inflation are projected, and if expected inflation rates for sales prices and input costs differ materially, such an adjustment must be made.

SUMMARY

This chapter has dealt with several issues in capital budgeting, including risk, equipment replacement decisions, the comparison of projects with unequal lives, and the effects of inflation.

Our analysis of risk focused on two issues: a given project's effect on the firm's beta coefficient (*beta risk*) and the project's effect on the probability of large losses (*corporate risk*). Both types of risk are important. Although beta risk is theoretically more correct, CAPM theory itself is not completely valid, and it is more difficult to obtain the data necessary for applying the theory to projects than to stocks. Corporate risk affects the financial strength of the firm; this in turn influences its ability to use debt, to maintain smooth operations over time, and to avoid crises that might consume the energy of the firm's managers and disrupt its employees, customers, suppliers, and community.

The major difficulty in determining the beta risk of a given project is in establishing the project's beta coefficient. It is not really meaningful to be concerned about the beta of a particular asset like a truck or a machine, but it is meaningful to think about betas of divisions that are large enough to be operated as independent firms. Therefore, in practice, beta risk is estimated for large divisions of firms and used to establish divisional costs of capital, which are then scaled up or down in a somewhat ad hoc manner to reflect a given project's own risk.

The key to making good replacement decisions is developing accurate estimates of incremental cash flows — how large an investment will the replacement entail, and what net savings will it produce? If the present value of the net savings exceeds the cost of the equipment, the replacement should be undertaken. As noted in the chapter, however, if the various replacement alternatives have different lives, it is necessary to adjust to a common life before comparing them. This adjustment may be accomplished through the creation of replacement chains.

Inflation exists in the United States and most other economies, and it must be dealt with in capital budgeting analysis. If inflation is simply ignored, then (1) the cash flows in the numerator of the NPV equation are *not* adjusted for expected inflation, but (2) an adjustment is automatically (and usually unconsciously) made in the denominator, because market forces build inflation into the cost of capital. Thus the net result of ignoring inflation is the creation of a downward bias when evaluating projects (that is, rejecting projects that should be accepted). The best way of correcting for the bias is to build price increases based on expected inflation rates directly into the cash flows.

RESOLUTION TO DECISION IN FINANCE

Gambling on a State-of-the-Art Refinery

Despite the expense and riskiness of the venture, Valero went ahead with its plans to upgrade the Saber refinery. In its actions it followed the lead of numerous other U.S. refiners, who planned to spend a combined total of $7 billion on converting their facilities to run on less expensive, low-grade crude oils. By the fall of 1983 all were taking a second look at their calculations, and few were happy with what they saw. It seems that no one had anticipated the many changes that had hit the oil industry since the decision to upgrade had been made.

It took Valero three years to retool the Saber plant. By the time it was ready to begin operations, economic circumstances had vastly changed. Most unexpected and damaging was the price of resid, which had risen from $20 per barrel to $26. With lighter crude selling at $29 per barrel, the heavy crude was no longer the attractive bargain it had been in 1980. In addition, the price of gasoline had not risen as expected.

With gasoline selling at under $36 per barrel, Valero was lucky to squeeze out a gross margin of $8 per barrel. That was still twice the industry average, but Valero also had higher-than-av-

erage expenses. It cost the company more than $4 per barrel to service its $550 million debt. And the plant itself had high operating costs.

Although Valero claimed that the phasing in of its new operation was on schedule, industry sources contended that the company was having trouble getting its costly new plant to work. They speculated that one setback stemmed from the fact that constant processing of heavy crude can create refining problems. The usual solution would be to mix in lighter, more expensive crude, but that would have cut even further into Valero's margins. Also, in another snag, the plant was having trouble meeting federal air pollution standards.

Not surprisingly, the price of Valero's stock reflected the difficulties the company was having with its refining operations. Analysts and investors had been extremely enthusiastic when Valero first announced its plans in late 1980, sending the stock up to 43⅞ per share. But by fall 1983, the price had fallen below 30.

Throughout, Chairman Greehey remained optimistic, arguing that Valero's troubles were only temporary. According to him, the quality of available crude oil would steadily drop, eventually restoring the greater price spread between heavy and light crudes. "We will be right back where we started," he insisted. "Take your potshots now, because this thing will be profitable."

Source: "Valero Energy: Gambling on a State-of-the-Art Refinery," *Business Week,* October 24, 1983, 96; and "Heavy Crude Has Backfired on the Refiners," *Business Week,* November 7, 1983, 126, 130.

QUESTIONS

16-1   The focus of the capital budgeting discussion has been on operating cash flows rather than on accounting profits. What is the basis for this emphasis on cash flows as opposed to net income?

16-2   Think about the example of GCI's coffee bean roasting machine purchase, and answer these questions:
    a. Why is the salvage value of the new machine reduced for taxes?
    b. Why is depreciation on the old machine in effect deducted from the depreciation on the new machine in Table 16-2?
    c. How would the analysis be affected if the new machine permitted a reduction in working capital?

16-3   Distinguish between the beta risk and the corporate risk of a project being considered for inclusion in the capital budget. Which type do you think should be given the greater weight in capital budgeting decisions?

16-4   Suppose Gonzo Technologies, which has a high beta as well as a great deal of corporate risk, merged with E-Z Patterns, Inc. E-Z Patterns' sales rise during recessions, when people are more likely to make their own clothing; consequently, its beta is quite low but its corporate risk is relatively high. What would the merger do to the costs of capital in the consolidated company's technology division and in its patterns division?

SELF-TEST PROBLEMS

ST-1   You have been asked by the president of your company, Campsi Construction Company, to evaluate the proposed acquisition of a new earthmover. The earthmover's basic price is $50,000, and it will cost another $10,000 to modify it for Campsi's special use. The earthmover falls into the ACRS 5-year class. It will be sold after 3 years for $20,000. Use of the earthmover will require an increase in net working capital (spare parts inventory) of $2,000. The earthmover will have no effect on revenues, but it is expected to save Campsi $20,000 per year in before-tax operating costs, mainly labor. The firm's marginal tax rate is 40 percent.
    a. What is the net cost of the earthmover? (That is, what are the Year 0 cash flows?)
    b. What are the operating cash flows in Years 1, 2, and 3?
    c. What are the additional (nonoperating) cash flows in Year 3?
    d. If the project's cost of capital is 10 percent, should the earthmover be purchased?

ST-2   Wofford Novelty Plastics (WNP) currently uses an injection molding machine that was purchased several years ago. This machine is being depreciated on a straight line basis; it has 6 years of remaining life, and its current book value is $2,100. Thus the annual depreciation expense is $2,100/6 = $350 per year. The machine can be sold for $2,500 at this time.
       WNP has been offered a replacement machine that has a cost of $8,000, an estimated useful life of 6 years, and an estimated salvage value of $800. This machine falls into the ACRS 5-year class. It would permit an output expansion, so sales would rise by $1,000 per year; even so, its much greater efficiency would still cause operating expenses to decline by $1,500 per year. The new machine would require inventories to be increased by $2,000, but accounts payable would simultaneously increase by $500.

WNP's effective tax rate is 40 percent, and its cost of capital is 15 percent. Should it replace the old machine?

PROBLEMS

16-1 **Replacement decision.** Nortex Manufacturing is considering the purchase of a new machine to replace an obsolete one. The machine used in current operations has both a book value and a market value of zero. It is in good working order and will operate at an acceptable level for an additional 5 years. Nortex's engineers estimate that the proposed machine will perform operations so much more efficiently that if it is installed, labor, materials, and other direct costs of the operation will decline by $56,000 annually. The proposed machine costs $150,000 delivered and installed. The asset has a tax life of 5 years and will be depreciated by the straight line method over this period. The expected salvage value of the new machine is zero. The company's cost of capital is 12 percent and its tax rate is 40 percent.
a. What is the replacement project's annual cash flow?
b. What is the project's NPV?
c. What is the project's IRR?
d. Should the old machine be replaced?

16-2 **Replacement project.** Hobbes Equipment Company is considering replacing an old machine with a new one that will increase cash earnings before taxes by $30,000 annually. The new machine will cost $60,000 and will have an estimated life of 8 years with no salvage value. It will be depreciated over a 5-year tax life using the straight line method. The applicable corporate tax rate is 40 percent, and the firm's cost of capital is 10 percent. The old machine has been fully depreciated and has no salvage value. Calculate the net present value for the replacement project. Should the old machine be replaced by the new one?

16-3 **Replacement decision.** The Harrington-Wilson Corporation (HWC) currently uses an injection molding machine that was purchased several years ago. This old machine is being depreciated on a straight line basis. It has 5 years of remaining life with zero expected salvage value. Its current book value is $5,000, and it can be sold for $6,000 at this time.

HWC is offered a replacement machine that has a cost of $16,000, a tax and useful life of 5 years, and an estimated salvage value of $2,000. This machine is also depreciated on a straight line basis. The replacement machine will permit an output expansion, so sales will rise by $2,000 annually; yet the new machine's much greater efficiency will cause operating expenses to decline by $3,000 per year. The new machine will cause inventories to increase by $4,000 and accounts payable to increase by $1,000.

HWC's effective tax rate is 40 percent, and its cost of capital is 15 percent. Should it replace the old machine?

16-4 **Risk adjustment.** The risk-free rate of return is 7 percent, and the market risk premium ($k_M - R_F$) is 6 percent. The beta of the project under analysis is 1.5, with the expected after-tax net cash flows estimated at $2,000 annually for 5 years. The required investment outlay for the project is $6,550.
a. What is the required risk-adjusted return on the project?
b. What is the project's NPV?

    c. What is the project's IRR?

    d. Should this project be accepted?

16-5   **Required rate of return.** Modern Technology is considering investing in a 5-year project that has expected annual cash flows of $80,000. The project's cost is $250,000. Modern Technology bases its required return on the Security Market Line (SML). The risk-free rate is expected to be 7 percent, and the return on an average security in the market is forecast to be 11 percent. The firm's beta is 2.0.

    a. What is the firm's required return?

    b. What is the project's IRR?

    c. What is the project's NPV?

    d. Should the firm invest in this project?

16-6   **Risk adjustment.** Huffman Industries has two independent projects under consideration. Huffman's beta is 1.2. The average-risk security in the market has a return of 11 percent, and the risk-free rate is 6 percent. The Project E has the same risk as Huffman's current projects, whereas Project F has a beta of 1.8. Project E has a cost of $100,000 and expected after-tax cash flows of $25,700 annually for the next 5 years. Project F also has a cost of $100,000 and expected after-tax cash flows of $29,000 annually for 5 years.

    a. What is the required rate of return for each project?

    b. What is the NPV for each project?

    c. Which project(s) should Huffman accept?

16-7   **Replacement project.** Hinsdale Publishing Company is contemplating the replacement of one of its bookbinding machines with a newer and more efficient one. The old machine has a book value of $400,000 and a remaining useful life of 5 years. The firm does not expect to realize any return from scrapping the old machine in 5 years, but it can sell it now to another firm in the industry for $200,000. The old machine is being depreciated toward a zero salvage value, or by $80,000 per year, using the straight line method.

    The new machine has a purchase price of $1.2 million, an estimated useful life and ACRS class life of 5 years, and an estimated salvage value of $100,000. It is expected to economize on electric power usage, labor, and repair costs, as well as to reduce the number of defective bindings. In total, an annual saving of $200,000 will be realized if it is installed. The company is in the 40 percent marginal tax bracket, and it has a 10 percent cost of capital.

    a. What is the initial cash outlay required for the new machine?

    b. Calculate the annual depreciation allowances for both machines, and compute the change in the annual depreciation expense if the replacement is made. (Assume the appropriate ACRS depreciation percentages for a 5-year asset are: Year 1 = 20%; Year 2 = 32%; Year 3 = 20%; Year 4 = 14%; and Year 5 = 14%.)

    c. What are the cash flows in Years 1 to 5?

    d. What is the cash flow from the salvage value in Year 5.

    e. Should Hinsdale purchase the new machine? Support your answer.

    f. In general, how would each of the following factors affect the investment decision, and how should each be treated? (Give verbal answers.)

      1. The expected life of the existing machine decreases.

      2. The cost of capital is not constant but is increasing.

(Do Parts g, h, and i only if you are using the computerized problem diskette.)

g. Hinsdale Publishing may be able to purchase an alternative new bookbinding machine from another supplier. Its purchase price would be $900,000, and its salvage value would be $165,000. This machine would lower annual operating costs by $180,000. Should Hinsdale purchase this machine?

h. If the salvage value on the alternative new machine were $135,000 rather than $165,000, how would this affect the decision?

i. With everything as in Part h, assume that the cost of capital declined from 10 percent to 9.75 percent. How would this affect the decision?

16-8   **Unequal lives.** The Spartan Corporation has two mutually exclusive projects code-named Gold and White. The firm must determine which of the two projects to select. The following table provides the necessary information to evaluate the projects.

	Gold	White
Cost	$30,000	$30,000
Annual after-tax cash flow	$11,000	$ 7,000
Life	4 years	8 years

If the firm's cost of capital for the projects is 12 percent, which of the two projects should be selected for investment?

16-9   **Cash flow estimate and replacement analysis.** Wonder Bakers, whose motto is, "If it's good, it's a Wonder," is considering the replacement of its oven. The old oven, with a book value of $150,000, has a useful life of 3 years and is being depreciated using the straight line method to a salvage value of zero. If the old oven is sold today, its market value will be only $50,000. The new oven has a total cost, delivered and installed, of $180,000 and an expected salvage value of $30,000 at the end of its 3-year life. The firm uses the ACRS depreciation methodology and has a tax rate of 40 percent.

a. What are the incremental cash flows that would result from the replacement of the old oven?

b. If the firm's cost of capital is 15 percent, should Wonder replace the old oven? (Assume that the ACRS depreciation percentages for a 3-year asset are: Year 1 = 34%; Year 2 = 33%; and Year 3 = 33%.)

16-10   **Cash flow estimate and replacement analysis.** Boston Construction Company is considering replacing an old crane with a new one that will increase cash earnings before taxes by $30,000 per year. The new crane, which costs $60,000, will have an estimated useful life of 8 years and a salvage value of $8,000 at the end of that time. The new machine will be depreciated over its 5-year ACRS recovery period. The old crane, which has been in service since 1979, currently has a book value of $20,000 and a remaining life of 8 years. It is being depreciated by $2,500 per year toward a zero salvage value using the straight line method. The marginal tax rate is 40% for Boston Construction. If replaced, the old crane can be sold now for $15,000.

a. What are the incremental cash flows that occur each year as a result of the replacement decision?

b. If the firm's cost of capital is 12 percent, should the replacement be made? (Assume the appropriate ACRS depreciation percentages for a 5-year asset are: Year 1 = 20%; Year 2 = 32%; Year 3 = 20%; Year 4 = 14%; and Year 5 = 14%.)

16-11   **CAPM approach to risk adjustments.** Toledo Rubber Company has two divisions: (1) the Tire Division, which manufactures tires for new automobiles, and (2) the Recap Division, which manufactures recapping materials that are sold to independent tire recapping shops throughout the United States. Since auto manufacturing moves up and down with the general economy, the Tire Division's earnings contribution to Toledo's stock price is highly correlated with returns on most other stocks. If the Tire Division were operated as a separate company, its beta coefficient would be about 1.60. The sales and profits of the Recap Division, on the other hand, tend to be countercyclical, as recap sales boom when people cannot afford to buy new tires. Recap's beta is estimated to be 0.40. Approximately 75 percent of Toledo's corporate assets are invested in the Tire Division and 25 percent are in the Recap Division.

Currently, the rate of interest in Treasury securities is 10 percent, and the expected rate of return on an average share of stock is 15 percent. Toledo uses only common equity capital, and it has no debt outstanding.

a. What is the required rate of return on Toledo's stock?

b. What discount rate should be used to evaluate capital budgeting projects in each division? Explain your answer fully, and in the process illustrate your answer with a project that costs $104,322, has a 10-year life, and provides after-tax cash flows of $20,000 per year.

ANSWERS TO SELF-TEST PROBLEMS

ST-1   **a.** *Estimated Investment Requirements:*

Price	($50,000)
Modification	(10,000)
Net working capital	(2,000)
Total investment	($62,000)

b. *Operating Cash Flows:*

	Year 1	Year 2	Year 3
1. After-tax cost savings[a]	$12,000	$12,000	$12,000
2. Depreciation[b]	12,000	19,200	12,000
3. Depreciation tax savings[c]	4,800	7,680	4,800
Net cash flow (1 + 3)	$16,800	$19,680	$16,800

[a]Before-tax savings (1 − Tax rate) = $20,000(0.6) = $12,000.
[b]Depreciation in Year 1 = 0.20($60,000) = $12,000; depreciation percentages in Years 2 & 3 are 32% and 20% respectively.
[c]T(Depreciation) = Tax savings.

c. *End-of-Project Cash Flows:*

Salvage value	$20,000
Tax on salvage value[a]	(1,280)
Net working capital recovery	2,000
	$20,720

[a]Salvage value	$20,000	
Less: Book value	16,800	
Taxable income	$ 3,200	
Tax at 40%	1,280	

d. No, the project has a negative NPV.

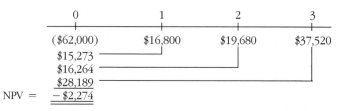

	0	1	2	3
	($62,000)	$16,800	$19,680	$37,520
	$15,273			
	$16,264			
	$28,189			
NPV =	− $2,274			

ST-2   First determine the net cash outflow at t = 0:

Purchase price	$8,000
Sale of old machine	(2,500)
Tax on sale of old machine	160[a]
Net working capital	1,500[b]
Total investment	$7,160

[a]The market value is $2,500 − $2,100 = $400 above the book value. Thus there is a $400 recapture of depreciation and WNP would have to pay 0.40($400) = $160 in taxes.
[b]The change in net working capital is a $2,000 increase in current assets minus a $500 increase in current liabilities, or $1,500.

Now examine the annual operating cash inflows:

Sales increase	$1,000
Cost decrease	1,500
Pretax operating revenue increase	$2,500

$$\text{After-tax operating revenue increase} = \$2,500(1 - T)$$
$$= \$2,500(0.60)$$
$$= \$1,500.$$

Depreciation:

	1	2	3	4	5	6
New[a]	$1,600	$2,560	$1,600	$1,120	$1,120	$ 0
Old	350	350	350	350	350	350
Depreciation	$1,250	$2,210	$1,250	$ 770	$ 770	(350)
Depreciation tax savings[b]	$ 500	$ 884	$ 500	$ 308	$ 308	($140)

[a]Depreciation expense each year equals depreciable basis times the assumed ACRS factor of 0.20 for Year 1, 0.32 for Year 2, 0.20 for Year 3, and 0.14 for Years 4 and 5.
[b]Depreciation tax savings = Depreciation(T).

Now recognize that, at the end of Year 6, WNP will recover its working capital investment of $1,500, and it will also receive $800 from the sale of the replacement machine. However, the firm will have to pay 0.40($800) = $320 in taxes on the sale of the machine since it had been depreciated to a zero book value.

Finally, place all the cash flows on a time line:

	0	1	2	3	4	5	6
Net cost	($7,160)						
After-tax revenue increase		$1,500	$1,500	$1,500	$1,500	$1,500	$1,500
Depreciation tax savings		500	884	500	308	308	(140)
Working capital recovery							1,500
Salvage value on new machine							800
Tax on salvage value							(320)
Net cash flow	($7,160)	$2,000	$2,384	$2,000	$1,808	$1,808	$3,340

The net present value of this incremental cash flow stream, when discounted at 15 percent, is $1,073. Thus the replacement should be made.

Part VI

LONG-TERM FINANCING

In the previous section we discussed means by which a firm can identify and evaluate investment opportunities. This section identifies the primary types of long-term capital and the analysis firms employ when deciding which combination of securities to use. We begin in Chapters 17 and 18 by examining the characteristics of long-term debt, preferred stock, and common stock. Portions of these chapters are dedicated to the determination of stock and bond values. These values are determined, in part, by the expected rate of return required by investors to provide capital to companies. In Chapter 19, we see how the investor's expected returns are combined to form the firm's weighted average cost of capital. Chapter 20 explains how the concepts of business and financial risk are used to determine the optimal capital structure — that is, the most appropriate mix of debt and equity for the firm. Finally, Chapter 21 examines the interaction between the financing and investment decisions which determine the firm's dividend policy.

Chapter 17

Bonds and Preferred Stock

 DECISION IN FINANCE

A Deal for All Seasons

In May 1981, 27-year-old investment banker Michael Hollis and his law-school buddy had a problem. They needed to raise more than $50 million to start an airline, but there appeared to be no shortage of obstacles for two corporate novices trying to break into an industry noted for its swift consumption of cash as well as gas. Then Hollis had a brainstorm. They would finance their venture, Air Atlanta, Inc., with zero coupon bonds.

The zero coupon bond is to bonds what the Mexican hairless is to dogs. It looks like the traditional model, but upon close inspection one feature is disturbingly missing. Although a hairless dog may appeal to only a small and select group, the zero is attractive to anyone trying to beat the high cost of money. The zero coupon bond (the term *coupon* refers to days past when payable drafts were literally snipped from the bond certificate itself and redeemed for cash) is the kind of ingenious win/win financial instrument only captalists could dream up.

The beauty of the zero is that it is designed so that the borrower does not have to service the debt through periodic cash payments. Instead, the original loan is discounted from par ($1,000 in bond parlance) so that when the borrower pays it back at par on the due date, it yields the equivalent of the missing interest. Extra incentives can be added to make the zero even more enticing to potentially reluctant lenders. These can include warrants that pro-

vide for buying yet more (and cheaper) stock, stock in another corporation, or dividend-bearing preferred stock.

The borrower does not have to make periodic interest payments (all interest paid at maturity). For the lender, the locked-up nature of the zero cements the rate of compound interest for the duration of the bond.

Although Air Atlanta managed to raise more than $5 million through the issue of common stock, as of year-end 1985 interest-free convertible debentures, or zeros, accounted for roughly $19 million of Air Atlanta's total funding of $54 million. This was exceeded as a single source only by a capital lease on its fleet of jets. Air Atlanta's reliance on zero coupon convertible bonds for its very sustenance is thought to be unique, not only in the airline industry but among new ventures anywhere.

How did Air Atlanta manage to sell its zeros to such demanding and traditionally conservative investors as Aetna Life Insurance, Equitable Life Assurance Society of the United States, and General Electric Credit, which together loaned more than $13 million via zero coupon bonds to the fledgling carrier that had only four routes, five planes, and no profits?

As you read this chapter, imagine that you are one of Air Atlanta's founders. How would you convince a corporate asset manager to buy zero coupon bonds to finance your company? What advantages could you offer the investor if your company were successful? What risks would a purchaser of zeros run if your airline venture failed to take off?

See end of chapter for resolution.

Most firms find it both necessary and desirable to use long-term debt financing, and some also use preferred stock. There are many types of fixed-income securities: secured and unsecured, marketable and nonmarketable, convertible and nonconvertible, and so on. Different groups of investors favor different types of securities, and their tastes change over time. An astute financial manager knows how to package securities at a given point in time to make them most attractive to the most potential investors, thereby keeping the firm's cost of capital to a minimum. This chapter first discusses long-term securities in general, then analyzes the three most important types of *fixed-income securities* — term loans, bonds, and preferred stocks. Later chapters deal with other types of long-term capital, whereas the proper mix of securities is discussed in Chapter 20.

FUNDED DEBT

funded debt

Long-term debt; "funding" refers to replacing short-term debt with longer maturity securities.

Long-term debt is often referred to as **funded debt.** When a firm is said to be planning to "fund" its floating debt, it is planning to replace short-term debt with securities of longer maturity. Funding does not imply placing money with a trustee or other repository; it is simply part of the jargon of finance and means "replacing short-term debt with permanent (long-term) capital." Tampa Electric Company provides a good example of funding. This company has a continuous construction program and typically uses short-term debt to finance construction expenditures. Once short-term debt has built up to about $100 million, however, the company sells stock or a bond issue, uses the proceeds to pay off (or fund) its bank loans, and starts the cycle again. There is a high fixed cost involved in selling stocks or bonds that makes it quite expensive to issue small amounts of these securities. The high fixed portion of the flotation charge, discussed in the next chapter, makes this process of funding the short-term debt by Tampa Electric very logical.

TERM LOANS

term loan

A loan, generally obtained from a bank or insurance company, with a maturity greater than one year.

A **term loan** is a contract under which a borrower agrees to make payments of interest and principal, on specific dates, to a lender.[1] Term loans usually are negotiated directly between the borrowing firm and a financial institution — generally a bank, an insurance company, or a pension fund. Although the maturities of term loans vary from two to thirty years, most are for periods in the three- to fifteen-year range.

---

[1]If the interest and maturity payments are not met on schedule, the issuing firm is said to have *defaulted* and can then be forced into *bankruptcy.* See Appendix 20A for a discussion of bankruptcy.

Advantages of Term Loans

Term loans have three major advantages over publicly issued securities—*speed, flexibility,* and *low issuance costs.* Because they are negotiated directly between the lender and the borrower, formal procedures are minimized. The key provisions of the loan can be worked out much more quickly and with more flexibility than can those for a public issue, and it is not necessary for a term loan to go through the Securities and Exchange Commission (SEC) registration process. A further advantage of term loans over publicly held debt securities has to do with future flexibility: if a bond issue is held by many different bondholders, it is difficult to obtain permission to alter the terms of the agreement, even though new economic conditions may make such changes desirable. With a term loan, the borrower usually can sit down with the lender and work out modifications in the contract.

Amortization

Most term loans are **amortized,** or paid off, in equal installments over the life of the loan. (At this point you should review the discussion of amortization in Chapter 13.) The purpose of amortization is to have the loan repaid gradually over its life rather than fall due all at once. Amortization forces the borrower to retire the loan slowly; this protects both the lender and the borrower against the possibility that the borrower will not make adequate provisions for its retirement during the life of the loan. Amortization is especially important whenever the loan is used to purchase a specific item of equipment; here the repayment schedule should be matched to the productive life of the equipment, with the payments being made from cash flows resulting from its use.

amortize
To liquidate on an installment basis; an amortized loan is one in which the principal amount of the loan is repaid in installments during the life of the loan.

Interest Rate

The interest rate on a term loan can be either fixed for the life of the loan or variable. If it is fixed, the rate used will be close to the rate on long-term bonds for companies of equivalent risk. If the rate is variable, it is usually set at a certain number of percentage points over the prime rate. Thus, when the prime rate goes up or down, so does the rate on the outstanding balance of the term loan.

BONDS

A **bond** is a long-term dead instrument under which a borrower contractually agrees to make payments of interest and principal, on specific dates, to the holder of the bond. Traditionally bonds have been issued with maturities of between 20 and 30 years, but in the early 1980s shorter maturities, such as 7 to 10 years, have been used to an increasing extent. Although bonds are similar to term loans, a bond issue is generally advertised, offered to all investors (the "public"), and actually sold to many different investors. Indeed, thousands of

bond
A long-term debt instrument.

individual and institutional investors may purchase bonds when a firm sells a bond issue, whereas there is usually only one lender in the case of a term loan. The bond is a debt contract; its **par value** represents the amount to be repaid at maturity, which typically is $1,000 for corporate bonds issued in the United States. With bonds, the interest rate, or **coupon rate** is generally fixed, although in recent years there has been an increase in the use of various types of floating rate bonds. There are a number of different types of bonds, the more important of which are discussed in this chapter.

Indenture and Trustee

An **indenture** is a legal document that spells out the rights and duties of both the bondholders and the issuing corporation. A **trustee** is an official (usually of a bank) who represents the bondholders and makes sure the terms of the indenture are carried out. The indenture may be several hundred pages in length, and it will cover such points as the conditions under which the issuer can pay off the bonds prior to maturity, the times-interest-earned ratio the issuer must maintain if it is to sell additional bonds, restrictions against the payment of dividends unless earnings meet certain specifications; and the like. The trustee monitors the situation and, in the event that the issuer violates any provision in the indenture, takes appropriate action on behalf of the bondholders. Exactly what constitutes "appropriate action" varies with the circumstances. It might be that to insist on immediate compliance would result in bankruptcy, which in turn might lead to large losses on the investors' bonds. In such a situation, the trustee may decide that the bondholders would be better served by giving the company a chance to work out its problems rather than by forcing it into bankruptcy.

The Securities and Exchange Commission approves indentures and makes sure that all indenture provisions are met before allowing a company to sell new securities to the public. It should be noted that the indentures of most larger corporations were actually written back in the 1930s or 1940s and that many issues of new bonds, all covered by this same indenture, have been sold down through the years. The interest rates on the bonds and perhaps their maturities will change from issue to issue, but bondholders' protections as spelled out in the indenture will be the same for all bonds in the class. Some of the more important provisions in most indentures are discussed in the following sections.

Bond Repayment Provisions

Sinking Fund. A **sinking fund** is a provision that facilitates the orderly retirement of a bond issue (or, in some cases, an issue of preferred stock). Typically, the sinking fund provision requires the firm to retire a portion of the bond issue each year. On rare occasions, the firm is required to deposit money with a trustee, who invests the money and then uses the accumulated sum to retire the bonds when they mature. Sometimes the stipulated sinking fund

---

par value
The nominal or face value of a stock or bond.

coupon rate
The stated rate of interest on a bond.

indenture
A formal contract between the issuer of a bond and the bondholders.

trustee
The representative of bondholders who acts in their interest and facilitates communication between them and the bond issuer.

sinking fund
A required annual payment designed to retire a bond or a preferred stock issue.

Chapter 17 Bonds and Preferred Stock 477

payment is tied to sales or earnings of the current year, but usually it is a mandatory fixed amount. If it is mandatory, a failure to meet the sinking fund requirement causes the bond issue to be thrown into default, which may force the company into bankruptcy. Obviously, then, a sinking fund can constitute a dangerous cash drain on the firm.

In most cases, the firm is given the right to handle the sinking fund in either of two ways:

1. It may call in for redemption a certain percentage of the bonds at a stipulated price each year — for example, 2 percent of the total original amount of the issue at a price of $1,000 per bond. The bonds are numbered serially, and the ones called for redemption are determined by a lottery.

2. It may buy the required amount of bonds on the open market.

The firm will take whichever action results in the greatest reduction of outstanding bonds for a given expenditure. Therefore, if interest rates have risen and bond prices have fallen, the company will elect to use the option of buying bonds at a discount in the open market.

Although sinking funds are designed to protect bondholders by insuring that an issue is retired in an orderly fashion, it must be recognized that they will, at times, work to the detriment of bondholders. If, for example, the bond carries a 14 percent interest rate, and if yields on similar securities are 10 percent, the bond will sell above par. A sinking fund call at par would greatly disadvantage the bondholders whose securities are called for retirement purposes.

On balance, securities that provide for a sinking fund and continuing redemption are likely to be offered initially on a lower-yield basis than securities without such funds. Since sinking funds provide additional protection to investors, bond issues that have them are likely to be issued with lower coupon rates than otherwise similar bonds without sinking funds.

Call Provision. A **call provision** gives the issuing corporation the right to call the bond for redemption. If it is used, the call provision generally states that the company must pay an amount greater than the par value for the bond, with this additional sum being termed the *call premium.* The call premium is typically set equal to one year's interest if the bond is called during the first year, with the premium declining at a constant rate each year thereafter. For example, the call premium on a $1,000 par value, 10-year, 9 percent coupon bond would generally be $90 if it were called during the first year, $81 if it were called during the second year (calculated by reducing the $90 call premium by one-tenth annually), and so on.

Suppose a company sold bonds or preferred stock when interest rates were relatively high. Provided the issue is callable, the company could sell a new issue of lower-yielding securities if interest rates drop. It could then use the proceeds to retire the high-rate issue and thus reduce its interest or, in the case of preferred stock, dividend expenses. In business this procedure is called

call provision
A provision in a bond contract that gives the issuer the right to redeem the bonds under specified terms before the normal maturity date.

a *refunding operation,* but the principle is quite familiar to a homeowner who refinances a high-interest home loan with a lower-interest loan.

The call privilege is valuable to the firm but potentially detrimental to the investor, especially if the bond is issued in a period when interest rates are cyclically high. Accordingly, the interest rate on a new issue of callable bonds will exceed that on a new issue of noncallable bonds. For example, on May 27, 1987, Great Plains Power Company sold an issue of A-rated bonds to yield 14.375 percent. These bonds were callable immediately. On the same day Midwest Electric sold an issue of A-rated bonds to yield 14.125 percent. Midwest's bonds were noncallable for ten years. (This is known as *deferred call.*) Investors were apparently willing to accept a 0.25 percent lower interest rate on Midwest's bonds for the assurance that the relatively high (by historic standards) rate of interest would be earned for at least 10 years. Great Plains, on the other hand, had to incur a 0.25 percent higher annual interest rate to obtain the option of calling the bonds in the event of a subsequent decline in interest rates.

Note that the call for refunding purposes is quite different from the call for sinking fund purposes. The call for sinking fund purposes generally has no call premium, but only a small percentage of the issue is callable each year.

Restrictive Covenants

restrictive covenant
A provision in a bond indenture or term loan agreement that requires the bond issuer to meet certain stated conditions.

A **restrictive covenant** is a provision in a bond indenture or term loan agreement that requires the issuer of the bond to meet certain stated conditions. Typical provisions include requiring that debt does not exceed a specific percentage of total capital, that the current ratio is maintained above a specific level, that dividends are not paid on common stock unless earnings are maintained at a given level, and so on. Overall, these covenants are designed to insure, insofar as possible, that the firm does nothing to cause the bonds' quality to deteriorate after they are issued. As with other provisions in the indenture, the trustee is responsible for making sure that the restrictive covenants are not violated or that violations are quickly corrected in the best interests of the bondholders or lenders.

TYPES OF BONDS

Mortgage Bonds

mortgage bond
A pledge of designated property (real assets) as security for a bond.

Under a **mortgage bond** the corporation pledges certain real assets as security for the bond. To illustrate, in 1987 Bio-tech Pharmaceuticals needed $15 million to purchase land and to build a major research and development center. Bonds in the amount of $7 million, secured by a mortgage on the property, were issued. (The remaining $8 million was financed with equity funds.) If Bio-tech defaults on the bonds, the bondholders can foreclose on the property and sell it to satisfy their claims.

If Bio-tech chose to, it could issue second mortgage bonds secured by the same $15 million plant. In the event of liquidation, the holders of these second mortgage bonds would have a claim against the property only after the first mortgage bondholders had been paid off in full. Thus second mortgages are sometimes called *junior mortgages* because they are junior in priority to the claims of senior mortgages, or *first mortgage bonds.*

The first mortgage indentures of most major corporations were written 20, 30, 40, or more years ago. These indentures are generally "open-ended," meaning that new bonds may be issued from time to time under the existing indenture. However, the amount of new bonds that can be issued is almost always limited by clauses in the indenture to a specified percentage of the firm's total "bondable property," which generally includes all plant and equipment. For example, Savannah Electric can issue first mortgage bonds in total up to 60 percent of its fixed assets. If fixed assets total $1 billion, and if the company has $500 million of first mortgage bonds outstanding, it can, by the property test, issue another $100 million of bonds (60% of $1 billion = $600 million).

In recent years, Savannah Electric has at times been unable to issue any new first mortgage bonds because of another indenture provision — its times-interest-earned (TIE) ratio has been below 2.5, the minimum coverage that it must maintain to sell new bonds. Savannah Electric passed the property test but failed the coverage test; hence it cannot issue the first mortgage bonds and has to finance with junior securities. Since first mortgage bonds carry lower rates of interest than junior long-term debt, this restriction is a costly one.

Savannah Electric's neighbor, Georgia Power Company, has more flexibility under its indenture; its interest coverage requirement is only 2.0. In hearings before the Georgia Public Service Commission, it was suggested that Savannah Electric change its indenture coverage to 2.0 so that it could issue more first mortgage bonds. However, this is simply not possible; the holders of the outstanding bonds would have to approve the change, and it is inconceivable that they would vote for a change that would seriously weaken their position.

Debentures

A **debenture** is an unsecured bond and, as such, provides no lien on specific property as security for the obligation. Debenture holders are therefore general creditors whose claims are protected by property not otherwise pledged. In practice, the use of debentures depends on the nature of the firm's assets and its general credit strength. An extremely strong company like IBM will tend to use debentures — it simply does not need to put up property as security for its debt issues. Debentures are also issued by industries in which it would not be practical to provide security through a mortgage on fixed assets. Examples of such industries are the large mail-order houses and finance companies, which characteristically hold most of their assets in the form of inventory or receivables, neither of which is satisfactory security for a mortgage bond.

debenture
A long-term debt instrument that is not secured by a mortgage on specific property.

Subordinated Debentures

The term *subordinate* means "below," or "inferior." Thus subordinated debt has claims on assets in the event of bankruptcy only after senior debt (usually mortgage bonds) has been paid off. Debentures may be subordinated to designated notes payable — usually bank loans — or to all other debt. In the event of liquidation or reorganization, holders of **subordinated debentures** cannot be paid until senior debt as named in the debentures' indenture has been paid. Precisely how subordination works, and how it strengthens the position of senior debtholders, is explained in Appendix 20A.

Other Types of Bonds

Several other types of bonds are used sufficiently often to warrant mention. First, **convertible bonds** are securities that are convertible into shares of common stock, at a fixed price, at the option of the bondholder. Basically, convertibles provide investors with a chance to receive capital gains in exchange for a lower coupon rate, while the issuing firm gets the advantage of that lower rate. Bonds issued with warrants are similar to convertibles. **Warrants** are options that permit the holder to buy stock for a stated price, thereby providing a capital gain if the price of the stock rises. Like convertibles, bonds that are issued with warrants carry lower coupon rates than straight bonds. Warrants and convertibles are discussed in detail in Appendix 18A.

Income bonds pay interest only when the interest is earned. This flexibility means that income bonds are similar to preferred stock in that there is no default if these obligations are not met. However, unlike a preferred stock dividend, the interest payment on an income bond is a tax-deductible expense, just as with any other business debt instrument. These bonds are often issued by companies in reorganization or by firms whose financial situation does not allow a fixed, inescapable interest charge common to all other classes of bonds. Thus although these securities cannot bankrupt a company, from an investor's perspective they are riskier than regular bonds, owing to the weakness of the issuing firm and the uncertainty of the timing of interest receipts.

RECENT BOND INNOVATIONS

Zero Coupon Bonds

The majority of all bonds pay interest periodically, generally semiannually or annually, and then pay the principal when the bond matures. However, a recent development in the corporate bond market is the issuance of bonds that do not make periodic interest payments. These securities are called **zero coupon bonds** (zeros), and they are unique in that, like many government bonds, they are sold at less than face value and mature at par, usually $1,000. Assume that a firm wishes to sell a 12 percent, 10-year, zero coupon bond. As found in Chapter 13, the present value of $1,000 to be received in 10 years and

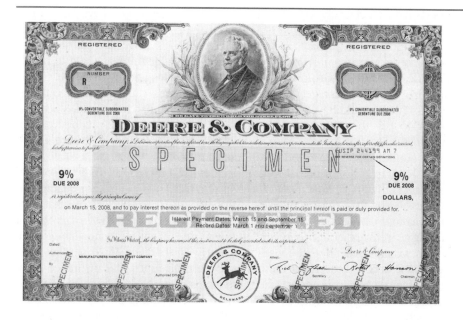

In this convertible subordinated debenture (or bond) issued by Deere & Company, the borrower (Deere) agrees to make payments of interest (on March 15 and September 15) to the holder of the bond. Terms of the bond are 9 percent; it is due in the year 2008. The term *convertible* means that this bond gives the bondholder the option of converting it into shares of common stock; the term *subordinated* means that, in the event of liquidation or reorganization, the bondholder would not be paid until senior debt has been paid off.

Source: Courtesy of Deere & Company.

discounted at 12 percent would equal $322 today. Thus, by using Equation 13-2a,

$$PV = FV(DF)$$
$$= \$1,000(0.322)$$
$$= \$322.00,$$

we can find the price an investor would pay for this zero coupon bond.

Zeros were first used in a major way in 1981. In recent years IBM, Alcoa, J.C. Penney, ITT, Cities Service, GMAC, Martin-Marietta, and many other companies have used them to raise billions of dollars. Moreover, investment bankers have in effect created zero coupon Treasury bonds. To understand what zeros are, consider J.C. Penney's $200 million par value issue of bonds that have no coupons and that pay no annual interest. These zero coupon bonds were sold in 1981 and mature after 8 years, in 1989, at which time holders will be paid $1,000. The bonds were sold at a discount below par for $322.41 per $1,000 bond. The compound interest rate that causes $322.41 to grow to $1,000 over 8 years is 14.76 percent. Penney received $66.482 million minus underwriting expenses for the issue, but it will have to pay back $200 million in 1989.

The advantages to Penney include the following: (1) no cash outlays are required for either interest or principal until the bonds mature; (2) these bonds have a relatively low yield to maturity (Penney would have had to pay approximately 15.25 percent versus the actual 14.76 percent had it issued regular coupon bonds at par); and (3) Penney receives an annual tax deduction equal to the yearly amortization of the discount, which means that the bonds provide a positive cash flow in the form of tax savings over their life. There are also two disadvantages to Penney: (1) the bonds simply are not callable, because they would have to be called at their $1,000 par value, and, since it is better to pay the $1,000 in 1989 than at some earlier date, Penney cannot refund the issue if interest rates should fall; and (2) Penney will have a very large nondeductible cash outlay coming up in 1989.

There are two principal advantages to the purchasers of zero coupon bonds: (1) they have no danger whatever of a call, and (2) they are guaranteed a "true" yield (14.76 percent in the Penney's case) irrespective of what happens to interest rates; the holders of these bonds do not have to worry about having to reinvest coupons received at low rates if interest rates should fall, which would result in a true yield to maturity of less than 14.76 percent. This second feature is extremely important to pension funds, life insurance companies, and other institutions that make actuarial contracts based on assumed reinvestment rates; for such investors the risk of declining interest rates, hence an inability to reinvest cash inflows at the assumed rates, is greater than the risk of an increase in rates and the accompanying fall in bond values.

Because of tax considerations (the difference between the purchase price and the maturity value for individuals is treated as amortized annual interest income and not as a capital gain), these bonds are best suited for tax-exempt organizations, especially pension funds. However, since pension funds are by far the largest purchasers of corporate bonds, the potential market for zero coupon bonds is by no means small.

Floating Rate Debt

In the early 1980s, inflation pushed interest rates up to unprecedented levels, causing sharp declines in the prices of long-term bonds. Even some supposedly "risk-free" U.S. Treasury bonds lost fully half their value, and a similar situation occurred with corporate bonds, mortgages, and other fixed rate, long-term securities. The lenders who held the fixed rate debt were, of course, hurt very badly. Bankruptcies (or forced mergers to avoid bankruptcy) were commonplace in the banking and especially the savings and loan industries. Insurance company reserves also plummeted, causing those companies severe problems, including the bankruptcy of Baldwin-United, a $9 billion diversified insurance firm. As a result, many lenders became reluctant to lend money at fixed rates on a long-term basis, and they would do so only at high rates.

There is normally a *maturity risk premium* embodied in long-term interest rates; this is a risk premium designed to offset the risk of declining bond prices if interest rates rise. Prior to the 1970s, this maturity risk premium on 30-year bonds was about one percentage point, meaning that under normal conditions, a firm might expect to pay about one percentage point more to borrow on a long-term than on a short-term basis. In the early 1980s, however, the maturity risk premium is estimated to have jumped to about three percentage points, which made long-term debt very expensive relative to short-term debt. Lenders were able and willing to lend on a short-term basis, but corporations were rightly reluctant to borrow short-term to finance long-term assets—such action is, as we have seen in Chapter 9, extremely dangerous. Therefore, there was a situation in which lenders did not want to lend on a long-term basis but corporations needed long-term money. The problem was solved by the introduction of *long-term, floating rate debt.*

A typical **floating rate bond** works as follows. The coupon rate is set for, say, the initial six-month period, after which it is adjusted every six months based on some market rate. For example, Gulf Oil sold a floating rate bond that was pegged at 35 basis points above the going rate on 30-year Treasury bonds. Other companies' issues have been tied to short-term rates. Many additional provisions have been included in floating rate issues; for example, some are convertible to fixed rate debt, whereas others have a stated minimum coupon rate as well as a cap on how high the rate can go.

floating rate bond
A bond whose interest rate fluctuates with shifts in the general level of interest rates.

Floating rate debt is advantageous to lenders because the interest rate moves up if market rates rise. This, in turn, causes the market value of the debt to be stabilized and provides lenders such as banks with more income to meet their own obligations (for example, a bank that owns floating rate bonds can use the interest it earns to pay interest on its own deposits). Moreover, floating rate debt is advantageous to corporations because by using it, they can obtain debt with a long maturity without committing themselves to paying an historically high rate of interest for the entire term of the loan. Of course, if interest rates increase after a floating rate note has been signed, the borrower would have been better off issuing conventional, fixed rate debt.

Junk Bonds

Another new type of bond is the **junk bond,** a high-risk, high-yield bond either issued to finance a leveraged buyout or a merger, or issued by a troubled company. For example, when Ted Turner attempted to buy CBS, he planned to finance the acquisition by issuing junk bonds to CBS's stockholders in exchange for their shares. Similarly, Merrill Lynch has helped Public Service of New Hampshire finance construction of its troubled Seabrook nuclear plant with junk bonds. In all junk bond deals, the debt ratio is extremely high, so the bondholders must bear as much risk as stockholders normally would. The bonds' yields reflect this fact — Ted Turner's bonds would have carried a coupon rate of about 16 percent, and Merrill Lynch has reported that it will have to set a coupon rate in the 25 to 30 percent range to sell the Public Service of New Hampshire bonds.

junk bond
A high-risk, high-yield bond used to finance mergers, leveraged buyouts, and troubled companies.

The emergence of junk bonds as an important type of debt is another example of how the investment banking industry adjusts to—and facilitates—

new developments in capital markets. In the 1980s, mergers and takeovers increased dramatically. People like T. Boone Pickens and Ted Turner thought that certain old-line, established companies were run inefficiently and financed too conservatively, and they wanted to take over these companies and restructure them. To help finance these takeovers, the investment banking firm of Drexel Burnham Lambert began an active campaign to persuade certain institutions to purchase high-yield bonds. Drexel developed expertise in putting together deals that were attractive to the institutions yet feasible in the sense that cash flows were sufficient to meet the required interest payments. The fact that interest on the bonds is tax deductible, combined with the much higher debt ratios of the restructured firms, also increased after-tax cash flows and helped make the whole deal feasible.

The development of junk bond financing has done as much as any single factor to reshape the U.S. financial scene. It has led directly to the loss of Gulf Oil and hundreds of other companies as independent entities, and it has led to major shake-ups in companies like CBS. It also allowed Drexel Burnham Lambert to leap from essentially nowhere in the 1970s to one of the top five investment banking firms by the mid-1980s.

BOND RATINGS

Since the early 1900s bonds have been assigned quality ratings that reflect their probability of going into default. The two major rating agencies are Moody's Investors Service and Standard & Poor's Corporation (S&P). These agencies' rating designations are shown in Table 17-1.[2]

The triple A bonds are extremely safe, and the double A and single A bonds are also strong enough to be held in conservative portfolios. The triple B rated bonds are strong enough to be termed *investment grade,* but they are the lowest-rated bonds that many banks and other institutional investors are permitted by law to hold. Double B bonds and lower-rated bonds are considered speculative grade securities, with increasingly higher probabilities of default as ratings decline. Many financial institutions are prohibited from buying these higher risk securities.

Although the rating assignments are judgmental, they are based on both qualitative and quantitative factors, some of which are the following:

- *Ratio analysis:* The firm's leverage position, liquidity, and debt coverage are among the first factors considered by the bond-rating agencies. We discuss in a later section two of the more important coverage ratios—the times-interest-earned and the fixed charge ratios.

- *Security provisions:* Whether the bond is backed by real assets (mortgage bond) or not (debenture), or by another firm (guaranteed bond), or

---

[2]In the discussion to follow, reference to the S&P code is intended to imply the Moody code as well. Thus, for example, *triple B bonds* means both BBB and Baa bonds, *double B bonds* both BB and Ba bonds, and so on.

Table 17-1 **Comparison of Bond Ratings**

	High Quality		**Investment Grade**		**Substandard**		**Speculative**
Moody's	Aaa	Aa	A	Baa	Ba	B	Caa to D
S&P	AAA	AA	A	BBB	BB	B	CCC to D

Note: Both Moody's and S&P use "modifiers" for bonds rated below triple A. S&P uses a plus and minus system; thus, A+ designates the strongest A-rated bonds and A− the weakest. Moody's uses a 1, 2, or 3 designation, with 1 denoting the strongest and 3 the weakest. Thus, within the double A category, Aa1 is the best, Aa2 is average, and Aa3 is the weakest.

whether funds are distributed to these bondholders after others receive theirs are important factors in the rating scheme.

- *Sinking fund:* If the issue has a sinking fund to insure systematic repayment, it is a plus factor to the rating agencies.

- *Maturity:* Other things being the same, a bond with a shorter maturity will be judged less risky than a longer-term bond, and this will be reflected in the rating.

- *Stability:* As a general rule, the more stable the firm's sales and earnings, the stronger the rating.

- *Legal actions:* Any major legal controversies such as antitrust suits could erode the ratings.

- *Pension liabilities:* If the firm has unfunded pension liabilities that could cause a problem, that fact is reflected in its bond ratings.

- *Other:* Many other factors enter into the bond-rating scheme used by agencies. A sample of other factors includes potential for labor problems, political unrest in host countries for multinational firms, and the regulatory climate for public utilities and other regulated industries.

Analysts at the rating agencies have consistently stated that no precise formula is used when setting a firm's rating; all the factors listed, plus others, are taken into account, but not in a mathematically precise manner. Statistical studies have borne out this contention; researchers who have tried to predict bond ratings on the basis of quantitative data have had only limited success, indicating that the agencies do indeed use a good deal of subjective judgment when establishing a firm's rating.[3]

Importance of Bond Ratings

Bond ratings are important both to firms and to investors. First, a bond's rating is an indicator of its risk; hence the rating has a direct, measurable influence on the bond's interest rate and the firm's cost of debt capital. Second, most

---

[3]See G. E. Pinches and K. A. Mingo, "A Multivariate Analysis of Industrial Bond Ratings," *Journal of Finance,* March 1973, 1–18; or Ahmed Belkaoui, *Industrial Bonds and the Rating Process* (London: Quorum Books, 1983).

bonds are purchased by institutional investors, not by individuals, and these institutions are generally restricted to investment-grade securities. Thus, if a firm's bonds fall below BBB, it will have a difficult time selling new bonds, as most of the potential purchasers will not be allowed to buy them.

Ratings also have an effect on the availability of debt capital. If an institutional investor buys BBB bonds and these bonds are subsequently downgraded to BB or lower, the institution's regulators will reprimand or perhaps impose restrictions on the institution if it continues to hold the bonds. However, since many other institutional investors cannot purchase the bonds, the institution that owns them will probably not be able to sell them except at a sizable loss. Because of this fear of downgrading, many institutions restrict their bond portfolios to at least A, or even AA, bonds. Some even confine purchases to AAA bonds. Thus the lower a firm's bond rating, the smaller the group of available purchasers for its new issues.

As a result of their higher risk and more restricted market, lower-grade bonds have much higher required rates of return, k_d, than do high-grade bonds. Figure 17-1 illustrates this point. In each of the years shown on the graph, U.S. Government bonds always have had the lowest yields, AAA bonds have been next, and the BBB bonds have had the highest yields of the three types. The figure also shows that the gaps between the yields on the three types of bonds vary over time; in other words, the cost differentials, or risk premiums, fluctuate from year to year.

This point is highlighted in Table 17-2, which gives the yields on the three types of bonds and the risk premiums for AAA and BBB bonds on various dates over nearly a quarter-century. Yields for all financial assets have been higher in recent years, but those yields grew dramatically from 1979 to 1981. Recall from Chapter 5 that the return on financial assets is based on the risk-free rate plus risk premiums for increasing risk. Government bonds are default-risk free, but because investors in these securities still face (and must be compensated for) inflation risk, the return on "risk-free" government securities must include an inflation risk premium. The government bond rate rose nearly 9 percentage points from 1963 to 1981, reflecting the increase in realized and anticipated inflation. However, this riskless rate has declined from 11.8 percent in March 1985 to below 8 percent in November 1986, reflecting the economic community's lower expectation about future inflation. Government bonds are considered to be free of default risk, but corporate bonds are not. AAA bonds have little default risk. BBB securities have a higher potential for default, so investors require a higher rate of return on these securities. Investors' risk aversion, as measured by the bonds' risk premium in Table 17-2, has grown significantly from 1963 to the present, reflecting the economic uncertainties of the times. However, interest rates dropped from 1985 to late 1986. Therefore, the penalty for having a low credit rating has varied over time. Occasionally, as in 1963, this penalty is quite small, but at other times, as in 1975, it is very large. These differences reflect investors' risk aversion; in 1975 the United States was emerging from a severe recession caused by a quadrupling of oil

Figure 17-1 **Yields on U.S. Government Bonds, AAA Corporates, and BBB Corporates, 1953–1987**

A bond's rating is an indicator of its risk. Because a lower-grade bond entails greater risk, it must pay a higher interest rate to attract investors. During the 34 years shown here, U.S. Government long-term bonds, which are considered default-free, paid the lowest interest rates. Corporate AAA bonds paid somewhat higher interest rates, while corporate BBB bonds paid the highest rates. The spreads between the curves indicate the risk premiums that corporate bond issuers had to pay to raise capital.

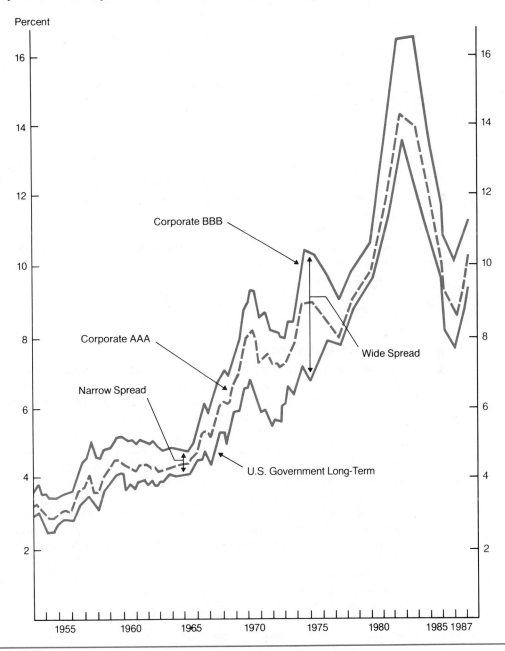

Sources: *Federal Reserve Board Historical Chart Book,* 1979, and *Federal Reserve Bulletin,* various issues.

Table 17-2 **Risk Premiums in Selected Economic Periods**

	Long-Term Government Bonds (Risk-Free) (1)	AAA Corporate Bonds (2)	BBB Corporate Bonds (3)	Risk Premiums	
				AAA (4) = (2) − (1)	BBB (5) = (3) − (1)
June 1963	4.00%	4.23%	4.84%	0.23%	0.84%
January 1975	6.68	8.83	10.62	2.15	3.94
May 1981	12.96	14.32	15.95	1.36	2.99
March 1985	11.77	12.47	13.51	0.70	1.74
November 1986	7.81	8.68	10.07	0.87	2.26

Source: *Federal Reserve Bulletin,* various issues.

prices in 1973 and 1974, and investors were afraid the economy would slip back into a slump. At such times people seek safety in bonds, Treasuries are in great demand, and the premium on low-quality over high-quality bonds increases.

These relationships for three selected time periods are graphically depicted in Figure 17-2. Note that the government bond return (the riskless rate) on the vertical axis has risen since 1963, reflecting the increase in expected and realized inflation. The slope of the line reflects investors' risk aversion. The increase in risk aversion was quite pronounced from 1963 to 1975 but fell somewhat by 1985.

Changes in Ratings

A change in a firm's bond rating will have a considerable effect on its ability to borrow long-term capital and on the cost of that capital. Rating agencies review outstanding bonds on a periodic basis, occasionally upgrading or downgrading a bond as a result of its issuer's changed circumstances. For example, in the spring of 1985, when Mobil Oil announced that it was planning to spin off its Montgomery Ward unit (Mobil had acquired Montgomery Ward in a diversification move back in the early 1970s), S&P immediately placed Ward on its *Credit Watch* list. (*Credit Watch* is a weekly publication that discusses developing situations that may lead to upgradings or downgradings.) The statement made in *Credit Watch* was that without Mobil's backing, Montgomery Ward's credit position might deteriorate to the point where its first mortgage bonds would have to be lowered from BBB to BB and its debentures from BB+ to some lower rating. The final outcome will depend on Ward's condition when Mobil does spin it off. Similarly, when it was announced that Chevron would buy Gulf in 1984, borrowing much of the money for the purchase, Chevron was immediately placed on the *Credit Watch* list with negative

Figure 17-2 **Relationship between Bond Ratings and Bond Yields, 1963, 1975, and 1985**

This figure takes a closer look at the relationship between bond ratings and bond yields. Between 1963 and 1985, the default-free rate of interest rose from 4.0 percent to 11.77 percent to reflect both realized and anticipated inflation. Corporate borrowers, of course, had to pay a risk premium in addition. In 1963 corporate AAA bonds paid a risk premium of 0.23 percent, and corporate BBB bonds paid a risk premium of 0.84 percent. In 1975 the risk premium rose to 2.15 percent for AAA bonds and to 3.94 percent for BBB bonds. In 1985 the risk premium dropped to 0.70 percent for AAA bonds and to 1.74 percent for BBB bonds. The risk premiums fluctuated to reflect changes in investors' attitudes toward assuming risk.

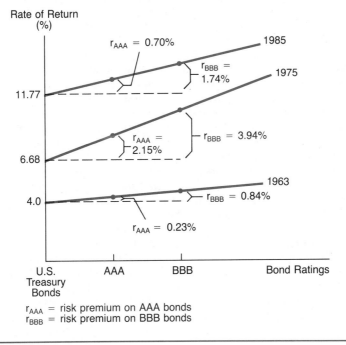

Source: Table 17-2.

implications, and its bonds were downgraded when it became clear that the deal was going through.

Coverage Ratios

One of the key elements in the analysis of corporate bonds is **coverage,** which measures a firm's ability to meet interest and principal payments and thus avoid default. The most commonly used coverage ratio is the *times interest*

coverage
The measure of a firm's ability to meet interest and principal payments; times interest earned is the most common coverage ratio.

INDUSTRY PRACTICE

Is Junk a Four-Letter Word?

Junk bonds, named more in jest than in malice, are corporate bonds rated as below investment grade by bond rating services. Relative newcomers to the financial scene, junk bonds first made their appearance in 1976, the brainchild of Michael Milken, the now legendary junk-bond doyen of Drexel Burnham Lambert. While studying for his MBA at Wharton, Milken decided that it is cash flow, not credit ratings, that determine a company's ability to pay back its debt. He argued that the risks associated with bonds issued by "fallen angels" (companies whose once-high ratings had been downgraded) could be offset by higher-than-average coupon payments and a thorough understanding on the part of the purchaser of the risks involved. As the idea took hold, new companies, as well as fallen angels, began raising money by issuing high-yield junk bonds.

"Junk bonds is a misnomer," says Richard E. Omohundro, Jr., manager of Merrill Lynch's high-yield bond group. "Many of these companies have bright or improving futures." Frequently, he explains, they get low ratings from Moody's and Standard & Poor's because they are emerging-growth companies with little or no credit history, or because they are established companies that have hit a cyclical downturn.

Obviously Omohundro is not alone in his views. In recent years investors have been pouring money into the market for junk bonds at an

ever-increasing rate. According to Edward I. Altman, professor of finance at New York University and a consultant to Morgan Stanley & Co., between June 1986 and April 1987 the high-yield debt market grew from $93 billion to over $125 billion. Junk bonds now approach almost 20 percent of the total corporate debt market, with fallen angels accounting for roughly 30 percent of the junk-bond market.

More than ever the junk-bond market has become a high-risk, high-reward place. Temptingly high yields, often 4 to 5 percent higher than government Treasury bonds and heavily loaded into the early years, often blind investors to the concomitant high risks involved in buying debt issued by companies that have below-investment-grade ratings. Indeed, as the junk-bond market has exploded, the default rate has risen accordingly. In 1986 the default rate was 3.39 percent of debt outstanding, considered high for a non-recession year.

However, as junk-bond proponents are quick to point out, more than 50 percent of that total was caused by the bankruptcy of steel giant LTV Corporation. This fact has made observers wonder whether the jump in defaults is the beginning of a trend or simply a one-time increase due to LTV. However, the question remains: How many more issuers of junk bonds will follow the example of LTV and file for protection under Chapter 11 of the bankruptcy laws?

The junk-bond market is now bigger, deeper, more liquid, and more controversial than ever. Some analysts claim that the market is heading for a tumble, especially if fueled by a recession. Again, the inclination of many investors to focus on junk's high yields while ignoring the concomitant risks is troubling. Analysts are also worried that although the market is large, in some ways it is quite thin. They are concerned

Source: Nick Gilbert, "Junk," *Financial World,* January 20, 1987, 20–23; Ben Weberman, "Low Quality, High Potential," *Forbes,* October 5, 1987, 237; Edward I. Altman, "The Anatomy of the High-Yield Bond Market," *Financial Analysts Journal,* July–August 1987, 12–25; "Junk Collecting," *Financial World,* February 15, 1983; and Christopher Farrell, Richard Melcher, and Ronald Grover, "Why Junk-Bond Investors Are Losing Sleep," *Business Week,* October 13, 1986, 151–152.

that when one scrutinizes this huge financial market, what emerges is some mutual funds, a couple of insurance companies and thrifts that specialize in junk bonds, and a handful of corporations that actively buy and sell each other's junk. A market accounting for 20 percent of corporate debt is composed of fewer than a 100 major players and dominated by one Wall Street firm, Drexel Burnham Lambert. Within Drexel, one man, Michael Milken, is the single most influential player in the market.

Drexel and Milken have taken their knocks of late. Both have been tarnished by the Boesky scandal, and the news that Milken had hired the nation's top three criminal lawyers to represent him in the wake of further investigations sent tremors through the market. However, Drexel spokespersons are quick to point out that a subpoena is not an indication of guilt and Milken is hardly a one-man band. Junk bonds, they assert, are here to stay.

Other analysts agree. They point out that the crash of the junk-bond market has been predicted every year since 1982 and has still failed to materialize. They point out that as the market has grown, so has the number of players. Tempted by juicy fees, Merrill Lynch, Morgan Stanley, Salomon Brothers, Shearson Lehman,

and First Boston have all entered the market as underwriters.

Not all junk bonds are created equal (even those with the same rating), but there are lucrative rewards to be garnered by those who are skilled at assessing risk. And although it may be difficult to predict whether a particular company that has financed itself with junk is going to come up a winner, a well-selected portfolio of high-risk, high-yield bonds may actually have a lower risk than a portfolio of long-term Treasurys. The reason, of course, is that the high coupon payments on the junk help offset the risk of interest rate fluctuations, as important component in calculating the risk of any bond.

Even if there is trouble in the junk market, chances are it will create as much opportunity as danger for investors. "The high-yield market is so large now," says Alan C. Peterson, portfolio manager of Cigna Corp.'s $250 million high-yield mutual fund, that there are "vast differences in quality." The market doesn't stand by itself anymore but is an integral part of the nation's financial system. In a market where some issues are offering more than 70 percent above government yields, there are many good buys for investors who really know how to evaluate risk.

earned (TIE). This ratio is defined in the following formula and illustrated with data for Carter Chemical Company (see Chapters 6 and 7 for the basic data):

$$\text{Times interest earned} = \frac{\text{Earnings before interest and taxes (EBIT)}}{\text{Interest}} = \frac{\$266}{\$66}$$

$$= 4.03 \text{ for Carter.}$$

$$\text{Industry average} = 6 \text{ times.}$$

The times-interest-earned ratio (TIE) depends on the level of interest payments, which in turn depends on the percentage of total capital represented by debt. For example, if Carter used twice as much debt (with a corresponding reduction in equity) and if the interest rate remained constant, its interest charges would be $66 \times 2 = \$132$. EBIT is not affected by changes in capital structure, so the increased use of debt would lower Carter's TIE to 2.02.

$$\text{TIE} = \frac{\$266}{\$132} = 2.02 \text{ times.}$$

As we will see in Chapter 20, the times-interest-earned ratio is given careful consideration when a firm establishes its target capital structure. The pro forma, or projected, TIE that would result under different financing plans is calculated, and care is taken to insure that the use of debt does not lower the TIE to an unacceptable level.

Another ratio that is often used to measure a company's ability to service its debt is the *fixed charge coverage ratio,* defined as follows:

$$\begin{aligned}\frac{\text{Fixed charge}}{\text{coverage ratio}} &= \frac{\text{EBIT} + \text{Lease payments}}{\text{Interest} + \left(\begin{array}{c}\text{Lease}\\\text{payments}\end{array}\right) + \left(\dfrac{\text{Sinking fund payment}}{1 - \text{Tax rate}}\right)}\\[2em]&= \frac{\$266 + \$28}{\$66 + \$28 + [\$20/(1 - 0.4)]}\\[1em]&= 2.3 \text{ times for Carter.}\end{aligned}$$

Industry average = 2.5 times.

Sinking funds were discussed earlier in this chapter; in essence, a sinking fund payment goes toward the retirement of the bond. Because sinking fund payments are not tax deductible, and the interest and lease payments are deductible, the sinking fund payment is divided by $(1 - \text{Tax rate})$ to find the before-tax income required to pay taxes and have enough left to make the sinking fund payment.

VALUATION OF BONDS

In Chapter 14 we indicated that the value of a capital budgeting project is its discounted future cash flow. What is true for the valuation of real assets is true for financial asset valuation as well. In other words, the value of a financial asset — a bond, a share of preferred stock, or a share of common stock — is equal to the cash returns provided by the security discounted back to the present.

A bond is a contractual debt instrument calling for the payment of a specified amount of interest for a stated number of years and for the repayment of the par value on the bond's maturity date.[4] Thus the bond's cash flow is rep-

---

[4]Actually, most bonds pay interest semiannually rather than annually, which would make it necessary to modify our valuation formula, Equation 17-1, slightly. We will use annual compounding at this point to avoid unnecessary detail; however, semiannual compounding was discussed in Appendix 13A. Also see Appendix 17A at the end of this chapter for a discussion of the valuation of bonds under semiannual compounding.

resented by an annuity plus a lump sum, and its value is found as the present value of this cash stream.

The following equation is used to find a bond's value:

$$\text{Value} = V = \sum_{t=1}^{n} I \left(\frac{1}{1 + k_d} \right)^t + M \left(\frac{1}{1 + k_d} \right)^n$$

$$= I(DF_a) + M(DF),$$ (17-1)

where

I = dollars of interest paid each year = coupon interest rate $\times$ par value.

M = the par value, or maturity value, which typically is $1,000.

k_d = the appropriate rate of interest on the bond.[5]

n = the number of years until the bond matures; n declines each year after the bond is issued.

We can use Equation 17-1 to find the value of Carter Chemical Company's bonds. Simply substitute $90 for I, $1,000 for M, and the values for DFa (found in Appendix D) and for DF (found in Appendix B) at 9 percent, Period 15:

$$V = \$90(8.0607) + \$1,000(0.2745)$$

$$= \$725.46 + \$274.50$$

$$= \$999.96 \cong \$1,000 \text{ when } k_d = 9\%.$$

Figure 17-3 gives a graphic view of the bond valuation process.

If k_d remained constant at 9 percent, what would the value of the bond be 1 year after it was issued? We can find this value using the same valuation formula, but now the term to maturity is only 14 years; that is, $n = 14$:

$$V = \$90(7.7862) + \$1,000(0.2992)$$

$$= \$999.96 \cong \$1,000.$$

This same result will hold for every year as long as the appropriate interest rate for the bond remains constant at 9 percent.

Now suppose that interest rates in the economy rose immediately after Carter's 9 percent bonds were issued, and as a result k_d increased from 9 to 12 percent. Of course, the interest and principal payments on the bonds are set, but now 12 percent values at 15 years for DF and DFa would be used in Equation 17–1. Thus the bond's value would be $795.68 if investors want a 12 percent return:

---

[5]An appropriate interest rate is determined by a number of factors. Most of these are reflected in the bond's rating, but they also include such factors as supply and demand in the capital markets.

Figure 17-3 **Time Line for Carter Chemical Company Bonds**

A bond's value is equal to the sum of its future interest payments and its final lump sum payment discounted to their present value. For example, the discounted cash flows from a 15-year, 9 percent Carter Chemical bond purchased in October 1987 totaled approximately $1,000; the first interest payment of $90.00 was discounted for one year in the future to $82.57, the second interest payment of $90.00 was discounted for two years in the future to $75.75, and so on.

$\dfrac{\text{Present}}{\text{Value}}$ = $999.97 = $1,000 when k_d = 9%. The difference is due to rounding.

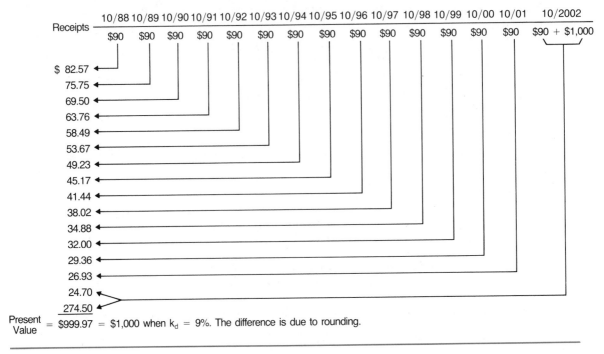

$\dfrac{\text{Present}}{\text{Value}}$ = $999.97 = $1,000 when k_d = 9%. The difference is due to rounding.

$$V = \$90(6.8109) + \$1,000(0.1827)$$

$$= \$612.98 + \$182.70$$

$$= \$795.68 \text{ when } k_d = 12\% \text{ and } n = 15.$$

The bond would sell at a *discount*—that is, at a price below its par value.

The arithmetic of the bond's price decrease should be clear, but what is the logic behind it? The reason for the decrease is simple. Carter Chemical's bondholders notice that other companies are issuing bonds, with the same risk characteristics as Carter's but with higher rates of return. Carter's bondholders, eager to receive the higher yield, sell Carter's 9 percent bonds in order to purchase the new 12 percent bonds. The drop in the demand for Carter's bonds means that the price of Carter's bond issue will fall. As investors sell

Carter's bonds, the price will be further depressed until at the price of $795.68, Carter's bonds will yield the same rate of return to a potential investor as the new 12 percent bonds.

Assuming that interest rates remain constant at 12 percent for the next 15 years, what would happen to the price of this Carter Chemical bond? It would rise gradually from $795.68 at present to $1,000 at maturity, when Carter Chemical must redeem each bond for $1,000. This point can be illustrated by calculating the value of the bond 1 year later, when it has 14 years to maturity:

$$V = \$90(6.6282) + \$1,000(0.2046)$$
$$= \$596.54 + \$204.60$$
$$= \$801.14 \text{ when } k_d = 12\% \text{ and } n = 14.$$

The value of the bond will have risen from $795.68 to $801.14, or by $5.46. If you were to calculate the value of the bond at other future dates, the price would continue to rise as the maturity date approached.

If interest rates had fallen from 9 to 6 percent when Carter Chemical Company's bonds had 15 years to maturity, the value of each bond would have risen to $1,291.40:

$$V = \$90(DFa) + \$1,000(DF)$$
$$= \$90(9.7122) + \$1,000(0.4173)$$
$$= \$874.10 + \$417.30$$
$$= \$1,291.40 \text{ when } k_d = 6\% \text{ and } n = 15.$$

In this case, the bond would sell at a *premium* above its par value. If interest rates remain at 6 percent for the next 15 years, the value of the bond would fall gradually from $1,291.40 to $1,000 at maturity.

Figure 17-4 graphs the value of the bond over time, assuming that interest rates in the economy remain constant at 9 percent, rise to 12 percent, or fall to 6 percent. Of course, if interest rates do *not* remain constant, the price of the bond will fluctuate. Regardless of what interest rates do, however, the bond's price will approach $1,000 as the maturity date comes nearer (barring bankruptcy, in which case the bond's value might drop to zero).

Figure 17-4 illustrates the following key points:

1. Whenever the going rate of interest (k_d) is equal to the coupon rate, a bond will sell at its par value.

2. Whenever the going rate of interest is above the coupon rate, a bond will sell below its par value. Such a bond is called a **discount bond.**

3. Whenever the going rate of interest is below the coupon rate, a bond will sell above its par value. Such a bond is said to sell at a **premium.**

4. An increase in interest rates will cause the price of outstanding bonds to fall, whereas a decrease in rates will cause bond prices to rise.

discount bond
A bond that sells below its par value, which occurs when the coupon rate is lower than the going rate of interest.

premium
The amount that a bond sells for above its par value, which occurs when the coupon rate is higher than the going rate of interest.

Figure 17-4 **Time Path of the Value of a 9% Coupon, $1,000 Par Value Bond When Interest Rates are 6%, 9%, and 12%**

The value of a bond fluctuates in response to changes in market interest rates. When a bond's coupon rate is equal to the market rate of interest, the bond sells at par. When the market rate falls below a bond's coupon rate, the bond sells above par. And when the market rate rises above a bond's coupon rate, the bond sells below par. This graph shows how the selling price of a 15-year, 9 percent bond with a par value of $1,000 will change if market interest rates rise to 12 percent or fall to 6 percent. Note that as the bond's maturity date approaches, its value fluctuates less and less until it finally reaches par.

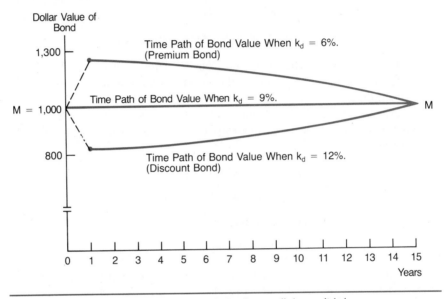

Note: The curves for 6% and 12% appear to be straight, but they actually have a slight bow.

5. The market value of a bond will approach its par value as its maturity date approaches.

These points are very important to investors, for they show that bondholders may suffer capital losses or make capital gains depending on whether interest rates rise or fall. And, as we saw earlier in this chapter, interest rates do indeed change over time.

Finding the Interest Rate on a Bond: Yield to Maturity

yield to maturity (YTM)
The rate of return earned on a bond if it is held to maturity.

Suppose you were offered a 14-year, 9 percent coupon, $1,000 par value bond at a price of $1,082.48. What rate of interest would you earn if you bought the bond and held it to maturity? This rate is defined as the bond's **yield to maturity,** and it is the interest rate discussed by bond traders when they talk about rates of return. To find the yield to maturity, often called the **YTM,** you could solve the following equation for k_d:

$$V = \$1,082.48$$

$$= \frac{\$90}{(1 + k_d)^1} + \frac{\$90}{(1 + k_d)^2} + \cdots + \frac{\$90}{(1 + k_d)^{14}} + \frac{\$1,000}{(1 + k_d)^{14}}$$

$$= \$90(DFa) + \$1,000(DF).$$

Just as we did in finding the IRR for a project in Chapter 14, we can substitute values of DFa and DF in the equation until we find a rate that *just equates* the present market price of the bond with the present value of its future cash flow of interest and principal. Thus

$$\$1,082.48 = \$90(DFa) + \$1,000(DF).$$

What would be a good interest rate to use as a starting point? First, referring to Point 3 in the preceding subsection, we know that since the bond is selling at a premium over its par value ($1,082.48 versus $1,000), the bond's yield is *below* the 9 percent coupon rate. Therefore, we might try a rate of 7 percent. Substituting in factors for 7 percent, we obtain

$$\$90(8.7455) + \$1,000(0.3878) = \$1,174.90 \neq \$1,082.48.$$

Our calculated bond value, $1,174.90, is *above* the actual market price, so the yield to maturity is *not* 7 percent. To lower the calculated value, we must *raise* the interest rate used in the process. Inserting factors for 8 percent, we obtain

$$V = \$90(8.2442) + \$1,000(0.3405)$$

$$= \$741.98 + \$340.50$$

$$= \$1,082.48.$$

This calculated value is exactly equal to the market price of the bond; thus 8 percent is the bond's yield to maturity.[6]

The yield to maturity is the total rate of return for an investor; this rate of return is equal to the bond's interest yield, if the bond is selling at par. If a bond is purchased at a price other than its par value, the YTM consists of the interest yield plus either a positive capital gains yield (if the bond was purchased at a discount) or a negative capital gains yield (if the bond was purchased at a premium). Note also that a bond's yield to maturity changes whenever interest rates in the economy change, and this is almost daily. An investor that purchases a bond and holds it until maturity will receive the YTM that

---

[6]There is also a formula that can be used to find the approximate yield to maturity on a bond:

$$k_d = YTM = \frac{I + (M - V)/n}{(M + V)/2}$$

In the situation where $I = \$90$, $M = \$1,000$, $V = \$1,082.48$, and $n = 14$,

$$k_d = \frac{\$90 + (\$1,000 - \$1,082.48)/14}{(\$1,000 + \$1,082.48)/2} = 0.0808 = 8.08\%.$$

This is close to the exact value, 8 percent. This formula can also be used to obtain a starting point for the trial-and-error method.

existed on the purchase date, but the bond's calculated YTM will change frequently between the date the bond is purchased and when it matures.

PREFERRED STOCK

preferred stock
A long-term equity security paying a fixed dividend.

Preferred stock is a *hybrid* — it is similar to bonds in some respects and to common stock in others. The hybrid nature of preferred stock becomes apparent when we try to classify it in relation to bonds and common stock. Like bonds, preferred stock has a par value. Preferred dividends are also similar to interest payments on bonds, in that they are fixed in amount and generally must be paid before common stock dividends can be paid. However, if the preferred dividend is not earned, the directors can omit (or "pass") it without throwing the company into bankruptcy. So, even though preferred stock has a fixed payment like bonds, a failure to make this payment will not lead to bankruptcy.

Preferred stock is sometimes treated like debt and sometimes like equity, depending on the type of analysis being made. If the analysis is being made by a common stockholder considering the fixed charge that must be paid ahead of common stock dividends, the preferred stock will be viewed much like debt. Suppose, however, that the analysis is being made by a bondholder studying the firm's vulnerability to failure because of a future decline in sales and income. Since the dividends on preferred stock are not a fixed charge in the sense that failure to pay them represents a default on an obligation, preferred stock provides an additional equity base. We see, then, that common stockholders view preferred stock much like debt, whereas creditors view it as being like equity.

Major Provisions of Preferred Stock Issues

Preferred stock has a number of features, the most important of which are covered in the following sections.

Priority in Assets and Earnings. Preferred stockholders have priority over common stockholders with regard to earnings and assets. Thus dividends must be paid on preferred stock before they can be paid on the common stock, and in the event of bankruptcy, the claims of the preferred shareholders must be satisfied before the common stockholders receive anything. To reinforce these features, most preferred stock certificates have coverage requirements, similar to those on bonds, which limit the amount of preferred stock a company can use; they also require that a minimum level of retained earnings is maintained before common dividends are permitted.

Par Value. Unlike common stock, preferred stock always has a par value (or its equivalent under some other name), and this value is a meaningful quantity. First, the par value establishes the amount due the preferred stockholders in the event of liquidation. Second, the preferred dividend is frequently stated as a percentage of the par value. For example, J. I. Case's preferred stock has a par value of $100 and a stated dividend of 7 percent of par. It would, of course, be just as appropriate for the Case preferred stock to simply call for an annual dividend of $7.

Cumulative Dividends. Most preferred stock provides for **cumulative dividends;** that is, all preferred dividends **arrearages** must be paid before common dividends can be paid. The cumulative feature is a protective device, for if the preferred stock dividends were not cumulative, a firm could avoid paying preferred and common stock dividends for, say, 10 years and thus "save" a large amount of earnings, and then pay a large common stock dividend but pay only the stipulated annual amount to the preferred stockholders. Obviously, such an action could be used to effectively void the preferred position that the preferred stockholders have tried to obtain, but the cumulative feature prevents such abuses.

cumulative dividends

A protective feature on preferred stock that requires all past preferred dividends to be paid before any common dividends.

arrearage

An omitted dividend on preferred stock.

Convertibility. Approximately 40 percent of the preferred stock that has been issued in recent years is convertible into common stock. For example, each share of InterNorth's $10.50 Class J preferred stock can be converted into 3.413 shares of its common stock at the option of the preferred shareholders. (Convertibility is discussed in more detail later, in Appendix 18A.)

Some Infrequent Provisions. Some other provisions occasionally encountered in preferred stocks include the following:

1. *Voting rights.* Sometimes preferred stockholders are given the right to vote for directors if the company has not paid the preferred dividend for a specified period, say, four, eight, or ten quarters. This feature certainly motivates management to make every effort to pay preferred dividends.

2. *Participating.* A rare type of preferred stock is one that participates with the common stock in sharing the firm's earnings. The following sequence generally relates to participating preferred stocks: (a) the stated preferred dividend is paid — for example, $5 a share; (b) income is allocated to common stock dividends up to an amount equal to the preferred dividend — in this case, $5; and (c) any remaining income is shared equally between the common and preferred stockholders.

3. *Sinking fund.* Some preferred issues have a sinking fund requirement, which ordinarily calls for the purchase and retirement of a given percentage of the preferred stock each year. For example, 2 percent, which is a common amount, gives the relevant preferred issue an average life of 25 years and a maximum life of 50 years.

4. *Maturity.* Preferred stocks almost never have maturity dates on which they must be retired. However, if the issue has a sinking fund, this effectively creates a maturity date.

5. *Call provision.* A call provision gives the issuing corporation the right to call in the preferred stock for redemption, as in the case of bonds. Call provisions generally state that the company must pay an amount greater than the par value of the preferred stock, and the additional sum is known as a **call premium.** For example, IBES Corporation's 12 percent, $100 par value preferred stock, issued in 1984, is noncallable for 10 years, but it may be called at a price of $112 after 1995.

call premium
The amount in excess of par value that a company must pay when it calls a security.

Evaluation of Preferred Stock

There are both advantages and disadvantages to financing with preferred stock. These are discussed in the following sections.

Issuer's Viewpoint. By using preferred stock, a firm can fix its financial costs and thus keep more of the potential future profits for its existing set of common stockholders, as with bonds, yet avoid the danger of bankruptcy if earnings are too low to meet these fixed charges. Also, because preferred stock typically has no maturity and often no sinking fund, this too reduces cash flow problems as compared with bonds. Finally, by selling preferred rather than common stock, the firm avoids sharing either control or earnings with the new investors.

However, preferred stock does have a major disadvantage from the issuer's standpoint: It has a higher after-tax cost of capital than debt. There are two reasons for this high cost. First, preferred stock often carries a higher coupon yield than bonds. Second, preferred dividends are not deductible as a tax expense, which makes the component cost of preferred stock much greater than that of bonds. The after-tax cost of debt is approximately two-thirds the stated coupon rate for profitable firms, whereas the cost of preferred stock is the full percentage amount of the preferred dividend. Of course, the deductibility differential is most important for issuers that are in relatively high tax brackets — if a company pays little or no taxes because it is unprofitable or because it has a great deal of accelerated depreciation, the deductibility of interest does not make much difference. Thus the higher a company's tax bracket, the less likely it is to use preferred stock financing.

Investor's Viewpoint. In designing securities, the financial manager must also consider the investor's point of view. Frequently it is asserted that preferred stock has so many disadvantages to both the issuer and the investor that it should never be issued. Nevertheless, preferred stock is issued in substantial amounts. It provides investors with reasonably steady and assured income plus a preference over common stockholders in the event of liquidation. In addition, 85 percent of the preferred dividends received by corporations are not taxable. For this reason, a large percentage of outstanding preferred stock is owned by corporations.

The principal disadvantage of preferred stock from an investor's standpoint is that although preferred stockholders bear a substantial portion of ownership risk, their returns are limited. In addition, preferred stockholders have no legally enforceable right to dividends, even if a company earns a profit. Also, companies often manage to avoid paying off all accumulated dividends when they emerge from a troubled, low-income period. Such companies frequently go through reorganization under the Bankruptcy Act, and preferred stockholders often do not fare well in these proceedings.

Valuation of Preferred Stock

Despite the fact that preferred stock dividends can be omitted without throwing the firm into bankruptcy, most financial managers attempt to pay these dividends without omission. Thus these dividends may reasonably be expected to be paid on time, and, because few preferred stock dividends are participating, these dividends should not change in value from period to period.

Just as bondholders value debt instruments as the present value of the bond's future cash flows, discounted at a required rate of return, k_d, preferred stockholders also discount future cash flows (in this case dividends) to arrive at a current market price for preferred stock:

$$P_p = \sum_{t=1}^{\infty} \frac{D_t}{(1 + k_p)^t} \qquad (17\text{-}2)$$

Where:

P_p = the market price of preferred stock today.
D_t = dividend payments each period for t periods.
k_p = the required rate of return on preferred stock.

Recalling that preferred stock dividends can be expected to remain at some constant amount in the future (that is, $D_1 = D_2 = D_3$ and so on), we can drop the subscripts and determine the value of preferred stock, P_p:

$$P_p = \frac{D}{(1 + k_p)^1} + \frac{D}{(1 + k_p)^2} + \cdots + \frac{D}{(1 + k_p)^n} + \cdots + \frac{D}{(1 + k_p)^\infty}.$$

$$(17\text{-}2a)$$

The value of the stock, P_p, can be determined by discounting each year's dividend back to the present. However, as we noted in Chapter 13, as the holding period, t, becomes infinitely large, the value of any no-growth security, perpetuity, may be simplified from Equation 17-2 (or Equation 17-2a) to:

$$P_p = D/k_p. \qquad (17\text{-}3)$$

Thus if Carter Chemical Company had a $100 par value preferred stock issue with a 12 percent dividend yield, the stock's price would be determined by the investors' required return, k_p. If investors were satisfied with a 12 percent rate of return, they would pay a price equal to the stock's par value:

$$P_p = \$12/0.12$$

$$= \$100.$$

Note that the value of the stock could have also been derived, with a great deal more effort, by discounting each year's dividend from Year 1 to infinity by the required rate of return, 12 percent.

If, however, investors desired a 14 percent rate of return, they would pay less than the preferred stock's par value:

$$P_p = \$12/0.14$$

$$= \$85.71.$$

Similarly, if rates on competing investment opportunities fall to 8 percent, the price of the preferred stock will rise to $150:

$$P_p = \$12/0.08$$

$$= \$150.$$

We could transpose the P_p and the k_p in Equation 17-3 and solve for k_p. We could then look up the price of the stock and the preferred dividend in the financial section of the newspaper, and the value of D/P_p would be the rate of return we could expect to earn if we bought the stock. Thus:

$$k_p = D/P_p. \qquad (17\text{-}4)$$

If we bought the preferred stock, which pays a constant dividend of $12, for $150, the stock's rate of return would be

$$k_p = \$12/\$150 = 0.08 = 8\%.$$

However, if investors are paying only $85.71 for a preferred stock that pays a constant $12 dividend, their required rate of return would be

$$k_p = \$12/\$85.71 = 0.14 = 14\%.$$

SUMMARY

This chapter described the characteristics, advantages, and disadvantages of the major types of long-term, fixed-income securities: *term loans, bonds,* and *preferred stocks.* The key difference between bonds and term loans is the fact that term loans are arranged directly by a corporate borrower with between one and twenty lenders, whereas bonds are generally sold to many public investors through investment bankers. Preferred stocks are similar to bonds in that they offer a fixed return. However, preferred stock is less risky than bonds from the corporation's viewpoint because (1) the dividend does not have to be paid if it is not earned, and (2) nonpayment of preferred dividends will not bankrupt the firm. From the investors' standpoint, however, preferred stocks are riskier than bonds because (1) firms are more likely to omit preferred dividends than to fail to pay interest, and (2) bonds have priority over preferred stock in the event of bankruptcy.

RESOLUTION TO DECISION IN FINANCE

A Deal for All Seasons

According to Daniel H. Kolber, a corporate attorney who worked with Air Atlanta's founders to design the company's zeros, the secret to selling the bonds was to keep sweetening the deal. Says Kolber, "Back then, the zero was getting a lot of press, and it seemed a perfect way to get money without paying periodic interest payments. It would still be accruing the interest, but we wouldn't have any cash outlay." The icing that Air Atlanta put on its cake was the rate at which the zeros could be converted into Air Atlanta stock at maturity. For Air Atlanta's purposes, because they had no stream of revenues to tap into to sweeten the deal, convertibility into stock was the most promising alternative. The decision was made. They would get the money first and worry about dilution of ownership when they had built something worth owning.

Although the advantages of the zero coupon bond offering for Air Atlanta were obvious for the lending companies, says Kolber, buying Air

Atlanta's zeros was a chance to speculate on a start-up, a capital position they would not usually take if it meant just putting up the cash for a new venture. "It's a ticket to play the game without looking like a venture capitalist," he remarks.

If Air Atlanta is a big hit, the pay-off for the coupon purchasers is owning a big chunk of a winning company. Still, a zero debenture like Air Atlanta's could easily end up being worth, literally, zero. The risk for the coupon holder is that because of accounting practices, even if Air Atlanta were on the verge of going under, the zeros would still be carried in the books as a debt in good standing. After all, there would be no missed payments.

"Doing a zero with start-up companies *is* a high risk," agrees Slivy Edmunds, Equitable's assistant vice president of corporate finance — but it is not an unexpected one. "You use it where you're willing to take an equity risk," he explains. "You should not evaluate the investment as debt. The determination would be whether or not you would take equity in the company. And to be comfortable with an equity risk, you have to be prepared to lose all your money."

Source: Robert A. Mamis, "A Deal for All Seasons," *Inc.,* January 1986, 105–110.

QUESTIONS

17-1   What effect would each of the following items have on the interest rate a firm must pay on a new issue of long-term debt? Indicate by a plus (+), minus (−), or zero (0) whether the factor will tend to raise, lower, or have an indeterminate effect on the firm's interest rate.

	Effect on Interest Rate

a. The firm uses bonds rather than a term loan. _____

b. The firm uses nonsubordinated debentures rather than first mortgage bonds. _____

c. The firm makes its bonds convertible into common stock. _____

d. The firm makes its debentures subordinated to its bank debt. What will the effect be:
(1) On the debentures? _____
(2) On the bank debt? _____
(3) On the average total debt? _____

e. The firm sells income bonds rather than debentures. _____

f. The firm must raise $100 million, all of which will be used to construct a new plant, and is debating the sale of mortgage bonds or debentures. If it decides to issue $50 million of each type, as opposed to $75 million of mortgage bonds and $25 million of debentures, how will this affect:
(1) The debentures? _____
(2) The mortgage bonds? _____
(3) The average cost of the $100 million? _____

g. The firm is planning to raise $25 million of long-term capital. Its outstanding bonds yield 9 percent. If it sells preferred stock, how will this effect the yield on the outstanding debt? _____

h. The firm puts a call provision on its new issue of bonds. _____

i. The firm includes a sinking fund on its new issue of bonds. _____

j. The firm's bonds are downgraded from A to BBB. _____

17-2 Rank the following securities from lowest (1) to highest (10) in terms of their riskiness for an investor. All securities (except the government bond) are for a given firm. If you think two or more securities are equally risky, so indicate.

	Rank (10 = Highest Risk)

a. Income bond _____

b. Subordinated debentures — noncallable _____

c. First mortgage bond — no sinking fund _____

d. Preferred stock _____

e. Common stock _____

f. U.S. Treasury bond _____

g. First mortgage bond — with sinking fund _____

h. Subordinated debentures — callable _____

i. Amortized term loan _____

j. Nonamortized term loan _____

17-3 A bond that pays interest forever and has no maturity date is a perpetual bond. In what respect is a perpetual bond similar to a share of preferred stock?

17-4 "The values of outstanding bonds change whenever the going rate of interest changes. In general, short-term interest rates are more volatile than long-term interest rates. Therefore, short-term bond prices are more sensitive to interest rate changes than are long-term bond prices." Is this statement true or false? Explain.

SELF-TEST PROBLEM

ST-1 A firm issued a new series of bonds on January 2, 1973. The bonds were sold at par ($1,000), have an 8 percent coupon, and mature 30 years after the date of issue. Interest is paid annually on December 31.

    a. What was the yield to maturity (YTM) of the bond on January 2, 1973?

    b. What was the price of the bond on January 2, 1978, five years later, assuming that the level of interest rates had risen to 10 percent?

    c. If, for this type of bond, interest rates had been 6 percent on January 2, 1978, what would investors have paid for the bond?

    d. Find the current yield and capital gains yield on the bond if interest rates as of January 2, 1978, were 6 percent, as in Part c.

    e. On January 2, 1983, the bond sold for $525.70. What was the YTM on that date?

    f. What was the current yield and capital gains yield for the bond under the conditions described in Part e?

    g. It is now January 2, 1988. The going rate of interest is 14 percent. How large a check must you write to buy the bond?

PROBLEMS

17-1 **Preferred stock valuation.** FSA Corporation has a $100 par, $8 dividend preferred stock outstanding. Investors require a 14 percent return on investments of this type.

    a. What is the current market price of FSA's preferred stock?

    b. Is the price you computed in Part a the same price that you would find if you discounted each future dividend back to the present using the 14 percent discount factors?

    c. If the investment community's required return fell for FSA's preferred stock, what would happen to the price?

17-2 **Yield computations.** Southwest Publications sold a 20-year, 10 percent coupon, $1,000 par bond 5 years ago. Today, with 15 years to maturity, the bond is selling for $754.32. What is the bond's:

    a. Nominal yield?

    b. Current yield?

    c. Yield to maturity?

17-3 **Bond valuation.** Americal sold a 15-year, 14 percent coupon bond at a par value of $1,000 in September 1983. In September 1988 the bond's yield to maturity is 12 percent. What is the current price of the bond?

17-4 **Bond valuation.**

    a. Audiomax Corporation's bonds pay $100 annual interest, mature in 10 years, and pay $1,000 on maturity. What will be the value of these bonds when the going rate of interest is: **(a)** 8 percent, **(b)** 10 percent, and **(c)** 12 percent?

    b. Now suppose that Audiomax has some other bonds that pay $100 interest per year, $1,000 at maturity, and mature in 1 year. What is the price of these bonds if the going rate of interest is: **(a)** 8 percent, **(b)** 10 percent, and **(c)** 12 percent? Assume there is only one more interest payment to be made.

    c. Why do the longer-term bond prices fluctuate more when interest rates change than do the shorter-term bond prices?

17-5   **Yield to maturity.** The Phillips Company's bonds have 5 years remaining to maturity. Interest is paid annually, the bonds have a $1,000 par value, and the coupon interest rate is 8 percent.

     a. What is the yield to maturity at a current market price of: **(1)** $924 and **(2)** $1,084? You may wish to use the approximation formula found in Footnote 6.

     b. Would you pay $924 for the bond described in Part a if you thought that the appropriate rate of interest for these bonds was 9 percent? Explain your answer.

17-6   **Bond valuation.** Suppose Olympic Industries sold an issue of bonds with a 10-year maturity, a $1,000 par value, and a 10 percent coupon rate paid annually.

     a. Suppose that 3 years after the issue, the going rate of interest had risen to 12 percent. At what price would the bonds sell?

     b. Suppose that the conditions in Part a continued (that is, interest rates remained at 12 percent throughout the bond's life). What would happen to the price of Olympic's bonds over time?

17-7   **Loan amortization.** Suppose that a firm is setting up an amortized term loan. What are the annual payments for a $2 million loan under the following terms:

     a. 9 percent, 5 years?

     b. 9 percent, 10 years?

     c. 12 percent, 5 years?

     d. 12 percent, 10 years?

17-8   **Amortization schedule.** Set up an amortization schedule for a $1 million, 3-year, 9 percent term loan.

17-9   **Amortization payments.** A company borrows $1 million on a 3-year, 9 percent, partially amortized term loan. The annual payments are to be set so as to amortize $700,000 over the loan's 3-year life and also to pay interest on the $300,000 nonamortized portion of the loan.

     a. How large must each annual payment be? (*Hint:* Think of the loan as consisting of two loans, one fully amortized for $700,000 and one on which interest only is paid each year until the end of the third year.)

     b. Suppose the firm requests a $1 million, 9 percent, 3-year loan with payments of $250,000 per year (interest plus some principal repayment) for the first 2 years and the remainder to be paid off at the end of the third year. How large must the final payment be?

17-10   **Yield to call.** (*Do this problem only if you are using the computerized problem diskette.*) It is now January 1, 1989, and you are considering the purchase of an outstanding Morgan Corporation bond that was issued on January 1, 1987. Morgan's bond has a 10.5 percent annual coupon and a 30-year original maturity (it matures in 2017). There was originally a 5-year call protection (until December 31, 1991), after which time the bond can be called at 110 (that is, at 110 percent of ar, or $1,100). Interest rates have declined since the bond was issued, and the boi is now selling at 115.174 percent of par, or $1,151.74. You want to determine bot' yield to maturity and the yield to call for this bond. (*Note:* The yield to call considers the impact of a call provision on the bond's probable yield. In the calculation, we assume that the bond will be outstanding until the call date, at which time it will be called. Thus the investor will have received interest payments for the call-protected period and then will receive the call price — in this case, $1,100 — on the call date.)

     a. What is the yield to maturity in 1989 for Morgan's bond? What is its yield to call?

b. If you bought this bond, which return do you think you would actually earn? Explain your reasoning.

c. Suppose that the bond had sold at a discount. Would the yield to maturity or the yield to call have been more relevant?

d. Suppose that the bond's price suddenly jumps to $1,250. What is the yield to maturity now, and what is the yield to call?

e. Suppose that the price suddenly falls to $800; now what would the YTM and the YTC be?

ANSWER TO SELF-TEST PROBLEM

ST-1   **a.** The bonds were sold at par. Therefore, the YTM equals the coupon rate, which is 8 percent. The coupon rate is also referred to as the *nominal yield* or *stated yield*.

b. We must find the PV of the 25 remaining interest payments of $80 each and the $1,000 lump sum payment of principal to be paid when the bond matures in 25 years. Therefore

$$\text{Bond value} = \$80(\text{DFa}_{10\%, 25 \text{ years}}) + \$1,000(\text{DF}_{10\%, 25n})$$

$$= \$80(9.0770) + \$1,000(0.0923)$$

$$= \$726.16 + \$92.30$$

$$= \$818.46.$$

c. Using the 6 percent discount factors, we find

$$\text{Bond value} = \$80(12.7834) + \$1,000(0.2330)$$

$$= \$1,022.67 + \$233.00$$

$$= \$1,255.67.$$

d. If interest rates were 6 percent on January 1, 1978, the bond's price was $1,255.67, as found in Part c. Thus

$$\text{Current yield} = \frac{\text{Coupon payment}}{\text{Price}}$$

$$= \frac{\$80}{\$1,255.67}$$

$$= 0.0637 = 6.37\%.$$

$$\text{Capital gains yield} = \text{Total yield} - \text{Current yield}$$

$$= 6\% - 6.37\% = -0.37\%.$$

e. Use the approximate YTM formula to get a starting point:

$$\text{Approximate YTM} = \frac{I + (M - V)/n}{(M + V)/2}$$

$$= \frac{\$80 + [(\$1,000 - \$525.70)/20]}{(\$1,000 + \$525.70)/2}$$

$$= \frac{\$103.715}{\$762.85}$$

$$= 13.6\%.$$

Because this approximation understates the true return, we will try a bit higher discount rate:

$$k_d = 16\%$$

$$V = I(DFa_{16\%,20}) + M(DF_{16\%,20})$$

$$= \$80(5.9288) + \$1,000(0.0514)$$

$$= \$474.30 + \$51.40$$

$$= \$525.70.$$

Therefore the YTM at the beginning of January 1983 was 16 percent.

f.
$$\text{Current yield} = \$80/\$525.70$$

$$= 15.22\%.$$

$$\text{Capital gains yield} = 16\% - 15.22\%$$

$$= 0.78.$$

g. The bond has 15 years until it matures; at 14 percent the price would be

$$V = \$80(6.1422) + \$1,000(0.1401)$$

$$= \$491.38 + \$140.10 = \$631.48.$$

Appendix 17A

Semi-Annual Compounding for Bonds

Although some bonds do pay interest annually, most actually pay interest semiannually. The same methodology discussed in Appendix 13A for multiple compounding periods applies to the valuation of bonds when interest is paid more than once each year. To evaluate semiannual payment bonds, we must modify the bond valuation model (Equation 17-1) as follows:

1. Divide the annual coupon interest payment by 2 to determine the amount of interest paid each 6 months.

2. Multiply the years to maturity, n, by 2 to determine the number of periods.

3. Divide the annual interest rate, k_d, by 2 to determine the semiannual interest rate.

By making these changes, we arrive at the following equation for finding the value of a bond that pays interest semiannually:

$$V = \sum_{t=1}^{2n} \frac{I}{2}\left(\frac{1}{1+\frac{k_d}{2}}\right)^t + M\left(\frac{1}{1+\frac{k_d}{2}}\right)^{2n} \tag{17-1a}$$

$$= I/2(DFa_{k_d/2,2n}) + M(DF_{k_d/2,2n}).$$

To illustrate, assume now that a firm, Super-Natural Foods, has a bond that has a 15 percent coupon, a par value of $1,000, and 15 years to maturity. If interest is paid semiannually, the firm will pay $75 interest per bond every 6 months rather than $150 at the end of each year. Thus each interest payment is only half as large, but there are twice as many of them. When the going rate of interest is 10 percent, the value of this 15-year bond is found as follows:

$$V = \$75(DFa_{5\%,30 \ periods}) + \$1,000(DF_{5\%,30 \ periods})$$

$$= \$75(15.3725) + \$1,000(0.2314)$$

$$= \$1,152.94 + \$231.40$$

$$= \$1,384.34.$$

If the bond has paid its interest annually, the bond's price would have been:

$$V = \$150(DFa_{10\%,15 \ periods}) + \$1,000(DF_{10\%,15 \ periods})$$

$$= \$150(7.6061) + \$1,000(0.2394)$$

$$= \$1,140.92 + \$239.40$$

$$= \$1,380.32.$$

The $1,384.34 value with semiannual interest payments is slightly larger than $1,380.32, the bond's value when interest is paid annually. The higher value occurs because interest payments are received somewhat faster and compounded more often under semiannual compounding.

When bonds pay interest semiannually, students sometimes want to discount the maturity value (M = $1,000) at 10 percent over 15 periods, rather than at the correct 5 percent over 30 six-month periods. This is *incorrect*; logically, all cash flows in a given contract must be discounted on the same basis — semiannually in this instance. For consistency, bond traders *must* apply semiannual compounding to the maturity value, and they do.

Chapter 18

Common Stock

Fred Adler's Big Giveaway

In 1983 Biotechnology General Corporation (BTC) was like a lot of other small genetic engineering companies: it did research only and did not as yet have any products ready to market. During its three years of existence, BTG had lost $5.86 million, and it now badly needed a new infusion of capital.

BTG's chairman was Fred Adler, a venture capitalist with a reputation for backing hot new businesses. To raise the needed capital, Adler, who owned 60 percent of the company's stock, decided to sell shares to the public.

Adler's original plan was to sell 1 million shares of common stock at $15 to $17 per share. Because of unpredictable market conditions, however, he reduced the offering to 800,000 shares at $13 each. Adler could have chosen to delay the offering until the market for new issues improved, but he preferred to go ahead, as the market had been generally good that year. From his point of view, his job as a venture capitalist was to fund his company, not try to figure out when the market would be ripe. "If the company does a good job, its stock price will eventually reflect that," Adler observed.

According to Robert Doolittle, corporate finance manager at BTG's lead underwriter, J. C. Bradford & Co., orders for the stock looked solid after the reduction. No one could have predicted what happened next.

Trouble began the first day the stock was issued. Because Adler's name was involved, a lot of people rushed to buy BTG stock. But when the price didn't rise rapidly, as had been expected, they began selling back to the syndicate. Under so much pressure, the syndicate was unable to maintain the stock's price, which fell from 13 to 10¼.

A week later, things got even worse. BTG conducted its research in Israel. When a currency crisis hit that country, nervous BTG investors sold off their stock, knocking the price down to 8¼. At that point Adler decided he should do something nice for his remaining shareholders.

As you read this chapter, consider the pros and cons of Adler's decision to issue BTG stock despite a highly volatile market. How were investors, the investment banking syndicate, and BTG each affected by the decision? What could Adler do to compensate his shareholders for their losses?

See end of chapter for resolution.

Common stock — or, for unincorporated businesses, the proprietors' or partners' capital — represents the ownership of a firm. In earlier chapters we discussed the legal and accounting aspects of common stock and the markets in which it is traded. Now we consider some of the rights and privileges of equity holders, the process by which investors establish the value of equity shares in the marketplace, and the procedures involved when firms raise new capital by issuing additional shares of stock.

LEGAL RIGHTS AND PRIVILEGES OF THE COMMON STOCKHOLDERS

The common stockholders are the owners of the corporation, and as such they have certain rights and privileges. The most important of these are discussed in this section.

Control of the Firm

The stockholders have the right to elect the firm's directors, who in turn select the officers who manage the business. In a small firm the major stockholder typically assumes the positions of president and chairman of the board of directors. In a large, publicly owned firm the managers typically have some stock, but their personal holdings are insufficient to exercise voting control; thus the management of a publicly owned firm can be removed by the stockholders if the stockholder group decides that the management is not effective.

Various state and federal laws stipulate how stockholder control is to be exercised. Corporations must hold an election of directors periodically, usually once a year, with the vote taken at the annual meeting. Frequently, one third of the directors are elected each year for a three-year term. Each share of stock has one vote; thus the owner of 1,000 shares has 1,000 votes. Stockholders can appear at the annual meeting and vote in person, or they can transfer their right to vote to a second party by means of an instrument known as a **proxy.** Management always solicits stockholders' proxies and usually gets them. However, if earnings are poor or stockholders are otherwise dissatisfied, an outside group may solicit the proxies in an effort to overthrow management and take over control of the business. This is known as a **proxy fight.**

The question of control has become a central issue in finance in recent years. The frequency of proxy fights has increased, as have attempts by one corporation to take over another by purchasing a majority of the outstanding stock. This latter action, which is called a *takeover,* is discussed in detail in Chapter 22. Some well-known examples of recent takeover battles include DuPont's acquisition of Conoco, Chevron's acquisition of Gulf Oil, and CBS's successful defense of a takeover attempt by Ted Turner — although CBS's management later lost control to a group headed by Lawrence Tisch.

Managers who do not have majority control of their firm's stock (over 50 percent) are very concerned about takeovers, and many of them are attempting

proxy
A document giving one person the authority to act for another; typically, it is the authority to vote shares of common stock.

proxy fight
An attempt by a person, group, or company to gain control of a company by getting the stockholders to vote a new management into office.

to get stockholder approval for changes in their corporate charters that would make takeovers more difficult. For example, a number of companies in the 1980s have moved to get their stockholders to agree (1) to elect only one third of the directors each year (rather than to elect all directors each year) and (2) to require 75 percent of the stockholders (rather than 50) percent to approve a merger. Managements seeking such changes generally indicate a fear of the firm's being picked up at a bargain price, but some stockholders wonder whether concern about their jobs may not be an even more important consideration.

The Right to Purchase New Stock: The Preemptive Right

Common stockholders often have the right, called the **preemptive right,** to purchase, on a pro rata basis, any additional shares sold by the firm. In some states the preemptive right is made a part of every corporate charter; in others it is necessary to insert the preemptive right specifically into the charter.

    The purpose of the preemptive right is twofold. First, it protects the power of control of present stockholders. If it were not for this safeguard, the management of a corporation under criticism from stockholders could prevent stockholders from removing it from office by issuing a large number of additional shares and purchasing these shares itself. Management would thereby secure control of the corporation to frustrate the will of the current stockholders.

    The second, and by far the more important, protection that the preemptive right affords stockholders regards dilution of value. For example, assume that 1,000 shares of common stock, each with a price of $100, are outstanding, making the total market value of the firm $100,000. An additional 1,000 shares are sold at $50 a share, or for $50,000, thus raising the total market value of the firm to $150,000. When the total market value is divided by the new total shares outstanding, a value of $75 a share is obtained. If such an event occurred, the original stockholders would lose $25 per share whereas the new stock purchasers would have an instant profit of $25. Thus selling common stock at below-market values dilutes the stock's price and is detrimental to the initial stockholders and beneficial to those who purchase the new shares. The preemptive right prevents such a loss of wealth for the original stockholders.[1]

Types of Common Stock

Although most firms have only one type of common stock, in some instances **classified stock** is created to meet the special needs of the company. Generally, when different types of stock are used, one type is designated *Class A,* the second *Class B,* and so on. Small, new companies seeking to acquire funds

preemptive right
A provision contained in the corporate charter and bylaws that gives holders of common stocks the right to purchase on a pro rata basis new issues of common stock (or securities convertible into common stock).

classified stock
Common stock that is given special designations, such as Class A, Class B, and so forth, to meet special needs of the company.

---

[1]The procedure for issuing stock to existing stockholders, called a *rights offering,* is discussed in detail in Eugene F. Brigham and Louis Gapenski, *Intermediate Financial Management,* 2nd ed., Chapter 12.

Stock certificates, such as this sample from The Boeing Company, are issued to common stockholders as owners of the corporation. The certificate states the value of the stock (in this case $5 each) and the number of shares purchased, which would be shown in the boxed area in the upper right corner. Note the similarity of this certificate to that of the bond in Chapter 17. The intricate border designs of both are done to make counterfeiting difficult (as with U.S. dollar bills).

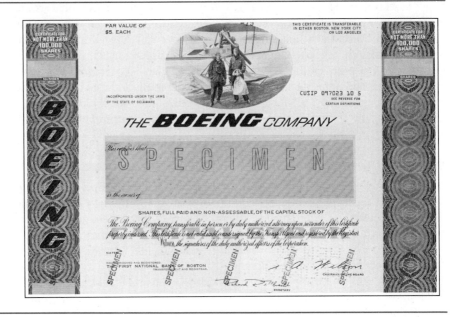

Source: Courtesy of The Boeing Company.

from outside sources sometimes use different types of common stock. For example, when Silicon Systems went public in 1987, its Class A stock was sold to the public, and although this stock classification pays a dividend, it provides no voting rights to the purchasers until 1994. The Class B stock, which maintains all voting privileges, was retained by the organizers of the company. However, this stock classification will not receive any dividends until the company has established its earning power by building up retained earnings to a designated level. By the use of classified stock, the public can take a position in a conservatively financed growth firm without sacrificing dividend income. The Class B stock, in similar situations, is often called **founders' shares** and is given *sole* voting rights in the firm's formative years. This permits the organizers of the firm to maintain complete control of the operations in the crucial early stages of the firm's development. At the same time, other investors are protected against excessive withdrawals of funds by the original owners.

founders' shares

Classified stock that has sole voting rights and restricted dividends; it is owned by the firm's founders.

Columbia Electric provides an example of yet another type of classification. This company has Class A common that pays a $3.16 annual dividend versus $2.75 for the Class B common. If earnings increase and the dividend on the Class B stock is raised to a level above $3.16, the Class A stockholders can convert to Class B. Conversion from A to B will occur automatically in 1991, if voluntary conversion has not occurred earlier. The reason for selling the Class A was quite simple; although Columbia needed money badly in 1981, it could not sell debt because of indenture restrictions, it could not sell preferred stock because of other restrictions, and it could not sell regular common because the market would not absorb it without depressing the price very badly. The Class A common was the only feasible alternative.

Note that "Class A," "Class B," and so on have no standard meanings. Most firms have no classified shares. Also, one firm may designate its Class B shares as founders' shares and its Class A shares as those sold to the public. Another firm can reverse these designations. Other firms, like Columbia Electric, can use the A and B designations for entirely different purposes.

COMMON STOCK VALUATION

As we have noted, a share of common stock represents participation in the ownership of a firm. To the majority of shareholders, however, it is more valued for the returns that can be gained from its purchase. These returns come from two sources:

1. **Cash dividends.** The owner of common stock is entitled to dividends, but there is no guarantee that they will be paid in any given period. In order for common stock dividends to be paid, the firm must first generate earnings from which dividends can be paid, and then management must decide to pay dividends rather than retain after-tax earnings.[2] Interest payments on debt, on the other hand, are fixed legal obligations that *must* be paid. Failure to pay interest when it comes due means that the firm is actually bankrupt.

2. **Capital gains.** When purchasers of common stock buy their securities, they generally expect that the stock's price will increase in the future. If the stock is sold later at a price above its purchase price, the investor receives a *capital gain.* Of course, the investor can expect a capital gain but end up with a capital loss instead.

Definitions of Terms Used in the Stock Valuation Models

An asset's value is determined by the benefits that the asset provides a purchaser. Financial assets provide *cash flows,* and their value is equal to the present value of those cash flows. The value of a share of common stock is determined by the present value of its cash flows, which consist of dividends as long as ownership in the stock is maintained, and, if the stock is sold, expected capital gains.

We have learned in Chapter 1 that the goal of financial management is to maximize the wealth of the owners of the firm. To accomplish this goal, financial managers seek to maximize the value of their investors' stock. Through their actions, managers affect the stream of cash flows to the investors as well as the riskiness of these cash flows. Therefore, financial managers must learn

---

[2]We note in Chapter 21 that although most companies will make extraordinary efforts to pay dividends regularly and not let the dollar amount of those dividends decline, this effort does not guarantee the firm's ability to maintain its dividends.

how their actions will affect stock prices. At this point we develop some models to better understand how the value of a share of stock is determined under several different sets of conditions. We begin by defining the following terms:

D_t = the dividend the stockholder expects to receive at the end of Year t. D_0 is the most recent dividend, which has already been paid; D_1 is the next dividend, which will be paid at the end of this year; D_2 is the dividend expected at the end of two years; and so on.

P_t = the price of the stock at the end of each year t. P_0 is the price of the stock today; P_1 is the price expected at the end of one year; and so on.

g = the expected rate of growth in the stock price. (In most of our models, g is also the expected rate of growth in earnings and dividends. In addition, we assume that g will be constant over time.)

required rate of return
The minimum rate of return on common stock that stockholders consider acceptable.

k_s = the minimum acceptable or **required rate of return** on the stock, considering both its riskiness and the returns available on other investments.

expected rate of return
The rate of return on common stock that an individual stockholder actually expects to receive.

$\hat{k}_s$ = (pronounced "k hat") the **expected rate of return** that the individual who buys the stock actually expects to receive. The caret, or "hat," is used to indicate that $\hat{k}_s$ is a predicted value. $\hat{k}_s$ could be above or below k_s, but one would buy the stock only if $\hat{k}_s$ were equal to or greater than k_s.

dividend yield
The ratio of the current dividend to the current price of a share of stock.

D_1/P_0 = the expected **dividend yield** on the stock during the coming year. If the stock is expected to pay a dividend of $1 during the next 12 months, and if its current price is $10, the dividend yield is $1/$10 = 0.10 = 10%.

capital gains yield
The capital gain during any one year divided by the beginning price.

$\dfrac{P_1 - P_0}{P_0}$ = the expected **capital gains yield** on the stock during the coming year. If the stock sells for $10 today, and if it is expected to rise to $10.50 at the end of one year, the expected capital gain is $P_1 - P_0 = \$10.50 - \$10.00 = \$0.50$, and the expected capital gains yield is $0.50/$10 = 0.05 = 5%. If the stock price grows at a constant rate, then the growth rate, g, is equal to the capital gains yield.

Total return = Dividend yield + Capital gains yield = k_s = 10% + 5% = 15%.

Expected Dividends as the Basis for Stock Values

As we mentioned before, the value of any financial or real asset that we will study is the present value of its cash flows. For example, in our discussion of capital budgeting, the present value of a project was equal to the project's cash flow (consisting of the project-related net income and depreciation) discounted back to the present:

$$V = \sum_{t=1}^{n} \frac{CF_t}{(1 + k)^t}.$$

Similarly, in Chapter 17 we found the value of a bond to be the present value of its stream of payments, in this case the present value of the interest payments over the life of the bond plus the present value of the bond's maturity or par value:

$$V = \frac{I}{(1 + k_d)^1} + \frac{I}{(1 + k_d)^2} + \cdots + \frac{I}{(1 + k_d)^n} + \frac{M}{(1 + k_d)^n}.$$

Therefore, if all other assets are valued at the present value of their future expected cash returns, one should not expect the valuation model for common stock to be any different. Common stock values are determined by the present value of a stream of cash flows associated with owning the stock. But what is the stream of cash flows that a corporation provides its stockholders? As long as an individual owns stock, the only cash received is in the form of *dividends.* Thus the value of a share of common stock is calculated as the present value of an infinite stream of dividends:

Value of stock $= P_0 =$ PV of expected future dividends

$$= \frac{D_1}{(1 + k_s)^1} + \frac{D_2}{(1 + k_s)^2} + \cdots + \frac{D_\infty}{(1 + k_s)^\infty}. \quad \textbf{(18-1)}$$

What about a more reasonable case, one in which stock is purchased to be held for a shorter, finite period? Will the value of the stock change? In a word, *no.* Assume that you plan to hold a share of stock for only five years. The value of the stock will equal the present value of the dividends over the five-year period plus the present value of the stock's selling price in the fifth year:

$$P_0 = \sum_{t=1}^{5} \frac{D_t}{(1 + k_s)^t} + \frac{P_5}{(1 + k_s)^5}. \quad \textbf{(18-2)}$$

The next question is: What would a rational investor pay for the stock in that future year? The rational investor would be willing to pay only the present value of the future flows that are expected during the future ownership period. What are those flows? Dividends, of course! Therefore

$$P_5 = \sum_{t=6}^{\infty} \frac{D_t}{(1 + k_s)^t}. \quad \textbf{(18-3)}$$

If we substitute into Equation 18-2 the value of the stock in Year 5, found in Equation 18-3, it is obvious that even when the stock is sold at some future date *the value of the stock is still determined by the general model of discounted future cash flows presented in Equation 18-1.* To see this, recognize that for any individual investor, the expected cash flows consist of expected dividends plus the expected sale price of the stock. However, the sale price the current investor receives will be dependent upon the dividends some future investor expects to receive. Therefore, for *all* present and future investors expected cash flows must be based on expected future dividends. To put it another way, unless a firm is liquidated or sold to another concern, the cash flows it provides to its stockholders consist only of a stream of dividends, so the value of a share of its stock must be established as the present value of that expected dividend stream.

Equation 18-1 is a generalized stock valuation model in the sense that the pattern of dividend payments can be anything; D_t can be rising, falling, or constant, or it can even be fluctuating randomly, and Equation 18-1 will still hold. Even so, it is often difficult, even for professionals, to estimate future dividend payments beyond a few periods. In the next section we develop a simplified stock valuation model, based on the concepts from Equation 18-1, which makes only two simplifying assumptions: (1) that the growth in earnings and dividends for the firm will progress at a constant rate into the future, and (2) that $k_s > g$.

"Normal," or Constant, Growth

As firms stabilize in the maturity phase of their life cycles, the growth of their earnings and dividends tends to stabilize as well. This period of stability is not one of stagnation but rather one of moderate growth. In general, this growth is expected to continue into the foreseeable future at about the same rate as that of the nominal gross national product (real GNP plus inflation). On this basis, it is expected that a "normal" or constant growth company will grow at a rate of approximately 5 to 10 percent a year.

If we wish to determine next year's dividend, D_1, for a firm whose future growth is expected to be constant, we need only multiply last year's dividend, D_0, by the expected growth rate. Thus, if Carter Chemical Company has just paid a dividend of $1.87 and investors expect a 7 percent growth rate for the company throughout the foreseeable future, next year's dividend, D_1, may be found in the following manner:

$$D_1 = D_0(1 + g)$$

$$= \$1.87(1.07)$$

$$= \$2.00.$$

Equation 18-1 describes the valuation of a share of common stock as the present value of all future cash flows, and for common stock that flow is dividends. If those dividends are expected to grow *at a constant rate, g,* Equation 18-1 can be simplified as follows.[3]

---

[3]We spare the reader the mathematical proof of our assertion. For those who are interested, the derivation of Equation 18-4 is provided in Eugene F. Brigham and Louis Gapenski, *Intermediate Financial Management,* 2nd ed., Appendix 3A.

$$P_0 = \frac{D_1}{k_s - g}. \qquad\qquad (18\text{-}4)$$

If investors require a 12 percent return from an investment in Carter's common stock, k_s, the value of the firm's common stock can be determined by substituting into Equation 18-4 the values for next year's dividend, the required return on Carter's equity, and the firm's expected growth rate:

$$P_0 = \frac{D_1}{k_s - g}$$

$$= \frac{\$2.00}{0.12 - 0.07}$$

$$= \frac{\$2.00}{0.05} = \$40.00.$$

Recall that we can come to the same conclusion — the price of Carter's common stock is $40 — by utilizing the more cumbersome Equation 18-1. The simplification provided by Equation 18-4 is often referred to as the *Gordon Model,* after Professor Myron J. Gordon, who did much to develop and popularize it.

The concept underlying the valuation process in Equation 18-4 is presented graphically in Figure 18-1. The top dashed curve represents the dollar value of Carter's dividends growing at a 7 percent rate. The bottom dashed line plots the present value of those dividends. The value of the firm's common stock may be obtained by adding the present value of each future year's dividend, as suggested by Equation 18-1, or, because the dividends are growing at a constant rate, the value may be found by utilizing Equation 18-4. In either case the result will be *exactly the same.*

Constant growth of future dividends is a necessary condition that must be observed when utilizing Equation 18-4. For this equation to have any economic validity, another important condition is that the constant growth rate, g, must always be less than the required rate of return, k_s. Although there are several excellent economic reasons to assert that k_s will never be smaller than g, the model has no rational meaning if $g \geq k_s$. For example, if Carter's $k_s = 12\%$, $D_1 = \$2.00$, but $g = 15\%$, then

$$P_0 = \frac{\$2.00}{0.12 - 0.15}$$

$$= \frac{\$2.00}{-0.03}$$

$$= -\$66.67.$$

This result indicates that a present owner of Carter's equity would be willing to give you a share of the stock *and* $66.67 to induce you to take it. A highly

Figure 18-1 **Growing Dividend Stream and
Present Value of the Stream:**
$$D_0 = \$1.87, g = 7\%, k_s = 12\%$$

This figure illustrates a stock valuation model. The value of a share of common stock equals the present value of all future dividends. This example assumes that these dividends will grow at a constant rate. The $2.00 dividend for the first year (D_1) has a present value (PV) of $1.87. At a growth rate (g) of 7 percent and an expected rate of return (k_s) of 12 percent, we can plot the growing dividend stream both in actual dollar amounts and in present values into infinity. Adding discounted future dividends yields the present value of the firm's stock.

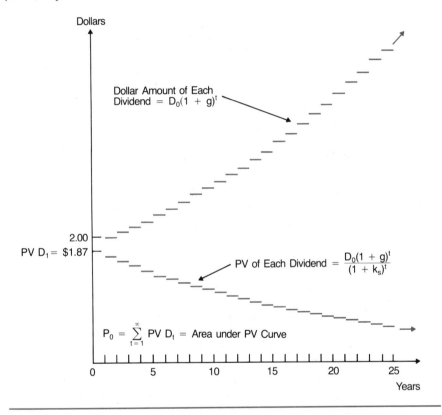

unlikely scenario! Therefore, the Gordon Model, Equation 18-4, always requires a constant rate of growth, g, and further requires that $k_s > g$.[4]

---

[4]Note that the growth rate in Equation 18-4 can be equal to zero. If growth was equal to zero, Equation 18-4 would simplify to $P = D/k_s$. Because the firm is not growing, there would be no difference in dividends in any period, so $D_0 = D_1 = D_2$, etc. As we will see in Chapter 21, since there are no growth opportunities for the firm, the firm would pay out all earnings as dividends, so $E_1 = D_1 = E_2$, etc. Therefore, an alternative measure of the stock price of a *no-growth* firm is $P = E/k_s$.

It should be made clear that the constant-growth valuation model is intended to price the equity shares of a company that has normal or constantly growing earnings and dividends. However, for a firm that is in the early stages of its life cycle or in a highly variable economic environment, Equation 18-4 may not provide an effective means of equity valuation. Equation 18-4 would be a poor choice to use in evaluating the share price of a new high-technology firm, but it would probably provide an excellent approximation of the economic value of a mature company. Therefore, the more variable the growth rate in earnings and hence dividends, the less satisfactory job the model represented by Equation 18-4 will do in valuing a firm.

Expected Rate of Return for a Constant Growth Stock

When investors purchase stock that they expect to sell in the future, their expected rate of return is determined by the stock's expected dividend yield and the expected capital gains yield. We can demonstrate this relationship by algebraically rearranging Equation 18-4 into Equation 18-5:

$$\text{Expected rate of return} = \begin{array}{c} \text{Expected dividend} \\ \text{yield} \end{array} + \begin{array}{c} \text{Expected capital} \\ \text{gains yield} \end{array}$$

$$\hat{k}_s = \frac{D_1}{P_0} + g. \tag{18-5}$$

Thus, if you buy a stock for a price $P_0 = \$40.00$, and if you expect the stock to pay a dividend $D_1 = \$2.00$ one year from now and to grow at a constant rate $g = 7\%$ in the future, your expected rate of return is 12 percent:

$$\hat{k}_s = \frac{\$2.00}{\$40.00} + 7\% = 5\% + 7\% = 12\%.$$

In this form, we see that $\hat{k}_s$ is the *expected total return* and that it consists of an *expected dividend yield,* $D_1/P_0 = 5\%$, plus an *expected growth rate* or *capital gains yield,* $g = 7\%$.

Suppose that the previously described analysis had been conducted on January 1, 1988, so $P_0 = \$40.00$ is the January 1, 1988, stock price and $D_1 = \$2.00$ is the dividend expected at the end of 1988 (or the beginning of 1989). What should the stock price be at the end of 1988 (or the beginning of 1989)? We would again apply Equation 18-4, but this time we would use the 1990 dividend, $D_2 = D_1(1 + g) = \$2.00(1.07) = \$2.14$:

$$\hat{P}_{1/1/1989} = \frac{D_{1990}}{k_s - g} = \frac{\$2.14}{0.12 - 0.07} = \$42.80.$$

Now notice that $\$42.80$ is 7 percent greater than P_0, the $\$40.00$ price on January 1, 1988:

$$\$40.00(1.07) = \$42.80.$$

Thus you would expect to make a capital gain of $42.80 - $40.00 = $2.80 during the year, and a capital gains yield of 7 percent:

$$\text{Capital gains yield} = \frac{\text{Capital gain}}{\text{Beginning price}} = \frac{\$2.80}{\$40.00} = 0.07 = 7\%.$$

We could extend the analysis on out, and in each future year the expected capital gains yield would always equal g, the expected dividend growth rate. The dividend yield in 1989 can be estimated as follows:

$$\text{Dividend yield}_{1989} = \frac{D_{1990}}{\hat{P}_{1989}} = \frac{\$2.14}{\$42.80} = 0.05 = 5\%.$$

The dividend yield for 1990 could also be calculated, and again it would be 5 percent. Thus, *for a constant growth stock,* these conditions will hold:

1. The dividend is expected to grow at a constant rate, g.

2. The stock price is expected to grow at the same rate.

3. The expected dividend yield is a constant.

4. The expected capital gains yield is also a constant, and it is equal to g.

5. The expected total rate of return, $\hat{k}$, is equal to the expected dividend yield plus the expected growth rate.

Supernormal, or Nonconstant, Growth

supernormal (non-constant) growth
The part of the life cycle of a firm in which its growth is much faster than that of the economy as a whole.

Firms typically go through *life cycles.* During the early part of the cycles, their growth is much faster than that of the economy as a whole; then they match the economy's growth; and finally their growth is slower than that of the economy. Automobile manufacturers in the 1920s and computer software firms like Lotus in the 1980s are examples of firms in the early part of the cycle, and these firms are called **supernormal,** or **nonconstant, growth** firms. Figure 18-2 illustrates such nonconstant growth and compares it with normal growth, zero growth, and negative growth.

In the figure, the dividends of the supernormal growth firm are expected to grow at a 30 percent rate for 3 years, after which the growth rate is expected to fall to 10 percent, the assumed norm for the economy. The value of this firm, like any other, is the present value of its expected future dividends as determined by Equation 18-1. In the case in which D_t was growing at a constant rate, we simplified Equation 18-1 to $P_0 = D_1/(k_s - g)$. In the supernormal case, however, the expected growth rate is not a constant; it declines at the end of the period of supernormal growth. To find the value of such a stock, or any nonconstant growth stock when the growth rate will eventually stabilize, we proceed in three steps:

Figure 18-2 **Illustrative Dividend Growth Rates**

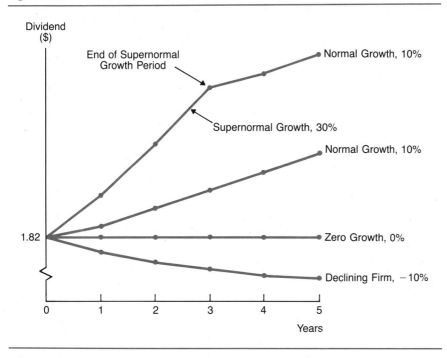

1. Find the present value (PV) of the dividends during the period of nonconstant growth.

2. Find the price of the stock at the end of the nonconstant growth period, at which point it has become a constant growth stock, and then discount this price back to the present.

3. Add these two components to find the intrinsic value of the stock, P_0.

To illustrate the process for valuing nonconstant growth stocks, suppose the following facts exist:

k_s = stockholders' required rate of return = 16%.
N = years of supernormal growth = 3.
g_s = rate of growth in both earnings and dividends during the supernormal growth period = 30%.
g_n = rate of growth after the supernormal period = 6%.
D_0 = last dividend the company paid = $1.82.

The valuation process is graphed in Figure 18-3 and explained in the steps that follow.

Figure 18-3 **Time Line for Finding the Value of a Supernormal Growth Stock**

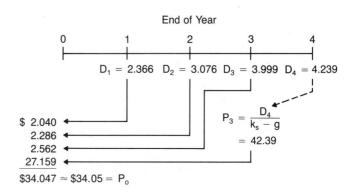

Note: P_3, the stock price expected at the end of Year 3, is the sum of the PVs of dividends in Years 4 to infinity; hence $P_3 = D_4/(k_s - g_n)$.

Step 1. Find the PV of dividends paid (PV D_t) at the end of Years 1 to 3 using this procedure:

D_0	×	$FVIF_{30\%,t}$	=	D_t	×	$PVIF_{16\%,t}$	=	$PV\ D_t$
D_1: $1.82	×	1.3000	=	$2.366	×	0.8621	=	$2.040
D_2: 1.82	×	1.6900	=	3.076	×	0.7432	=	2.286
D_3: 1.82	×	2.1970	=	3.999	×	0.6407	=	2.562

Sum of PVs of supernormal period dividends = $6.888

Step 2. Find the PV of the dividends expected in Year 4 and thereafter. This requires that we (a) first find the expected value of the stock at the end of Year 3 and (b) then find the present value of the Year 3 stock price:

a.
$$P_3 = \frac{D_4}{k_s - g_n} = \frac{D_0(1 + g_s)^3(1 + g_n)}{k_s - g_n} = \frac{D_3(1 + g_n)}{0.16 - 0.07}$$

$$= \frac{\$3.999(1.06)}{0.16 - 0.06} = \frac{\$4.239}{0.10} = \$42.39.$$

b. $PV\ P_3 = \$42.39(PVIF_{16\%,3\ years}) = \$42.39(0.6407) = \$27.16.$

Step 3. Find P_0, the value of the stock today:

$$P_0 = \$6.89 + \$27.16 = \$34.05.$$

EVALUATION OF COMMON STOCK AS A SOURCE OF FUNDS

So far this chapter has covered the main characteristics of common stock and how its price is determined. Now we will appraise the advantages and disadvantages of stock financing from the viewpoint of the corporation and its creditors.

Advantages of Common Stock Financing

There are several advantages to the corporation associated with common stock financing:

1. Common stock does not carry a fixed obligation to pay periodic dividends to stockholders. When a firm uses debt, it incurs a legal obligation to pay interest on it, regardless of its operating conditions, its cash flows, and so on. When the company uses equity financing, however, it can pay common stock dividends if it generates earnings and has no pressing internal needs for them.

2. Common stock, unlike debt issues, never matures; hence it never has to be repaid at some future date.

3. Common stock provides a cushion against losses from the creditors' viewpoint. Therefore, the sale of common stock increases the proportion of equity financing and thus the firm's creditworthiness. This, in turn, should raise the firm's bond rating, lower its cost of debt, and increase its future ability to use debt.

4. When a company's prospects look bright, common stock can often be sold on better terms than debt. Stock appeals to certain groups of investors because (a) it carries a higher expected total return (dividends plus capital gains) than preferred stock or debt and (b) since stock represents the ownership of the firm, it provides the investor with a better hedge against unanticipated inflation than does preferred stock or bonds. Ordinarily, common stock increases in value when the firm's real asset values rise during inflationary periods.

5. When a company is having operating problems, it often needs new funds to overcome its problms. However, investors are reluctant to supply equity capital to a troubled company. From a practical standpoint, this means that a firm that is experiencing problems can often obtain new capital only by issuing debt, which is safer from the investor's standpoint. Corporate treasurers are well aware of this, so they often choose to finance with common stock so as to maintain a reserve borrowing capacity. Indeed, surveys have indicated that maintenance of an adequate reserve of borrowing capacity is the primary consideration in most financing decisions.

Disadvantages of Common Stock Financing

Disadvantages to a company that issues common stock include the following:

1. The sale of common stock extends voting rights, and therefore perhaps control, to new stockholders. For this reason, additional equity financing is often avoided by managers who are concerned about maintaining control.

The use of classified stock or founders' shares can, however, mitigate this problem.

2. Common stock gives new owners the right to share in the income of the firm. If profits soar, the new stockholders get to share in this bonanza, whereas if debt had been used, new investors would have received only a fixed return no matter how profitable the company became.

3. As we shall see, the costs of underwriting and distributing common stock are usually higher than those for underwriting and distributing preferred stock or debt. Flotation costs associated with the sale of common stock are characteristically higher, because the costs of investigating an equity security investment are higher than those for a comparable debt security. Also, because stocks are riskier than debt, investors must diversify their equity holdings, which in turn means that a given dollar amount of new stock must be sold to a larger number of purchasers than the same amount of debt.

4. As we will learn in Chapter 19, the cost of capital for equity is greater than the cost of debt. Therefore, if the firm has more equity than required for its optimal capital structure, the average cost of capital will be higher than necessary. Therefore, a firm will not want to sell stock to the point where its equity ratio exceeds this optimal level.

5. Under current tax laws, common stock dividends are not deductible as an expense for calculating the corporation's taxable income, but bond interest is deductible. As we will also see in Chapter 19, the impact of this factor is reflected in an even lower effective cost of debt.

THE DECISION TO GO PUBLIC

As we noted in Chapter 2, most businesses begin their lives as proprietorships or partnerships, but as they grow, they find it desirable to convert at some point to a corporation. The ownership of these young corporations is often kept in the hands of the founders, a few key employees, and perhaps a limited number of investors who are not actively involved in management. As the firm grows, it will probably outgrow its ability to finance its equity needs through internal sources or the increased investment of the owners. Whenever a closely held firm offers stock to the public for the first time, it is said to be **going public.** The advantages and disadvantages of public ownership are discussed next.

going public
The act of selling stock to the public for the first time by a closely held corporation or its principal stockholders.

Advantages of Going Public

Facilitates Stockholder Diversification. As a company grows and becomes more valuable, its founders often have most of their wealth tied up in the company. By selling some of their stock in a public offering, the founders can diversify their holdings and thereby reduce somewhat the riskiness of their personal portfolios.

Increases Liquidity. The stock of a closely held firm is illiquid and cannot be easily sold because no ready market exists for it. If an owner wishes to sell some shares to raise cash, it is hard to find potential buyers, and even if a buyer is located, there is no established price at which to complete the transaction. These problems do not exist with publicly owned firms.

Facilitates Raising New Corporate Cash. If a privately held company wants to raise cash by a sale of new stock, it must either go to its existing owners, who may not have any money or may not want to put any more eggs into this particular basket, or shop around for wealthy investors who are willing to make an investment in the company. However, it is usually difficult to get outsiders to put money into a closely held company, because of low diversification, low liquidity, and the disadvantages new shareholders face if they hold less than 50 percent of the stock. The inside stockholders-managers can pay or not pay dividends, pay themselves exorbitant salaries, have private deals with the company, and so on. Similarly, insiders can even keep the outsiders from knowing the company's actual earnings or its real worth. There are not many positions more vulnerable than that of an outside stockholder in a closely held company, and for this reason it is hard for closely held companies to raise new equity capital. Going public, which brings with it disclosure and regulation by the Securities and Exchange Commission (SEC) greatly reduces these problems and makes people more willing to invest in the company.

Establishes a Value for the Firm. For a number of reasons, it is often useful to establish a firm's value in the marketplace. For one thing, when the owner of a privately owned business dies, state and federal inheritance tax appraisers must set a value on the company for estate tax purposes. Often these appraisers set too high a value, which creates all sorts of problems. However, a company that is publicly owned has its value established, with little room for argument. Similarly, if a company wants to give incentive stock options to key employees, it is useful to know the exact value of these options; employees much prefer to own stock, or options on stock, that is publicly traded, because public trading increases liquidity.

Disadvantages of Going Public

Cost of Reporting. A publicly owned company must file quarterly and annual reports with the SEC or various state officials (or both). These reports can be costly, especially for small firms.

Disclosure. Management may not like the idea of reporting operating data, because such data will then be available to competitors. Similarly, the owners of the company may not want people to know their net worth. Since publicly owned companies must disclose the number of shares owned by officers, directors, and major stockholders, it is easy enough for anyone to multiply number of shares held by price per share to estimate the insiders' net worth.

Self-dealings. The owners-managers of closely held companies have many opportunities for various types of questionable but legal self-dealings, including the payment of high salaries, nepotism, personal transactions with the business (such as a leasing arrangement), excellent retirement programs, and not-truly-necessary fringe benefits. Such self-dealings are much harder to arrange if a company is publicly owned; they must be disclosed, and the managers are also subject to stockholder suits.

Inactive Market/Low Price. If a firm is very small, and if its shares are not traded with much frequency, its stock will not truly be liquid, and the market price may not be representative of the stock's real value. Security analysts and stockbrokers simply will not follow the stock, because there will not be sufficient trading activity to generate enough sales commissions to cover the analysts' or brokers' costs of keeping up with it.

Control. Because of the dramatic increase in tender offers and proxy fights in the 1980s, the managers of publicly owned firms who do not have at least 50 percent of the stock must be concerned about maintaining control. Further, there is pressure on such managers to produce annual earnings gains, even when it is in the shareholders' best long-term interest to adopt a strategy that may penalize short-run earnings but leads to higher earnings in future years. These factors have led a number of public companies to "go private" in leveraged buyout deals in which the managers borrow the money to buy out the nonmanagement stockholders.

Conclusions on Going Public

It should be obvious from this discussion that there are no hard and fast rules about whether or when a company should go public. It is an individual decision that should be made on the basis of the company's and its stockholders' unique circumstances.

If a company does decide to go public, either by the sale of newly issued stock to raise new capital for the corporation or by the sale of stock by the current owners, one key issue is that of setting the price at which shares will be offered to the public. The company and its current owners want to set the price as high as possible — the higher the offering price, the smaller the fraction of the company the current owners will have to give up to obtain any specified amount of money. On the other hand, potential buyers will want the price set as low as possible. The valuation models presented earlier in this chapter aid investment bankers in determining the initial selling price.

THE INVESTMENT BANKING PROCESS

The role of investment bankers was discussed in general terms in Chapter 3. There we saw (1) that the major investment banking houses are often divisions of large financial service corporations engaged in a wide range of activities and

(2) that these bankers help firms issue new securities in the primary markets and also operate as brokers in the secondary markets. Sears, Roebuck is one of the largest financial services corporations; in addition to its insurance and credit card operations, it owns a large brokerage house and a major investment banking house. Similarly, Merrill Lynch has a brokerage department that operates thousands of offices as well as an investment banking department that helps companies issue securities. Of course, Merrill Lynch's and Sears's brokers also sell securities that have been issued through their investment banking departments. In this section we describe how securities are issued and explain the role of investment bankers in this process.

Company Decisions

The firm itself makes some initial, preliminary decisions on its own, including the following:

1. *Dollars to be raised.* How much new capital is needed?

2. *Type of securities used.* Should stock, bonds, or a combination be used? Further, if stock is to be issued, should it be offered to existing stockholders or sold directly to the general public?

3. *Selection of an investment banker.* Which investment banker should the firm use? Older firms that have "been to market" before will have already established a relationship with an investment banker, although it is easy enough to change bankers if the firm is dissatisfied. A firm that is just going public will have to choose an investment banker, and different investment banking houses are better suited for different companies. Some investment banking houses specialize in new issues, whereas others are not well suited to handle new issues because their brokerage clients are relatively conservative.

Joint Decisions

After the firm has decided to issue new securities, there are still decisions to be made jointly by the firm and its selected investment banker, including the following:

1. *Reevaluating the company's initial decisions.* The firm and its banker will reevaluate the firm's initial decisions about the size of the issue and the type of securities to use. For example, the firm may have initially decided to raise $50 million by selling common stock, but the investment banker may convince management that it would be better off, in view of current market conditions, to limit the stock issue to $25 million and to raise the other $25 million as debt.

2. *Best efforts or underwritten issues.* The firm and its investment banker must decide whether the banker will work on a best efforts basis or underwrite the issue. Under a **best efforts** arrangement, the banker does not guarantee that the securities will be sold or that the company will get the

best efforts
Agreement for the sale of an issue of securities in which the investment banker handling the transaction gives no guarantee that the securities will be sold.

full underwriting
Agreement for the sale of an issue of securities in which the investment banker guarantees the sale of the securities, thus agreeing to bear any risks involved in the transaction.

cash it needs. Under a **full underwriting** arrangement, the company does get a guarantee, so the banker bears significant risks in such an offering. For example, the same day that IBM signed an agreement to sell $1 billion of bonds in 1979, interest rates rose sharply and bond prices fell. IBM's investment bankers lost somewhere between $10 million and $20 million. Had the offering been on a best efforts basis, IBM would have been the loser.

3. *Issuance costs.* The investment banker's fee must be negotiated, and the firm must also estimate the other expenses it will incur in connection with the issue — lawyers' fees, accountants' costs, printing and engraving, and so on. Usually, the banker will buy the issue from the company at a discount below the price at which the securities are to be offered to the public, and this **spread** covers the banker's costs and provides a profit.

spread
The difference between the price a security dealer pays for securities and the sale price that the dealer receives.

flotation costs
The cost of issuing a new stock or bond issue.

Table 18-1 gives an indication of the **flotation costs** associated with public issues of bonds, preferred stock, and common stock. As the table shows, costs as a percentage of the proceeds are higher for stocks than for bonds, and costs are also higher for small than for large issues. The relationship between size of issue and flotation costs is primarily the result of fixed costs. Certain costs must be incurred regardless of the size of the issue, so the percentage of flotation costs is quite high for small issues.

Also, it should be noted that when relatively small companies go public to raise new capital, the investment bankers frequently take part of their compensation in the form of options to buy stock in the firm. For example, when Data Technologies, Inc., went public with a $10 million issue in 1986 by selling 1 million shares at a price of $10, its investment bankers (1) bought the stock from the company at a price of $9.75, so the direct underwriting fee was only 1,000,000($10.00 − $9.75) = $250,000 or 2.5 percent, and (2) received a 5-year option to buy 200,000 shares at a price of $10. If the stock goes up to $15, which the bankers expect it to do, they will make a $1 million profit on top of the $250,000 underwriting fee.

4. *Setting the offering price.* If the company is already publicly owned, the offering price will be based on the existing market price of the stock or the yield on the bonds. For common stock, the most typical arrangement calls for the investment banker to buy the securities at a prescribed number of points below the closing price on the last day of registration.

If the company is going public for the first time, there will be no established price, so the investment bankers will have to estimate the *equilibrium price* at which the stock will sell after issue. Note that if the offering price is set below the true equilibrium price, the stock will rise sharply after issue and the company and its original stockholders will have given away too much stock to raise the required capital. If the offering price is set above the true equilibrium price, either the issue will fail or, if the bankers succeed in selling the stock, their investment clients will be unhappy when the stock subsequently falls to its equilibrium level. Therefore, it is important that the equilibrium price is approximated as closely as possible.

Table 18-1 **Costs of Flotation for Underwritten, Nonrights Offerings (Expressed as a Percentage of Gross Proceeds)**

Size of Issue (Millions of Dollars)	Bonds			Preferred Stock			Common Stock		
	Underwriting Commission	Other Expenses	Total Costs	Underwriting Commission	Other Expenses	Total Costs	Underwriting Commission	Other Expenses	Total Costs
Under 1.0	10.0%	4.0%	14.0%	—	—	—	13.0%	9.0%	22.0%
1.0–1.9	8.0	3.0	11.0	—	—	—	11.0	5.9	16.9
2.0–4.9	4.0	2.2	6.2	—	—	—	8.6	3.8	12.4
5.0–9.9	2.4	0.8	3.2	1.9%	0.7%	2.6%	6.3	1.9	8.2
10.0–19.9	1.2	0.7	1.9	1.4	0.4	1.8	5.1	0.9	6.0
20.0–49.9	1.0	0.4	1.4	1.4	0.3	1.7	4.1	0.5	4.6
50.0 and over	0.9	0.2	1.1	1.4	0.2	1.6	3.3	0.2	3.5

Notes:
1. Small issues of preferred are rare, so no data on preferred issues below $5 million are given.
2. Flotation costs tend to rise somewhat when interest rates are cyclically high; because money is in relatively tight supply, the investment bankers will have a difficult time placing issues with permanent investors. Thus, the figures shown here represent averages, and actual flotation costs vary somewhat over time.

Sources: Securities and Exchange Commission, *Cost of Flotation of Registered Equity Issues* (Washington, D.C.: U.S. Government Printing Office, December 1974); Richard H. Pettway, "A Note on the Flotation Costs of New Equity Capital Issues of Electric Companies," *Public Utilities Fortnightly,* March 18, 1982; Robert Hansen, "Evaluating the Costs of a New Equity Issue," *Midland Corporate Finance Journal,* Spring 1986; and informal surveys of common stock, preferred stock, and bond issues conducted by the authors.

Selling Procedures

Once the company and its investment bankers have decided how much money to raise, the type of securities to issue, and the basis for pricing the issue, they will prepare and file an SEC registration statement and a prospectus. It generally takes about 20 days for the issue to be approved by the SEC. The final price of the stock (or the interest rate on a bond issue) is set at the close of business the day the issue clears the SEC, and the securities are offered to the public the following day.

Investors are not required to pay for the stock until ten days after they place their buy orders, but the investment bankers must pay the issuing firm within four days of the time the offering officially begins. Typically, the bankers sell the stock within a day or two after the offering begins, but on occasion they miscalculate, set the offering price too high, and are unable to move the issue. At still other times the market declines during the offering period, forcing the bankers to reduce the price of the stock. In either instance, on an underwritten offering the firm receives the price that was agreed upon, and the bankers must absorb any losses that are incurred.

Because they are exposed to potentially large losses, investment bankers typically do not handle the purchase and distribution of an issue singlehandedly unless it is a very small one. If the amount of money involved is large and the risk of price fluctuations substantial, investment bankers form **underwriting syndicates** in an effort to minimize the amount of risk each one

underwriting syndicate
A syndicate of investment firms formed to spread the risk associated with the purchase and distribution of a new issue of securities.

carries. The banking house that sets up the deal is called the lead, or managing, underwriter.

In addition to the underwriting syndicate, on larger offerings still more investment bankers are included in a **selling group,** which handles the distribution of securities to individual investors. The selling group includes all members of the underwriting syndicate plus additional dealers who take relatively small participations (or shares of the total issue) from the syndicate members. Thus the underwriters act as wholesalers, whereas members of the selling group act as retailers. The number of houses in a selling group depends partly on the size of the issue; for example, the one set up when Communications Satellite Corporation (Comsat) went public consisted of 385 members.

Maintenance of the Secondary Market

In the case of a large, established firm like Carter Chemical Company, the investment banking firm's job is finished once it has disposed of the stock and turned the net proceeds over to the issuing firm. However, in the case of a company going public for the first time, the investment banker is under some obligation to maintain a market in the shares after the issue has been completed. Such stocks are typically traded in the over-the-counter market, and the principal underwriter generally agrees to "make a market" in the stock so as to keep it reasonably liquid. The company wants a good market to exist for its stock, as do the stockholders. Therefore, if the banking house wants to do business with the company in the future, keep its own brokerage customers happy, and have future referral business, it will hold an inventory and help to maintain an active secondary market in the stock.

SUMMARY

Common stock represents ownership shares in the firm. The common stockholders are the owners of the firm and enjoy all rights and privileges associated with control of the firm.

However, most purchasers buy common stock for its investment qualities. Some buy stock to hold for the foreseeable future, depending on the dividend income for their major source of returns. Others are less interested in current dividend income but are concerned with potential capital gains. This chapter has emphasized that even though the goals of these two types of investors are different, each investor should evaluate a potential investment in the same manner. Despite all the folklore associated with pricing common stock (ranging from Uncle Bernie's "inside tips" to the "bigger fool theory"), this chapter has stressed that common stock valuation is no different than the valuation of any other financial or real asset. The value of any asset is the present value of the cash flows associated with the asset's acquisition. The only cash flows that are available to the common shareholder, as long as the stock is held, are dividends. Therefore the value of a share of common stock is the present value of all of its future dividends. If the stock is subsequently sold, its value at that future date is the present value of future cash flows (dividends) that the buyer will receive from that point on.

The chapter concluded with a discussion of the advantages and disadvantages of going public and the process by which common stock is sold by the firm. The functions of the investment banker in this capital accumulation process were also evaluated.

 RESOLUTION TO DECISION IN FINANCE

Fred Adler's Big Giveaway

Because the market for Biotechnology General's stock deteriorated so rapidly, it was impossible for Fred Adler to cancel the offering before things got too far out of hand. As a result, stockholders, BTG's investment bankers, and Adler himself all lost money. Obviously, investors who bought at the original offering price of $13 and then panicked and sold at a lower price lost money in proportion to their original investments.

Investment bankers like to price an issue to maximize the amount of money raised while simultaneously allowing room for about 15 to 20 percent market appreciation in the first day or two. Because an underwriting syndicate purchases a stock offering from the issuing company at a fixed price, it stands to benefit if the stock price rises, but it also must absorb any losses that occur if the stock sells below the expected price. BTG's underwriters had to buy back stock that investors didn't want, were

forced to lower the stock's price, and then were left with unsold shares. Although underwriters never disclose their losses, it's a good bet that members of BTG's syndicate lost a substantial amount.

Fred Adler didn't like to see his public shareholders suffer, so he came up with an unorthodox plan to compensate them for their losses: he would give them five shares of BTG stock for every four shares they held. Such a generous act would only be possible for a company like BTG, where one person controlled the majority of stock and needed the agreement of only a small group of insiders. And before Fred Adler, no one had ever done such a thing.

Although Fred Adler's extraordinary giveaway didn't send BTG stock prices soaring, the stock has been steady since then, and it is doing as well as its major competitor. Adler is optimistic about the future because some of BTG's products could become commercially available very soon. Industry analysts remain cautious, however; with so many promising bio-tech companies working on similar products, it may take time for the winners to surface.

Source: "Fred Adler's One-Time-Only Stock Giveback," *Venture,* February 1984, 102.

QUESTIONS

18-1   Two investors are investigating the common stock of Multiple Basic Industries (MBI) for possible purchase. MBI is in the mature stage of its life cycle, and its earnings and dividends are growing at a constant rate. The investors agree on the expected value of D_1 and also on the expected future dividend growth rate. However, one investor normally holds stock for 2 years, whereas the other holds stock for 10 years. Based on the analysis presented in this chapter, they should both be willing to pay the same price for MBI's stock. True or false? Explain.

18-2   As we discussed in this chapter, purchasers of common stock typically expect to receive dividends plus capital gains. Would the distribution between dividends and capital gains be influenced by the firm's decision to pay more dividends rather than to retain and reinvest more of its earnings? Explain your answer.

18-3   The firm's dividend yield is defined as the next expected dividend, D_1, divided by the current price of the stock, P_0. What is the relationship between the dividend yield, the total yield, and the remaining years of supernormal growth for a supernormal growth firm?

18-4   The following expression can be used to determine the value of a constant growth stock:

$$P_0 = D_0/k_s + g.$$

Is this statement true or false? Explain your answer.

18-5   The SEC attempts to protect investors who are purchasing newly issued securities by making sure that the information put out by a company and its investment bankers is correct and is not misleading. However, the SEC *does not* provide any information about the real value of the securities; hence an investor might pay too much for some new stock and consequently lose heavily. Do you think the SEC should, as a part of every new stock or bond offering, render an opinion to investors as to the proper value of the securities being offered? Explain.

18-6   Draw a Security Market Line graph. Put dots on the graph to show (approximately) where you think a particular company's **(a)** common stock and **(b)** bonds would lie. Now where would you add a dot to represent the common stock of a riskier company?

18-7   Goss Enterprises is going public and is selling shares of its common stock for the first time. The firm sells research materials to the medical community. Because of the critical importance of their product, the firm's existence is guaranteed for many years. The firm's founder, Kendric Goss, has just announced that the firm will *never* pay a dividend. As a financial analyst, determine the price you would consider appropriate for the firm's stock.

SELF-TEST PROBLEMS

ST-1   You are considering buying the stock of two very similar companies. Both companies are expected to earn $4.50 per share this year. However, Alliance Manufacturing (AM) is expected to pay all of its earnings out as dividends, whereas Bascombe Industries (BI) is expected to pay out only one third of its earnings, or $1.50. AM's stock price is $30. Which of the following is most likely to be true?

a. BI will have a faster growth rate than AM. Therefore, BI's stock price should be greater than $30.

b. Although BI's growth rate should exceed AM's, AM's current dividend exceeds that of BI, and this should cause AM's price to exceed BI's.

c. An investor in AM will get his or her money back faster because AM pays out more of its earnings as dividends. Thus, in a sense, AM's stock is like a short-term bond, and BI's is like a long-term bond. Therefore, if economic shifts cause k_d and k_s to increase, and if the expected streams of dividends from AM and BI remain constant, AM's and BI's stock prices will both decline, but AM's price should decline further.

d. AM's expected and required rate of return is $\hat{k}_s = k_s = 15$ percent. BI's expected return will be higher because of its higher expected growth rate.

e. Based on the available information, the best estimate of BI's growth rate is 10 percent.

ST-2 You can buy a share of the Crown Company's stock today for 33⅛. Crown's last dividend was $2.50. In view of Crown's low risk, its required rate of return is only 14 percent. If dividends are expected to grow at a constant rate, g, in the future, and if k is expected to remain at 14 percent, what is Crown Company's expected stock price 5 years from now?

ST-3 TGI Group, Inc. is experiencing a period of rapid growth. Earnings and dividends are expected to grow at a rate of 18 percent during the next 2 years and 15 percent in the third year, then at a constant rate of 6 percent thereafter. TGI's last dividend was $1.15, and the required rate of return on the stock is 12 percent.
a. Calculate the price of the stock today.
b. Calculate P_1 and P_2.
c. Calculate the dividend yield and capital gains yield for Years 1, 2, and 3.

PROBLEMS

18-1 **Constant growth stock valuation.** Rakes Radiator Repair, Inc., has enjoyed many years of growth through franchising. Financial analysts now believe that the firm is moving into a mature, constant-growth phase of its life cycle. Next year's dividend is expected to be $3.00, and dividends and earnings are expected to grow at a constant 7 percent in the future. What price should investors pay for a share of Rakes Radiator if they require a 12 percent rate of return on their investment?

18-2 **Constant growth stock valuation.** Home Products Corporation's last dividend was $5.00($D_0 = \$5.00$). Home Product's growth is expected to remain at a constant 6 percent. If investors demand a 14 percent rate of return, what is Home Product's current market price?

18-3 **Constant growth stock valuation.** What would you expect Home Product's (Problem 18-2) stock price to be in three years? That is, solve for P_3. Assume that growth projections and investor-required returns will remain constant.

18-4 **Zero growth stock valuation.** Pittsburg Properties has been paying a $6.00 dividend for several years. Growth prospects for higher earnings are dim, but the company's treasurer is confident that the firm can continue to provide the current dividend into the foreseeable future. If investors require a 12 percent return, what is the current market price of the stock?

18-5   Return on common stock. Chicago Forge and Steel's earnings and dividends have grown at a constant 5 percent over the past few years. This growth rate is expected to continue at a constant rate into the future. The firm's current dividend, D_0, is $2.38, and the current market price of the firm's stock is $25.

a. What is the firm's dividend yield?

b. What rate of return are the firm's investors expecting?

18-6   Calculating the growth rate. You can buy a share of Carolina Tobacco today for $48. Last year's dividend was $3.20. The market rate of return for stocks in Carolina's risk class is 12 percent. Earnings and dividends are expected to grow at a constant rate, g, in the future, and k is also expected to remain at 12 percent.

a. What rate of growth in earnings and dividends is Carolina expecting?

b. What is Carolina Tobacco's expected stock price 4 years from now?

18-7   Calculating the growth rate. Birmingham Industries will pay a $5 dividend next year, in 1989. Seven years ago, in 1982, its dividend was $2.74. This growth in dividends is expected to remain constant in the future. If investors expect a 15 percent return, what is Birmingham's common stock price today?

18-8   Constant growth stock valuation. Trinity Valley Corporation paid a dividend of $4.00 last year. The dividend is expected to grow at a constant rate of 7 percent into the future. You plan to buy the stock today, hold it for 3 years, and then sell it — if indeed you do decide to purchase it.

a. What is the expected dividend for each of the next three years? That is, calculate D_1, D_2, and D_3. Note that $D_0 = $4.00.

b. If the appropriate discount rate is 15 percent, and the first of these dividend payments will occur one year from today, what is the present value of the dividend stream? That is, calculate the PV of D_1, D_2, and D_3, and sum these PVs.

c. You expect the price of the stock to be $65.54 three years from now; that is, you expect P_3 to equal $65.54. Discounted at a 15 percent rate, what is the present value of this future stock price? In other words, calculate the PV of $65.54.

d. If you plan to buy the stock, hold it for 3 years, and then sell it for $65.54, what is the most you should pay for it if your minimum required return is 15 percent?

e. Use Equation 18-4 to calculate the present value of this stock. Assume that the rate of growth is a constant 7 percent.

f. Is the value of this stock to you dependent on how long you plan to hold it? In other words, if your planned holding period were 2 years or 5 years rather than 3 years, would this affect the value of the stock today, P_0?

18-9   Return on common stock. Gulf and Pacific's current market price is $27. Your stock broker has determined that the firm's dividends will be $2.70 next year, $2.916 in two years, and $3.149 in three years. Although your broker expects that the dividends will continue to grow at the same growth rate in the future, she recommends that you sell the stock for $34 at the end of three years.

a. Calculate the growth rate in dividends.

b. Calculate the stock's dividend yield.

c. If the growth rate continues as expected, what is this stock's expected rate of return? Confirm your answer using Equation 18-4.

18-10   Constant growth stock valuation.

a. Investors require a 15 percent rate of return on Montoya Company's stock ($k_s = 15\%$). At what price will the stock sell if the previous dividend was $D_0 = $2 and investors expect dividends to grow at a constant compound rate of (1) minus 5 percent, (2) 0 percent, (3) 7 percent, (4) 10 percent, and (5) 14 percent? [*Hint:* Use $D_1 = D_0 (1 + g)$, not D_0, in the formula.]

b. In Part a, what is the "formula price" for Montoya's stock if the required rate of return is 15 percent and the expected growth rate is **(1)** 15 percent or **(2)** 20 percent? Are these results reasonable? Explain.

18-11 **Declining growth stock valuation.** Ewing Oil Company's oil and gas reserves are being depleted, and the costs of recovering a declining amount of crude petroleum products are rising each year. As a result, the company's earnings and dividends are declining at the rate of 10 percent per year. If $D_0 = \$7.50$ and $k_s = 13.5\%$, what is the value of Ewing Oil's stock?

18-12 **Supernormal growth stock valuation.** Concord Computer Company (CCC) has been growing at a rate of 20 percent per year in recent years. This same growth rate is expected to last another 3 years. After that time CCC's financial manager expects the firm's growth to slow to a constant 7 percent.

a. Assuming that $D_0 = \$1$ and that the firm's required return, k_s, is 16 percent, what is CCC's stock worth today?

b. Calculate the dividend yield and capital gains yield for Years 1, 2, and 3.

c. Now assume that CCC's period of supernormal (20 percent) growth will last for 6 years rather than 3 years. Describe how this longer supernormal growth period will affect the stock's price, dividend yield, and capital gains yield.

18-13 **Supernormal growth stock valuation.** The earnings per share of Mission Motors are currently $2.00 ($E_0 = \$2.00$). These earnings are expected to grow at 25 percent for the next two years and at 12 percent for the following three years, then to slow to a sustainable growth rate of 6 percent thereafter. The firm has previously had a policy of paying zero dividends because of its rapid growth. However, since its growth will be slower in the future, the payout policy will change. Payout for the next two years will remain at zero but will increase to 25 percent for the following three years. The payout will be 75 percent after Year 5. Mission's shareholders require a 14 percent rate of return. What is the current market price for Mission Motors?

18-14 **Equilibrium stock price.** The risk-free rate of return, R_F, is 8 percent; the required rate of return on the market, k_M, is 13 percent; and Walsh-Saunders Company's stock has a beta coefficient of 1.6.

a. If the dividend expected during the coming year, D_1, is $4.00, and if $g = $ a constant 5%, at what price should Walsh-Saunders's stock sell?

b. Now suppose that the Federal Reserve Board increases the money supply, causing the riskless rate to drop to 7 percent. What would this do to the price of the stock?

c. In addition to the change in Part b, suppose that investors' risk aversion declines; this fact, combined with the decline in R_F causes k_M to fall to 11 percent. At what price would Walsh-Saunders's stock sell?

d. Now suppose that Walsh-Saunders has a change in management. The new group institutes policies that increase the expected constant growth rate to 6 percent. Also, the new management stabilizes sales and profits and thus causes the beta coefficient to decline from 1.6 to 1.3. After all these changes, what is Walsh-Saunders's new equilibrium price? (*Note:* D_1 goes to $4.04.)

18-15 **Beta coefficients.** Suppose Norfolk Shipping Company's management conducts a study and concludes that if Norfolk expanded its consumer products division (which is less risky than its primary business, industrial chemicals), the firm's beta would decline from 1.2 to 0.9. However, consumer products have a somewhat lower profit margin, and this would cause Norfolk's constant growth rate in earnings and dividends to fall from 7 to 5 percent.

a. Should management make the change? Assume the following: $k_M = 12\%$; $R_F = 9\%$; $D_0 = \$2$.

b. Assume all the facts as given previously except the change in the beta coefficient. What would the beta have to equal to cause the expansion to be a good one? (*Hint:* Set P_0 under the new policy equal to P_0 under the old one, and find the new beta that will produce this equality.)

18-16 **Stock pricing.** The Atherton Company is a small jewelry manufacturer. The company has been successful and has grown. Now Atherton is planning to sell an issue of common stock to the public for the first time, and it faces the problem of setting an appropriate price on its common stock. The company and its investment bankers believe that the proper procedure is to select firms similar to it with publicly traded common stock and to make relevant comparisons.

Several jewelry manufacturers are reasonably similar to Atherton with respect to product mix, size, asset composition, and debt/equity proportions. Of these, Gemex and Dimson are most similar. Data are given in the following table. When analyzing these data, assume that 1983 and 1988 were reasonably normal years for all three companies; that is, these years were neither especially good nor bad in terms of sales, earnings, and dividends. At the time of the analysis, R_F was 10 percent and k_M was 15 percent. Gemex is listed on the American Exchange and Dimson on the NYSE, whereas Atherton will be traded in the OTC market.

	Gemex	**Dimson**	**Atherton (Totals)**
Earnings per share			
1988	$4.50	$ 7.50	$1,200,000
1983	3.00	5.50	816,000
Price per share			
1988	$36.00	$65.00	———
Dividends per share			
1988	$ 2.25	$ 3.75	$ 600,000
1983	1.50	2.75	420,000
Book value per share			
1988	$30.00	$55.00	$9,000,000
Market/book ratio			
1988	120%	118%	———
Total assets, 1988	$28 million	$ 82 million	$20 million
Total debt, 1988	$12 million	$ 30 million	$11 million
Sales, 1988	$41 million	$140 million	$37 million

a. Assume that Atherton has 100 shares of stock outstanding. Use this information to calculate earnings per share (EPS), dividends per share (DPS), and book value per share for Atherton. (*Note:* Since there are only 100 shares outstanding, your results may seem a bit large.)

b. Based on your answer to Part a, do you think Atherton's stock would sell at a price in the same "ballpark" as Gemex's and Dimson's—that is, sell in the range of $25 to $100 per share?

c. Assuming that Atherton's management can split the stock so that the 100 shares could be changed to 1,000 shares, 100,000 shares, or any other number, would such an action make sense in this case? Why?

d. Now assume that Atherton did split its stock and has 400,000 shares. Calculate new values for EPS, DPS, and book value per share.

e. What can you say about the relative growth rates of the three companies?

f. What can you say about their dividend payout policies?

g. Return on equity (ROE) can be measured as EPS/book value per share, or as total earnings/total equity. Calculate ROEs for the three companies.

h. Calculate debt/total assets ratios for the three companies.

i. Calculate P/E ratios for Gemex and Dimson. Are these P/Es consistent with the growth and ROE data? If not, what other factors could explain the relative P/E ratios?

j. Now determine a range of values for Atherton's stock, with 400,000 shares outstanding, by applying Gemex's and Dimson's P/E ratios, price/dividends ratios, and price/book value ratios to your data for Atherton. For example, one possible price for Atherton's stock is (P/E Gemex)(EPS Atherton) = (8)($3) = $24 per share. Similar calculations would produce a range of prices based on both Gemex and Dimson data.

k. Using the equation $k = D_1/P_0 + g$, find approximate k values for Gemex and Dimson. Then use these values in the constant growth stock price model to find a price for Atherton's stock.

l. At what price do you think Atherton's shares should be offered to the public? You will want to find the *equilibrium price* (i.e., a price that will be low enough to induce investors to buy the stock, but not so low that it will rise sharply immediately after it is issued). Think about relative growth rates, ROEs, dividend yields, and total returns ($k = D/P + g$). Also, as you think about the appropriate price, recognize that when Howard Hughes let the Hughes Tool Company go public, different investment bankers proposed prices that ranged from $20 to $30 per share. Hughes naturally accepted the $30 price, and the stock jumped to $40 almost immediately. Nobody's perfect!

m. Would your recommended price be different if the offering was by the Atherton family, selling some of its 400,000 shares, or if it was new stock authorized by the company? For example, another 100,000 shares could be authorized, which when issued would bring the outstanding shares up to 500,000, with 400,000 shares owned by the Athertons and 100,000 shares held by the public. If the Athertons sell their own shares, they receive the proceeds as their own personal funds. If the company sells newly issued shares, the company receives the funds and presumably uses the money to expand the business.

n. If the price you selected in Part l actually was established as the price at which the stock would be offered to the public, approximately how much money, in total, would the Atherton Company actually receive?

18-17 **Supernormal growth stock valuation.** The Donnolly Corporation has been growing at a rate of 25 percent per year in recent years. This same growth rate is expected to last for another 2 years.

a. If $D_0 = \$2$, $k = 14\%$, and $g_n = 6\%$, what is Donnolly's stock worth today? What are its current dividend yield and capital gains yield?

b. Now assume that Donnolly's period of supernormal growth is 5 years rather than 2 years. How does this affect its price, dividend yield, and capital gains yield? Answer in words only.

c. What will be Donnolly's dividend yield and capital gains yield the year after its period of supernormal growth ends? (*Hint:* These values will be the same regardless of whether you examine the case of 2 or 5 years of supernormal growth; the calculations are trivial.)

d. Of what interest to investors is the changing relationship between dividend yield and capital gains yield over time?

(Do Parts e and f only if you are using the computerized problem diskette.)

e. What will be Donnolly' stock price, dividend yield, and capital gains yield if the supernormal growth period is 5 years?

f. What will be the price, dividend yield, and capital gains yield if the required rate of return is 16 percent and the supernormal growth period is 2 years?

ANSWERS TO SELF-TEST PROBLEMS

ST-1 a. This is not necessarily true. Since BI plows back two thirds of its earnings, its growth rate should exceed that of AM, but AM pays higher dividends ($4.50 versus $1.50). We cannot say which stock should have the higher price.

b. Again, we just do not know which price would be higher.

c. This is false. The changes in k_d and k_s would have a greater effect on BI's stock— its price would decline more.

d. Once again, we just do not know which expected return would be higher. The total expected return for AM is $k_{AM} = D_1/P_0 + g = 15\% + 0\% = 15\%$. The total expected return for BI will have D_1/P_0 less than 15 percent and g greater than 0 percent, but k_{BI} could be either greater or less than AM's total expected return, 15 percent.

e. We have eliminated a, b, c, and d, so e must be correct. Based on the available information, AM's and BI's stocks should sell at about the same price, $30. Thus $k_s = \$4.50/30 = 15\%$ for both AM and BI. BI's current dividend yield is $\$1.50/\$30 = 5\%$. Therefore $g = 15\% - 5\% = 10\%$.

ST-2 The first step is to solve for g, the unknown variable, in the constant growth equation. Since D_1 is unknown, substitute $D_0(1 + g)$ as follows:

$$P_0 = \frac{D_0(1 + g)}{k_s - g}$$

$$\$33.125 = \frac{\$2.50(1 + g)}{0.14 - g}$$

Solving for g, we find the growth rate to be 6 percent. The next step is to use the growth rate to project the stock price 5 years hence:

$$P_5 = \frac{D_0(1 + g)^6}{k_s - g}$$

$$= \frac{\$2.50(1.06)^6}{0.14 - 0.06}$$

$$= \$44.33.$$

[Alternatively, $P_5 = \$33.125(1.06)^5 = \$44.33$.]

Therefore, Crown Company's expected stock price 5 years from now, P_5, is $44.33.

ST-3 **a.** *Step 1:* Calculate the PV of the dividends paid during the supernormal growth period:

$$D_1 = \$1.1500(1.18) = \$1.3570.$$

$$D_2 = \$1.3570(1.18) = \$1.6013.$$

$$D_3 = \$1.6013(1.15) = \$1.8415.$$

$$PV\ D = \$1.3570(0.8929) + \$1.6013(0.7972) + \$1.8415(0.7118)$$

$$= \$1.2117 + \$1.2766 + \$1.3108$$

$$= \$3.7991 \cong \$3.80.$$

Step 2: Find the PV of the stock's price at the end of Year 3:

$$P_3 = \frac{D_4}{k_s - g} = \frac{D_3(1 + g)}{k_s - g}$$

$$= \frac{\$1.8415(1.06)}{0.12 - 0.06}$$

$$= \$32.53.$$

$$PV\ P_3 = \$32.53(0.7118) = \$23.15.$$

Step 3: Sum the two components to find the price of the stock today:

$$P_0 = \$3.80 + \$23.15 = \$26.95.$$

b.
$$P_1 = \$1.6013(0.8929) + \$1.8415(0.7972) + \$32.53(0.7972)$$

$$= \$1.4298 + \$1.4680 + \$25.9329$$

$$= \$28.8307 \cong \$28.83.$$

$$P_2 = \$1.8415(0.8929) + \$32.53(0.8929)$$

$$= \$1.6443 + \$29.0460$$

$$= \$30.6903 \cong \$30.69.$$

c.

Year	Dividend Yield	Capital Gains Yield	Total Return
1	$\dfrac{\$1.3570}{\$26.95} = 5.04\%$	$\dfrac{\$28.83 - \$26.95}{\$26.95} = 6.98\%$	$\cong 12\%$
2	$\dfrac{\$1.6013}{\$28.83} = 5.55\%$	$\dfrac{\$30.69 - \$28.83}{\$28.83} = 6.45\%$	12
3	$\dfrac{\$1.8415}{\$30.69} = 6.00\%$	$\dfrac{\$32.53 - \$30.69}{\$30.69} = 6.00\%$	12

Appendix 18A

Warrants and Convertibles

In Chapter 18 we discussed the sale of equity securities to investors. It happens at times that a company may wish to sell equity but its management determines that market conditions are not favorable for an immediate equity issue. In such a situation, the company may decide to sell equity indirectly through convertible securities or securities with warrants attached. Additionally, the use of warrants and convertibles can make a company's securities attractive to an even broader range of investors, thereby increasing the supply of capital and decreasing its cost. Reducing the cost of capital, as we learn in Chapter 20, helps to maximize the value of the firm's stock. Because warrants and convertibles are rapidly gaining popularity, a knowledge of these instruments is especially important today.

Warrants

warrant

An option to buy a stated number of shares of common stock at a specified price.

option

A contract giving the holder the right to buy or sell an asset at some predetermined price within a specified period of time.

A **warrant** is an **option** to buy a stated number of shares of stock at a specified price. Generally, warrants are distributed with debt, and they are used to induce investors to buy a firm's long-term debt at a lower interest rate than would otherwise be required. For example, when Florida Atlantic Airlines (FAA) wanted to sell $50 million of 20-year bonds in 1987, the company's investment bankers informed the financial vice president that the bonds would be difficult to sell and that an interest rate of 14 percent would be required. As an alternative, the bankers suggested that investors might be willing to buy the bonds at a rate as low as 10⅜ percent if the company would offer 30 warrants with each $1,000 bond, each warrant entitling the holder to buy one share of common stock at a price of $22 per share. The stock was selling for $20 per share at the time. The warrants would expire in 1997 if not exercised before then.

Why would investors be willing to buy Florida Atlantic's bonds at a yield of only 10⅜ percent just because warrants were also offered as part of the package? It is because the lure of higher values of the warrants in the future offset the low interest rate on the bonds and thus makes the entire package of below-market bonds plus warrants attractive to investors.

Initial Market Price of a Bond with Warrants

If the FAA bonds had been issued as straight debt, they would have carried a 14 percent interest rate. With warrants attached, however, the bonds were sold to yield 10⅜ percent. Someone buying one of the bonds at its $1,000 initial offering price would thus have been receiving a package consisting of a 10⅜ percent, 20-year bond plus 30 warrants. Because the going interest rate on bonds as risky as those of FAA is 14 percent, we can find the straight-debt value of the bonds, assuming an annual coupon, as follows:

$$\text{Value} = \sum_{t=1}^{20} \frac{\$103.75}{(1.14)^t} + \frac{\$1,000}{(1.14)^{20}}$$

$$= \$103.75(\text{PVIFA}_{14\%,20}) + \$1,000(\text{PVIF}_{14\%,20})$$

$$= \$687.15 + \$72.80$$

$$= \$759.95 \approx \$760.$$

Table 18A-1 **Formula and Actual Values of FAA Warrants at Different Market Prices of Common Stock**

Price of Stock	Formula Value	Actual Warrant Price	Premium
$ 20.00	$ − 2.00	$ 8.00	$10.00
22.00	0.00	9.00	9.00
23.00	1.00	9.75	8.75
24.00	2.00	10.50	8.50
33.67	11.67	17.37	5.70
52.00	30.00	32.00	2.00
75.00	53.00	54.00	1.00
100.00	78.00	78.50	0.50
150.00	128.00	Not available	—

Thus a person buying the bonds in the initial underwriting period would pay $1,000 and receive in exchange a straight bond worth about $760 plus warrants presumably worth about $1,000 − $760 = $240.

Formula Value of a Warrant. Warrants have both a **formula,** or **exercise, value,** which is equal to the value of the warrant if it were exercised today, and an actual price that is determined in the marketplace. The formula value is found by using the following equation:

$$\begin{matrix} \text{Formula,} \\ \text{or exercise,} \\ \text{value} \end{matrix} = \left(\begin{matrix} \text{Market price} \\ \text{of common} \\ \text{stock} \end{matrix} - \begin{matrix} \text{Option} \\ \text{price} \end{matrix} \right) \times \left(\begin{matrix} \text{Number of shares} \\ \text{each warrant entitles} \\ \text{owner to purchase} \end{matrix} \right).$$

For instance, FAA warrant entitles the holder to purchase one share of common stock at $22 a share. If the market price of the common stock rises to $64.50, the formula value of the warrant will be

$$(\$64.50 - \$22) \times 1.0 = \$42.50.$$

The formula gives a negative value when the stock is selling for less than the option price. For example, if FAA stock is selling for $20, the formula value of the warrants is minus $2.

Actual Price of a Warrant. *Generally, warrants actually sell at prices above their formula values.* When FAA stock sold for $20, the warrants had a formula value of minus $2 but were selling at a price of $8. This represented a premium of $10 above the formula value.

FAA stock rose substantially after the bonds with warrants were issued in 1987. A set of FAA stock prices, together with actual and formula warrant values, is given in Table 18A-1 and plotted in Figure 18A-1. At any stock price below $22, the formula value of the warrants is negative; beyond $22, each $1 increase in the price of the stock brings with it a $1 increase in the formula value of the warrants. The actual market price of the warrants lies above the formula value at each price of the common stock. Notice, however, that the premium of market price over formula value declines as the price of the common stock increases. For example, when the common stock sold for $22 and the warrants had a zero formula value, their actual price, and the premium,

formula, or exercise, value

The theoretical value of a warrant if it were exercised today. The actual value of a warrant is determined in the marketplace.

Figure 18A-1 **Formula and Actual Values of FAA Warrants at Different Common Stock Prices**

Warrants have both a formula value (value if exercised today) and an actual market value, which are compared graphically in this figure. As the formula warrant value increases dollar for dollar with the stock price, the premium of market warrant price over formula value declines. At low formula values, premiums are high because the investor has large gain and small loss potentials. As stock prices (and formula values) rise, this leverage effect is diminished, causing the premium to decrease.

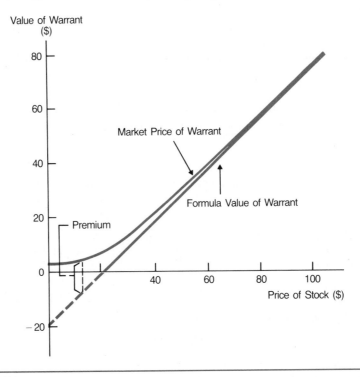

was $9. As the price of the stock rises, the *formula value* of the warrants matches the increase dollar for dollar, but for a while the *market price* of the warrants climbs less rapidly and the premium declines. The premium is $9 when the stock sells for $22 a share, but it declines to $1 by the time the stock price has risen to $75 a share. Beyond this point the premium virtually seems to disappear.

Why does this pattern exist? Why should the warrant ever sell for more than its formula value, and why does the premium decline as the price of the stock increases? The answer lies in the speculative appeal of warrants — they enable a person to gain a high degree of personal leverage when buying securities. To illustrate, suppose FAA warrants sold for exactly their formula value. Now suppose you are thinking of investing in the company's common stock at a time when it is selling for $25 a share. If you buy a share and the price rises to $50 in a year, you have made a 100 percent capital gain.

However, had you bought the warrants at their formula value ($3 when the stock sells for $25), your capital gain would have been $25 on a $3 investment, or 833 percent. At the same time, your total loss potential with the warrant is only $3, whereas the loss potential from the purchase of the stock is $25. The huge capital gains potential, combined with the loss limitation, is clearly worth something — the exact amount it is worth to investors is the amount of the premium.

But why does the premium decline as the price of the stock rises? The answer is that both the leverage effect and the loss protection feature decline at high stock prices. For example, if you are thinking of buying the stock at $75 a share, the formula value of the warrants is $53. If the stock price doubles to $150, the formula value of FAA warrants goes from $53 to $128. The percentage capital gain on the stock is still 100 percent, but the percentage gain on the warrant is now only 142 percent versus 833 percent in the earlier case. Moreover, notice that the loss potential on the warrant is much greater when the warrant is selling at a high price. These two factors, the declining leverage impact and the increasing danger of losses, explain why the premium diminishes as the price of the common stock rises.

Use of Warrants in Financing. In the past, warrants have generally been used by small, rapidly growing firms as "sweeteners" when selling either debt or preferred stocks. Such firms are frequently regarded by investors as being highly risky. Their bonds could be sold only if they were willing to pay extremely high rates of interest and to accept very restrictive indenture provisions. To avoid this, firms like Florida Atlantic often offered warrants along with the bonds. In the early 1970s, however, AT&T raised $1.57 billion by selling bonds with warrants. This was the largest financing of any type ever undertaken by a business firm, and it marked the first use ever of warrants by a large, strong corporation.

Obtaining warrants along with bonds enables investors to share in the company's growth if it does in fact grow and prosper; therefore investors are willing to accept a lower bond interest rate and less restrictive indenture provisions. A bond with warrants has some characteristics of debt and some characteristics of equity. It is a hybrid security that offers the financial manager an opportunity to expand the firm's mix of securities, thus appealing to a broader group of investors and possibly lowering the firm's cost of capital.

Warrants can also bring in additional funds. The option price is generally set at from 10 to 30 percent above the market price of the stock at the time of the bond issue. If the firm does grow and prosper, and if its stock price rises above the option price at which shares may be purchased, warrant holders will surrender their warrants and buy stock at the stated price.

Convertible Securities

Convertible securities are bonds or preferred stocks that can be exchanged for common stock at the option of the holder and under specified terms and conditions. Unlike the exercise of warrants, which brings in additional funds to the firm, converting a bond does not bring in additional capital; debt on the balance sheet is simply replaced by common stock. Of course, this reduction of the debt ratio will make it easier to obtain additional debt capital, but this is a separate action.

One of the most important provisions of a convertible bond is the number of shares of stock a bondholder receives upon conversion, defined as the **conversion ratio, R.** Related to the conversion ratio is the **conversion price, P_c,** which is the

convertible securities
Bonds or preferred stocks that are exchangeable at the option of the holder for common stock of the issuing firm.

conversion ratio, R
The number of shares of common stock that may be obtained by converting a convertible bond or share of convertible preferred stock.

conversion price, P_c
The effective price paid for common stock when the stock is obtained by converting either convertible preferred stocks or convertible bonds.

effective price paid for the common stock when conversion occurs. The relationship between the conversion ratio and the conversion price is illustrated by the Adams Electric Company's convertible debentures, issued at their $1,000 par value in 1978. At any time prior to maturity on July 1, 1998, a debenture holder can turn in a bond and receive in its place 20 shares of common stock; therefore R = 20. The bond has a par value of $1,000, so the holder is giving up this amount upon conversion. Dividing the $1,000 par value by the 20 shares received gives a conversion price of $50 a share:

$$\text{Conversion price} = P_c = \frac{\text{Par value of bond}}{\text{Shares received}},$$

or

$$P_c = \frac{\$1,000}{R} = \frac{\$1,000}{20} = \$50.$$

Therefore

$$R = \frac{\$1,000}{P_c} = \frac{\$1,000}{\$50} = 20 \text{ shares.}$$

Once R is set, this establishes the value of P_c, and vice versa.

Like warrant option prices, the conversion price is characteristically set at from 10 to 30 percent above the prevailing market price of the common stock at the time the convertible issue is sold. Exactly how the conversion price is established can best be understood after examining some of the reasons firms use convertibles.

Advantages of Convertibles. Convertibles offer advantages to corporations as well as to individual investors by functioning in the following two ways:

1. As a "sweetener" when selling debt. A company can sell debt with lower interest rates and less restrictive convenants by giving investors a chance to share in potential capital gains. Convertibles, like bonds with warrants, offer this possibility.

2. To sell common stock at prices higher than those currently prevailing. Many companies actually want to sell common stock, not debt, but believe that the price of their stock is temporarily depressed. Management may know, for example, that earnings are depressed because of a strike but may think that earnings will snap back during the next year and pull the price of the stock up with them. To sell stock now would require giving up more shares to raise a given amount of money than management thinks is necessary. However, setting the conversion price 10 to 30 percent above the present market price of the stock will require giving up 10 to 30 percent fewer shares when the bonds are converted than would be required if stock were sold directly.

Notice, however, that management is counting on the stock's price rising above the conversion price to make the bonds attractive in conversion. If the stock price does not rise and conversion does not occur, the company is saddled with debt.

call provision

A provision in a bond contract that gives the issuer the right to redeem the bonds under specified terms prior to the normal maturity date.

How can the company be sure that conversion will occur when the price of the stock rises above the conversion price? Typically, convertibles contain a **call provision** that enables the issuing firm to force bondholders to convert. Suppose that the conversion price is $50, the conversion ratio is 20, the market price of the common stock has risen to $60, and the call price on the convertible bond is $1,050. If the company calls the bond, bondholders either can convert into common stock with a market value of

$1,200 or can allow the company to redeem the bond for $1,050. Naturally, bondholders prefer $1,200 to $1,050, so conversion occurs. The call provision therefore gives the company a means of forcing conversion, provided the market price of the stock is greater than the conversion price.

Disadvantages of Convertibles. From the standpoint of the issuer, convertibles have two important disadvantages. First, although the convertible bond does give the issuer the opportunity to sell common stock at a price 10 to 30 percent higher than the price at which it could otherwise be sold, if the common stock greatly increases in price, the issuing firm may find that it would have been better off if it had waited and simply sold the common stock. Second, if the company truly wants to raise equity capital, and if the price of the stock does not rise sufficiently after the bond is issued, the company is stuck with debt. This debt will, however, have a low interest rate.

Decisions on the Use of Warrants and Convertibles

Accuron, an electronic circuit and component manufacturer with assets of $60 million, illustrates a typical case in which convertibles proved useful. Accuron's profits had been depressed as a result of its heavy expenditures on research and development (R&D) for a new product. This situation held down the growth rate of earnings and dividends; the price/earnings ratio was only 18 times, as compared with an industry average of 22. At the current $2 earnings per share and P/E of 18, the stock was selling for $36 a share. The Perkins family owned 70 percent of the 1,500,000 shares outstanding, or 1,050,000 shares. It wanted to retain majority control but could not buy more stock.

The heavy R&D expenditures had resulted in the development of a new type of printed circuit that management believed would be highly profitable. Twenty-five million dollars was needed to build and equip new production facilities, but profits were not expected to flow into the company for some 18 months after construction on the new plant was started. Accuron's debt amounted to $27 million, or 45 percent of assets, well above the 25 percent industry average. Its debt indenture provisions restricted the company from selling additional debt unless the new debt was subordinated to outstanding debt.

The company's investment bankers informed Patricia Perkins, the financial vice president, that subordinated debentures could not be sold at any reasonable interest rate unless they were convertible or had warrants attached. The investment bankers were willing to sell either convertibles or bonds with warrants at a 10 percent interest rate. They concluded that the convertible bonds would have a conversion price of $43.48. If bonds were sold with warrants attached, investors would be allowed to buy 20 new shares of Accuron's common stock at a special exercise price of $40 during the next 5 years. On the other hand, if the firm chose to sell common stock directly, it would net, after flotation costs, $33 a share. The effect of each of these financing options is presented in Table 18A-2. Note that there is no difference on the balance sheet between the convertible debt and the debt with warrants attached as long as the options are unexercised.

Which of the alternatives should Accuron choose? First, note that if common stock were used, the company would have to sell 757,576 shares ($25 million divided by $33). Combined with the 450,000 shares already held outside the family, this amounts to 1,207,576 shares versus the family holdings of 1,050,000. Thus the family would lose majority control if common stock were sold.

Table 18A-2 **Financing Options Available to Accuron Prior to
Conversion or Exercise of Warrants (in Thousands of Dollars)**

Original Position

	Current liabilities	$10,000
	Long-term debt	17,000
	Common stock ($2)	3,000
	Paid-in capital	10,000
	Retained earnings	20,000
Total assets $60,000	Total claims on assets	$60,000

Shares outstanding	= 1.50 million.
Family-controlled shares	= 1.05 million.
Family control (%)	= 70%.
Debt ratio (D/TA)	= 45%.

Equity Option

	Current liabilities	$10,000
	Long-term debt	17,000
	Common stock ($2)	4,515
	Paid-in capital	33,485
	Retained earnings	20,000
Total assets $85,000	Total claims on assets	$85,000

Shares outstanding	= 2.26 million.
Family-controlled shares	= 1.05 million.
Family control (%)	= 47%.
Debt ratio (D/TA)	= 32%.

Debt Option[a]

	Current liabilities	$10,000
	Long-term debt	42,000
	Common stock ($2)	3,000
	Paid-in capital	10,000
	Retained earnings	20,000
Total assets $85,000	Total claims on assets	$85,000

Shares outstanding	= 1.50 million.
Family-controlled shares	= 1.05 million.
Family control (%)	= 70%.
Debt ratio (D/TA)	= 61%.

[a]The balance sheet will not differ under either the convertible or the debt-with-warrants option before exercise of the options.

However, if the 10 percent convertible bonds were sold, conversion would yield only 575,000 new shares. In this case the family would have 1,050,000 shares versus 1,025,00 for outsiders. If bonds with warrants were sold, the results would be much the same with respect to control. If all warrants were exercised, 500,000 new shares would be created, meaning the family would still control 52.5 percent of the common stock. Thus, in either of the debt options, the Perkins family could retain absolute control.

In addition to assuring family control, using the convertibles or warrants would also benefit earnings per share in the long run. The total number of shares would be smaller because fewer new shares would be issued to obtain the $25 million, so earnings per share would be greater. Before conversion or exercise, however, the firm

Table 18A-3 **Accuron after Conversion of Debt or Exercise of Warrants (in Thousands of Dollars)**

After Debt Conversion

	Current liabilities	$10,500
	Long-term debt	17,000
	Common stock ($2)	4,150
	Paid-in capital	33,850
	Retained earnings[a]	22,000
Total assets $87,500	Total claims on assets	$87,500

Shares outstanding	= 2.075 million.
Family-controlled shares	= 1.050 million.
Family control (%)	= 50.6%.
Debt ratio (D/TA)	= 31%.

After Exercise of Warrants

	Current liabilities	$ 10,500
	Long-term debt	42,000
	Common stock ($2)	4,000
	Paid-in capital	29,000
	Retained earnings[b]	22,000
Total assets $107,500	Total claims on assets	$107,500

Shares outstanding	= 2.00 million.
Family-controlled shares	= 1.05 million.
Family control (%)	= 52.5%.
Debt ratio (D/TA)	= 48.8%.

[a]The change in retained earnings is the result of prior years' profitability and is not the result of the conversion of debt into equity.
[b]Again, the change in retained earnings is due to operations and not to the exercise of warrants.

would have a considerable amount of debt outstanding. Because adding $25 million would raise the total debt to $52 million against new total assets of $85 million, the debt ratio would be over 61 percent versus the 25 percent industry average. This could be dangerous. If delays were encountered in bringing the new plant into production, if demand failed to meet expectations, if the company experienced a strike, if the economy went into a recession — if any of these things occurred — the company would be extremely vulnerable because of its high debt ratio.

In the present case the decision was made to sell the 10 percent convertible debentures. Two years later earnings climbed to $3 a share, the P/E ratio to 20, and the price of the stock to $60. The bonds were called, and, of course, conversion occurred. After conversion, debt amounted to approximately $27.5 million against total assets of $87.5 million (some earnings had been retained), so the debt ratio was down to a more reasonable 31 percent. The effect of conversion on Accuron's balance sheet, along with the effect of warrant exercise (if that option had been chosen), is presented in Table 18A-3.

Convertibles were chosen rather than bonds with warrants for the following reason. If a firm has a high debt ratio and its near-term prospects are favorable, it can anticipate a rise in the price of its stock and thus be able to call the bonds and force conversion. Warrants, on the other hand, have a stated life, and even though the price of the firm's stock rises, the warrants may not be exercised until near their expiration date. If, subsequent to the favorable period (during which convertibles could have been called), the firm finds itself in a less favorable position and the price of its stock falls, the warrants lose their value and may never be exercised. The heavy debt burden will then become aggravated. Therefore, the use of convertibles gives the firm greater control over the timing of future capital structure changes. This factor is of particular importance to the firm if its debt ratio is already high in relation to the risks in its line of business.

Reporting Earnings if Warrants or Convertibles Are Outstanding

If warrants or convertibles are outstanding, a firm could theoretically report earnings per share in three ways:

1. *Simple EPS,* in which earnings available to common stockholders are divided by the average number of shares actually outstanding during the period.

2. *Primary EPS,* in which earnings available are divided by the average number of shares that would have been outstanding if warrants and convertibles "likely to be converted in the near future" had actually been exercised or converted. The accountants have a formula that basically compares the conversion or option price with the actual market value of the stock to determine the likelihood of conversion, and they also add interest on the convertible bonds back into earnings.

3. *Fully diluted EPS,* which is similar to primary EPS except that *all* warrants and convertibles are assumed to be exercised or converted, regardless of the likelihood of exercise or conversion.

Simple EPS is virtually never reported by firms that have warrants or convertibles likely to be exercised or converted, but the SEC requires that primary and fully diluted earnings be shown. For firms with large amounts of option securities outstanding, there can be a substantial difference between the two EPS figures. The purpose of the provision is, of course, to give investors a more accurate picture of the firm's true profit position.

Summary

Both warrants and convertibles are forms of options used to finance business firms. The use of such long-term options is encouraged by an economic environment in which either recessions or booms can occur. The senior position of the securities protects against recessions, while the option feature offers the opportunity for participation in rising stock markets.

Both convertibles and warrants are used as "sweeteners." The option privileges they grant may make it possible for small companies to sell debt or preferred stock that otherwise could not be sold. For large companies the sweeteners result in lower costs of the securities sold.

The conversion of bonds by their holders does not provide additional funds to the company, whereas the exercise of warrants does provide such funds. The conversion of securities results in reduced debt ratios. The exercise of warrants also strengthens the equity position, but it still leaves the debt or preferred stock on the balance sheet. A firm with a high debt ratio should probably choose to use convertibles rather than senior securities carrying warrants. A firm with a moderate or low debt ratio may choose to employ warrants. Note, however, that if the securities with warrants or convertibles attached were issued in a period of low interest, the low-interest-rate debt remains outstanding when warrants are exercised, but the firm loses this advantage when convertibles are converted.

PROBLEM

18A-1 The Maloney Manufacturing Company has grown rapidly during the past 5 years. Recently its investment bankers urged the company to consider increasing its permanent financing. Its bank loan under a line of credit has risen to $250,000, carrying 8 percent interest. Maloney has been 30 to 60 days late in paying trade creditors.

Discussions with the investment bankers have resulted in the decision to raise $500,000 at this time. The investment bankers have assured Maloney that the following alternatives are feasible (flotation costs will be ignored):

1. Sell common stock at $8.

2. Sell convertible bonds at an 8 percent coupon, convertible into 100 shares of common stock for each $1,000 bond (that is, the conversion price is $10 per share).

3. Sell debentures at an 8 percent coupon, each $1,000 bond carrying 100 warrants to buy common stock at $10.

Tom Prestwich, the president, owns 80 percent of the common stock of Maloney Manufacturing Company and wishes to retain control of the company. One hundred thousand shares are outstanding. Additional information is given in the tables that follow.

a. Show the new balance sheet under each alternative. For Alternatives 2 and 3, show the balance sheet after conversion of the debentures or exercise of the warrants. Assume that one half of the funds raised will be used to reduce the bank loan and one half to increase total assets.

b. Show Prestwich's control position under each alternative, assuming that he does not purchase additional shares.

c. What is the effect on earnings per share of each alternative if it is assumed that profits before interest and taxes will be 20 percent of total assets?

d. What will be the debt ratio under each alternative?

e. Which of the three alternatives would you recommend to Prestwich, and why?

Maloney Manufacturing Company: Balance Sheet

	Current liabilities	$400,000
	Common stock, par $1	100,000
	Retained earnings	50,000
Total assets $550,000	Total claims	$550,000

Maloney Manufacturing Company: Income Statement

Sales	$1,100,000
All costs except interest	990,000
Gross profit	$ 110,000
Interest	20,000
Profit before taxes	$ 90,000
Taxes at 50%	45,000
Profits after taxes	$ 45,000
Shares	100,000
Earnings per share	$0.45
Price/earnings ratio	19×
Market price of stock	$8.55

Chapter 19

The Cost of Capital

 DECISION IN FINANCE

Capital Outlays: Business on the Hot Seat

When President Reagan used his 1987 State of the Union address to make rebuilding American "competitiveness" a national priority, he put the spotlight on this country's declining economic prowess. In the ensuing fingerpointing, American business found itself consistently blamed for its failure to make the capital investment necessary to meet the competitive threat from overseas, specifically the threat from the booming economies of Germany and Japan.

Trade deficits have been setting records each year, and the U.S. share of such major export markets as capital equipment, consumer durables, and textiles has declined. Business capital investment — the key to increased productivity — has been lackluster. The Commerce Department has, in fact, recently revised downward its capital investment figures for the 1980s to an annual average increase of just 2.7 percent from 3.1 percent. This is particularly disturbing because even during the inflation/recession-ravaged 1970s, capital outlays grew at an annual rate of 3.7 percent.

Not only has capital investment been weak, but it has been sporadic as well. Business spending on new plant and equipment boomed in the early years of the business expansion of the 1980s, fired by the massive tax cuts of 1981. In 1985, however, capital spending slowed sharply, and in 1986 it actually declined by 2.3 percent, according to the Commerce Department.

Among the seven big industrial nations, the U.S. ranks last in the share of GNP devoted to capital spending. If the nation is to regain its competitive edge, more of the country's resources must be channeled into new plant and equipment. Says William C. Freund, chairman of the Graduate Business School of Pace University: "If the gross business investment to GNP ratio could be raised by approximately one percentage point . . . productivity could be raised by at least one-third of a percentage point."

Recently, the amount of resources devoted to capital spending has been shrinking. In the first half of 1987, business fixed investment as a percentage of GNP dropped to 9.7 percent from 10.5 percent the previous year, according to Data Resources, Inc. This is the lowest level since 1964. "You expect that kind of capital investment figure only in recessions," notes Data Resources vice president Christopher Caton.

Given the low level of investment, it is hardly surprising that the amount of capital stock (i.e., plant and equipment in place) has been growing at a painfully slow pace. Says Freund: "Net investment — spending that increases capacity because it is more than just replacement investment — is still seriously lacking."

As you read this chapter, try to think of some of the factors that might account for the low rate of capital investment among American businesses. How might this trend affect the performance of an individual corporation? What should business and government do to reverse this trend?

See end of chapter for resolution

The cost of capital is critically important in finance for several reasons. First, capital budgeting decisions have a major impact on a firm, and proper capital budgeting procedures require an estimate of the cost of capital. Second, many other types of decisions, including those related to leasing, to bond refunding, and to working capital policy, require estimates of the cost of capital. Finally, maximizing the value of a firm requires that the costs of all inputs, including capital, be minimized, and to minimize the cost of capital one must be able to calculate it.[1]

This chapter first explains the logic of the weighted average cost of capital. Next, we consider the costs of the major components of the capital structure. Third, the individual component costs are brought together to form a weighted average cost of capital. Finally, the relationship between capital budgeting and the cost of capital is discussed.

THE LOGIC OF THE WEIGHTED AVERAGE COST OF CAPITAL

When we discussed capital budgeting, we assumed that equity was the only source of financing used by the firm. We made this assumption so that we could concentrate on the investment decision without being concerned about how the project was to be financed. Of course, few firms are financed entirely with equity. Most finance a substantial portion of their new assets with debt and some use preferred stock as well. In that case, the firm's cost of capital must reflect the diversity of financing sources and financing costs for the long-term funds it uses, not just its cost of equity.

Precision Associates (PA), a subcontractor of engineering systems to many of the nation's largest aerospace firms, has a cost of debt of 11 percent and a cost of equity of 16 percent. Suppose that the firm decides to finance all of next year's projects with debt. The argument is sometimes made that the cost of capital for a project financed exclusively with debt is equal to the cost of debt. However, this position is *incorrect*. To finance a particular set of projects exclusively with debt implies that the firm is also using up some of its potential for obtaining new low-cost debt in the future. As the firm continues to expand in subsequent years, PA will at some point find it necessary to use additional equity financing to prevent the debt ratio from becoming too large.

To illustrate, suppose that PA borrows heavily at 11 percent during 1988 to finance projects yielding 12 percent, using up its debt capacity in the pro-

---

[1]The cost of capital is also vitally important in regulated industries, including electric, gas, telephone, railroad, airline, and trucking companies. In essence, regulatory commissions seek to measure a utility's cost of capital, then set prices so that the company will earn just this rate of return. If the estimate is too low, the company will not be able to attract sufficient capital to meet long-range demands for service, and the public will suffer. If the estimate of capital costs is too high, customers will pay too much for service.

cess. In 1989 it has new projects available that yield 15 percent, well above the return of the 1988 projects, but PA cannot accept them because they would have to be financed with 16 percent equity money. To avoid this problem, the firm should be viewed as an ongoing concern, and the cost of capital used in captial budgeting should be calculated as a weighted average, or composite, of the various types of funds it uses, regardless of the specific financing used to fund a particular project.

BASIC DEFINITIONS

Capital components are the long-term items on the right-hand side of the balance sheet: various types of debt, preferred stock, and common equity. Capital is a necessary factor of production, and, like any other factor, it has a cost. The cost of each component is defined as the *component cost* of that particular type of capital. For example, if Precision Associates can borrow money at 11 percent, the component cost of debt is defined as 11 percent. Throughout most of this chapter we concentrate on debt, retained earnings, and new issues of common stock. These are the major capital structure components; their component costs are identified by the following symbols:

capital components
The long-term items on the right-hand side of the balance sheet: various types of long-term debt, preferred stock, and common equity.

k_d = interest rate on the firm's new debt = component cost of debt, before tax.

$k_d(1 - t)$ = component cost of debt, after tax, where t is the marginal tax rate. The term $k_d(1 - t)$ is the debt cost used to calculate the weighted average cost of capital.

k_p = component cost of preferred stock.

k_s = component cost of retained earnings (or internal equity). This k_s is identical to the k_s developed in Chapters 15 and 18 and defined there as the required rate of return on common stock.

k_e = component cost of external capital obtained by issuing new common stock. As we shall see, it is necessary to distinguish between equity raised by retaining earnings versus that raised by selling new stock. This is why we distinguish between k_s and k_e.

k_a = the average, or composite, cost of capital. It is also called the weighted average cost of capital, WACC, so k_a = WACC. If a firm raises $1 of new capital to finance asset expansion, and if it is to keep its capital structure in balance (that is, if it is to keep the same percentage of debt, preferred stock, and common stock equity funds), it must raise part of its new funds as debt, part as preferred stock, and part as common equity (with equity coming either from earnings retention or from the issuance of new common stock).[2]

These definitions and concepts are explained in detail in the remainder of the chapter, where we seek to accomplish two goals: (1) to develop a marginal cost of capital schedule (k_a = MCC) that can be used in capital budgeting and (2) to determine the mix of types of capital that will minimize the firm's cost of capital and thereby maximize its value.

MINIMUM REQUIRED RETURN

Any source of funds that the company uses has an implicit cost associated with it. As we learned in the chapters on capital budgeting, the firm raises money to invest in productive assets, which provide a cash flow to the firm. The cash flow must cover not only the project's *operating expenses* but the *financial obligations* arising from the acceptance of the project as well.

In Chapters 17 and 18 we explored the various forms of return associated with each financing vehicle. With debt financing, the project's cash flow must cover the periodic interest payments. If the company is financed in part with preferred stock, preferred dividends must be paid. Finally, the required return on common stock equity financing must also be met through the project's cash flow. The firm will determine the portion of after-tax earnings that will be paid in the form of dividends to shareholders and the portion that will be reinvested to insure the firm's future growth. Remember, even if a particular project is financed entirely with debt, the appropriate required return for the project is the firm's weighted average cost of capital. Therefore the project's cash flow must be large enough to cover these explicit financial costs (interest and dividends) as well as implicit financial costs (earnings retention for growth).

The minimum acceptable rate of return a project can earn is that rate which just satisfies all sources of financing. Perhaps a simple example will clarify this point. Heath Publishing Company is planning to begin operations by purchasing a new printing press and other necessary operating assets for $5 million. The company will raise funds for the new machine in proportion to the industry's average capital structure, 40 percent debt and 60 percent equity. The lenders will require a 13 percent return, whereas equity investors, including the firm's founders, expect to receive a 16 percent return on their investment. Let us also suppose, for simplicity's sake, that the after-tax cash returns from the firm will continue at their current planned level forever and that all residual earnings will be paid out in the form of dividends. If the

---

[2]Firms try to keep their debt, preferred stock, and common equity in optimal proportions; we will see how they establish these proportions in Chapter 20. However, firms do not try to maintain any proportional relationship between the common stock and retained earnings accounts as shown on the balance sheet — common equity is common equity, whether it is represented by common stock or by retained earnings.

company's marginal tax rate is 40 percent, what minimum cash flow *after* operating expenses (net income plus depreciation) must be produced to justify the creation of the firm? In essence, the question becomes: What return must the firm produce to satisfy all sources of financing?

In Chapter 6, we discussed the expenses that a firm must cover if it is to make a profit. However, satisfying only the claims arising from operations (labor and materials costs, for example) and the claims of the government for taxes still leaves one group, the firm's financing partners, without their rightful return. Therefore, the successful firm must cover interest payments and dividends (or capital gains required by equity investors), as well as operating costs and taxes. Hence, the project's required cash flow after operating expenses is equal to the amount of financing times the required return of each financing source:

$$\text{Required cash flow} = \text{Required after-tax return on debt} \times \text{Amount of debt}$$
$$+ \text{Required return on equity} \times \text{Amount of equity}$$

$$= (0.13)(1 - t)(\$2,000,000) + (0.16)(\$3,000,000)$$

$$= (0.13)(1 - 0.4)(\$2,000,000) + (0.16)(\$3,000,000)$$

$$= \$156,000 + \$480,000$$

$$= \$636,000.$$

Thus

$$\frac{\text{Minimum acceptable}}{\text{rate of return}} = \frac{\text{Required cash flow}}{\text{Investment}}$$

$$= \frac{\$636,000}{\$5,000,000}$$

$$= 12.72\%.$$

As we shall demonstrate with Equation 19-6, the cost of capital for a company is the weighted average of the component cost of each source of capital. In the present example, with a capital structure composed of 40 percent debt and 60 percent equity,

$$\text{Cost of capital} = \text{After-tax cost of debt} \times \text{Proportion of debt in}$$
$$\text{the capital structure} + \text{Cost of equity} \times$$
$$\text{Proportion of equity in the capital structure}$$

$$= (0.13)(1 - 0.4)(0.4) + (0.16)(0.6)$$

$$= 0.0312 + 0.096$$

$$= 0.1272, \text{ or } 12.72\%.$$

Thus it should be clear that for either a project or a firm (which is a combination of projects), the minimum acceptable cash flow is one that just satisfies each of the suppliers of capital. Therefore the minimum acceptable rate of return for a project or the firm as a whole is the cost of capital. In Chapter 14, we found this to be the point where the project's net present value (NPV) equaled zero. At this point the claims of all contributors to the project's success have been satisfied. Operating costs for labor, materials, and so on, have been paid, taxes have been paid, and the required rates of return for each of the various suppliers of capital have been met. Thus the true break-even point for the firm is where all of its projects' NPVs = $0.[3] Recall from Chapter 14 that firms do not seek projects whose NPV = $0, but, rather, firm's actively seek projects that have positive NPVs. This reflects the fact that once all claims from operations have been satisfied, the owners of the firm — the investors in the firm's common stock — receive a return in excess of their required return. Naturally a firm would reject any project with an anticipated NPV that is negative, since the cash flows from the project would not be sufficient to meet the needs of either expenses from operations, tax obligations, or the firm's suppliers of capital.

Now that we have analyzed the basic concept behind the cost of capital and its use as the minimum acceptable rate of return for investment proposals, we will turn to a more complete definition of how each source of capital is computed.

COST OF DEBT

The component cost used to calculate the weighted cost of capital is the interest rate on debt, k_d, multiplied by $(1 - t)$, where t is the firm's marginal tax rate:[4]

$$\text{Component cost of debt} = k_d(1 - t). \qquad \textbf{(19-1)}$$

For example, if a firm can borrow at a rate of 14 percent, and if it has a tax rate of 40 percent, its **after-tax cost of debt** is

$$k_d(1 - t) = 14\%(0.6) = 8.4\%.$$

after-tax cost of debt, $k_d(1 - t)$
The relevant cost to the firm for new debt financing, since interest is deductible from taxable income.

The reason for making the tax adjustment is as follows. The value of the firm's stock, which we want to maximize, depends on *after-tax* income. Inter-

---

[3]In Chapter 20 we will introduce an operating breakeven point where EBIT = $0, that is, where all operating costs are just satisfied. As we will explain there, this breakeven point can be expanded to include the payment of fixed financial charges such as interest (that is, where EBT = $0). Yet these definitions of breakeven are incomplete because they do not contain a provision for meeting the return of the firm's owners, the investors in the firm's common stock.

[4]In our discussion of the required return on equity, flotation costs (or the cost of selling equity through an investment banker) will be an integral part of the *cost of equity.* However, when we evaluate the *cost of debt,* flotation costs will be ignored. The flotation cost for a debt issue, sold through investment bankers in the capital markets, is usually quite low as a percentage of the issue. In fact, most debt is placed directly with banks, insurance companies, pension funds, and the like, and therefore has virtually no flotation cost. Thus, although the costs associated with the sale of both debt and equity by investment bankers are real, only the cost of selling equity will be considered in this chapter.

est is a deductible expense. The effect of this is as if the taxing authorities were paying part of the interest charges. Therefore, to put the costs of debt and equity on a comparable basis, we adjust the interest rate downward to account for the preferential tax treatment of debt.

The importance of the tax deductibility of interest may be observed in the following example. Suppose a firm with a 50 percent tax rate has the choice of financing with debt or preferred stock. Interest is paid before taxes (thus it is tax deductible), whereas preferred stock dividends are paid after taxes and therefore are not tax deductible. If we assume the interest *or* preferred dividend payment is equal to $1,000, the result is as follows:

	Debt Option	**Preferred Option**
EBIT	$5,000	$5,000
−I	−1,000	− 0
EBT	4,000	5,000
−T	−2,000	−2,500
EAIT	2,000	2,500
−Pfd	− 0	−1,000
NI	$2,000	$1,500

Note that because of the tax deductibility of interest, the preferred dividend would have to fall by the amount of the tax subsidy on interest — 50 percent in this example — for the net income under the preferred-stock-financed income stream to equal the debt-financed stream's net income. Therefore, the effective cost of debt capital to the business is not the interest rate on debt but, rather, the after-tax cost determined by Equation 19-1.

Our primary concern with the cost of capital is to use it in a decision-making process — to determine the minimum acceptable return on new capital budgeting or other investment projects. Thus the appropriate cost of debt is the cost for new borrowing, not the historical interest rates on old, previously outstanding debt. In other words, we are interested in the cost of the next dollar borrowed, or the *marginal* cost of debt. Whether the firm borrowed at a high or low rate in the past is irrelevant for this purpose.

COST OF PREFERRED STOCK

The component **cost of preferred stock, k_p,** that is used to calculate the weighted cost of capital is the preferred dividend, D_p, divided by the net issuing price, P_n, or the price the firm receives after deducting flotation costs:

$$\text{Component cost of preferred stock} = k_p = \frac{D_p}{P_n} \qquad \textbf{(19-2)}$$

cost of preferred stock, k_p
The preferred dividend, D_p, divided by the net issuing price, P_n.

Equation 19-2 assumes that the dividend from the preferred stock remains constant — that is, that the dividend will always be paid and that the preferred stock is not a participating preferred issue.

Phoenix Power and Light has preferred stock that pays a $12 dividend and sells for $100 per share in the market. If the company issues new shares of preferred, it will incur an underwriting (or flotation) cost of 2.5 percent, or $2.50 per share, so it will net $97.50 per share. Therefore, the cost of preferred stock would be 12.31 percent:

$$k_p = \$12.00/\$97.50 = 12.31\%.$$

Equation 19-2 can also be used to determine the cost of preferred stock if an issue is already outstanding. Suppose the price of Phoenix Power's preferred stock falls to $80 per share. This is a signal to the firm that investors will no longer accept a return of 12.3 percent; now they will require a 15 percent return:

$$k_p = \$12.00/\$80.00 = 15\%.$$

Of course, the investors' required return is the firm's cost of capital for that source of financing. Note also that no tax adjustments are made when calculating k_p because, unlike interest on debt, dividends are not tax deductible.

COST OF RETAINED EARNINGS, k_s

cost of retained earnings, k_s
The rate of return stockholders require on the firm's common stock based on alternative investment opportunities that stockholders could make if no earnings were retained.

opportunity cost
The rate of return on the best alternative investment available; the highest return that will *not* be earned if the funds are invested in a particular project.

The costs of debt and preferred stock are based on the returns investors require on these securities. Similarly, the **cost of retained earnings, k_s,** is the rate of return stockholders require on the firm's common stock.[5]

At one time many managers believed that retained earnings were a costless source of funds. However, managers now realize that retained earnings are not cost-free. The reason that a cost of capital must be assigned to retained earnings can be explained by the principle of **opportunity cost.** The firm's after-tax earnings literally belong to the stockholders. Bondholders are compensated by interest payments and preferred stockholders by preferred dividends, but the earnings remaining after interest and preferred dividends belong to the common stockholders and serve to compensate them for the use of their capital. Management may pay out earnings in the form of dividends, or earnings can be reinvested in the business. If management decides to retain earnings, there is an opportunity cost involved — stockholders could have received the earnings as dividends and invested these funds in other stocks, in bonds, in real estate, or in anything else. Thus the firm must earn on the retained earnings at least as much as stockholders themselves could earn in alternative investments of comparable risk.

What rate of return do stockholders expect to earn on equivalent risk investments? For example, assume that Mission Electronic's investors expect to earn a return of $k_s = 17\%$ on their money. If a stockholder received $10,000

---

[5]The term *retained earnings* can be interpreted to mean either the balance sheet item "retained earnings," consisting of all the earnings retained in the business throughout its history, or the income statement item "additions to retained earnings." The latter definition is used in this chapter. For our purpose, *retained earnings* refers to the period's *changes in retained earnings* or, in other words, to that part of the period's earnings not paid out in dividends and hence available for reinvestment in the business during the period.

from any source — from savings, from dividends paid by Mission, or from any-where else — he or she could buy more stock in Mission or some company with similar risk and expect to earn $k_s = 17\%$. *Therefore, if the firm cannot invest retained earnings and earn at least k_s, it should pay these funds to its stockholders and let them invest directly in other assets that do provide this return.*

FINDING THE BASIC REQUIRED RATE OF RETURN ON COMMON EQUITY

In the United States the majority of business firms have a debt-to-total-assets ratio that is less than 50 percent. Thus common stock equity provides the largest proportion of financing in the average firm's capital structure. Unfortunately, the cost of equity is the most difficult of the components of the cost of capital to compute.

Other sources of capital have periodic fixed or semifixed payment sched-ules, such as debt's interest and principal payments, which are contractual ob-ligations, and preferred stock's dividends, which are not contractually guaran-teed but are generally treated as fixed obligations by financial managers. The amount and timing of cash flows from these financing sources can be forecast with a high degree of certainty, making investors' required return (and hence the cost of capital from these sources) easy to determine. Unlike these securi-ties, however, the cash flows resulting from the purchase of common stock generally have been difficult to forecast. Although it is not at all easy to mea-sure k_s, we can employ the principles developed in Chapters 15 and 18 to produce reasonably good cost of equity measures.

It is obvious by now that the basic rate of return investors require on a firm's common equity, k_s, is an important yet elusive quantity. This re-quired rate of return is the cost of retained earnings, and it forms the basis for the cost of capital obtained from new stock issues. How is this all-important quantity estimated? To begin with, we know that for stocks in equilibrium (which is the typical situation), the required rate of return, k_s, is also equal to the expected rate of return, $\hat{k}_s$. Further, the required return is equal to a risk-less rate, R_F, plus a premium for all risks, RP, and the expected return on a con-stant growth stock is equal to a dividend yield, D_1/P_0, plus an expected growth rate, g:

$$\text{Required rate of return} = \text{Expected rate of return}$$

$$k_s = R_F + RP = D_1/P_0 + g = \hat{k}_s.$$

Therefore, k_s can be estimated either directly as $k_s = R_F + RP$ or indirectly as $k_s = \hat{k}_s = D_1/P_0 + g$. Actually, we can use three methods for finding the cost of retained earnings: (1) the discounted cash flow (DCF) approach, which was introduced in Chapter 18, (2) the CAPM approach, which was introduced in Chapter 15, and (3) the bond yield plus risk premium approach. These three approaches are discussed in the following sections. In Chapter 18 we saw that the expected rate of return on a share of common stock ultimately depends on the dividends paid on the stock:

$$P_0 = \frac{D_1}{(1 + \hat{k}_s)} + \frac{D_2}{(1 + \hat{k}_s)^2} + \cdots + \frac{D_\infty}{(1 + \hat{k}_s)^\infty}. \qquad \textbf{(18-1)}$$

Here P_0 is the current price of the stock; D_t is the dividend expected to be paid at at the end of Year t; and $\hat{k}_s$ is the expected rate of return. If dividends are expected to grow at a constant rate, then, as we saw in Chapter 18, Equation 18-1 reduces to the following expression:

$$P_0 = \frac{D_1}{\hat{k}_s - g}. \qquad \textbf{(19-3)}$$

We can solve for $\hat{k}_s$ to obtain the expected rate of return on common equity, which in equilibrium is also equal to the required rate of return.[6]

$$\hat{k}_s = \frac{D_1}{P_0} + \text{Expected g}. \qquad \textbf{(19-4)}$$

Thus investors expect to receive a dividend yield, D_1/P_0, plus a capital gains yield (a measure of the expected growth in the firm's value), g, for a total expected return of $\hat{k}_s$.

To illustrate, suppose a business, Hadaway Industries, begins to retain some earnings rather than paying them all out as dividends. The stock is in equilibrium, it sells for $30.00, the next expected dividend is $2.70, and the expected growth rate is now 7 percent. The firm's expected and required rate of return, and hence its cost of retained earnings, is

$$\hat{k}_s = k_s = \frac{\$2.70}{\$30.00} + 7\% = 9\% + 7\% = 16\%.$$

Thus 16 percent is the minimum rate of return that Hadaway Industries' management must be able to earn on the equity financed projects to justify retaining earnings and plowing them back into the business rather than paying them out to stockholders as dividends. Henceforth in this chapter we assume that equilibrium exists and use the terms k_s and $\hat{k}_s$ interchangeably.

It is relatively easy to determine the dividend yield, but it is difficult to establish the proper growth rate. If past growth rates in earnings and dividends have been relatively stable, and if investors appear to be projecting a continuation of past trends, then g may be based on the firm's historical growth rate. *However, if the company's past growth rate has been abnormally high or low, either because of its own unique situation or because of general economic*

---

[6]Note, however, that if a firm's growth rate is not expected to remain constant, Equations 19-3 and 19-4 will not hold.

conditions, investors will not project the past growth rate into the future. Remember, an investor is purchasing the firm's *future, not its past,* cash flows.

In practice, security analysts regularly make forecasts of the growth in both dividends and earnings, looking at such factors as projected sales, profit margins, and competitive factors. An individual making a cost of capital estimate can obtain some analysts' forecasts, average them, use the average as a proxy for the growth expectations of investors in general, and then combine the forecast growth with the current dividend yield to estimate the cost of equity capital, as follows:

$$k_s = D_1/P_0 + \text{growth rate, g, as projected by security analysts.}$$

Again, note that this estimate of k_s is based on the assumption that g is expected to remain constant in the future.[7]

The CAPM Approach

The Capital Asset Pricing Model (CAPM) as developed in Chapter 15 can be used to help estimate k_s as follows:

Step 1 Estimate the riskless rate, R_F, generally taken to be either the Treasury bond rate or the 30-day Treasury bill rate.

Step 2 Estimate the stock's beta coefficient, b, and use this as an index of the stock's risk.

Step 3 Estimate the rate of return on the market or on an average stock. Designate this return k_M.

Step 4 Estimate the required rate of return on the firm's stock as follows:

$$k_s = R_F + b(k_M - R_F).$$

This equation shows that the CAPM estimate of k_s begins with the risk-free rate, R_F, to which is added a risk premium that is equal to the premium on an average security, $k_M - R_F$, scaled up or down to reflect the stock's relative risk by multiplying by its beta coefficient.

---

[7]Analysts' growth rate forecasts are usually for five years into the future, and the rates provided represent the average growth rate over that 5-year horizon. Studies have shown that analysts' forecasts represent the best source of growth data for DCF cost of capital estimates. See Robert Harris, "Using Analysts' Growth Rate Forecasts to Estimate Shareholder Required Rates of Return." *Financial Management,* Spring 1986, pp. 58–67.

It is also worth noting that another method for estimating g used by financial analysts involves first projecting the firm's average future dividend payout ratio and its complement, the *retention rate,* and then multiplying the retention rate by the company's average future projected rate of return on equity (ROE):

$$g = (\text{Retention rate})(\text{ROE}) = (1.0 - \text{Payout rate})(\text{ROE}).$$

Security analysts often use this procedure when they estimate growth rates, but their real skill as forecasters is in accurately estimating the payout rate and the future ROE.

To illustrate the CAPM approach, assume that $R_F = 6\%$, $k_M = 10\%$, and $b = 0.7$ for a given stock. The stock's k_s is calculated as follows:

$$k_s = 6\% + 0.7(10\% - 6\%) = 6\% + 2.8\% = 8.8\%.$$

Had b been 1.8, indicating that the stock was riskier than average, k_s would have been

$$k_s = 6\% + 1.8(4\%) = 6\% + 7.2\% = 13.2\%.$$

For an average-risk security,

$$k_s = k_M = 6\% + 1.0(4\%) = 6\% + 4\% = 10\%.$$

It should be noted that even though the CAPM approach appears to yield accurate, precise estimates of k_s, there actually are several problems with it. First, as we saw in Chapter 15, if a firm's stockholders are not well diversified, they may be concerned with total risk rather than market risk only; in that case the firm's true investment risk will not be measured by beta, and the CAPM procedure will understate the correct value of k_s. Further, even if the CAPM method is valid, it is hard to obtain correct estimates of the inputs required to make it operational, such as the forecasts of the risk-free rate, the firm's future beta, and the market risk premium. This latter problem has been particularly vexing in the 1980s, because the riskiness of stocks versus bonds has been changing, making the market risk premium unstable.

Bond Yield plus Risk Premium Approach

Although it is essentially an ad hoc, subjective procedure, analysts often estimate a firm's cost of common equity by adding a risk premium of from three to five percentage points to the interest rate on the firm's long-term debt. For example, if a firm's bonds yield 9 percent, its cost of equity may be estimated as follows:

$$k_s = \text{Bond rate} + \text{Risk premium} = 9\% + 4\% = 13\%.$$

This 4 percent risk premium is a judgmental estimate, so the estimated value of k_s is also judgmental.[8] A judgmental estimate is not likely to result in a very accurate measure of the cost of equity capital — about all that it can do is "get us into the right ballpark." Low premiums occur when interest rates are quite high and people are reluctant to invest in long-term bonds for fear of runaway inflation, further increases in interest rates, and losses on bond investments. High premiums occur when interest rates are relatively low.

---

[8]Analysts who use this procedure often cite studies of historical returns on stocks and bonds and use the difference between the average yield (dividends plus capital gains) on stocks and the average yield on bonds as the risk premium of stocks over bonds. The most frequently cited study is R. G. Ibbotson and R. A. Sinquefield, "Stocks, Bonds, Bills, and Inflation: Year-By-Year Historical Returns (1926–1974)," *Journal of Business,* January 1976, pp. 11–47.

Conclusions on the Cost of Equity Capital

Which of the methods to determine the cost of equity is correct? The answer is, of course, that all are correct within their limiting assumptions. Then, which ones should be used in business situations? Many business firms use all of these methods or more to approximate the cost of equity. In fact, the Du Pont Corporation uses five different methods to evaluate and approximate the cost of equity capital to the firm. Therefore, we suggest that in practical work it is best to use all three of the methods discussed here and then to apply judgment when the methods produce differing results. Managers experienced in estimating equity capital costs recognize that both careful analysis and some very fine judgments are required. *It would be nice to pretend that these judgments are unnecessary and to be able to specify an easy, precise way of determining the exact cost of equity capital. Unfortunately, this is not possible. Finance is in large part a matter of judgment, and we simply must face this fact.*

COST OF NEWLY ISSUED COMMON STOCK, OR EXTERNAL EQUITY, k_e

cost of external equity, k_e
The cost of retained earnings adjusted for flotation costs.

The cost of new common stock, or external equity capital, k_e, is higher than the cost of retained earnings, k_s, because of flotation costs involved in selling new common stock. What rate of return must be earned on funds raised by selling stock in order to make this action worthwhile? To put it another way, what is the cost of new common stock?

For a firm with a constant growth rate, the answer is found by applying the following formula:

$$k_e = \frac{D_1}{P_0(1 - F)} + g. \qquad \textbf{(19-5)}$$

Here **F** is the percentage **flotation cost** incurred in selling the issue, so $P_0(1 - F)$ is the net price per share received by the company when it sells new shares.

flotation cost, F
The percentage cost of issuing new common stock.

Recall that Hadaway Industries had a required return of 16 percent on its currently issued common stock equity. If the firm wishes to issue new equity, however, there will be a flotation cost charged by the investment banker that will affect the cost of equity. If the flotation charge for Hadaway's new issue is 10 percent, the cost of new outside equity is computed as follows:

$$k_e = \frac{\$2.70}{\$30(1 - 0.10)} + 7\%$$

$$= \frac{2.70}{\$27} + 7\%$$

$$= 10\% + 7\%$$

$$= 17\%.$$

Investors require a return on equity shares that consists of a current dividend yield, D_1/P_0, and a growth or capital gains component, g. For Hadaway this required return, k_s, was 16 percent. However, because of flotation costs, the company *must earn more* than 16 percent on funds obtained by selling common stock to provide this 16 percent return. What causes this seeming contradiction? Specifically, the firm will have to provide the $2.70 in dividends next year and maintain a 7 percent growth with $27 a share, not $30. The firm must meet these investor expectations with only 90 percent of the issue, 10 percent goes to the investment banker for services in selling the stock. Therefore, if Hadaway earns less than 17 percent on the new equity-financed project, the investment will be unable to provide the required dividend of $2.70 and the anticipated 7 percent growth. Such a decline in either dividends or growth or both would cause the value of the stock to decline. Conversely, if the project earns more than 17 percent, the firm's dividend and/or growth will be larger than required and the price of Hadaway stock will rise.

WEIGHTED AVERAGE, OR COMPOSITE, COST OF CAPITAL, WACC = k_a

target capital structure

The optimal capital structure; the percentage of debt, preferred stock, and common equity that will maximize the price of the firm's stock.

As we shall see in Chapter 20, each firm has a **target capital structure,** which is that mix of debt, preferred stock, and common equity that causes the firm's stock price to be maximized. Therefore, a rational, value-maximizing firm will establish its optimal capital structure and then raise new capital in a manner that will keep the actual capital structure on target over time. In this chapter we assume that the firm has identified its optimal capital structure, that it uses this optimum as the target, and that it finances so as to remain constantly on target. How the target is established will be examined in Chapter 20.

weighted average cost of capital, WACC = k_a

A weighted average of the component costs of debt, preferred stock, and common equity.

The target proportions of debt, preferred stock, and common equity, along with the component costs of capital, are used to calculate the firm's **weighted average cost of capital, WACC = k_a.** To illustrate, suppose Environmental Design Systems, Inc. (EDS) has a target capital structure calling for 30 percent debt and 70 percent common stock equity. Other key data are as follows:

$P_0 = \$80.00$.

$D_0 = \$5.09 =$ Dividends per share in the *last* period. (D_0 has already been paid, so an investor purchasing this stock today would *not* receive D_0 but, rather, would receive D_1, the *next* dividend.)

$g = 10\%$.

$$k_s = \frac{D_1}{P_0} + g = \frac{D_0(1 + g)}{P_0} + g$$

$$= \frac{\$5.09(1.1)}{\$80} + 0.10$$

$$= 0.07 + 0.10 = 0.17$$

$$= 17\%.$$

$$k_d = 12\%.$$

$$t = 40\% = 0.4.$$

$$k_d(1 - t) = 12\%(0.6) = 7.2\%.$$

Now suppose that the company needs to raise $3 million. To keep its capital structure on target, it must obtain 0.3($3,000,000) = $900,000 as debt and 0.7($3,000,000) = $2,100,000 as equity. The weighted average cost of the new capital is calculated as follows:

Component	Weight	Component Cost	Product
Debt	0.3	7.2%	2.16%
Equity	0.7	17.0%	11.90%
		Weighted average cost = k_a =	14.06%

The calculations in the preceding table can also be thought of in an equation format:

$$k_a = \left(\begin{array}{c}\text{Fraction} \\ \text{of debt in} \\ \text{capital} \\ \text{structure}\end{array}\right)\left(\begin{array}{c}\text{Interest} \\ \text{rate}\end{array}\right)\left(1 - \text{Tax rate}\right) + \left(\begin{array}{c}\text{Fraction} \\ \text{of equity} \\ \text{in capital} \\ \text{structure}\end{array}\right)\left(\begin{array}{c}\text{Cost of} \\ \text{equity}\end{array}\right)$$

$$= w_d(k_d)(1 - t) + w_s(k_s) \tag{19-6}$$

$$= 0.3(12\%)(0.6) + 0.7(17\%)$$

$$= 2.16\% + 11.9\%$$

$$= 14.06\%.$$

Using either method, we see that every dollar of new capital consists of 30 cents of debt with an after-tax cost of 7.2 percent and 70 cents of equity with a cost of 17 percent. The average cost of the whole dollar is 14.06 percent.

Preferred Stock

Environmental Design Systems does not use preferred stock. However, if it did, the cost of preferred stock would be included in the calculation of the composite cost of capital as follows:

1. Estimate the component cost of the preferred stock, k_p:

$$k_p = D_p/P_n.$$

Here D_p is the dividend that EDS would have to pay on the preferred stock (remember, the dividend is constant and generally is not skipped, because no common dividends may be paid if preferred dividends are omitted), and P_n is the net (after flotation costs) price per share that the company would receive. If $D_p = \$3.25$ and $P_n = \$25$, then

$$k_p = \$3.25/\$25 = 0.13 = 13\%.$$

Since preferred dividends are not deductible, no tax adjustment is needed.

2. Determine the target capital structure percentages, or weights. We assume that EDS has decided to use $w_d = 35$ percent debt, $w_p = 10$ percent preferred stock, and $w_s = 55$ percent common stock equity.

3. Combine the component costs with the capital structure weights to determine the weighted average cost of capital, using an expanded version of Equation 19-6. We have already assumed that $k_d = 12\%$, $k_p = 13\%$, and $k_s = 17\%$, so

$$k_a = w_d(k_d)(1 - t) + w_pk_p + w_sk_s$$

$$= 0.35(12\%)(0.6) + 0.10(13\%) + 0.55(17\%)$$

$$= 2.52\% + 1.3\% + 9.35\%$$

$$= 13.17\%.$$

Thus, if EDS decided to use preferred stock in addition to debt and common stock, the average cost of each dollar raised would fall slightly to 13.17 percent.

CHANGES IN THE COST OF CAPITAL

marginal cost of capital (MCC)
The cost of obtaining another dollar of new capital; the weighted average cost of capital at a particular dollar value of new capital.

The cost of capital changes as the proportion of debt and equity in the capital structure changes. As a general rule, a different **marginal cost of capital (MCC)**[9] will exist for every possible capital structure; *the optimal capital structure is the one that produces the lowest MCC*. Could EDS raise an unlimited amount of new capital at the 14.06 percent cost as long as its capital structure is maintained at 30 percent debt and 70 percent equity? The answer is *no*. As companies raise larger and larger sums during a given time period, the costs of both the debt and the equity components begin to rise, and as this occurs, the weighted average cost of obtaining new capital rises.

This increase in the cost of capital occurs for several reasons. First, even if the proportions of debt and equity remain the same, the level of interest payments must increase as the debt increases. As the fixed interest payments increase, the financial risk increases, as evidenced by lower coverage ratios. Certainly, as the financial risk increases, the suppliers of debt capital will require higher interest rates to offset the greater risk. Second, generating larger amounts of equity means that the firm will exhaust its internal equity and will have to turn to more expensive new equity. Another factor that would affect

---

[9]Recall that the marginal cost of a dollar is defined as the cost of obtaining another dollar of new capital. For our purposes the terms *marginal* and *weighted average* cost of capital will be used synonymously.

the cost of capital is that the firm's risk profile may change with rapid growth, because the company's management may be pressed beyond its capabilities or the firm may take on more risky projects than before.

Where will these cost increases or breaks in the **MCC schedule** occur? Although it is difficult to tell in practice, we can provide some insights into the determination of these points by utilizing the data generated in discussing the cost of capital for Environmental Design Systems. Additionally, we need to assume the following:

1. The firm wishes to maintain the same 30%/70% debt/equity capital structure under all financing plans.

2. The company will not invest in any project that is riskier than current projects.

3. EDS can borrow up to $45,000 at the current 12 percent interest rate, with additional debt costing 15 percent.

4. The firm has a total of $84,000 in undistributed profits for this period, which management has decided to retain rather than use for dividends. (Note that this money was earned this year and not retained previously.) A 20 percent flotation charge will be incurred if new common stock is sold.

5. $k_s = D_1/P_0 + g = \$5.60/\$80 + 10\% = 17\%$.

$k_e = D_1/P_0(1 - F) + g = \$5.60/\$80(1 - 0.20) + 10\% = 18.75\%$,

where

D_1 = next year's dividend,

P_0 = current common stock price for EDS's shares,

F = percentage flotation cost for new equity shares,

g = expected growth rate.

6. The marginal tax rate will remain a constant 40 percent for these computations.

EDS's weighted average cost of capital is calculated in Table 19-1, which first shows the new retained earnings (earnings retained this year, not in the past) and then the new common stock. We see that the weighted average cost of each dollar, or the marginal cost of capital, is 14.06 percent as long as retained earnings are used, but the average cost jumps to 15.29 percent as soon as the firm exhausts its internal financing and is forced to sell new common stock.

How much new capital can EDS raise before it exhausts its retained earnings and is forced to sell new common stock; that is, where will the **break, or jump, in the MCC schedule** occur? The question becomes one of how much *total financing* — debt plus the $84,000 in retained earnings — can be done before retained earnings are exhausted and the firm is forced to sell new

MCC schedule
A graph or table that relates the firm's weighted average cost of capital to the amount of new capital raised.

break, or jump, in the MCC schedule
A change in the weighted average cost of capital that occurs when there is a change in a component cost of capital.

Table 19-1 **EDS's Marginal Cost of Capital Using:**
(1) New Retained Earnings and (2) New Common Stock

Source	Weight	×	Component Cost	=	Product
(1) MCC When Equity Is Obtained Internally (from Retained Earnings)					
Debt	0.3		7.2%[a]		2.16%
Equity	0.7		17.0		11.90
	1.0				14.06%
(2) MCC When Equity Is Obtained Externally (from Sale of New Stock)					
Debt	0.3		7.20%		2.16%
Equity	0.7		18.75%		13.13
	1.0				15.29%

[a]Recall that the cost of debt = $k_d(1 - t) = 12\%(0.6) = 7.2\%$.

common stock. Seventy percent of the total financing will be made with the $84,000 of retained earnings. Therefore, if X equals total financing allowable with no new equity, then

$$0.7X = \text{Retained earnings} = \$84,000.$$

break point
The dollar value of new capital raised that corresponds to a jump in the MCC schedule.

Solving for X, we obtain the **break point:**

$$\text{Break point} = X = \frac{\text{Retained earnings}}{0.7} = \frac{\$84,000}{0.7} = \$120,000.$$

Thus EDS can raise $120,000, consisting of $84,000 of retained earnings and $36,000 ($120,000 − $84,000 = $36,000) of new debt supported by these new retained earnings, without altering its capital structure:

30% — new debt supported by retained earnings	$ 36,000
70% — retained earnings	84,000
Total expansion supportable by retained earnings, or break point for retained earnings in the MCC schedule	$120,000

We have noted that there will be other possible breaks in the MCC schedule when the cost of any component source of capital changes. One such possible change for EDS would be the increase in the cost of debt if more than $45,000 is needed. If additional debt (over the $45,000 level) is required, it can be acquired, but at a cost of 15 percent. This will result in a second break point in the MCC schedule at the level where the $45,000 of cheaper, 12 percent debt is exhausted. At what amount of *total financing* will the 12 percent debt be used up? If we let Y represent the total financing at this second break point, then

$$0.3Y = \$45,000,$$

and, solving for Y, we obtain

$$Y = \frac{12\% \text{ debt}}{0.3} = \frac{\$45,000}{0.3} = \$150,000 = \text{Break point for debt.}$$

Thus there will be another break in the MCC schedule after EDS has raised a total of $150,000. As we demonstrated previously, up to $120,000 the MCC is 14.06 percent and just beyond $120,000 the MCC rises to 15.29 percent. Now we see that the MCC rises again at $150,000, to 15.83 percent.

Source	Weight	×	Component Cost	=	Product
Debt	0.3		9.00%[a]		2.70%
Equity	0.7		18.75		13.13
	1.0				15.83%

[a]The cost of debt = $k_d(1 - t) = 15\% (1 - 0.4) = 9.0\%$.

In other words, the next dollar beyond $150,000 will consist of 30 cents of 15 percent debt (9 percent after taxes) and 70 cents of new common stock (retained earnings were used up much earlier), and this marginal dollar will have an average cost of 15.83 percent.

The effect of this new MCC increase is shown in Figure 19-1. EDS now has two breaks, one caused by using up all of the retained earnings and the other caused by using up all of the 12 percent debt. With the two breaks, there are three different MCCs: $MCC_1 = 14.06\%$ for the first $120,000 of new capital; $MCC_2 = 15.29\%$ in the interval between $120,000 and $150,000; and $MCC_3 = 15.83\%$ for all new capital beyond $150,000.

There could, of course, be still more break points. For example, debt costs could continue to rise, or the flotation costs on new common stock could increase above 20 percent as larger amounts of stock are sold. These changes would cause more breaks in the MCC.

The easiest sequence for calculating MCC schedules is as follows:

1. Identify the points where breaks occur. A break will occur any time the cost of one of the capital components rises. (However, it is possible that two capital components could both increase at the same point.)

2. Determine the cost of capital for each component in the intervals between breaks.

3. Calculate the weighted averages of these costs; the weighted averages are the MCCs in each interval.

Notice that if there are n separate breaks, there will be n + 1 different MCCs. For example, in Figure 19-1 we see two breaks and three different MCCs.

Before concluding this section, we should note again that a different MCC schedule would result if a different capital structure were used. The optimal capital structure produces the lowest MCC.

Figure 19-1 **Marginal Cost of Capital Schedule for EDS Using Retained Earnings, New Common Stock, and Debt**

Even though a business may maintain a constant optimal capital structure, it cannot count on raising an unlimited amount of new capital at the same cost. For example, EDS can expect to encounter two breaks, or increases, in its marginal cost of capital (MCC). The first occurs at $120,000 in total financing, when retained earnings are exhausted and the firm issues new common stock. The second break comes at $150,000, when cost of debt increases, bringing the MCC to 15.83 percent. A break will thus occur whenever costs of either debt or equity increase.

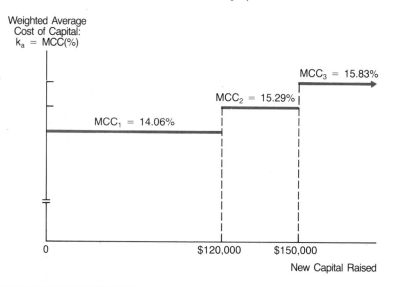

COMBINING THE MCC AND THE INVESTMENT OPPORTUNITY SCHEDULE (IOS)

Now that we have calculated the MCC schedule, we can use it to determine the discount rate used in the capital budgeting process; that is, *we can use the MCC schedule to find the cost of capital for use in determining projects' net present values (NPVs) as discussed in Chapter 14.*

To understand how the MCC is used in capital budgeting, assume that EDS has three financial executives: a financial vice president, a treasurer, and a director of capital budgeting. Of course, if the firm were smaller, the steps we will outline would still be carried out, but by the financial officer — perhaps with the aid of the firm's president — rather than with a staff as in the case of a larger firm.

For EDS, the financial vice president first asks the treasurer to develop the firm's MCC schedule, as we have done in Figure 19-1. Next, the financial vice

Table 19-2 **Potential Capital Budgeting Projects Available to EDS**

Project	Cost	Annual Inflows	Project Life (Years)	IRR (or Discount Rate at Which NPV = 0)
A	$30,000	$ 8,950	5	15.0%
B	23,000	5,864	7	17.0
C	35,000	6,710	10	14.0
D	52,000	15,250	6	19.0
E	30,000	6,907	8	16.0
F	35,000	16,097	3	18.0

president asks the director of capital budgeting (DCB) to determine the dollar amounts of potentially acceptable projects, using the IRR method (or using the NPV method at a number of different discount rates). The DCB has a listing of all the firm's potential projects, including the cost of each project and its projected annual net cash inflows. This listing is shown in Table 19-2.

The DCB would first calculate each project's IRR, as shown in the last column of Table 19-2, then plot the data given there as the **investment opportunity schedule (IOS)** shown in Figure 19-2. The figure also reproduces EDS's MCC schedule as plotted in Figure 19-1. The IOS shows how much money EDS could invest at different rates of return. If the cost of capital were above 19 percent, none of the available projects would have a positive NPV; hence none of them should be accepted. In that case EDS would simply not expand. If the cost of capital were 19 percent, EDS should take on only Project D, and its capital budget would call for the company to raise and invest $52,000. If the cost of capital were 18 percent, the firm should take only Projects D and F, raising a total of $87,000. Successively lower costs of capital call for larger and larger investment outlays.

Just how far down its IOS curve should the firm go? In other words, which of its available projects should it accept? The answer is that the firm should accept the four projects (D, F, B, and E) that have rates of return in excess of the cost of capital that would be required to finance them. Projects A and C should be rejected, because they would have to be financed with capital that has a cost of 15.83 percent, and at that cost of capital, A and C have negative NPVs and IRRs that are below their costs of capital. Therefore Environmental Design Systems should have a capital budget of $140,000.

In the plotting of the IOS and MCC schedules, their intersection should be noted — in our example the MCC is 15.29 percent at that point. If the firm uses 15.29 percent to evaluate all projects, then Projects D, F, B, and E will be accepted, whereas A and C will be rejected. Thus *the cost of capital used in the capital budgeting process as discussed in Chapter 14 is actually determined at the intersection of the IOS and MCC schedules.* If this intersection rate is used, the firm will make correct accept/reject decisions, and its level of financ-

investment opportunity schedule (IOS)
A listing or graph of the firm's investment opportunities ranked in order of the projects' rates of return.

Figure 19-2 **Combining EDS's MCC and IOS Curves to Determine Its Optimal Capital Budget**

This figure shows how the MCC schedule is used in capital budgeting. The investment opportunity schedule (IOS) indicates how much EDS can afford to invest at different rates of return. The two schedules intersect at an MCC of 15.29 percent, indicating the cost of capital that should be used in evaluating projects in capital budgeting. Projects D, F, B, and E, which have returns in excess of the cost of capital, would thus be accepted, making the total optimal capital budget $140,000. Because Projects A and C would have to be financed at 15.83 percent, they should be rejected.

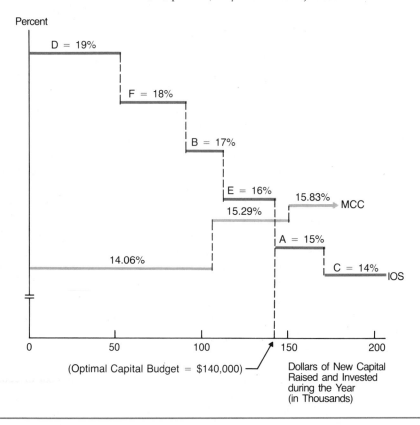

ing and investment will be optimal. If it uses any other rate, its capital budgeting will not be optimal.

DIVISIONAL COSTS OF CAPITAL

In Chapter 16 we learned that capital budgeting can affect a firm's beta risk, its corporate risk, or both. We have also seen that it is exceedingly difficult to quantify either effect. In other words, although it may be possible to reach the

SMALL BUSINESS

Cost of Equity Capital for Small Firms

Three techniques for estimating the cost of equity capital have been discussed in this chapter. They all have serious limitations when applied to small firms, increasing the need for the small firm's manager or owner to use judgment.

The first technique is the application of Gordon's constant growth model in the formula

$$k = D_1/P_0 + g,$$

where k is the cost of capital, D_1 is the expected dividend next period, P_0 is the market price of the stock, and g is the expected constant growth rate of the firm to perpetuity. That model will normally be impossible to apply to small firms because:

1. They pay no dividends;

2. They are not publicly traded and hence no market price can be observed; and

3. They are likely to have an unusual growth rate early in their life compared to later (i.e., g is not constant).

For such firms, the constant-growth dividend discount model is not useful, and, in fact, it is hard to imagine *any* dividend-based model that would be.

The second technique takes the yield on the firm's bonds and adds a risk premium of some amount, such as 4 or 5 percent. Of course, the small firm probably has no publicly traded bonds. Although it might be reasonable to add a risk premium to the interest rate applied to the firm's bank debt or other private debt, to do so is to employ a great deal of judgment. The third suggested approach is based on the CAPM. If the small firm is not a public corporation, there are no market prices to use in computing returns to estimate the beta.

Two alternatives can be attempted. One is the use of a *pure-play technique,* which requires identifying another firm in the same line of business with similar characteristics that does have a public equity issue. Such a firm is likely to be larger than the small firm, and because its equity is publicly traded, it has some degree of liquidity that the smaller firm doesn't have. The small firm's illiquidity means that one must add a risk premium above that implied by the CAPM.

Another alternative is to use accounting betas, which are betas estimated by using the firm's accounting data, to find a number to compare with the return on the market portfolio. For example, one could use the firm's accounting rate of return on equity as a measure of equity return. Two problems with this approach are that, unless the small firm is unusual, it probably produces complete accounting statements less often than large firms, and it may have only a short history. For example, financial statements done annually for only, say, three years, would not be adequate. Furthermore, the small firm is often dynamic; because it is changing rapidly, its historical data are not very useful for predicting the future.

On balance, the pure-play technique often is the most practical alternative.

Flotation Costs for Small Issues. When external equity capital is raised, the flotation costs increase the cost of equity capital beyond what it would be for internal funds. These external flotation costs are especially significant for smaller issues and may substantially affect capital budgeting decisions involving external equity funds.

To illustrate this point, consider a firm that is expected to pay constant dividends forever. In this case, if F is the percentage flotation cost, then the cost of equity capital is $D_1/[P_0(1 - F)]$. The higher the flotation cost, the higher the cost of external equity.

How big is F? According to a study made by the Securities and Exchange Commission in

1974, the average flotation cost of large common stock offerings (over $50 million) is only about 4 percent. If a firm is expected to pay a 20 percent return on equity (that is, $D_1/P_0 = 20\%$), for a large offering the cost of equity is $20\%/(1 - 0.04)$, or 20.8 percent.

The SEC's data for small offerings (less than $1 million) suggest that flotation costs for small offerings average about 21 percent. Thus the cost of equity capital in the previous example would be $20\%/(1 - 0.21)$, or about 25.3 percent. Compared to the 20.8 percent for large offerings, it is clear that a small firm will have a considerably higher hurdle rate for the same project than would a large firm. The small firm is therefore at a substantial disadvantage because of the effects of flotation costs.

The Small Firm Effect. A number of researchers have observed that portfolios of small-firm stocks have consistently higher average returns than portfolios of large-firm stocks. On the surface, it may seem to be beneficial for small firms to appear to produce average returns that are higher than those of large firms. In reality, it is bad news for the small firms. What it means is that the capital market demands higher returns for small firms' stocks than for otherwise similar stocks of large firms. The cost of equity capital is higher for small firms, even ignoring the flotation costs at the time of issuance.

It might be argued that the stocks of small firms are riskier than the stocks of large firms, thereby accounting for the differences in returns. It is true that research usually finds that betas are higher on average for small firms. However, the larger returns for small firms remain larger even after taking out the effects of higher risks — at least the higher risks in observed beta values.

The small-firm effect is an anomaly; that is, it is not consistent with presently available theory. In other words, we don't understand why small firms have higher returns, we just know that they do. Until a satisfactory explanation can be found for the small-firm effect, we can say only that the required returns (and cost of equity capital) are greater for small firms than for similar large firms. The manager of a small firm should take this factor into account when estimating the cost of equity capital. In general, the cost of equity capital appears to be about 4 percent higher per annum for small firms (those with market values of less than $20 million) than for large firms of similar risk characteristics.

general conclusion that one project is riskier than another (in either the beta or the corporate sense), it is difficult to develop a really good measure of project risk. Further, this lack of precision in measuring project risk makes it difficult to specify risk-adjusted rates of return, or project costs of capital, with which to evaluate individual projects. It is generally agreed, however, that riskier projects should be evaluated with a higher cost of capital than the overall corporate cost, whereas for lower-risk projects a lower cost of capital should be used. Unfortunately, there is no good way of specifying exactly how much higher or lower these cost rates should be; given the present state of the art, risk adjustments are necessarily judgmental and somewhat arbitrary.

Debt effects must also be taken into account. For example, one division may own a substantial amount of real estate, which is well suited as collateral for loans, whereas another division may have most of its capital tied up in special-purpose machinery, which is not good collateral. As a result, the division with the real estate may have a higher *debt capacity* than the machinery division. In this case, the first division might calculate its overall, or weighted average, cost of capital using a higher debt ratio than the second division.

Although the process is not exact, Environmental Design Systems (and many other companies) develops **risk-adjusted discount rates** for use in capital budgeting in a two-step process: (1) divisional costs of capital are established for each of the major operating divisions on the basis of the divisions' estimated risk and capital structures, and (2) within each division, all projects are classified into three categories — high risk, average risk, and low risk. Each of EDS's divisions then uses its basic divisional cost of capital as the discount rate for average-risk projects, reduces the discount rate by one percentage point when evaluating low-risk projects, and raises the rate by two percentage points for high-risk projects.

For example, if a division's basic cost of capital is estimated to be 10 percent, a 12 percent discount rate would be used for high-risk projects and a 9 percent rate for low-risk ones. Average-risk projects, which constitute about 80 percent of most of its divisions' capital budgets, would be evaluated at the 10 percent divisional cost of capital. This procedure is not very elegant, but at least it recognizes that different divisions have different characteristics and hence different costs of capital, and it acknowledges differential project riskiness within divisions. EDS's financial staff believes that these adjustments are in the right direction and that they result in better decisions than would be obtained if no adjustments were made.

risk-adjusted discount rate
The discount rate that applies to a particular risky (uncertain) stream of cash flows; the riskless rate plus a risk premium appropriate to the level of risk attached to a particular project's income stream.

SUMMARY

This chapter has explained how the MCC schedule is developed and used in the capital budgeting process. First the cost of each capital structure component is estimated. The *after-tax cost of debt* is simply $k_d(1 - t)$. The first increment of *common equity* is raised by *retaining earnings*, whose cost, k_s, may be estimated in one of three ways: (1) by the CAPM equation, $k_s = R_F + b(k_M - R_F)$; (2) by the dividend growth model, $k_s = D_1/P_0 + g$; or (3) by adding a risk premium of about 3 to 5 percent to the firm's cost of long-term debt. Once retained earnings have been exhausted, the firm must sell new common stock, or *external equity*, the cost of which is $k_e = D_1/[P_0(1 - F)] + g$ in the case of a constant-growth stock.

The component costs are then combined to form a *weighted average cost of capital, k_a*. The weights used to develop k_a should be based on the firm's target capital structure. If these weights are used, the stock price will be maximized and the cost of capital will simultaneously be minimized.

Capital usually has a higher cost if the firm expands beyond certain limits. This means that the MCC curve turns up beyond some point. We used the *break point concept* to develop a step-function MCC schedule, which was then combined with the IOS to determine both the optimal capital budget and the cost of capital that should be used in capital budgeting.

The concepts developed here are extended in Chapter 20, where we consider the effect of the firm's capital structure on the cost of capital.

RESOLUTION TO DECISION IN FINANCE

Capital Outlays: Business on the Hot Seat

Many American businesses say that a string of unexpected events, such as the collapse of oil prices and the near depression in the computer industry, distort the overall picture of capital spending and make its long-term record look worse. They also point to gyrations in federal tax policy that played havoc with business investment plans for most of the 1980s.

Huge federal deficits have also been a drag on investment. For most of this decade, Washington's rivers of red ink have helped push interest rates much higher than they would have been otherwise. High interest rates, of course, raise the cost of financing capital investment and offer attractive alternative investment opportunities. "Business has faced an enormous amount of uncertainty in this decade, which helps explain why so much money has been poured into high-yielding financial assests rather than physical assets," maintains Jerry Jordan, chief economist for First Interstate Bancorp. Adds Harvard economist Dale Jorgenson: "The cost of capital in the U.S. is much higher than in other countries, and high interest rates caused by mammoth budget deficits are a big reason."

The economy of the 1980s has also put a damper on capital investment. The decade began with one of the worst recessions in the postwar period. Growth has averaged only about 2.5 percent in the 1980s, compared with about 3.5 to 4 percent in the 1960s and 1970s. "So long as growth is weak, business will be reluctant to invest heavily," says Lawrence Chi-

merine, president of Wharton Econometrics Inc.

But these defenses aren't particularly persuasive because Japan and West Germany have also been subject to the same economic uncertainties, yet their capital investment has far outpaced that of the U.S. Many economists argue that the slide in the U.S. position began at least fifteen years ago and that business is now using the economic uncertainties of the 1980s as an excuse for its inaction. "Why did it take us so long to catch on to the competitive threat from Japan?" asks Chimerine. "You have to say that it was in part simply [management] complacency."

Complacency, of course, is usually bred by lack of competition. For twenty years after World War II, the U.S. economy dominated the world, and American business began to believe that its preeminence was permanent. Such attitudes are hard to shake, even when the reality has changed.

In the early twentieth century, the British also believed that their economic superiority was invincible and that others could do most of the grubbier aspects of manufacturing. Their long decline set in soon after.

Whatever the reason for business's reluctance to invest, the falling value of the dollar relative to other currencies puts U.S. corporations in a strong position to fight back. But if the trade deficit doesn't show much improvement and the pace of capital spending doesn't pick up, the old complaints of an overstrong dollar, an overpriced and underproductive workforce, and an intrusive government simply won't wash anymore. The fallout could be a sharp reversal of the pro-business climate of the Reagan years.

Source: Edward Mervosh, "Capital Outlays: Business Is on the Hot Seat," *Business Month*, September 1987, 50–54.

QUESTIONS

19-1 In what sense is the marginal cost of capital an average cost?

19-2 How would each of the following affect a firm's cost of debt, $k_d(1 - t)$; its cost of equity, k_s; and its average cost of capital, k_a? Indicate by a plus ($+$), a minus ($-$), or a zero (0) if the factor would raise, lower, or have an indeterminate effect on the items in question. Assume other things are held constant. Be prepared to justify your answer, but recognize that several of the parts probably have no single correct answer; these questions are designed to stimulate thought and discussion.

	Effect on		
	$k_d(1 - t)$	k_s	k_a
a. The corporate tax rate is lowered.	____	____	____
b. The Federal Reserve tightens credit.	____	____	____
c. The firm uses more debt; that is, it increases the debt/assets ratio.	____	____	____
d. The dividend payout ratio is increased.	____	____	____
e. The firm doubles the amount of capital it raises during the year.	____	____	____
f. The firm expands into a risky new area.	____	____	____
g. The firm merges with another firm whose earnings are countercyclical to those of the first firm and to the stock market.	____	____	____
h. The stock market falls drastically, and our firm's stock falls along with the rest.	____	____	____
i. Investors become more averse to risk.	____	____	____
j. The firm is an electric utility with a large investment in nuclear plants. Several states propose a ban on nuclear power generation.	____	____	____

19-3 Suppose a firm estimates its MCC and IOS schedules for the coming year and finds that they intersect at the point 10%, $10 million. What cost of capital should be used to evaluate average-risk projects, high-risk projects, and low-risk projects?

SELF-TEST PROBLEM

ST-1 L. H. Clore, Inc., has the following capital structure, which it considers to be optimal:

Debt	25%
Preferred stock	15
Common equity	60
	100%

Clore's expected net income this year is $171,428.60; its established dividend payout ratio is 30 percent; its federal-plus-state tax rate is 40 percent; and investors expect earnings and dividends to grow at a constant rate of 9 percent in the future. Clore paid a dividend of $3.60 per share last year. Its stock currently sells at a price of $60 per share.

Clore can obtain new capital in the following ways:

- *Common:* New common stock would have a flotation cost of 10 percent for up to $60,000 of new stock and of 20 percent for all common over $60,000.

- *Preferred:* New preferred can be sold to the public at a price of $100 per share, with a dividend of $11. However, flotation costs of $5 per share will be incurred for up to $37,500 of preferred, rising to $10, or 10 percent, on all preferred over $37,500.

- *Debt:* Up to $25,000 of debt can be sold at an interest rate of 12 percent; debt in the range of $25,001 to $50,000 must carry an interest rate of 14 percent; and all debt over $50,000 will have an interest rate of 16 percent.

Clore has the following investment opportunities:

Project	Cost at t = 0	Annual Net Cash Flow	Project Life	IRR
A	$50,000	$10,956	7 years	12.0%
B	$50,000	15,772	5	17.4
C	$50,000	10,851	8	14.2
D	$100,000	18,947	10	13.7
E	$100,000	27,139	6	

a. Find the break points in the MCC schedule.
b. Determine the component costs of capital for each capital structure component.
c. Calculate the weighted average cost of capital in the interval between each break in the MCC schedule.
d. Calculate the IRR for Project E.
e. Construct a graph showing the MCC and IOS schedules.
f. Which projects should L. H. Clore accept?

PROBLEMS

19-1 **After-tax cost of debt.** Calculate the after-tax cost of debt under each of the following conditions:
a. Interest rate = 14%; tax rate = 0 percent.
b. Interest rate = 14%; tax rate = 34 percent.
c. Interest rate = 14%; tax rate = 40 percent.
d. Interest rate = 14%; tax rate = 60 percent.

19-2 **After-tax cost of debt.** Iowa Enterprises can sell a bond with a 13.5 percent coupon. Analysts believe the company can sell the bond at a price that will provide a yield to maturity of 13.5 percent. If the tax rate is 40 percent, what is the firm's after-tax cost of debt?

19-3 **Cost of debt.** Michigan Motors has a 9 percent, $1,000 par bond issue outstanding with 15 years left to maturity.

a. If investors require a 10 percent return (yield to maturity), what is the current market price of the bond?

b. If the company wishes to sell a new issue of equal-risk bonds at par, what coupon rate will the investors require?

19-4 **Cost of preferred stock.** Cleveland Power plans to issue some $50 par value preferred stock with a 12 percent dividend. To issue the stock, the utility must pay flotation costs of 8 percent to the investment bankers. What is the cost of capital for this preferred stock?

19-5 **Cost of preferred stock.** Kansas Electric Authority sold an issue of $6.50 preferred stock to the public at its par value of $100 several years ago. Since that original sale, the stock's price has dropped to $46.43.

a. What is the current component cost of preferred stock to Kansas Electric Authority?

b. If the firm's tax rate is 40 percent, what is the after-tax component cost of preferred stock to Kansas Electric Authority?

19-6 **Cost of debt.** Milo Bloom Publishing has a bond issue outstanding with the following financial characteristics: 16 percent coupon; 5 years to maturity; $1,000 par value; and $1,144 current market price.

a. Using the formula found in Footnote 6 of Chapter 17, calculate the bond's approximate yield to maturity.

b. With the information obtained in Part a, determine the bond's exact yield to maturity.

c. What is the relationship between the yield to maturity on outstanding bonds and the cost of debt for new debt securities the firm wishes to issue?

19-7 **Cost of retained earnings.** M. C. Walker and Associates paid a dividend of $2.50 per share recently; that is, $D_0 = \$2.50$. The company's stock sells for $35.71 per share. The expected growth rate is 10 percent. Calculate Walker's cost of retained earnings.

19-8 **Cost of retained earnings.** Ohio Athleticwear's EPS 5 years ago was $3.25; its EPS today is $5.00. The company pays out 35 percent of its earnings as dividends, and the firm's stock sells for $23.88.

a. Calculate the firm's growth rate. (Assume that the growth rate and payout rate have been constant over the 5-year period.)

b. Calculate the expected dividend, D_1. (*Note:* $D_0 = 0.35(\$5.00) = \$1.75$.) Assume that the payout rate and past growth rate will continue into the foreseeable future.

c. What is the cost of retained earnings for the firm?

19-9 **Cost of retained earnings.** The risk-free rate is 9 percent and the required return on an average-risk security in the market is 13 percent. Calculate the firm's cost of retained earnings if the following conditions occur:

a. Beta = 1.6.

b. Beta = 0.7.

c. Beta = 1.0.

19-10 **Cost of retained earnings.** The earnings, dividends, and stock price of Empire State, Inc., are expected to grow at a rate of 5 percent into the foreseeable future. Empire's common stock sells for $37.33 per share, and its last dividend, D_0, was $3.20.

a. Using the discounted cash flow approach, what is the firm's cost of retained earnings?

b. The firm's beta is 1.3, the risk-free rate is 7 percent, and the average return in the market is 12 percent. What is the firm's cost of retained earnings as computed by the CAPM approach?

c. If Empire State's bonds yield 10.5 percent, what is k_s, according to the bond yield plus risk premium approach?

d. Based on the results in Parts a through c, what would you estimate Empire State's cost of retained earnings to be?

19-11 **Cost of equity.** Trinity Industries' last dividend was $2.71, its growth rate is 7 percent (which is expected to continue at a constant rate), and the stock now sells for $32.22. New stock can be sold to net the firm $29.64 after flotation costs.

a. What is Trinity Industries' cost of retained earnings?

b. What is Trinity Industries' percentage flotation cost, F?

c. What is Trinity Industries' cost of new common stock, k_e?

19-12 **Return on common stock.** Air Atlantic's common stock is currently selling for $27.50 per share. The firm is expected to earn $5.00 and to pay a year-end dividend of $2.75. The airline's return on assets is 6 percent, but 60 percent of its assets are financed with debt.

a. What is the firm's return on equity (ROE)?

b. What is the firm's expected growth rate? (*Hint:* $g = b(ROE)$, where b = the fraction of earnings that are retained.)

c. What is the firm's cost of equity capital?

19-13 **Cost of equity.** You have been hired as the treasurer of Cook Resources. The firm's president has asked you to compute the firm's cost of capital. You have gathered all pertinent financial data to make her calculations. Cook's EPS this year will be $10, whereas 7 years ago EPS was $2.79. The firm's expected dividend, D_1, will be $5.50, and Cook's market price is $61.11. The risk-free rate is 8 percent, and the return on an average security is 13 percent. Cook's beta is 1.4. Its bond issue is currently selling to yield investors 11 percent to maturity.

a. Using all three approaches, calculate the firm's cost of equity capital.

b. What conclusions can be drawn from your calculations? What is your best estimate of Cook Resources cost of equity capital? Explain your findings to the firm's president, Ruth Cook.

19-14 **Break point calculations.** Pier 39 Imports, Inc., expects earnings of $20 million next year. Its dividend payout ratio is 30 percent, and its debt/assets ratio is 40 percent. The firm uses no preferred stock.

a. How much will the firm pay in dividends next year?

b. What amount of additional retained earnings does the firm expect next year?

c. At what amount of equity financing will there be a break point in the MCC schedule?

d. The firm can borrow $15 million at an interest rate of 10 percent, but additional borrowing up to $25 million will require a rate of 12 percent, and above $25 million, additional debt will cost 15 percent. At what points will rising debt costs cause breaks in the MCC schedule?

19-15 **Required cash flow.** Kemp Electronics is making final calculations on the purchase of a new production assembler. The equipment is valued at $600,000. It will be in service for 5 years and will be depreciated at $120,000 annually. There is no salvage value. Additional annual costs include the following:

Labor	$ 75,000
Materials	100,000
Building lease	60,000
Overhead	25,000

If all costs are constant during the five year period, what is the minimum level of sales that will allow Kemp to earn at least its 15 percent cost of capital? Kemp's marginal tax rate is 40 percent.

19-16 **Weighted average cost of capital.** Travis Trucking Company has the following capital structure, which is considered optimal:

Debt	$ 80,000
Preferred stock	30,000
Common stock equity	90,000
Total assets	$200,000

The cost of debt is 13 percent, the cost of preferred stock is 15 percent, and the cost of equity is 18 percent. The firm's marginal tax rate is 34 percent. What is Travis Trucking's cost of capital?

19-17 **Optimal capital budget.** Gaylord Manufacturing's earnings per share have been growing at a steady 7 percent during the last 10 years. The firm's stock, 500,000 shares outstanding, is now selling for $80 a share, and the expected dividend for next year, D_1, is $7.20. The firm pays out 48 percent of its earnings in dividends. The current interest rate on new debt is 12 percent. The firm's marginal tax rate is 40 percent. The firm's capital structure, considered to be optimal, is as follows:

Debt	$ 5,000,000
Common equity	5,000,000
Total capital	$10,000,000

a. Calculate the after-tax costs of new debt and of common equity, assuming that new equity comes only from retained earnings. Because the historical growth rate is expected to continue, we may calculate the cost of equity as $k_s = D_1/P_0 + g$.
b. Find the marginal cost of capital, again assuming that no new common stock is to be sold.
c. If this year's addition to retained earnings is $3.9 million, how much can be spent for capital investments before external equity must be sold?
d. What is the marginal cost of capital (cost of funds raised in excess of the amount calculated in Part c) if new common stock can be sold to the public at $80 a share to net the firm $72 a share after flotation costs? The cost of debt is constant.
e. We have assumed that the capital structure is optimal. What would happen if the firm deviated from this capital structure? Use a graph to illustrate your answer.

19-18 **Optimal capital budget.** On January 1 the total assets of Gainesville Printing were $70 million. During the year the company plans to raise and invest $30 million. The firm's present capital structure, shown below, is considered to be optimal. Assume that there is no short-term debt.

Debt	$28,000
Common equity	42,000
Total capital	$70,000

New bonds will have an 11 percent coupon rate and will be sold at par. Common stock, currently selling at $50 a share, can be sold to net the company $42.50 a share. The stockholders' required rate of return is estimated to be 15 percent, consisting of a dividend yield of 6 percent and an expected growth rate of 9 percent. (The next expected dividend is $3, so $3/$50 = 6%.) Retained earnings for the year are estimated to be $6 million (ignore depreciation). The marginal corporate tax rate is 40 percent.

a. Assuming that all asset expansion (gross expenditures for fixed assets plus related working capital) is included in the capital budget, what is the dollar amount of the capital budget? (Ignore depreciation.)

b. To maintain the present capital structure, how much of the capital budget must be financed by common equity?

c. How much of the needed new common equity funds will be generated internally? Externally?

d. Calculate the cost of each of the common equity components.

e. At what level of capital expenditures will there be a break in the MCC schedule?

f. Calculate the MCC **(1)** below and **(2)** above the break in the schedule.

g. Plot the MCC schedule. Also, draw in an investment opportunity schedule that is consistent with both the MCC schedule and the projected capital budget. Any IOS that is consistent will do.

19-19 **Optimal capital budget.** JJK Group has the following capital structure, which it considers to be optimal under present and forecasted conditions:

Debt (long-term only)	40%
Common equity	60%
Total liabilities and equity	100%

For the coming year, management expects after-tax earnings of $2 million. JJK's past dividend policy of paying out 60 percent of earnings will continue. Present commitments from its banker will allow JJK to borrow according to the following schedule:

Loan Amount	Interest Rate
$0 to $500,000	10% on this increment of debt
$500,001 to $900,000	12% on this increment of debt
$900,001 and above	14% on this increment of debt

The company's average tax rate is 40 percent, the current market price of its stock is $24 per share, its *last* dividend was $2.05 per share, and the expected growth rate is 6 percent. External equity (new common) can be sold at a flotation cost of 15 percent.

JJK has the following investment opportunities for the next year:

Project	Cost	Annual Cash Flows	Project Life	IRR
1	$ 900,000	$186,210	10 years	
2	1,200,000	316,904	6	15.0%
3	500,000	303,644	2	
4	750,000	246,926	4	12.0
5	1,000,000	194,322	8	11.0

Management asks you to help determine which projects (if any) should be undertaken. You proceed with this analysis by answering the following questions as posed in a logical sequence:

a. How many breaks are there in the MCC schedule?

b. At what dollar amounts do the breaks occur, and what causes them?

c. What is the weighted average cost of capital, k_a, in each of the intervals between the breaks?

d. What are the IRR values for Projects 1 and 3?

e. Graph the IOS and MCC schedules.

f. Which projects should JJK's management accept?

g. What assumptions about project risk are implicit in this problem? If you learned that Projects 1, 2, and 3 were of above-average risk, yet JJK chose the projects that you indicated in Part f, how would this affect the situation?

h. The problem stated that JJK pays out 60 percent of its earnings as dividends. In words, how would the analysis change if the payout ratio were changed to zero, to 100 percent, or somewhere in between? If you are using the computerized problem diskette, re-analyze the firm's capital budgeting decision using dividend payout ratios of zero, 100 percent, and 40 percent.

(Do Parts i through l only if you are using the computerized problem diskette.)

i. Suppose JJK's tax rate fell to zero, with other variables remaining constant. How would that affect the MCC schedule and the capital budget?

j. Return the tax rate to 40 percent. Now assume that the debt ratio is increased to 65 percent, causing all interest rates to rise by 1 percentage point, to 11 percent, 13 percent, and 15 percent, and causing g to increase from 6 percent to 7 percent. What happens to the MCC schedule and the capital budget?

k. New information becomes available. Change the Part j scenario to assume earnings of only $1,000,000 but a growth rate of 9 percent. How does that affect the capital budget?

l. Would it be reasonable to use the model to analyze the effects of a change in the payout ratio without changing other variables?

ANSWER TO SELF-TEST PROBLEM

ST-1   **a.** A break point will occur each time a low-cost type of capital is used up. We establish the break points as follows, after first noting that Clore has $120,000 of retained earnings:

$$\text{Retained earnings} = (\text{Total earnings})(1.0 - \text{Payout})$$

$$= \$171,428.60(0.7)$$

$$= \$120,000.$$

$$\text{Break point} = \frac{\text{Total amount of low-cost capital of a given type}}{\text{Fraction of this type of capital in the capital structure}}.$$

Capital Used Up	Break Point Calculation		Break Number
Retained earnings	$BP_{RE} = \dfrac{\$120,000}{0.60}$	$= \$200,000$	2
10% flotation common	$BP_{10\%E} = \dfrac{\$120,000 + \$60,000}{0.60}$	$= \$300,000$	4
5% flotation preferred	$BP_{5\%P} = \dfrac{\$37,500}{0.15}$	$= \$250,000$	3
12% debt	$BP_{12\%D} = \dfrac{\$25,000}{0.25}$	$= \$100,00$	1
14% debt	$BP_{14\%D} = \dfrac{\$25,000 + \$25,000}{0.25}$	$= \$200,000$	2

Summary of Break Points

1. There are three common equity costs (and hence two changes and two equity-induced breaks) in the MCC. There are two preferred costs and hence one preferred break. There are three debt costs and hence two debt breaks.

2. The numbers in the third column of the table designate the sequential order of the breaks, determined after the break points had been calculated. Note that the second debt break and the break for retained earnings both occur at $200,000.

3. The first break point occurs at $100,000, when 12 percent debt is used up. The second break point, $200,000, results from using up both retained earnings and the 14 percent debt. The MCC curve also rises at $250,000 and $300,000 as preferred stock with a 5 percent flotation cost and common stock with a 10 percent flotation cost, respectively, are used up.

b. Component costs within indicated total capital intervals are as follows:
Retained earnings (used in interval $0 to $200,000):

$$k_s = \frac{D_1}{P_0} + g = \frac{D_0(1 + g)}{P_0} + g$$

$$= \frac{\$3.60(1.09)}{\$60} + 0.09$$

$$= 0.0654 + 0.09 = 15.54\%$$

Common with F = 10% ($200,001 to $300,000):

$$k_e = \frac{D_1}{P_0(1.0 - F)} + g = \frac{\$3.924}{\$60(0.9)} + 9\% = 16.27\%.$$

Common with F = 20% (over $300,000):

$$k_e = \frac{\$3.924}{\$60(0.8)} + 9\% = 17.18\%.$$

Preferred with F = 5% ($0 to $250,000):

$$k_p = \frac{\text{Preferred dividend}}{P_n} = \frac{\$11}{\$100(0.95)} = 11.58\%.$$

Preferred with F = 10% (over $250,000):

$$k_p = \frac{\$11}{\$100(09)} = 12.22\%.$$

Debt at k_d = 12% ($0 to $100,000):

$$k_d(1 - T) = 12\%(0.6) = 7.20\%.$$

Debt at k_d = 14% ($100,001 to $200,000):

$$k_d(1 - T) = 14\%(0.6) = 8.40\%.$$

Debt at k_d = 16% (over $200,000):

$$k_d(1 - T) = 16\%(0.6) = 9.60\%.$$

c. WACC calculations within indicated total capital intervals:
   1. $0 to $100,000 (debt = 7.2%, preferred = 11.58%, and RE = 15.54%):

$$WACC_1 = w_d k_d(1 - T) + w_p k_p + w_s k_s$$
$$= 0.25(7.2\%) + 0.15(11.58\%) + 0.60(15.54\%) = 12.86\%.$$

   2. $100,001 to $200,000 (debt = 8.4%, preferred = 11.58%, and RE = 15.54%):

$$WACC_2 = 0.25(8.4\%) + 0.15(11.58\%) + 0.60(15.54\%) = 13.16\%.$$

   3. $200,001 to $250,000 (debt = 9.6%, preferred = 11.58%, and equity = 16.27%):

$$WACC_3 = 0.25(9.6\%) + 0.15(11.58\%) + 0.60(16.27\%) = 13.90\%.$$

   4. $250,001 to $300,000 (debt = 9.6%, preferred = 12.22%, and equity = 16.27%):

$$WACC_4 = 0.25(9.6\%) + 0.15(12.22\%) + 0.60(16.27\%) = 14.00\%.$$

   5. Over $300,000 (debt = 9.6%, preferred = 12.22%, and equity = 17.18%):

$$WACC_5 = 0.25(9.6\%) + 0.15(12.22\%) + 0.60(17.18\%) = 14.54\%.$$

d. IRR calculation for Project E:

$$PVIFA_{k,6} = \frac{\$100,000}{\$27,139} = 3.6847.$$

This is the factor for 16 percent, so IRR_E = 16%.

e. See the graph of the MCC and IOS schedules for Clore on the following page.

MCC and IOS Schedules for L. H. Clore, Inc.

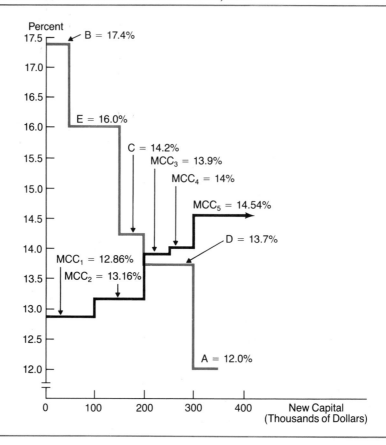

f. Clore clearly should accept Projects B, E, and C. It should reject Projects A and D, because their IRRs do not exceed the marginal costs of funds needed to finance them. The firm's capital budget would total $200,000.

Chapter 20

Leverage and the Target Capital Structure

 DECISION IN FINANCE

Putting Citicorp on Firmer Footing

When John Reed took over as Citicorp's chairman, he had some big shoes to fill. Walter Wriston, his mentor and predecessor, had turned Citibank into the nation's largest bank with the most aggressive expansion program the industry had ever seen. The eighties are turbulent times for banking. Citicorp faces strong challenges from cash-rich Japanese banks, as well as from U.S. financial institutions that continue to crowd into corporate lending — once banking's exclusive domain. Worse still, 80 percent of Citicorp's primary capital is equal to its loans to developing Latin American nations, many of which continue to flirt with default.

Reed also took the helm of a bank that had grown too fast for its underlying capital structure. When Wriston left, Citibank's capital cushion against bad loans was a sickly 0.88 percent, compared with an industry average of 1.25 percent. Its primary capital rate was also weak, 5.9 percent compared with an industry average of 6.3 percent. Since he has been chairman, Reed has nearly doubled Citibank's buffer against bad loans and boosted its primary capital ratio to 6.82 percent.

See end of chapter for resolution.

Although few fault Reed's fortifying Citibank's capital structure, his methods have financial analysts squawking. Rather than follow the traditional route of selling off high-value, nonessential assets, Reed has chosen to divert income to create capital. He has systematically allocated funds that could have been used to create loans and has used them to boost the bank's loan-loss reserve fund.

As Reed works to rebuild Citicorp's capital safety net, the bank's performance has fallen off. Analysts cite disappointing earnings, concern about the bank's huge Latin American loan exposure, and dissatisfaction with Reed's program to build up loan reserves at the expense of operating earnings.

As you read this chapter, consider whether Reed is doing a better job than Wriston in seeking a capital structure that strikes a balance between risk and return. Is he maximizing the price of the bank's stock and minimizing the firm's cost of capital? Think about the difficulties inherent in changing the established capital structure of a large corporation like Citicorp. Do you agree with Reed's policy of building capital at the expense of the corporation's present earnings?

In Chapter 19 when we calculated the weighted average cost of capital for capital budgeting purposes, the proportions of debt and equity in the capital structure were assumed to be appropriate. However, changing the proportion of debt and equity in the capital structure influences the firm's risk and thus its cost of capital. Naturally, as the firm's cost of capital changes, the universe of acceptable projects will change as well. A lower cost of capital would increase the number of acceptable projects, whereas a higher cost of capital would reduce the set of acceptable projects. The firm's cost of capital is determined by investors' required rates of return. A change in the riskiness of the firm affects the value of the firm's securities and thereby affects the value of the firm. Therefore, the choice of a capital structure, or the mix of securities the firm uses to finance its assets, has important ramifications for the shareholders' wealth. As we will see, a number of factors must be considered in determining the **target capital structure.** This target may change over time as conditions vary, but at any given moment the firm's management does have a specific capital structure in mind, and individual financing decisions should be consistent with this target. If the actual debt ratio is below the prescribed ratio, expansion capital will probably be raised by issuing debt, whereas if the debt ratio is above the target level, stock will probably be sold.

Capital structure policy involves a trade-off between risk and returns. Using more debt raises the riskiness of the firm's earnings stream, but more debt generally means a higher expected rate of return. Higher risk tends to lower the stock's price, but a higher expected rate of return raises it. *The optimal capital structure strikes a balance between risk and return, which maximizes the price of the stock and simultaneously minimizes the firm's overall cost of capital.* Because stock price maximization and capital cost minimization occur simultaneously, the problem of finding the optimal capital structure can be approached as either value maximization or cost minimization.

TYPES OF RISK

Throughout this text we have emphasized many different facets of the concept of risk. For example, in Chapter 15 we distinguished between *beta or market risk,* which cannot be diversified away and is measured by the beta coefficient, and *corporate or total risk,* which includes market risk *and* an element of risk that can be eliminated by diversification. In Chapter 16 we viewed risk specifically from the firm's viewpoint, considering how capital budgeting decisions affect the riskiness of the firm. Here we distinguished between *beta risk* (the effect of a project on the firm's beta risk) and *corporate risk* (the effect of the project on the firm's total risk).

In Chapter 5 we introduced the concept of risk and return. There we indicated that a security's returns are determined by the pure rate of interest plus appropriate risk premiums, which include a *default risk premium.* Now we introduce two dimensions of the default risk premium: (1) **business risk,**

target capital structure
The optimal capital structure; the capital structure that will minimize the firm's cost of capital and thereby maximize the price of its stock.

business risk
The risk associated with future operating income; the risk that would exist even if the firm's operations were all equity financed.

which is the riskiness of the firm's operations that would exist even if the firm were all equity financed, and (2) **financial risk,** which is the additional risk placed on the common shareholders as a result of the decision to use debt. Conceptually, the firm has a certain amount of risk inherent in its operations; this is its business risk. In the absence of debt in the capital structure, business risk equals total risk. When debt is used, total risk is apportioned, with most of it being allotted to one class of investors — the common stockholders. However, the common stockholders must be compensated by a higher *expected* rate of return.

financial risk
The portion of total corporate risk over and above the basic business risk that results from using debt.

BUSINESS RISK

The uncertainty associated with forecasting and realizing future **operating income** — earnings before interest and taxes (EBIT) — has been termed *business risk*. The element of uncertainty associated with business risk includes both the chance of not reaching a positive level of operating profits and the problems associated with fluctuating returns. Year-to-year fluctuations can be caused by many factors — booms or recessions in the national economy, successful new products introduced either by the firm or by its competitors, labor strikes, price controls, changes in the prices of raw materials, or disasters such as fires, floods, and the like.

operating income
Earnings before interest and taxes (EBIT).

Business risk varies not only from industry to industry but also among firms within a given industry. Furthermore, business risk can change over time. For example, a business considered at one time to be fairly safe was the railroad industry; this was before the advent of truck and airline competition for freight and passengers. More recently, electric utilities, regarded for years as having very little business risk, were affected by a combination of events in the 1970s and 1980s that drastically altered the situation, producing sharp declines in their operating income and greatly increasing the industry's business risk. Today food processors and grocery retailers are frequently given as examples of industries with low business risk, whereas cyclical manufacturing industries such as steel are regarded as having especially high business risks. Factors other than industry affiliation also play a role in determining business risk. For example, smaller companies or companies dependent on a single product or customer are often regarded as having a high degree of business risk.

Business risk depends on a number of factors, the more important of which are the following:

1. Demand variability. The more stable the demand for a firm's products, other things held constant, the lower its business risk.

2. Output price variability. Firms whose products are sold in highly volatile markets are exposed to more business risk than similar firms whose output prices are more stable.

3. Input price variability. Firms whose input prices are highly uncertain are exposed to a high degree of business risk.

4. Ability to adjust output prices for changes in input prices. Some firms are better able to raise their own output prices when input costs rise than others. The greater the ability to adjust output prices, the lower the degree of business risk, other things held constant. This factor has become increasingly important in the past decade because of inflation.

5. The extent to which operating costs are fixed — operating leverage. If a high percentage of a firm's operating costs are fixed, hence do not decline when demand falls off, the firm is exposed to a relatively high degree of business risk. This factor is called *operating leverage,* and it is discussed at length in the next section.

Each of these factors is determined partly by the firm's industry characteristics, but each of them is also controllable to some extent. For example, most firms can, through their marketing policies, take actions to stabilize both unit sales and sales prices. However, this stabilization may require firms to spend a great deal on advertising or price concessions to get their customers to commit to purchasing fixed quantities at fixed prices in the future. Similarly, firms may reduce the volatility of future input costs by negotiating long-term labor and materials supply contracts, but they may have to agree to pay prices above the current spot price level to obtain these contracts.

OPERATING LEVERAGE

As noted previously, business risk exists even if the firm has no fixed operating charges. However, when the firm has some fixed operating expenses, as the majority of firms do, a change in sales results in a greater than proportional change in operating profits. Business risk is intensified to the extent that a firm builds fixed costs into its operations. If fixed costs are high, even a small decline in sales can lead to a large decline in EBIT; thus, other things held constant, the higher a firm's operating fixed costs, the greater its business risk. Higher fixed operating costs are generally associated with more highly automated, capital intensive firms and industries. Also, businesses that employ highly skilled workers who must be retained and paid even during business recessions have relatively high fixed costs.

operating leverage
The extent to which fixed costs are used in a firm's operation.

If a high percentage of a firm's total operating costs are fixed, the firm is said to have a high degree of **operating leverage.** In physics, leverage implies the use of a lever to raise a heavy object with a small force. In politics, if individuals have leverage, their smallest word or action can accomplish a great deal. *In business terminology, a high degree of operating leverage, other things held constant, implies that a relatively small change in sales will result in a* *large change in operating income.* The common element in all of these examples is that a small initiating change is followed by a proportionally greater effect.

Figure 20–1 illustrates this concept by comparing the results that All-Technology Manufacturing (ATM) can expect if it uses different degrees of operating leverage. Option 1 calls for a relatively small amount of fixed charges, which will be accomplished by using less automated equipment. Depreciation, maintenance, property taxes, and so on will be lower than in the case of the other operating option. Note, however, that under Option 1 the total cost line in Figure 20–1 has a relatively steep slope, indicating that variable costs are higher per unit than if the firm were to use more operating leverage. Option 2 calls for a higher level of fixed costs in order to reduce variable costs per unit. Here the firm uses more automated equipment, thereby requiring fewer workers to make its product. Automation allows an operator to turn out few or many products at the same labor cost. Therefore, to reduce variable cost per unit, ATM's Option 2 raises fixed costs.

The differences in the ways fixed and variable costs are apportioned between Option 1 and Option 2 result in a **breakeven point** that is higher under Option 2; breakeven occurs at 40,000 units under Option 1 versus 60,000 units under Option 2.

We have seen that changing the level of fixed and variable costs changes the breakeven point. But how does operating leverage affect business risk? Other things held constant, *the higher a firm's operating leverage, the higher its business risk.* Since Option 2 requires a higher proportion of fixed to total costs, we can conclude that ATM will have higher business risk if it adopts that plan. This point is demonstrated numerically in the lower part of Figure 20-1 and graphically in Figure 20-2.

The top section of Figure 20-2 gives the **probability distribution** of sales. This distribution depends on how demand for the product varies, not on whether the product is manufactured under Option 1 or Option 2. Therefore the same sales probability distribution applies to both production plans, and expected sales for the next period are $200,000, with a range from zero to about $500,000, under either plan.

If we had actually specified the sales probability distribution, we could have used this information, together with the operating profit (EBIT) at each sales level as shown in the lower part of Figure 20-1, to develop probability distributions for EBIT under Options 1 and 2. Typical EBIT distributions are shown in the lower part of Figure 20-2. At the expected sales level of $200,000, Option 2's operating profits are higher than those for Option 1. Unfortunately, chances for losses are also greater for Option 2 than for Option 1. Therefore, Option 2, the one with more fixed costs and a higher degree of operating leverage, is riskier. *Holding other things constant, the higher the degree of operating leverage, the greater the degree of business risk as measured by the variability of EBIT.*

breakeven point
The level of operations at which total costs equal total revenues and therefore profits equal zero.

probability distribution
A listing of all possible outcomes or events, with a probability (the chance of the event's occurrence) assigned to each outcome.

Figure 20-1 **Effect of Operating Leverage on All-Technology Manufacturing**

This figure demonstrates that higher operating leverage (i.e., higher fixed costs) will create higher business risk and greater potential for large swings in profits. Both plans project sales of 100,000 units at $2.00 each, but Option 1 has one-third the fixed costs of Option 2. As a result Option 2 has a higher breakeven point. As both graphs and tables show, the further sales move on either side of the breakeven point, the faster profits or losses under Option 2 outstrip those under Option 1.

Selling price = $2.00	Selling price = $2.00
Fixed costs = $20,000	Fixed costs = $60,000
Variable costs = $1.50Q	Variable costs = $1.00Q

Option 1

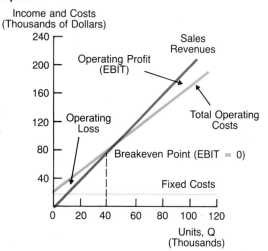

Option 2

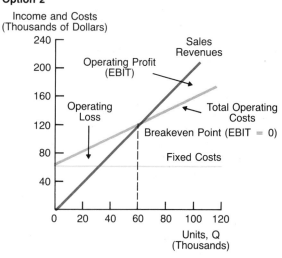

Expected level of sales under either production plan is 100,000 units.

Units Sold, Q	Sales	Operating Costs	Operating Profit (EBIT)	Units Sold, Q	Sales	Operating Costs	Operating Profit (EBIT)
0	$ 0	$ 20,000	$ −20,000	0	$ 0	$ 60,000	$ −60,000
40,000	80,000	80,000	0	40,000	80,000	100,000	−20,000
60,000	120,000	110,000	10,000	60,000	120,000	120,000	0
80,000	160,000	140,000	20,000	80,000	160,000	140,000	20,000
100,000	200,000	170,000	30,000	100,000	200,000	160,000	40,000
110,000	220,000	185,000	35,000	110,000	220,000	170,000	50,000
160,000	320,000	260,000	60,000	160,000	320,000	220,000	100,000
180,000	360,000	290,000	70,000	180,000	360,000	240,000	120,000
220,000	440,000	350,000	90,000	220,000	440,000	280,000	160,000

Figure 20-2 **Analysis of Business Risk**

Under both Option 1 and Option 2, expected sales are 100,000 units, as shown in the top probability curve. Taking the information from such a curve together with the profit amounts at each level from the lower part of Figure 20-1, it is possible to create probability distributions for profits under Options 1 and 2, as shown in the lower curve of this figure. Again the greater volatility of Option 2 is evident.

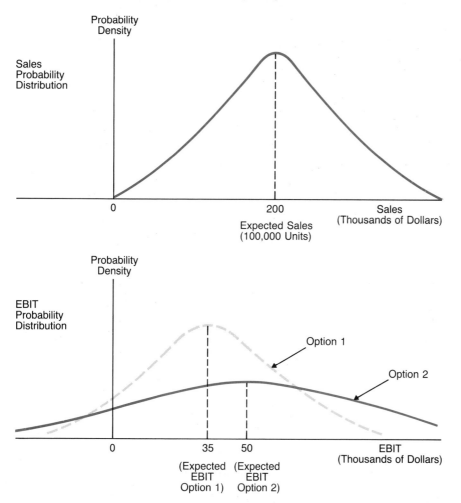

The breakeven point is the level of sales that just covers all operating costs, both fixed and variable. Therefore

$$\text{Total revenues} = \text{Total costs}$$

$$QP = QV + F,$$

where

Q = number of units produced and sold,

P = selling price per unit,

QP = level of sales in dollars,

V = variable cost per unit produced,

F = fixed operating cost.

If we combine terms,

$$QP - QV = F.$$

Factoring out Q leads to

$$Q(P - V) = F.$$

Dividing both sides of the equation by (P − V), we have

$$Q = \frac{F}{(P - V)}. \tag{20-1}$$

Equation 20-1 is the breakeven point, stated in terms of units of the company's product that must be sold to reach the threshold of profits. We can solve Equation 20-1 for the breakeven quantity, Q:

For Option 1,

$$Q_{O1} = \$20,000/(\$2.00 - \$1.50)$$

$$= 40,000 \text{ units.}$$

For Option 2,

$$Q_{O2} = \$60,000/(\$2.00 - \$1.00)$$

$$= 60,000 \text{ units.}$$

We can describe the risk associated with operating leverage in a different fashion, utilizing the sales and operating profit levels from Figure 9-1. But first note that if ATM had no fixed costs, an increase of 25 percent in sales would lead to a proportional 25 percent increase in operating profits. With fixed operating costs, however, there would be a larger than proportional change in operating profits, given a change in sales. For example, if current sales were $160,000 and increased by 25 percent to $200,000, profits under Option 1 would increase by 50 percent, from $20,000 to $30,000. On the other hand, under the larger operating leverage inherent in Option 2, the same 25 percent

Table 20-1 **Degree of Operating Leverage at $160,000 in Sales for ATM**

$$DOL_1 = \frac{Q(P - V)}{Q(P - V) - F}$$

$$= \frac{80,000(\$2.00 - \$1.50)}{80,000(\$2.00 - \$1.50) - \$20,000}$$

$$= \frac{\$40,000}{\$20,000}$$

$$= 2.$$

$$DOL_2 = \frac{Q(P - V)}{Q(P - V) - F}$$

$$= \frac{80,000(\$2.00 - \$1.00)}{80,000(\$2.00 - \$1.00) - \$60,000}$$

$$= \frac{\$80,000}{\$20,000}$$

$$= 4.$$

increase in sales would result in a 100 percent increase in operating profits. A problem with operating leverage arises when sales decline, however. Just as profits increase at a greater rate when sales are increasing, losses when sales decline are also magnified by the existence of fixed operating costs. For example, a 25 percent decline in sales from a level of 80,000 units would result in a 50 percent decline in operating profits under Option 1 but results in a much larger loss of 100 percent under Option 2!

The degree of operating leverage provides a more general way to measure the reaction of profits to changes in the volume of sales. The **degree of operating leverage (DOL)** is the ratio of the percentage change in operating income to the percentage change in sales. Equation 20-2 can be used to calculate the degree of operating leverage:

degree of operating leverage (DOL)
The ratio of the percentage change in operating income to the percentage change in sales.

$$DOL = \frac{Q(P - V)}{Q(P - V) - F}. \tag{20-2}$$

The symbols are the same as those developed earlier in this chapter:

Q = units of output.

P = sales price.

V = variable cost per unit.

F = fixed operating cost.

Using Equation 20-2, we determine in Table 20-1 the degree of operating leverage for Option 1 (DOL_1) and Option 2 (DOL_2) at a particular level of sales — in this case $160,000 in sales.[1] A DOL of 2 means that with a percentage change in sales, a doubled percentage change in EBIT will result under the operating leverage provided by Option 1. Thus a 10 percent increase in sales will result in a twice as large (20 percent) increase in operating profits. As we

---

[1] A word of caution: the degree of operating leverage changes as the level of sales changes. For example, in Table 20-1 we found that at sales of $160,000 the DOL_1 = 2 and the DOL_2 = 4. However, at the expected sales level of $220,000 the DOL_1 = 1.57 and the DOL_2 = 2.2.

already saw for Option 1, a 25 percent change in sales was doubled to a 50 percent change in operating profits. For Option 2 the DOL of 4 means that a percentage change in sales will result in a quadrupled change in operating profits. A 5 percent decline in sales will result in a four times larger (20 percent) decline in operating profits. Thus, before adopting Option 2, the financial planners at ATM will wish to consider the probability of future sales fluctuations.[2]

To what extent can firms control their operating leverage? For the most part, operating leverage is determined by technology. Electric utilities, telephone companies, airlines, steel mills, and chemical companies simply *must* have heavy investments in fixed assets; this results in high fixed costs and operating leverage. Grocery stores, on the other hand, generally have substantially lower fixed costs, hence lower operating leverage. Still, all firms have some control over their operating leverage. For example, an electric utility can expand its generating capacity by building either a nuclear reactor or a coal-fired plant. The nuclear generator would require a larger investment in fixed assets, which would involve higher fixed costs, but its variable operating costs would be relatively low. The coal plant would require a smaller investment in fixed assets and would have lower fixed costs, but the variable costs (for coal) would be high. Thus by its capital budgeting decisions a utility (or any other company) can influence its operating leverage and, hence, its basic business risk.

The concept of operating leverage was, in fact, originally developed for use in making capital budgeting decisions. Alternative methods for producing a given product often have different degrees of operating leverage and, therefore, different breakeven points and degrees of risk. Companies regularly undertake some type of breakeven analysis as part of their evaluation of proposed new projects. Still, once established, the degree of operating leverage, and hence the degree to which future operating profits will be uncertain, is the most important factor in determining the firm's capital structure.

FINANCIAL RISK

financial leverage
The extent to which fixed-income securities (debt and preferred stock) are used in a firm's capital structure.

Financial risk is the additional risk placed on the common shareholders as a result of **financial leverage.** Whereas operating leverage refers to the use of fixed operating costs, financial leverage refers to the use of fixed income securities — debt and preferred stock.[3] In this section we show how financial

---

[2]It is interesting to note that ATM chose neither Option 1 nor Option 2 for its operating leverage. Rather, as is often the case, the firm reached a compromise between the two options. Recall that Option 1 had the higher variable-cost ratio (75 percent of sales) but a lower level of fixed costs, $20,000, and Option 2 had lower variable costs (50 percent of sales) but higher fixed costs, $60,000. The compromise option selected a mid-level for both costs, with variable costs as 60 percent sales and fixed operating costs of $40,000, as we shall see in the next section.

[3]Preferred stock also adds to financial risk; however, to simplify matters somewhat, we will only consider the use of debt and equity in this chapter.

Table 20-2 **Data on All-Technology Manufacturing**

I. Balance Sheet on 12/31/88

Current assets	$100,000	Debt	$	0
Net fixed assets	100,000	Common equity (10,000 shares		
		outstanding)		200,000
Total assets	$200,000	Total claims		$200,000

II. Income Statement for 1988

Sales		$200,000
Fixed operating costs	$ 40,000	
Variable operating costs	120,000	160,000
Earnings before interest and taxes (EBIT)		$ 40,000
Interest		0
Taxable income		$ 40,000
Taxes (40%)		16,000
Net income after taxes		$ 24,000

III. Other Data
1. Earnings per share = EPS = $24,000/10,000 shares = $2.40.
2. Dividends per share = DPS = $24,000/10,000 shares = $2.40. (Thus ATM pays all of its earnings out as dividends. Alternatively stated, ATM has a 100 percent payout ratio.)
3. Book value per share = $200,000/10,000 shares = $20.
4. Market price per share = P_0 = $20. Thus the stock sells at its book value.
5. Price/earnings ratio = P/E = $20/$2.40 = 8.33 times.
6. Variable operating cost equals 60 percent of sales.

leverage affects a firm's expected earnings per share, the riskiness of these earnings, and consequently the price of the firm's stock. As we will see, the value of a firm that has no debt first rises as it substitutes debt for equity, then hits a peak, and finally declines as the use of debt becomes excessive. The objective of our analysis is to determine the point at which value is maximized; this point is then used as the *target capital structure.*

Determining the Optimal Capital Structure

At the present time All-Technology Manufacturing has no debt financing and is thus 100 percent equity financed (as shown in Table 20-2). Should it continue this policy of using no debt, or should it start using financial leverage? And if ATM does decide to substitute debt for equity, how far should it go? As in all such decisions, the correct answer is that *it should choose the capital structure that maximizes the price of its stock.*

Because the price of a share of stock is the present value of the stock's expected future dividends, if the use of financial leverage is to affect the stock's

Table 20-3 **Interest Rates for ATM with Different Debt/Assets Ratios**

Amount Borrowed	Debt/Assets Ratio[a]	Interest Rate, k_d, on All Debt
$20,000	10%	8.0%
$40,000	20	8.3
$60,000	30	9.0
$80,000	40	10.0
$100,000	50	12.0
$120,000	60	15.0

[a]We assume that the firm must borrow in increments of $20,000. We also assume that ATM is unable to borrow more than $120,000, or 60 percent of assets, because of restrictions in its corporate charter.

price, it must do so by changing either the expected dividend stream or the required rate of return on equity, k_s, or both. We first consider the effect of capital structure on earnings and dividends; then we examine its effect on k_s.

The Effect of Financial Leverage on Expected EPS

Changes in the use of debt will cause changes in earnings per share (EPS) and consequently in the stock price. To understand the relationship between financial leverage and EPS, consider first Table 20-3, which shows how ATM's cost of debt would vary if it used different percentages of debt in its capital structure. Naturally, the higher the percentage of debt, the riskier the debt, and hence the higher the interest rate lenders will charge.

Table 20-4 shows how expected EPS varies with changes in financial leverage. The top third of the table shows EBIT at sales of $100,000, $200,000, and $300,000. EBIT is independent of financial leverage — although it does depend on operating leverage, *EBIT does not depend on financial leverage.*

The middle third of Table 20-4 goes on to show the situation if ATM continues to use no debt. Net income after taxes is divided by the 10,000 shares outstanding to calculate EPS. If sales are as low as $100,000, EPS will be zero, but at sales of $300,000, EPS will rise to $4.80.

The EPS at each sales level is next multiplied by the probability of that sales level to calculate the expected EPS, which is $2.40 if ATM uses no debt. We also calculate the standard deviation of EPS to get an idea of the firm's risk at a zero debt ratio: $\sigma_{EPS} = \$1.52.$[4]

The lower third of the table shows the financial results that would occur if the company financed with a debt/assets ratio of 50 percent. In this situation $100,000 of the $200,000 total capital would be debt. The interest rate on the

---

[4]The procedure for calculating the standard deviation is explained in Chapter 15.

Table 20-4 ATM: EPS with Different Amounts of Financial Leverage (Thousands of Dollars except Per-Share Figures)

Probability of Indicated Sales	0.2	0.6	0.2
Sales	$100.0	$200.0	$300.0
Fixed costs	40.0	40.0	40.0
Variable costs (60% of sales)	60.0	120.0	180.0
Total costs (except interest)	$100.0	$160.0	$220.0
Earnings before interest and taxes (EBIT)	$ 0.0	$ 40.0	$ 80.0
Debt/Assets (D/A) = 0%			
Less: Interest	0.0	0.0	0.0
Earnings before taxes	0.0	40.0	80.0
Taxes (40%)	0.0	(16.0)	(32.0)
Net income after taxes	$ 0.0	$ 24.0	$ 48.0
Earnings per share on 10,000 shares (EPS)	$ 0.0	$ 2.40	$ 4.80
Expected EPS		$ 2.40	
Standard deviation of EPS		$ 1.52	
Debt/Assets (D/A) = 50%			
Less: Interest (0.12 × $100,000)	$ 12.0	$ 12.0	$ 12.0
Earnings before taxes	(12.0)	28.0	68.0
Taxes (40%)	4.8[a]	(11.2)	(27.2)
Net income after taxes	($ 7.2)	$ 16.8	$ 40.8
Earnings per share on 5,000 shares (EPS)	($1.44)	$ 3.36	$ 8.16
Expected EPS		$ 3.36	
Standard deviation of EPS		$ 3.04	

[a]Assumes tax credit on losses.

debt, 12 percent, is taken from Table 20-3. With $100,000 of 12 percent debt outstanding, the company's interest expense is shown in Table 20-4 to be $12,000 per year. This is a fixed cost, and it is deducted from EBIT as calculated in the top section. Next, taxes are taken out, to derive total net income. Then we calculate EPS = Net income after taxes ÷ Shares outstanding. With debt = 0, there are 10,000 shares outstanding. However, if half the equity is replaced by debt (debt = $100,000), there will be only 5,000 shares outstanding, and this fact is used to determine the EPS figures that will result at each sales level. With a debt/assets ratio of 50 percent, EPS will be a negative $1.44 if sales are as low as $100,000; it will rise to $3.36 if sales are $200,000; and it will soar to $8.16 if sales are as high as $300,000.

    The EPS distributions under the two financial structures are graphed in Figure 20-3, where we use continuous distributions to approximate the discrete distributions contained in Table 20-4. Although expected EPS is much higher if financial leverage is employed, the graph makes it clear that the risk of low or even negative EPS is also higher if debt is used.

Figure 20-3 **ATM: Probability Distribution of EPS with Different Amounts of Financial Leverage**

Financial leverage (debt via fixed-income securities) affects a firm's expected earnings per share and thus the price of its stock. With zero financial leverage, expected EPS is lower than expected EPS with 50 percent debt ($2.40 versus $3.36). Simultaneously, the probability of attaining $2.40 in EPS with zero debt is much higher than the probability of attaining $3.36 in EPS with 50 percent debt. In addition, with greater leverage, the probability of lower or even negative earnings is increased. Clearly, increased financial leverage carries with it both higher expected earnings and greater risk.

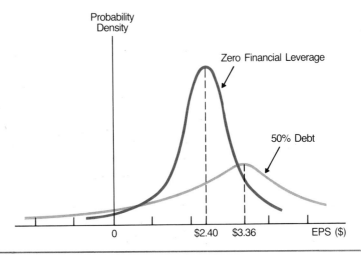

The relationships among expected EPS, risk, and financial leverage are extended in Table 20-5 and graphed in Figure 20-4. Here we see that expected EPS rises for a while as the use of debt increases; interest charges rise, but a smaller number of shares outstanding as debt is substituted for equity still causes EPS to increase. However, EPS peaks at a debt ratio of 50 percent. Beyond this ratio, interest rates rise so fast that EPS is depressed in spite of the falling number of shares outstanding. Risk, as measured by the standard deviation of EPS, rises continuously and at an increasing rate as debt is substituted for equity.

We see, then, that using leverage involves a risk/return trade off; higher leverage increases expected earnings per share (at least for a while), but it also increases the firm's risk. Exactly how this trade-off should be resolved is discussed in the next section.

The Effect of Financial Leverage on Stock Prices

As we saw in the preceding section, ATM's EPS is maximized at a debt/assets ratio of 50 percent. Does this mean that ATM's optimal capital structure is 50

Table 20-5 **ATM: Expected EPS and Standard Deviation with Different Degrees of Financial Leverage**[a]

Debt/Assets Ratio	Expected EPS	Standard Deviation of EPS
0%	$2.40	$1.52
10	2.56	1.69
20	2.75	1.90
30	2.97	2.17
40	3.20	2.53
50	3.36	3.04
60	3.30	3.79

[a]Values for D/A = 0 and 50 percent are taken from Table 20-4. Values at other D/A ratios are calculated similarly.

Figure 20-4 **ATM: Relationships among Expected EPS, Risk, and Financial Leverage**

As shown on the right side of this figure, financial risk rises at an increasing rate with each addition of financial leverage. Earnings per share, on the other hand, rise only to a certain point, as shown on the left. Beyond this peak, interest rates become prohibitive and EPS begins to fall.

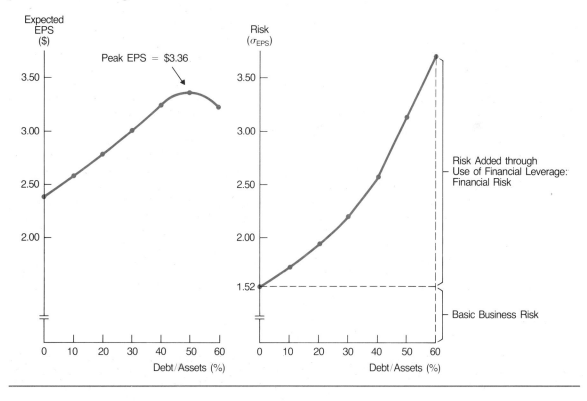

Table 20-6 ATM: Stock Price Estimates with Different Debt/Assets Ratios

Debt/ Assets (1)	k_d (2)	EPS (and DPS)[a] (3)	Estimated Beta (4)	$k_s = [R_F + b(k_M - R_F)]$[b] (5)	Implied Price[c] (6)	Resulting P/E Ratio (7)	Weighted Average Cost of Capital (8)[d]
0%	—	$2.40	1.50	12.0%	$20.00	8.33	12.00%
10	8.0	2.56	1.55	12.2	20.98	8.20	11.46
20	8.3	2.75	1.65	12.6	21.83	7.94	11.08
30	9.0	2.97	1.80	13.2	22.50	7.58	10.86
40	10.0	3.20	2.00	14.0	**22.86**	7.14	**10.80**
50	12.0	**3.36**	2.30	15.2	22.11	6.58	11.20
60	15.0	3.30	2.70	16.8	19.64	5.95	12.12

[a]We assume that ATM pays all of its earnings out as dividends; hence EPS = DPS.
[b]We assume that R_F = 6% and k_M = 10%. Therefore, at debt/assets = 0, k_s = 6% + 1.5(10% − 6%) = 6% + 6% = 12%. Other values of k_s are calculated similarly.
[c]In Chapter 18 we learned that under certain conditions the value of a share of stock is equal to $P = D_1/(k − g)$. We have already noted that ATM's payout is 100 percent; thus dividends and earnings are equivalent. If all earnings are paid out as dividends, no retained earnings will be plowed back into the firm, and growth in earnings and dividends will be zero. Thus, in this special case, D = E and g = 0. Therefore, at debt/assets = 0,

$$P_0 = \frac{E}{k_s}$$

$$P_0 = \frac{\$2.40}{0.12} = \$20.$$

Other prices are calculated similarly.
[d]Column 8 is found by using the weighted average cost of capital (WACC) equation developed in Chapter 19:

$$WACC = k_a = W_d k_d (1 - T) + w_s k_s$$
$$= (D/A)(k_d)(1 - T) + (1 - D/A)k_s.$$

For example, at D/A = 40%,

$$k_a = 0.4(10\%)(0.6) + 0.6(14.0\%) = 10.80\%.$$

percent debt, 50 percent equity? Not necessarily. *The optimal capital structure is the one that maximizes the price of the firm's stock, and this may call for a debt ratio different from the one that maximizes EPS.*

This statement is demonstrated in Table 20-6, which develops ATM's estimated stock price at different debt/assets ratios. The data in Columns 1, 2, and 3 are taken from Tables 20-3 and 20-5. The beta coefficients shown in Column 4 were estimated. Recall from Chapter 15 that beta measures a stock's relative volatility as compared to an average stock. It has been demonstrated both theoretically and empirically that a firm's beta increases with its degree of financial leverage. The exact nature of this relationship for a given firm like ATM is difficult to estimate, but the values in Column 4 do show the approximate relationship.

Assuming that the riskless rate of return, R_F, is 6 percent and that the required return on an average stock, k_M, is 10 percent, we use the CAPM equation to develop the required rates of return for ATM as shown in Column 5.

Here we see that k_s is 12 percent if no financial leverage is used but that k_s rises to 16.8 percent if the company finances with 60 percent debt.

The "zero growth" stock valuation model in footnote c of Table 20-6 is used, along with the Column 3 values of dividends and earnings per share and the Column 5 values of k_s, to develop the implied stock prices shown in Column 6. Here we see that the expected stock price first rises with financial leverage, hits a peak of $22.86 at a debt/assets ratio of 40 percent, and then begins to decline. Thus ATM's optimal capital structure calls for 40 percent debt.

The price/earnings ratios shown in Column 7 were calculated by dividing the implied price in Column 6 by the expected earnings given in Column 3. We use the pattern of P/E ratios as a check on the reasonableness of the other data. As a rule, P/E ratios do decline as the riskiness of a firm increases. Also, at the time the example was developed, the P/Es shown here were generally consistent with those of zero growth companies with varying amounts of financial leverage. Thus the data in Column 7 reinforce our confidence that the implied prices shown in Column 6 are reasonable.

Finally, Column 8 shows ATM's weighted average cost of capital, WACC = k_a, calculated as described in Chapter 19, at different capital structures. If the firm continues to use zero debt, its capital is all equity financed; hence ATM's WACC = k_a = k_s = 12%. As the firm begins to employ lower-cost debt, its weighted average cost of capital declines. As the debt ratio increases, however, the costs of both debt and equity rise, and the increasing costs of the two components begin to offset the fact that a larger proportion of the lower-cost debt component is being used. At 40 percent debt, the weighted average cost of capital reaches a minimum, and it rises if more debt is used.

The EPS, cost of capital, and stock price data in Table 20-6 are plotted in Figure 20-5. As the graph shows, the debt/assets ratio that maximizes ATM's expected EPS is 50 percent. However, the expected stock price is maximized, and the cost of capital is minimized at a 40 percent debt ratio. *Thus the optimal capital structure calls for 40 percent debt, 60 percent equity.* Management should set its target capital structure at these ratios, and if the present ratios are off target, it should move toward the target when new security offerings are made.

DEGREE OF LEVERAGE

Earlier in this chapter, we investigated the effect of fixed operating charges on ATM's operating profits under two proposed options. At that time we made no mention of financial leverage, and when we discussed financial leverage, we assumed operating leverage was given. Actually the two types of leverage are interrelated. For example, firms with high operating leverage often choose low levels of debt to reduce the overall variability of their cash flows. For firms with little operating leverage, however, the optimal capital structure might con-

Figure 20-5 **ATM: Relationships among Debt/Assets Ratio, EPS, Cost of Capital, and Estimated Stock Prices**

The amount of financial leverage that maximizes a firm's earnings per share is not necessarily the amount that will maximize its stock price. In this example, with data plotted from Table 20-6, the stock price is maximized and the cost of capital is minimized at a debt/assets ratio of 40 percent, even though EPS would be higher at 50 percent. This firm will thus seek to target its capital structure at 40 percent debt, 60 percent equity.

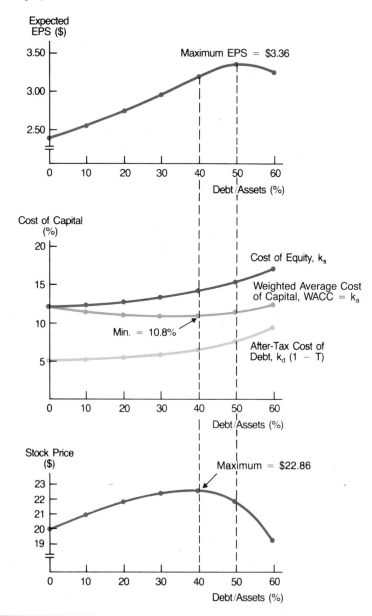

tain more debt. Thus there is a trade-off between operating risk and financial risk.

Unfortunately, the theory of finance has not been developed to the point where we can actually specify simultaneously the optimal levels of operating and financial leverage. We can gain a better understanding of how operating and financial leverage interact through an analysis of the degree of leverage concept.

Degree of Operating Leverage (DOL)

We have already investigated the ramifications of the two operating leverage options for ATM. Actually, the DOL can be computed in several different ways. For example, we chose to compute the DOL at a particular level of sales using Equation 20-2:

$$DOL = \frac{Q(P - V)}{Q(P - V) - F}. \qquad \textbf{(20-2)}$$

Alternatively we could have reached the same conclusion based on dollar sales rather than on units,

$$DOL = \frac{S - VC}{S - VC - F}. \qquad \textbf{(20-2a)}$$

Here, QP, the number of units sold times the sales price, equals sales, S, and QV, the variable cost per unit times the number of units, equals the amount of variable cost, VC.

Applying the equation to the compromise position for ATM's operating leverage, found in Table 20-2 for the expected sales level of $200,000, we find the degree of operating leverage to be 2.0; thus an X percent increase in sales will produce a 2X percent increase in EBIT when the base level of sales is $200,000:

$$DOL = \$200,000 - \$120,000/\$200,000 - \$120,000 - \$40,000$$

$$= 2.0.$$

Therefore, a 50 percent increase in sales, starting from sales of $200,000, would result in a 50% × 2.0 = 100% increase in EBIT. This result can be confirmed by examining the top section of Table 20-4, where we see that a 50 percent increase in sales, from $200,000 to $300,000, causes EBIT to double, from $40,000 to $80,000. Notice, however, that the DOL is specific to the beginning sales level. If we evaluate the DOL from a sales base of $300,000, there will be a different DOL:

$$DOL = \$300,000 - \$180,000/\$300,000 - \$180,000 - \$40,000$$

$$= 1.5.$$

Degree of Financial Leverage (DFL)

Operating leverage affects earnings before interest and taxes (EBIT), whereas financial leverage affects earnings after interest and taxes, or the earnings available to common stockholders. In terms of Table 20-4, operating leverage affects the top section of the table, financial leverage the lower section. Thus, if ATM had more operating leverage, its fixed costs would be higher than $40,000, its variable cost ratio would be lower than 60 percent of sales, and earnings before interest and taxes would vary with sales to a greater extent. Financial leverage takes over where operating leverage leaves off, further magnifying the effect on earnings per share of a change in the level of sales. For this reason, operating leverage is sometimes referred to as *first-stage leverage* and financial leverage as *second-stage leverage*.

degree of financial leverage

The percentage change in earnings available to common shareholders that is associated with a given percentage change in earnings before interest and taxes.

The **degree of financial leverage** (DFL) is defined as the percentage change in earnings available to common shareholders that is associated with a given percentage change in earnings before interest and taxes (EBIT). Where fixed financial charges exist, a change in EBIT will result in a greater than proportional change in earnings per share for the firm. An equation has been developed as an aid in calculating the degree of financial leverage[5] for any given level of EBIT and financing charges, I:

$$\text{Degree of financial leverage} = \frac{\text{EBIT}}{\text{EBIT} - \text{I}}. \qquad (20\text{-}3)$$

For ATM at sales of $200,000 and EBIT of $40,000, the degree of financial leverage with a 50 percent debt ratio is

$$\text{DFL at 50\% debt} = \frac{\$40,000}{\$40,000 - \$12,000}$$

$$= 1.43.$$

Therefore, a 20 percent increase in EBIT would result in a 20%(1.43) = 28.6% increase in earnings per share. If no debt were used, I in Equation 20-3 would equal zero, and the DFL would equal 1.0. Thus, in the absence of fixed financial charges such as interest, a 20 percent increase in EBIT would produce a proportional 20 percent increase in EPS. This can be confirmed in the center section of Table 20-4.

---

[5]Utilizing the same symbols as those used earlier in the chapter, we have

$$\text{DFL} = \frac{Q(P - V) - F}{Q(P - V) - F - I}.$$

However, since EBIT = Q(P − V) − F, Equation 20-3 represents a less cumbersome statement of DFL. Even though we have ignored preferred stock, its presence in the firm's financial structure also will increase the firm's financial leverage and hence the DFL.

Combining Operating and Financial Leverage

We have seen that operating leverage causes a change in sales volume to have a magnified effect on EBIT, and if financial leverage is superimposed on operating leverage, changes in EBIT will have a magnified effect on earnings per share. Therefore, if a firm uses a considerable amount of both operating leverage and financial leverage, even small changes in the level of sales will produce wide fluctuations in EPS.

Equation 20-2 (for the degree of operating leverage) can be combined with Equation 20-3 (for financial leverage) to show the **total leverage effect** of a given change in sales on earnings per share:[6]

total leverage effect The combination of operating leverage and financial leverage that results in a magnified effect on earnings per share from any change in sales.

$$\text{Degree of total leverage (DTL)} = \frac{Q(P - V)}{Q(P - V) - F - I}. \quad \textbf{(20-4)}$$

For ATM, at sales of $200,000 the degree of total leverage, using 50 percent debt, is

$$
\begin{aligned}
\text{DTL} &= \frac{\$200,000 - \$120,000}{\$200,000 - \$120,000 - \$40,000 - \$12,000} \\
&= \frac{\$80,000}{\$28,000} \\
&= 2.86.
\end{aligned}
$$

Therefore, a 40 percent increase in sales would lead to a 2.86 × larger increase in earnings, or a 40%(2.86) = 114 percent increase in ATM's net income. Table 20-7 illustrates that a small increase in sales, 20 percent, leads to a much larger increase in ATM's earnings.

The usefulness of the degree of leverage concept lies in the fact that, first, it enables us to specify the precise effect of a change in sales volume on earnings available to common stock and, second, that it permits us to show the interrelationship between operating and financial leverage. For example, if ATM could *reduce* its degree of operating leverage, it probably could *increase* its use of financial leverage. On the other hand, if the company decided to use more operating leverage, its optimal capital structure would probably call for a lower debt ratio. As we said before, there is a trade-off between operating risk and financial risk.

---

[6]The degree of total leverage, DTL, is equal to the product of the DOL and DFL:

$$\text{DFL} = \frac{Q(P - V)}{Q(P - V) - F} \times \frac{Q(P - V) - F}{Q(P - V) - F - I} = \frac{Q(P - V)}{Q(P - V) - F - I}$$

and thus DTL = DOL × DFL.

Table 20-7 **Operating, Financial, and Total Leverage Effects for ATM with a 20 Percent Increase in Sales**

Income Statement		Previous Status	Percentage Increase	Resulting Status
DTL { DOL {	QP = Sales	$200,000	20%	$240,000
	QV = Variable operating costs (60% of sales)	120,000		144,000
	F = Fixed operating costs	40,000		40,000
	EBIT = Operating profits	40,000	40	56,000
DFL {	−I = Fixed financing charges[a]	12,000		12,000
	EBT = Earnings before taxes	28,000		44,000
	−T = Taxes (40%)	11,200		17,600
	NI = Net income	$ 16,800	57[b]	$ 26,400
	Common stock equity shares outstanding	5,000		5,000
	Earnings per share	$3.36	57[c]	$5.28

[a]Fixed financing charges include interest or a tax-adjusted preferred dividend equivalent or both. Since preferred dividends are paid after taxes and interest is a pretax expense, preferred dividends must be modified for the tax effect. Thus:

Pretax equivalent preferred dividend = Preferred dividend/(1 − Tax rate).

In this case all financing costs result from interest charges.
[b]Note that EBT also increases by the same 57 percent. Since taxes are a variable cost in this example, they do not affect the degree of leverage.
[c]Note that because of operating leverage (DOL = 2.0), a 20 percent increase in sales will result in twice as large a change in operating profits. Similarly, the effects of the combination of operating and financial leverage cause a change in sales to be magnified by 2.86×. Recall that DOL = 2.0 and DFL = 1.43; therefore 2.0 × 1.43 = 2.86, and if sales increase by 20 percent, 0.20(2.86) = 57 percent increase in EBT, NI, and EPS. Unfortunately, a 20 percent decrease in sales will likewise be magnified into a 57 percent decline in EBT, NI, and EPS!

TAXES, BANKRUPTCY COSTS, AND THE VALUE OF THE FIRM

Why does the expected stock price first rise as the firm begins to use financial leverage, then hit a peak, and finally decline when leverage becomes excessive? This pattern occurs primarily because of *corporate income taxes* and *bankruptcy costs*. Because interest on debt is tax deductible, the more debt a firm has, the greater the proportion of its operating income that flows through to investors, and hence the higher the value of the firm. On the other hand, the larger the debt, the greater the risk of bankruptcy. At very high levels of debt, the odds are very great that bankruptcy will occur, and if this happens, lawyers may end up with almost as much of the firm's assets as the investors.[7]

---

[7]See Appendix 20A for a discussion of actual bankruptcy costs.

Figure 20-6 **ATM: Effects of Tax Deductions and Bankruptcy Costs on Stock Value**

When a firm uses financial leverage, its expected stock price first rises and then falls. The initial rise occurs because the interest payments on corporate debt are tax-deductible. Thus, as a firm's debt load increases, more of its operating income escapes taxation and flows through to investors. As levels of debt increase, however, so does the risk of bankruptcy. Consequently, at point D_1, when investors begin to worry about the effects of debt, the potential risk of bankruptcy begins to offset the benefits of the tax-deductible interest. At point D_2 the balance between the benefits of leverage and the potential cost of bankruptcy is reached and the firm's capital structure is optimized. Beyond point D_2 the potential cost of bankruptcy overshadows the benefits of leverage and the stock's price falls.

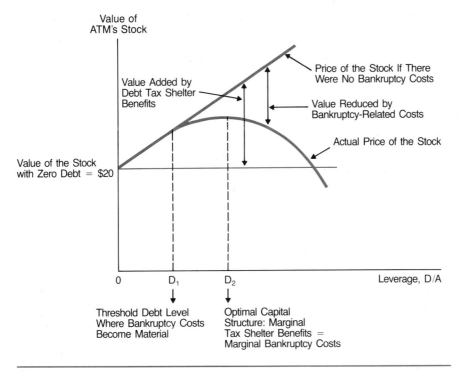

Figure 20-6 illustrates this concept. When ATM has zero debt, the value of its stock is $20 per share. As it begins to use debt, the stock price begins to rise because of the tax shelter benefits of debt. Prior to D_1, potential bankruptcy costs are insignificant. However, at D_1 investors begin to worry about the effects of debt, so *potential* bankruptcy costs begin to offset the debt's tax shelter benefits. At D_2 the marginal tax shelter benefits are equal to the marginal potential bankruptcy costs, and the value of the stock is maximized. Beyond D_2 potential bankruptcy costs more than offset the benefits of additional debt, so further increases in leverage reduce the price of the stock. Thus D_2 represents the optimal capital structure.[8]

LIQUIDITY AND CASH FLOW ANALYSIS

There are some difficult problems with the type of analysis described thus far in the chapter. Included are the following:

1. Because of the difficulties in determining exactly how P/E ratios and equity capitalization rates (k_s values) are affected by different degrees of financial leverage, management rarely, if ever, has sufficient confidence in this type of analysis to use it as the sole determinant of the target capital structure.

2. Many firms are not publicly owned. If the owners do not plan to ever have the firm go public, potential market value data are irrelevant. However, an analysis based on implied market values for a privately owned firm is useful if the owner is interested in knowing how the market value of the firm would be affected by leverage should the decision be made to go public.

3. Even for publicly owned firms, the managers may be more or less conservative than the average stockholder; hence they may set a somewhat different target capital structure than the one that would maximize the stock price. The managers of a publicly owned firm would never admit this, for unless they owned voting control, they would quickly be removed from office. However, in view of the uncertainties about what constitutes the value-maximizing structure, management could always say that the target capital structure employed is, in its judgment, the value-maximizing structure, and it would be difficult to prove otherwise.

4. Managers of large firms, especially those providing vital services such as electricity or telephones, have a responsibility to provide *continuous* service, so they must refrain from using leverage to the point where the firm's long-run viability is endangered. Long-run viability may conflict with maximizing short-run earnings per share.

For all of these reasons, managers are very much concerned with the effects of financial leverage on the risk of bankruptcy, so an analysis of this factor is an important input in the capital structure decision. Accordingly, managements give considerable weight to such ratios as the *times-interest-earned ratio (TIE)*. The lower this ratio, the higher the probability that a firm will default on its debt and be forced into bankruptcy.

---

[8]This entire concept — including (1) the reasons the tax shelter benefits cause a linear increase in value, (2) the specific elements that make up bankruptcy-related costs, and (3) the effects of personal income taxes on capital structure decisions — is discussed in Eugene F. Brigham and Louis Gapenski, *Intermediate Financial Management,* 2nd ed., Chapter 5.

Table 20-8 **ATM: Expected Times-Interest-Earned Ratio at Different Debt/Assets Ratios**

Debt/Assets	TIE[a]
0%	Undefined
10	25.0
20	12.1
30	7.4
40	5.0
50	3.3
60	2.2

[a]TIE = EBIT/Interest. For example, if debt/assets = 50%, then TIE = $40,000/$12,000 = 3.3. Data are from Tables 20-3 and 20-4.

Table 20-8 shows how ATM's expected TIE ratio declines as the debt/assets ratio increases. When the debt/assets ratio is only 10 percent, the expected TIE is a high 25 times, but the interest coverage ratio declines rapidly as debt rises. Note, however, that these coverages are the expected values; the actual TIE will be higher if sales exceed the expected $200,000 level but lower if sales fall below $200,000. The variability of the TIE ratios is highlighted in Figure 20-7, which shows the probability distributions of these ratios at debt/assets ratios of 40 percent and 60 percent. The expected TIE is much higher if only 40 percent debt is used. Even more important, with less debt there is a much lower probability of a TIE of less than 1.0, the level at which the firm is not earning enough to meet its required interest payments and is seriously exposed to the threat of bankruptcy.

CAPITAL STRUCTURE AND MERGERS

One of the more exciting developments in the financial world during the 1980s has been the high level of merger activity, especially takeovers. A *takeover* occurs when one firm buys out another over the opposition of the acquired firm's management. Because the acquired firm's stock is considered to be undervalued, the acquiring firm is willing to pay a premium of perhaps 50 percent to gain control. Mergers are discussed at length in Chapter 22, but it is useful to make these points now: (1) very often the acquiring firm issues debt and uses it to buy the target firm's stock; (2) this action effectively changes the enterprise's capital structure; and (3) if the acquired firm is operating below its optimal capital structure, the value enhancement resulting from the use of debt may be sufficient to cover the premium offered for the stock and still leave a profit for the acquiring company.

The recognition of the validity of the type of analysis described in this chapter led to the creation of companies whose major function was to acquire other companies. The managers of these acquiring companies (often called *conglomerates*) frequently made huge personal fortunes. Shrewd individual

Figure 20-7 **ATM: Probability Distributions of Times-Interest-Earned Ratios with Different Capital Structures**

The times-interest-earned ratio is an important indicator of bankruptcy risk. The lower the TIE, the greater the potential for bankruptcy. Management will be especially concerned about keeping TIE above 1.0, the point below which a firm's earnings will not cover its required interest payments. This figure shows that a 60 percent capital structure not only creates an overall lower TIE than a 40 percent structure but also results in a much higher probability of a TIE below 1.0.

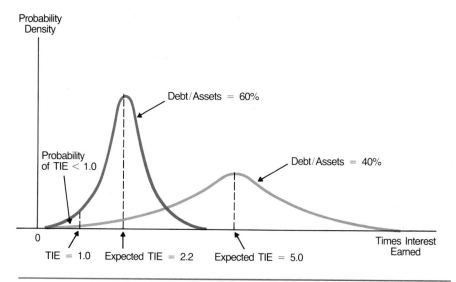

investors, including a few professors, selected stock portfolios heavily weighted with prime acquisition targets and did well in the market. Of course, the managements of firms with low leverage ratios that did not want to be taken over could be expected to react by attempting to find their optimal debt levels and then issuing debt and repurchasing stock. By doing so they would be raising the price of their firms' stock and making their companies less attractive acquisition targets.

The game is far from over — indeed, it can never end, because economic shifts lead to continuing changes in optimal capital structures. This makes it especially important that the lessons to be learned from this chapter are thoroughly understood by everyone actively involved in financial management.

CHECKLIST OF FACTORS THAT INFLUENCE CAPITAL STRUCTURE DECISIONS

The factors listed and briefly discussed in this section all have an important, though hard to measure, bearing on a firm's choice of a target capital structure.

1. Sales stability. If its sales are relatively stable, a firm can safely take on more debt and incur higher fixed charges than a company with unstable sales. For example, utility companies, because of their stable demand, are able to undertake more debt financing than the average industrial firm.

2. Asset structure. Firms whose assets are suitable as security for loans tend to use debt rather heavily. Thus real estate companies tend to be highly leveraged, whereas manufacturers with heavy investments in specialized machinery and work-in-process inventories employ less debt.

3. Operating leverage. Other things held constant, a firm with less operating leverage is better able to employ financial leverage. Earlier in this chapter we discussed how operating and financial leverage interact to determine the overall effect of a decline in sales on operating income and earnings per share.

4. Growth rate. Other things held constant, faster-growing firms must rely more heavily on external capital (see Chapter 8). Furthermore, the flotation costs involved in selling common stock exceed those incurred when selling debt. Thus, to minimize financing costs, rapidly growing firms tend to use somewhat more debt than slower-growing companies.

5. Profitability. One often observes that firms with very high rates of return on investment use relatively little debt. Although there is no theoretical justification for this fact, the practical reason seems to be that very profitable firms like IBM and 3M simply do not need to do much debt financing—their high profit margins enable them to do most of their financing with retained earnings.

6. Taxes. Interest is a deductible expense, whereas dividends are not deductible. Hence the higher a firm's corporate tax rate, the greater the advantage of using debt. This point was discussed in Chapter 19.

7. Control. The effect that debt or stock financing might have on a management's control position may influence its capital structure decision. If management has voting control (51 percent of the stock) but is not in a position to buy any more stock, debt may be the choice for new financings. On the other hand, a management group that is not concerned about voting control may decide to use equity rather than debt if the firm's financial situation is so weak that the use of debt might subject the firm to risk of default; if the firm goes into default, the managers will almost surely lose their jobs. If too little debt is used, however, management runs the risk of a takeover attempt; here another company or management group tries to persuade stockholders to turn over control to the new group, which may plan to boost earnings by using financial leverage. In general, control considerations do not necessarily suggest the use of debt or equity, but if management is at all insecure, the effects of capital structure on control will certainly be taken into account.

8. Management attitudes. In the absence of proof that one capital structure will lead to higher stock prices than another, management can exercise its own judgment about a proper capital structure. Some managements tend to be more (or less) conservative than others and thus use less (or more) debt than the average firm in their industry.

9. Lender and rating agency attitudes. Regardless of managers' own analyses of the proper leverage factors for their firms, there is no question that lenders' and rating agencies' attitudes are frequently important determinants of financial structures. In the majority of cases, the corporation discusses its financial structure with lenders and rating agencies and gives much weight to their advice. But when management is so confident of the future that it seeks to use leverage beyond the norms for its industry, lenders may be unwilling to accept such debt increases or may do so only at high price.

10. Market conditions. Conditions in the stock and bond markets undergo both long- and short-run changes, which can have an important bearing on a firm's optimal capital structure. For example, during the credit crunch in the winter of 1982, there was simply no market at any reasonable interest rate for new long-term bonds rated below A. Low-rated companies that needed capital were forced to go to the stock market or to the short-term debt market. Actions like this could represent either changes in these firms' target capital structures or temporary departures from these targets, but the important point is that stock and bond market conditions at a point in time do influence the type of securities used for a given financing.

11. The firm's internal conditions. A firm's own internal conditions also have a bearing on its target capital structure. For example, suppose that a firm has just successfully completed a research and development program and projects higher earnings in the immediate future. However, these new earnings are not yet anticipated by investors and hence are not reflected in the price of the stock. This company would not want to issue stock; it would prefer to finance with debt until the higher earnings materialized and were reflected in the stock price, at which time it might want to sell an issue of common stock, retire the debt, and return to its target capital structure.

12. Financial flexibility. It has been noted that firms can earn a great deal more money from good capital budgeting and operating decisions than they can from good financing decisions. Indeed, we really are not sure how (or even if) financing decisions affect stock prices, but we do know that having to turn down a large order because funds are not available for buying the raw materials or equipment needed to fill it will lower profits. For this reason, many treasurers' primary goal is always having the ability to raise the capital needed to support operations. We also know that when times are good, firms can raise capital with either stock or bonds, but when times are bad, suppliers of capital are much more willing to make funds available if they are given a secured position, and this means bonds.

Putting these two thoughts together gives rise to the goal of maintaining financial flexibility, which from an operational viewpoint means maintaining

Table 20-9 **Capital Structure Percentages, 1986:**
Selected Industries Ranked by Common Equity Ratios

Industry	Common Equity (1)	Preferred Stock (2)	Total Debt (3)	Long-Term Debt (4)	Short-Term Debt (5)	Times-Interest-Earned Ratio (6)
Drugs	78%	—	22%	13%	9%	9.1×
Electrical/electronics	75	1	23	15	8	6.9
Automotive	74	2	24	19	5	7.6
Retailing	52	1	47	32	15	3.1
Utilities (electric, gas, and telephone)	45	7	48	46	2	3.2
Steel	44	3	53	49	4	0.9
Composite (average of all industries, not just those listed above)	47%	3%	50%	32%	18%	2.3×

Note: These ratios are based on accounting (or book) values. Stated on a market value basis, the results would be somewhat different. Most important, the equity percentage would rise, because most stocks sell at prices that are much higher than their book values.
Source: *Industrial Compustat* data tape, 1986.

adequate reserve borrowing capacity. What constitutes "adequate" reserve borrowing capacity is judgmental, but it clearly depends on the factors mentioned previously in the chapter, including the firm's forecasted need for funds, predicted capital market conditions, management's confidence in these forecasts, and the consequences of a capital shortage.

VARIATIONS IN CAPITAL STRUCTURES AMONG FIRMS

As might be expected, wide variations in the use of financial leverage occur both among industries and among the individual firms in each industry. Table 20-9 illustrates this point. Retailers make heavy use of debt, especially short-term debt used to carry inventories. Manufacturing companies as a group use less debt, especially short-term debt. Within manufacturing, small firms with limited access to the stock market employ the most debt, and again the bulk of their liabilities are short-term. The data in the table are not broken down sufficiently to so indicate, but the majority of the debt shown for small manufacturers represents trade credit.

Financing mixes also vary widely among manufacturing sectors. Aircraft companies are highly leveraged, borrowing heavily on a short-term basis to finance the construction of airplanes. Because of their long production cycle, they have large work-in-process inventories that must be financed. Aircraft manufacturers receive advances from their customers, and these advances are shown as current liabilities. Like the aircraft companies, manufacturers of electrical equipment also have long construction periods—for example, nuclear

SMALL BUSINESS

Capital Structure in the Small Firm

Small businesses rely heavily on banks and other suppliers of debt funds for a large portion of their capital. As we mentioned before, small firms have relatively limited access to the public equity markets, which means that they must turn either to private equity or to debt. Debt financing is very important to small businesses.

In spite of debt's importance to small firms, there are many factors that may limit the extent to which the owner-manager of a small firm may wish to use the debt markets. These factors include the risk of debt financing to the owner-manager, the increased likelihood and relative cost of bankruptcy, and the effect of taxes.

Earlier in the chapter we noted that as financial leverage increases, EPS becomes more sensitive to changes in sales or operating profits. This variability in earnings may be even more pronounced (and thus more important) for small firms than for larger ones. In addition, small firms generally have narrower product lines and smaller, less diversified customer bases. Since their sales are poorly diversified, there is more uncertainty in predicting a smaller firm's earnings. Of course, a small customer base could be an advantage if the firm's key customers are willing to make long-term commitments to purchase the firm's output. Such commitments would be a definite plus in the eyes of a credit officer considering the firm for a loan. Normally, however, a small customer base makes earnings less predictable.

Financial theorists argue that EPS variability by itself is of no concern in making the capital structure decision. One argument, for example, is that shareholders can "undo" the firm's leverage by buying debt securities, which offset the firm's debt. Or, if the firm has too little debt, the shareholders can lever their own portfolios by borrowing. These arguments neglect the facts of life in a small business, however. The owner-manager may have virtually all of his or her wealth tied up in the business in order to maintain control, which leaves the owner little or no financial flexibility. The firm's capital structure is, in effect, the owner's capital structure. In such a setting, the owner's desire to avoid risk (or accept risk) must match the risk posture assumed by the business. Also, the owner's ability to remove cash from the firm will be influenced by the level and terms of debt employed by the firm. Therefore, owner-managers in small firms may be especially sensitive to the level of debt employed.

Bankruptcy costs are thought by many researchers to be an important factor in limiting the debt used by a firm. Two considerations that influence capital structure decisions are: (1) the *actual costs* of bankruptcy, if it occurs, and (2) the *probability* that bankruptcy will occur. As we have already mentioned, the probability of earnings fluctuation is greater in smaller firms, and greater earnings variability means higher risk of failure. The probability of bankruptcy would therefore normally be higher in a small firm, other things being equal.

Another disadvantage to the smaller firm is that some of the costs of bankruptcy are fixed. Although normally the larger the firm, the higher the bankruptcy costs, these costs are proportionately higher for small firms. Such concerns probably reduce the amount of debt financing that managers of small firms would consider optimal.

One of the obvious benefits of debt financing is that the interest payments on debt are tax deductible, making the after-tax cost of debt smaller. However, firms with lower earnings pay taxes at a lower marginal rate than do firms with higher earnings. This is not meant to suggest that higher taxes are beneficial but rather to indicate that the tax deductibility of interest is of greater advantage to firms with higher marginal tax rates. If most of the debt available in the financial markets is demanded by firms in high tax brackets, that debt may be priced with interest rates that are relatively unattractive to smaller, less profitable firms. As a result, the relative desirability of debt may be much less in a smaller firm when the cost of that debt is correctly measured on an after-tax basis.

There are certain factors that may make debt more attractive to small firms, such as their limited access to equity markets. A number of programs exist that make it easier for small firms to borrow money. Perhaps the best-known programs that assist small businesses in obtaining debt funds are those of the Small Business Administration (SBA). In addition to the SBA making direct loans to small businesses, it also guarantees small-business loans made by commercial banks and small-business investment companies. These loans, which are generally made on more attractive terms than conventional loans, are made to businesses that would otherwise have difficulty qualifying for loans.

One final point has to do with incorporation. If the small business has not incorporated, the owners are personally liable for all debt incurred by the firm. A corporation has, in theory, only limited liability; the owner's liability is limited to the investment made in the firm. In practice, however, the owner of a small business that takes out a substantial loan will probably find that he or she must agree to assume the liability out of personal net worth if the corporation defaults. Limited liability is thus a fiction for such owner-managers.

Small businesses face a dilemma. Because access to other sources of funds is difficult, the small firm is motivated to make heavy use of debt financing in its capital structure. On the other hand, factors that influence the target level of debt financing generally bias the small firm toward a *lower* use of debt than would otherwise be indicated. The owner-manager's dilemma is to balance these conflicting pressures when selecting a method of financing the firm. In achieving such a balance, the use of small-business debt sources that are unavailable to larger firms may be a help.

reactors take years to build—and short-term credit is often used to finance this construction. The drug companies, on the other hand, do not use much leverage. Their production period is short, and the uncertainties inherent in an industry that is both oriented toward research and development and exposed to lawsuits arising from adverse reactions to its products render the heavy use of leverage unwise.

SUMMARY

The concepts of business risk (which includes operating leverage) financial leverage, and target, or optimal, capital structure were discussed in this chapter. Business risk refers to the variability of operating profits, and operating leverage refers to the use of fixed costs in operations. Financial leverage refers to the use of fixed financial costs in the firm's capital structure. The common element for both types of leverage is that the higher the leverage, the greater the variability in earnings and hence the greater the firm's overall risk. There is ample evidence to suggest that the variability of operating income, EBIT, is the single most important determinant of a firm's target capital structure. Most

RESOLUTION TO DECISION IN FINANCE

Putting Citicorp on Firmer Footing

John Reed and his team at Citibank clearly think of their role in historic terms. Their time frame is not quarters, but decades. "We're not in a position here where anyone feels compelled to demonstrate short-term performance," says Lawrence M. Small, head of corporate banking. "This is a young management team that wants to leave behind a bank that's very solidly based and carefully crafted, not something that's slapped together."

In pursuing his long-term plan for the bank, Reed has been adamant about diverting income to boost loan-loss reserves and has flatly refused to sell any of the bank's valuable assets, such as Citicorp Center in New York. Says Reed, "If I'm wrong, it's not as if I spent the money buying a building or anything like that. It's there, and if I'm wrong, we've got a nice pot of money."

John Reed has not acted like a man concerned by his critics. While analysts have grown vocal and impatient waiting for Citibank to cash in on its impressive earnings potential, Reed has

in fact embarked on a buying spree. Citicorp paid $680 million for Quotron Systems, Inc., the company that provides stock quotations and other financial data to 80,000 users through desktop computer terminals. It has also recently acquired banks in Arizona, Utah, and Nevada in an effort to lessen Citicorp's dependence on the highly competitive New York consumer market for deposits. Reed also has picked up banks in Italy, Spain, and Belgium and is said to be shopping for a medium-sized Japanese bank in order to make Citicorp less vulnerable to fluctuations in the dollar.

Although some analysts think that Reed should either cool his spending or sell off some of the bank's high-value assets to pay for his acquisitions, Citibank's management team remains nonplussed. Says financial controller Thomas Jones, "We are *not* burning desks to keep the boilers going."

Whether Reed is building his dream house or a house of cards will be determined over the next several years. Citibank's reliance on Latin American loans has even Reed nervous. Walt Wriston coined the phrase, "countries don't go broke," and his critics quickly tacked on the rejoinder, "but those who lend to them do." Reed pointedly reminds colleagues that both sides of the statement are true.

Source: Suzanna Andrews, "John Reed Builds His Dream House," *Institutional Investor,* March 1987, 107–118; Sarah Bartlett, "John Reed's Citicorp," *Business Week,* December 8, 1986, 90–96; and "John Reed's Falling Star," *Bankers Monthly,* March 1987, 13–18.

financial managers view the target capital structure as a trade-off between business and financial risk.

The effects of leverage on stock prices, earnings per share, and the cost of capital were examined. The analysis suggests that some optimal capital structure exists that simultaneously maximizes the firm's stock price and minimizes its average cost of capital. Yet, although it is theoretically possible to determine the optimal capital structure, as a practical matter this structure cannot be estimated with precision. Accordingly, financial executives generally consider the optimal capital structure as a range (for example, 40 to 50 percent debt) rather than a precise point. In addition, they analyze the effects of different capital structures on expected earnings per share and interest coverage ratios rather than concentrating exclusively on imprecisely estimated stock prices. Firms also analyze factors such as sales stability, asset structure, effects on control, and so on, and the final target capital structure is determined in a more quantative manner.

QUESTIONS

20-1 The uncertainty inherent in projections of future operating income is called what?

20-2 "One type of leverage affects both EBIT and EPS. The other type affects only EPS." Explain what the statement means.

20-3 What is the relationship between market (or beta) risk and leverage?

20-4 Why is the following statement true? "Other things being the same, firms with relatively stable sales are able to carry relatively high debt ratios."

20-5 Why do public utility companies usually pursue a different financial policy than that of retail firms?

20-6 Some economists believe that swings in business cycles will not be as wide in the future as they have been in the past. Assuming that they are correct in their analysis, what effect might this added stability have on the types of financing used by firms in the United States? Would your answer be true for all firms?

20-7 Why is EBIT generally considered to be independent of financial leverage? Why might EBIT actually be influenced by financial leverage at high debt levels?

20-8 How might increasingly volatile inflation rates, interest rates, and bond prices affect the optimal capital structure for corporations?

20-9 If a firm went from zero debt to successively higher levels of debt, why would you expect its stock price to first rise, then hit a peak, and then begin to decline?

20-10 Why is the debt level that maximizes a firm's expected EPS generally higher than the debt level that maximizes its stock price?

20-11 In public utility rate cases, a utility's riskiness is a key issue, as utilities are supposed to be allowed to earn the same rate of return on common equity as unregulated firms of comparable risk. The difficulty is in specifying in quantitative terms the riskiness of utilities and nonutilities. Describe how the degree of leverage concepts (DOL, DFL, and DTL) might be used as indicators of risk in a rate case.

SELF-TEST PROBLEMS

ST-1 Visical, Inc., produces medical test equipment for ophthalmologists, which sells for $500 per unit. Visical's fixed costs are $1 million; 5,000 units are produced and sold each year; profits total $250,000; and the firm's assets (all equity financed) are $2,500,000. Visical estimates that it can change its production process, thereby adding $2 million to investment and $250,000 to fixed operating costs. This change will reduce variable costs per unit by $50 and increase output by 2,000 units, but the sales price on all units will have to be lowered to $475 to permit sales of the additional output. Visical has tax loss carry-forwards that cause its tax rate to be zero. It uses no debt, and its average cost of capital is 10 percent.

a. Should Visical make the change?

b. Would Visical's operating leverage as measured by DOL increase or decrease if it made the change? What about its breakeven point?

c. Suppose the investment totaled $4 million, and Visical had to borrow $2 million at an interest rate of 7 percent. Find the ROE on the $2 million incremental equity investment. Should Visical make the change if debt financing must be used?

ST-2 Brosky Production's situation is as follows: (1) EBIT = $2.86 million; (2) tax rate = t = 40%; (3) debt outstanding = D = $4 million; (4) k_d = 9%; (5) k_s = 12%; and (6) shares of stock outstanding = 500,000. Since Brosky's product market is stable and the company expects no growth, all earnings are paid out as dividends. The debt consists of perpetual bonds.

a. What are Brosky's earnings per share (EPS) and its price per share (P_0)?

b. What is Brosky's weighted average cost of capital (k_a)?

c. Brosky can increase its debt by $4 million, to a total of $8 million, using the new debt to buy back and retire some of its shares at the current price. Its interest rate on debt will be 12 percent (it will have to call and refund the old debt), and its cost of equity will rise from 12 percent to 15 percent. EBIT will remain constant. Should Brosky change its capital structure?

d. What is Brosky's TIE coverage ratio under the original situation and under the conditions in Part c?

PROBLEMS

20-1 **Combined leverage effects.** Rochester Associates has a DOL of 2.5 and a DFL of 4.0. If sales increase by 10 percent, what will happen to net income?

20-2 **Operating leverage effects.** Consolidated Electric Company has a single product, which sells for $30 and has a variable cost of $20 per unit. Fixed costs are $500,000.

a. What is the firm's breakeven point in units?

b. What is the firm's breakeven point in sales dollars?

c. What is the firm's DOL if sales are 10,000 units above breakeven?

d. What is the firm's EBIT if Consolidated Electric's sales are 5,000 units below the breakeven point for the period?

20-3 **Operating leverage effects.** Now assume that Consolidated Electric (Problem 20-2) has begun an impressive modernization program. To reduce its per-unit variable costs to $10 per unit, the company's fixed costs have been allowed to rise to $1.4 million annually. Under these new conditions:

a. What is the firm's breakeven point in units?

b. What is the firm's breakeven point in sales dollars?

c. What is the firm's DOL if sales are 10,000 units above breakeven?

d. What is the firm's EBIT if Consolidated Electric's sales are 5,000 units below the breakeven point for the period?

e. What are the financial implications of the new level of operating leverage as compared to Consolidated's operating leverage before modernization?

20-4 **Operating leverage.** York Manufacturing is selling 600,000 units of its only product at $100 per unit. Variable costs are $40 per unit, whereas annual fixed operating costs are $30 million.

a. What is the firm's operating profit?

b. What is the firm's DOL?

c. If sales increase by 10 percent, what is the resulting operating profit? Use the DOL to answer this question.

d. Confirm your answer in Part c by preparing an income statement showing the dollar level of sales, fixed and variable costs, and operating profit after the 10 percent growth in sales.

e. What would happen to operating profits if sales decline by 10 percent? Confirm your answer with a pro forma income statement.

20-5 **Operating leverage.** Refer to Figure 20-1.

a. Calculate the degree of operating leverage for Options 1 and 2 at sales of $40,000, $120,000, and $240,000. The degree of operating leverage for other levels of sales are as follows:

Sales	DOL$_1$	DOL$_2$
$ 80,000	Undefined (or ∞)	−2.0
160,000	2.0	4.0
220,000	1.57	2.2

b. Is it true that the DOL is approximately equal to infinity just above the breakeven point, implying that a very small increase in sales will produce a huge percentage increase in EBIT, but that the DOL declines when calculated at higher levels of sales?

c. Is it true for both options for all sales levels where DOL > 0 that DOL$_2$ < DOL$_1$? Explain.

20-6 **Breakeven analysis.** Phoenix Industries will produce 200,000 outdoor gas grills this year. Variable costs are $40 per unit and fixed operating costs are $9,500,000. What selling price is required for Phoenix to obtain operating profits of $500,000 if all 200,000 units are sold?

20-7 **Combined leverage effects.** Sweetser's Candy has sales of $8 million, and variable cost is 65 percent of sales. Fixed operating costs are $1.5 million. The firm just received a $7 million loan with an interest rate of 11 percent.

a. What is the firm's DOL?

b. What is the firm's DFL?

c. What is the firm's DTL?

20-8 **Combined leverage effects.** Nebraska Novelty has a single product, which it sells for $50. Variable costs per unit are $35 and total fixed costs are $750,000, which include interest payments of $150,000. The firm plans to produce and sell 60,000 units this year.

a. What is the firm's DOL?

b. What is the firm's DFL?

c. What is the firm's DTL?

20-9 **Combined leverage effects.** Nixon's Tape Centers expects sales of $12 million this year. Variable costs are 45 percent of sales, and fixed operating costs are $6 million. The firm has debt of $8 million on which it pays 9 percent interest.

a. What is the firm's DOL?

b. What is the firm's DFL?

c. What is the firm's DTL?

20-10   **Financial leverage.** Turner Toys has annual sales of $3.7 million, variable costs are 40 percent of sales, and fixed operating costs are $2 million. The firm's DFL = 4.0. How much interest does the firm pay annually?

20-11   **Combined leverage effects.** Moses Engineering has the following financial characteristics:

> Sales in units = 50,000.
> Unit sales price = $100.
> Variable cost per unit = $55.
> Fixed operating cost = $1.5 million.
> Annual interest charges = $250,000.

    a. Determine the firm's EPS if sales increase by 20 percent next year. Use the DTL equation as the basis of your computations.

    b. Confirm your answer in Part a by preparing a projected income statement. The firm has 200,000 shares of common stock outstanding, and its marginal tax rate is 40 percent.

20-12   **Combined leverage effects.** Tennessee Manufacturing Incorporated (TMI) is a new firm that will manufacture and sell replacement parts for equipment to construction firms. The firm must determine the operating and financial leverage under which it will operate. TMI can use a low operating leverage (LOL) plan under which variable costs are $15 per unit (75 percent of sales) and fixed operating costs are $200,000. Alternatively, TMI can use high operating leverage (called the HOL plan) under which the variable costs are $10 per unit (50 percent of sales) and fixed operating costs are $600,000. Whichever production plan is implemented, the firm's product will sell for $20 per unit.

    a. Calculate the degree of operating leverage (DOL) for the LOL and HOL production plans at sales of $1.2 million and $1.6 million.

    b. Assume that the LOL and HOL plans can be financed in either of the following ways: (1) no debt, or (2) $900,000 debt at 10 percent interest. Calculate the degree of financial leverage (DFL) for the LOL plan at sales levels of both $1.2 and $1.6 million. The DFLs for the HOL plan at $900,000 debt and these sales levels are 0 and 1.82, respectively.

    c. Calculate the degree of total leverage (DTL) under the LOL plan with debt at sales of $1.2 and $1.6 million. The DTLs for the HOL plan at these same sales levels are −6.67 and 7.27, respectively.

    d. At the sales level of $1.2 million, the DTL for the HOL plan was negative (DTL_{HOL} = −6.67). Does a negative degree of operating leverage imply that an increase in sales will *lower* profits?

20-13   **Changing capital structure.** Mercury Papers is an all-equity firm that is considering changing its capital structure to include debt. The return on an average security in the market, k_M, is 14 percent, and the risk-free rate, R_F, is 9 percent. Mercury's beta is 0.9. If Mercury borrows to the extent that 30 percent of its total financing is debt financed, its beta will rise to 1.2. What is the cost of equity for Mercury Papers before and after the proposed change?

20-14   **Changing capital structure.** Edwardsville Supply Company is an all-equity firm with $20 million in assets and 400,000 shares of common stock outstanding. The firm's president is considering an expansion of the facilities, which will increase operating profits to $4 million. The cost of the plant expansion is $10 million. The funds may be obtained in one of three ways: (1) a common stock issue at $100 per share, resulting in 100,000 new shares of common; (2) a debt issue with a 9 percent coupon rate; or (3) a preferred stock issue with an 8 percent dividend. The company's tax rate is expected to be 40 percent.

a. Which alternative provides the highest EPS?

b. Edwardsville Supply has determined the P/E multiples of firms with capital structures similar to those proposed:

Financing	P/E Multiple
Equity	14
Debt issue	10
Preferred stock	12

What is the stock price that would be associated with the earnings from each financial plan?

c. How should the firm finance the proposed expansion?

20-15 **Financing alternatives.** The Fraser Company plans to raise a net amount of $180 million to finance new equipment and working capital in early 1988. Two alternatives are being considered: Common stock may be sold to net $40 per share, or debentures yielding 10 percent may be issued. The Fraser Company's balance sheet and income statement prior to financing are as follows:

The Fraser Company
Balance Sheet as of December 31, 1987
(Millions of Dollars)

Current assets	$600	Accounts payable	$115
Net fixed assets	300	Notes payable to bank	185
		Other current liabilities	150
		Total current liabilities	$450
		Long-term debt	185
		Common stock, $2 par	40
		Retained earnings	225
Total assets	$900	Total liabilities and equity	$900

The Fraser Company
Income Statement for Year Ended December 31, 1987
(Millions of Dollars)

Sales	$1,650
Operating costs	1,485
Earnings before interest and taxes (10%)	$ 165
Interest on debt	30
Earnings before taxes	$ 135
Federal-plus-state tax (40%)	54
Net income after tax	$ 81

The probability distribution for annual sales is as follows:

Probability	Annual Sales (Millions of Dollars)
0.30	$1,500
0.40	1,800
0.30	2,100

a. Assuming that EBIT is equal to 10 percent of sales, calculate earnings per share under both the debt financing and the stock financing alternatives at each possible level of sales. Then calculate expected earnings per share and σ_{EPS} under both debt and stock financing. Also calculate the debt ratio and the times-interest-earned (TIE) ratio at the expected sales level under each alternative. The old debt will remain outstanding. Which financing method would you recommend?

(Do Part b only if you are using the computerized problem diskette.)

b. Suppose each of the following happens, with other values held at the base-case (Part a) levels:

(1) The interest rate on new debt falls to 5 percent.
(2) The interest rate on new debt rises to 20 percent.
(3) The stock price falls to $20. (Return k_d to 0.10 = 10%.)
(4) The stock price rises to $70.
(5) With P_0 = $40 and k_d = 0.10 = 10%, now change the sales probability distribution to the following:

Sales	Probability		Sales	Probability
(a) $1,500	0	(b) $ 0	0.3
1,800	1.0		1,800	0.4
2,100	0		5,000	0.3

What are the implications of these changes?

ANSWERS TO SELF-TEST PROBLEMS

ST-1   **a. 1.** Determine the variable cost per unit at present, using the following definitions and equations:

P = average sales price per unit of output = $500.

F = fixed operating costs = $1 million.

Q = units of output (sales) = 5,000.

V = variable costs per unit, found as follows:

$$\text{Profit} = P(Q) - F - V(Q)$$

$$\$250,000 = \$500(5,000) - \$1,000,000 - V(5,000)$$

$$5,000V = \$1,250,000$$

$$V = \$250.$$

2. Determine the new profit level if the change is made:

$$\text{New profit} = P_2(Q_2) - F_2 - V_2(Q_2)$$

$$= \$475(7,000) - \$1,250,000 - \$200(7,000)$$

$$= \$675,000.$$

3. Determine the incremental profit:

$$\Delta\text{Profit} = \$675,000 - \$250,000 = \$425,000.$$

4. Estimate the approximate rate of return on the new investment:

$$\text{ROI} = \frac{\Delta\text{Profit}}{\text{Investment}} = \frac{\$425,000}{\$2,000,000} = 21.25\%.$$

Since the ROI exceeds Visical's average cost of capital, this analysis suggests that Visical should go ahead and make the investment.

b.

$$\text{DOL} = \frac{Q(P - V)}{Q(P - V) - F}$$

$$\text{DOL}_{\text{Old}} = \frac{5,000(\$500 - \$250)}{5,000(\$500 - \$250) - \$1,000,000} = 5.00.$$

$$\text{DOL}_{\text{New}} = \frac{7,000(\$475 - \$200)}{7,000(\$475 - \$200) - \$1,250,000} = 2.85.$$

This indicates that operating income will be less sensitive to changes in sales if the production process is changed, thus suggesting that the change would reduce risks. However, the change also would increase the breakeven point. Still, with a lower sales price, it might be easier to achieve the higher new breakeven volume:

$$\textit{Old:}\ Q_{BE} = \frac{F}{P - V} = \frac{\$1,000,000}{\$500 - \$250} = 4,000 \text{ units.}$$

$$\textit{New:}\ Q_{BE} = \frac{F_2}{P_2 - V_2} = \frac{\$1,250,000}{\$475 - \$200} = 4,545 \text{ units.}$$

c. The incremental ROE is:

$$\text{ROE} = \frac{\Delta\text{Profit}}{\Delta\text{Equity}}.$$

Using debt financing, the incremental profit associated with the equity investment is equal to that found in Part a minus the interest expense incurred as a result of the investment:

$$\Delta\text{Profit} = \text{New profit} - \text{Old profit} - \text{Interest}$$

$$= \$675,000 - \$250,000 - 0.07(\$2,000,000)$$

$$= \$285,000.$$

$$\text{ROE} = \frac{\$285,000}{\$2,000,000}$$

$$= 14.25\%.$$

The return on the new equity investment still exceeds the average cost of capital, so Visical should make the investment.

ST-2 **a.**

EBIT	$2,860,000
Interest ($4,000,000 × 0.09)	360,000
Net income before taxes	2,500,000
Taxes (40%)	1,000,000
Net income after taxes	$1,500,000

$$\text{EPS} = \$1,500,000/500,000 = \$3.00.$$

$$P_0 = \$3.00/0.12 = \$25.00.$$

b.

$$\text{Equity} = 500,000 \times \$25 = \$12,500,000$$

$$\text{Debt} = \$4,000,000$$

$$\text{Total capital} = \$16,500,000.$$

$$k_a = w_d k_d (1 - T) + w_s k_s$$

$$= (0.24)(9\%)(1 - 0.4) + (0.76)(12\%)$$

$$= 1.3\% + 9.12\%$$

$$= 10.42\%.$$

c.

EBIT	$2,860,000
Interest ($8,000,000 × 0.12)	960,000
Net income before taxes	$1,900,000
Taxes (40%)	760,000
Net income after taxes	$1,140,000

Shares bought and retired:

$$\Delta N = \Delta Debt/P_0 = \$4,000,000/\$25 = 160,000.$$

New outstanding shares:

$$N_1 = N_0 - \Delta N = 500,000 - 160,000 = 340,000.$$

New EPS:

$$\text{EPS} = \$1,140,000/340,000 = \$3.35.$$

New price per share:

$$P_0 = \$3.35/0.15 = \$22.33 \text{ versus } \$25.00.$$

Therefore, Brosky should not change its capital structure.

d.

$$\text{TIE} = \frac{\text{EBIT}}{\text{I}}.$$

$$\text{Original TIE} = \frac{\$2,860,000}{\$360,000} = 7.94.$$

$$\text{New TIE} = \frac{\$2,860,000}{\$960,000} = 2.98.$$

Appendix 20A[1]

Bankruptcy

In the event of bankruptcy, debtholders have a prior claim to a firm's income and assets over common and preferred stockholders. Because different classes of debtholders are accorded different treatments in bankruptcy settlements, it is important for one to know who gets what if the firm fails. These topics are discussed in this appendix.[2]

Federal Bankruptcy Laws

Bankruptcy actually begins when a debtor is unable to meet scheduled payments to creditors or when the firm's cash flow projections indicate that it will soon be unable to do so. As the bankruptcy proceedings go forward, the following central issues arise:

1. Is the inability to meet scheduled debt payments a temporary problem of technical insolvency or is it a permanent problem caused by asset values falling below debt obligations?

2. If the problem is a temporary one, an extension that gives the firm time to recover and to satisfy creditors will be worked out. If basic long-run asset values have truly declined, economic losses have occurred. In this event, who shall bear the losses? Two approaches exist: (1) the absolute priority doctrine, which states that claims must be paid in strict accordance with the priority of each claim, regardless of the consequence to other claimants, and (2) the relative priority doctrine, which is more flexible and which gives a more balanced consideration to all claimants.

3. Is the company "worth more dead than alive"? In other words, would the business be more valuable if it were maintained and continued in operation or if it were liquidated and sold off in pieces? Under the absolute priority doctrine, liquidations are more likely because this generally permits senior creditors to be paid off sooner, but often at the expense of junior creditors and stockholders. Under the relative priority doctrine, senior creditors are more likely to be required to wait for payment in order to increase the chances of providing some value to junior creditors and stockholders.

4. Who should control the firm while it is being liquidated or rehabilitated? The existing management may be left in control, or a *trustee* may be placed in charge of operations.

These are the issues that are addressed in the federal bankruptcy statutes.

The U.S. bankruptcy laws were first enacted in 1898, were modified substantially in 1938, were changed again in 1978, and were further fine-tuned in 1984. The 1978 act was a major revision designed to streamline and expedite proceedings, and it also represented a shift from the absolute priority doctrine toward the relative priority doctrine. (These doctrines should be thought of as a continuum, not as absolute points. The new laws represent a movement along the continuum, not a jump from one polar position to the other.)

---

[1]This appendix was coauthored by Arthur L. Hermann of the University of Hartford.
[2]Much of the current work in the area of bankruptcy is based on the writings of Edward I. Altman. For a summary of his work and that of others, see Edward I. Altman, "Bankruptcy and Reorganization," in *Financial Handbook,* ed. Edward I. Altman (New York: Wiley, 1981), Chapter 35.

The bankruptcy law consists of eight odd-numbered chapters. (The even numbers were eliminated by Congress in the rewrite.) Chapters 1, 3, and 5 contain general provisions applicable to the other chapters. Chapter 7 governs liquidations; Chapter 9 provides for financially distressed municipalities; Chapter 11 is the business reorganization chapter; Chapter 13 covers the adjustment of debts for "individuals with regular income"; and Chapter 15 sets up a system of trustees who help administer the act.

When you read in the paper that Texaco or some other company has "filed for Chapter 11," this means that the company is bankrupt and is trying to reorganize under Chapter 11 of the bankruptcy act. The 1978 act is quite flexible and contains provisions for informal negotiations between a company and its creditors and stockholders. Under this act, a case is started by filing a petition with the bankruptcy court. The petition may be either voluntary or involuntary; that is, it may be filed either by the firm's management or by its creditors. A committee of unsecured creditors is then appointed by the court to negotiate with management for a reorganization, which may include the restructuring of debt and other claims against the firm. A trustee may be appointed by the court if it is in the best interests of the creditors and stockholders; otherwise the existing management may stay in office. Under Chapter 11, if no fair and feasible reorganization can be worked out, the firm will be liquidated under the procedures spelled out in Chapter 7 of the act.

Financial Decisions in Reorganization

When a business becomes insolvent, a decision must be made whether to dissolve the firm through *liquidation* or to keep it alive through *reorganization*. Fundamentally, this decision depends on a determination of the value of the firm if it were rehabilitated as compared with the value of the assets if they were sold off individually. The procedure that promises higher returns to the creditors and owners will be adopted. Often the greater indicated value of the firm in reorganization versus its value in liquidation is used to force a compromise agreement among the claimants in a reorganization, even when each group believes that its relative position has not been treated fairly in the reorganization plan. Both the SEC and the courts are called upon to determine the *fairness* and the *feasibility* of proposed plans of reorganization.

Standard of Fairness. The basic doctrine of fairness states that claims must be recognized in the order of their legal and contractual priority. Carrying out this concept of fairness in a reorganization involves the following steps:

1. Future sales must be estimated.

2. Operating conditions must be analyzed so that the future earnings on sales can be predicted.

3. The capitalization rate to be applied to these future earnings must be determined.

4. This capitalization rate must be applied to the estimated future earnings to obtain an indicated value for the company.

5. Provision for distribution to the claimants must then be made.

Standard of Feasibility. The primary test of *feasibility* in a reorganization is whether the fixed charges after reorganization will be adequately covered by earnings. Adequate coverage generally requires an improvement in earnings or a reduction of fixed charges, or both. Among the actions that typically must be taken are the following:

1. Debt maturities usually must be lengthened, and some debt must be converted into equity.

2. When the quality of management has been substandard and inadequate for the task, a new team must be given control of the company.

3. If inventories have become obsolete or depleted, they must be replaced.

4. Sometimes the plant and the equipment must be modernized before the firm can operate and compete successfully on a cost basis.

Liquidation Procedures

If a company is too far gone to be reorganized, it must be liquidated. Liquidation should occur when the business is worth more dead than alive, or when the possibilities of restoring profitability are so remote that the creditors run a high risk of loss if operations are continued.

Chapter 7 of the Bankruptcy Reform Act of 1978 is designed to do three things: (1) provide safeguards against fraud by the debtor; (2) provide for an equitable distribution of the debtor's assets among the creditors; and (3) allow insolvent debtors to discharge all their obligations and to start new businesses unhampered by a burden of prior debt. Liquidation is time-consuming, it can be costly, and it results in the loss of the business.

The distribution of assets in a liquidation under Chapter 7 of the bankruptcy act is governed by the following priority of claims:

1. *Secured creditors, from the proceeds of the sale of specific property pledged for a lien or a mortgage.* If the proceeds from the sale of property do not fully satisfy the secured creditors' claims, the remaining balance is treated as a general creditor claim. See Item 8.

2. *Trustee's costs to administer and operate the bankrupt estate.*

3. *Expenses incurred after an involuntary case has begun but before a trustee is appointed.*

4. *Wages due workers if earned within three months prior to the filing of the petition in bankruptcy.* The amount of wages is not to exceed $2,000 per person.

5. *Claims for unpaid contributions to employee benefit plans.* These claims, plus wages in Item 4, are not to exceed the limit of $2,000 per wage earner.

6. *Unsecured claims for customer deposits, not to exceed a maximum of $900 per individual.*

7. *Taxes due the United States, state, county, and any other government agency.*

8. *Unfunded pension plan liabilities.* Pension plans have a claim above that of general creditors for an amount up to 30 percent of the common and preferred equity; any remaining unfunded pension claims rank with general creditors.

9. *General or unsecured creditors.* Trade credit, unsecured loans, the unsatisfied portion of secured loans, and debenture bonds are classed as general creditors. Holders of subordinated debt also fall into this category, but they must turn over required amounts to the holders of senior debt.

10. *Preferred stock.* The amount is not to exceed the stock's par value.

11. *Common stock.* Stockholders receive any remaining funds.

Table 20A-1 **Panhandle Drilling, Inc.: Balance Sheet**

Current assets	$80,000,000	Accounts payable	$20,000,000
Net property	10,000,000	Notes payable (due bank)	10,000,000
		Accrued wages, 1,400 at $500	700,000
		U.S. taxes	1,000,000
		State and local taxes	300,000
		Current debt	$32,000,000
		First mortgage	6,000,000
		Second mortgage	1,000,000
		Subordinated debentures[a]	8,000,000
		Long-term debt	$15,000,000
		Preferred stock	2,000,000
		Common stock	26,000,000
		Paid-in capital	4,000,000
		Retained earnings	11,000,000
		Total equity	$43,000,000
Total assets	$90,000,000	Total claims	$90,000,000

[a]Subordinated to $10 million notes payable to the First National Bank.

To illustrate how this priority of claims works out, consider the balance sheet of Panhandle Drilling, Inc., shown in Table 20A-1. Assets total $90 million. The claims are indicated on the right-hand side of the balance sheet. Note that the debentures are subordinated to the notes payable to banks.

Now assume that the assets are sold. The assets as reported in the balance sheet in Table 20A-1 are greatly overstated — they are, in fact, worth less than half of the $90 million at which they are carried. The following amounts are realized on liquidation:

Current assets	$28,000,000
Net property	5,000,000
Total receipts	$33,000,000

The order of priority for payment of claims is shown in Table 20A-2. The first mortgage is paid from the net proceeds of $5 million from the sale of fixed property, leaving $28 million available to other creditors. Next come the fees and expenses of administration, which are typically about 20 percent of gross proceeds; in this example they are assumed to be $6 million. Next in priority are wages due workers, which total $700,000. The total amount of taxes to be paid is $1.3 million. Thus far, the total of claims paid from the $33 million is $13 million, leaving $20 million for the general creditors.

The claims of the general creditors total $40 million. Since $20 million is available, claimants would each receive 50 percent of their claims before the subordination adjustment. This adjustment requires that the subordinated debentures turn over to the notes payable all amounts received until the notes are satisfied. In this situation the claim of the notes payable is $10 million, but only $5 million is available; the deficiency is therefore $5 million. After transfer by the subordinated debentures of $4 million, there remains a deficiency of $1 million, which will be unsatisfied.

Note that 90 percent of the bank claim is satisfied, whereas only 50 percent of other unsecured claims will be satisfied. These figures illustrate the usefulness of the

Table 20A-2 **Panhandle Drilling, Inc.: Order of Priority of Claims**

Distribution of Proceeds on Liquidation

1. Proceeds of sale of assets	$33,000,000
2. First mortgage, paid from sale of net property	5,000,000
3. Fees and expenses of administration of bankruptcy	6,000,000
4. Wages due workers earned 3 months prior to filing of bankruptcy petition	700,000
5. Taxes	1,300,000
6. Available to general creditors	$20,000,000

Claims of General Creditors	**Claim (1)**	**Application of 50 Percent (2)**	**After Subordination Adjustment (3)**	**Percentage of Original Claims Received (4)**
Unsatisfied portion of first mortgage	$ 1,000,000	$ 500,000	$ 500,000	92
Unsatisfied portion of second mortgage	1,000,000	500,000	500,000	50
Notes payable	10,000,000	5,000,000	9,000,000	90
Accounts payable	20,000,000	10,000,000	10,000,000	50
Subordinated debentures	8,000,000	4,000,000	0	0
	$40,000,000	$20,000,000	$20,000,000	56

Notes:
1. Column 1 is the claim of each class of creditor. Total claims equal $40 million.
2. From Line 6 in the upper section of the table we see that $20 million is available. This sum, divided by the $40 million of claims, indicates that general creditors will receive 50 percent of their claims. This is shown in Column 2.
3. The debentures are subordinated to the notes payable. Four million dollars is transferred from debentures to notes payable in Column 3.
4. Column 4 shows the results of dividing the Column 3 figure by the original amount given in Table 20A-1, except for the first mortgage, where $5 million paid on sale of property is included. The 56 percent total figure includes the first-mortgage transactions; that is, ($20,000,000 + $5,000,000) ÷ ($40,000,000 + $5,000,000) = 56%.

subordination provision to the security to which the subordination is made. Because no other funds remain, the claims of the holders of preferred and common stocks are completely wiped out. Studies of the proceeds in bankruptcy liquidations reveal that unsecured creditors receive, on the average, about 15 cents on the dollar, whereas common stockholders generally receive nothing.

PROBLEMS

20A-1   **Liquidation effects.** At the time it defaulted, Johnson Technologies had net current assets valued on the books at $40 million and net fixed assets valued at $50 million. At the time of final settlement its debts were as follows:

Current liabilities	$24 million
First-mortgage bonds	20 million
Second-mortgage bonds	10 million
Debenture bonds	8 million

None of the current liabilities have preferences in liquidation as provided for in the bankruptcy laws, and none have been secured by pledge of assets.

Assume that the amount shown for each of the four classes of liabilities includes all unpaid interest to the date of settlement. The fixed assets were pledged as security for the first-mortgage bonds and repledged for the second-mortgage bonds. Determine the appropriate distribution of the proceeds of liquidation under the following conditions:

a. Liquidation of current assets realizes $36 million, and $14 million is obtained from fixed assets.

b. Liquidation of current assets realizes $18 million, and $8 million is obtained from fixed assets.

20A-2   Liquidation effects. Agriculture Impliments (AI) is bankrupt and the firm's assets are to be sold to satisfy the claims of the firm's creditors. The firm's balance sheet follows.

Current assets	$4,200	Accounts payable	$ 900
Fixed assets	2,250	Notes payable (to bank)	450
		Accrued taxes	150
		Accrued wages	150
		Total current liabilities	$1,650
		First mortgage bonds	$ 750
		Second mortgage bonds	750
		Total mortgage bonds	$1,500
		Subordinated debentures	900
		Total debt	$4,050
		Preferred stock	300
		Common stock	2,100
Total assets	$6,450	Total claims and equity	$6,450

The debentures are subordinated only to the notes payable. Suppose that $1,100 is received from the sale of the fixed assets, which were pledged as security for the first and second mortgage bonds, and $2,000 is obtained from the sale of current assets.

a. How much will each class of investors receive?

(Do Part b only if you are using the computerized problem diskette.)

b. How much would each class of investors receive if:

1. $800 were received from the sale of fixed assets and $1,300 from the sale of current assets?

2. $1,400 were received from the sale of fixed assets and $2,700 from the sale of current assets?

Chapter 21

Determining the Dividend Policy

 DECISION IN FINANCE

The Last Conglomerate

In this era of businesses getting back to basics, Tenneco Inc. would seem to be a dinosaur. The corporate giant, which began as a gas pipeline company in the 1940s, has grown into one of the nation's largest and most varied enterprises. In addition to pipelines, the company also produces oil, gas, chemicals, packaging, auto parts, farm machinery, submarines, construction equipment, and aircraft carriers. "Diversity is right for us," insists James L. Ketelsen, Tenneco's CEO. "We are *not* portfolio managers. We are building businesses."

The problem is, not everyone is thrilled with the way that Ketelsen is going about building those businesses. In theory, the advantage of a conglomerate is that the businesses that are doing well can support those that are experiencing a slump. The reality, especially in Tenneco's case, is slightly more complicated, largely because both of Tenneco's biggest businesses — energy (oil and gas) and tractors — have been in a simultaneous downturn. The company lost $39 million in 1986. Cash flow, which was $2.2 billion in 1984, dropped to approximately $1.4 billion in 1986. To his critics' dismay, instead of selling off less-profitable divi-

sions, Ketelsen has insisted on expanding Tenneco's tractor business in the face of huge losses, piling up costly debt.

Worse, he has doggedly maintained Tenneco's generous dividend on its common stock. The annual rate is $3.04 a share for a current yield of more than 6½ percent — higher than the return on most oil-company stocks and an obvious attraction for many of the 185,000 shareholders. Unfortunately, Tenneco hasn't actually earned the dividend since 1984.

Ketelsen is hardly oblivious to the financial pressure his company is under. After all, he chopped capital spending in 1986 by about 37 percent, to $1 billion. Still, his critics contend that his insistence on maintaining the dividend at nearly one-third of cash flow is proving to be a major drain on assets. Critics suggest that the money would be better spent paying down debt, which is at a hefty 55 percent of total capitalization. Currently, about 20 percent of that debt is subject to floating rates, leaving the company vulnerable if interest rates go up.

As you read this chapter, try to think of reasons Ketelsen may think that it is important to maintain Tenneco's dividend policy. How would you feel about it if you were a Tenneco shareholder?

See end of chapter for resolution.

Dividend policy involves the decision to pay out earnings or to retain them for reinvestment in the firm. The basic stock price model, $P_0 = D_1/(k_s - g)$, shows that a policy of paying out more cash dividends will raise D_1, which will tend to increase the price of the stock. However, raising cash dividends means that less money is available for reinvestment, and plowing back less earnings into the business will lower the expected growth rate and depress the price of the stock. Thus dividend policy has two opposing effects, and the **optimal dividend policy** is the one that strikes a balance between current dividends and future growth and thereby maximizes the price of the firm's stock.

optimal dividend policy

The dividend policy that strikes a balance between current dividends and future growth and thereby maximizes the firm's stock price.

A number of factors influence dividend policy, among them the investment opportunities available to the firm, alternative sources of capital, and stockholders' preferences for current versus future income. The primary goal of this chapter is to show how these and other factors interact to determine the optimal dividend policy.

THE RESIDUAL THEORY OF DIVIDENDS

In the preceding chapters on capital budgeting and the cost of capital, we indicated that the marginal cost of capital and investment opportunity schedules generally must be combined before the cost of capital can be established. In other words, the optimal capital budget, the marginal cost of capital, and the marginal rate of return on investment are determined *simultaneously*. In this section we use this framework to develop what is called the **residual theory of dividends**, which states that a firm should follow these four steps: (1) determine the optimal capital budget, (2) determine the amount of equity needed to finance that budget, (3) use retained earnings to supply this equity to the greatest extent possible, and (4) pay dividends only if more earnings are available than are needed to support the capital budget. The word *residual* implies "left over," and the residual theory states that dividends should be paid only out of leftover earnings.

residual theory of dividends

The theory that dividends paid should equal the excess of earnings over retained earnings necessary to finance the optimal capital budget.

The basis of the theory is that *investors prefer to have the firm retain and reinvest earnings rather than pay them out in dividends if the return on reinvested earnings exceeds the rate of return the investors could obtain on other investments of comparable risk.* For example, if the corporation can reinvest retained earnings at a 15 percent rate of return, whereas the best rate stockholders can obtain if the earnings are passed on in the form of dividends is 12 percent, then stockholders will prefer to have the firm retain the profits.

We saw in Chapter 19 that the cost of retained earnings is an *opportunity cost* that reflects rates of return available to equity investors. If a firm's stockholders can buy other stocks of equal risk and obtain a 14 percent dividend-plus-capital-gains yield, then 14 percent is the firm's cost of retained earnings. The cost of new outside equity raised by selling common stock is higher because of the costs of floating the issue.

Because most firms have a target capital structure that calls for at least some debt, new financing is done partly with debt and partly with equity. As

Figure 21-1 **Marginal Cost of Capital**

The marginal cost of capital is the weighted average of the costs of equity (k_s) and debt (k_d), as shown on the left. The MCC will be 12 percent as long as the firm finances its equity needs through retained earnings. The right side of this figure shows that retained earnings of $60 million, with a 40 percent debt ratio, will allow the firm to raise $100 million at an MCC of 12 percent. Beyond $100 million, new stock must be issued, which means an increase in the cost of equity and a resultant rise in the MCC.

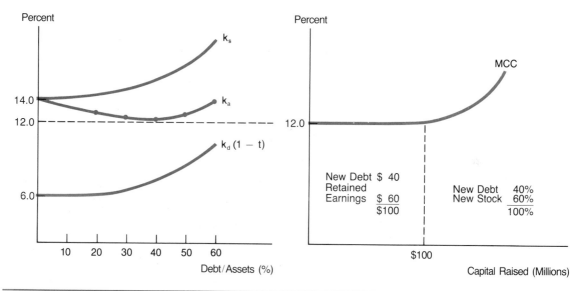

long as the firm finances with the optimal mix of debt and equity, and as long as it uses only internally generated equity (retained earnings), its marginal cost of each new dollar of capital will be minimized. Internally generated equity is available for financing a certain amount of new investment; beyond this amount the firm must turn to more expensive new common stock. At the point where new stock must be sold, the cost of equity and consequently the marginal cost of capital rises.

These concepts, which were developed in Chapter 19, are illustrated in Figure 21-1 with data from Georgia Paper Products (GPP). The firm has a marginal cost of capital of 12 percent as long as retained earnings are available, but the MCC begins to rise at the point where new stock must be sold. GPP has $60 million of net income and a 40 percent optimal debt ratio. Provided it does not pay cash dividends, GPP can make net investments (investments in addition to asset replacements financed from depreciation) of $100 million, consisting of $60 million from retained earnings plus $40 million of new debt supported by the retained earnings at a 12 percent marginal cost of capital.

Figure 21-2 **Investment Opportunity (or IRR) Schedules**

Investment opportunity schedules show which new investments are available to a firm at various rates of return. In this figure IOS_G represents a good year, IOS_N a normal year, and IOS_B a bad year. When investment opportunities are good, internal rates of return are higher and GPP can invest large amounts. When opportunities are poor, as in IOS_B, the firm will necessarily curtail its investment plans.

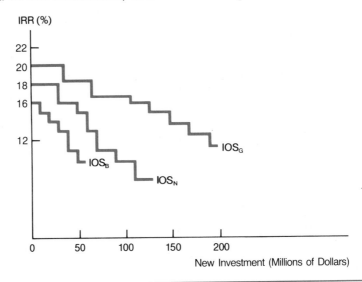

Therefore, its marginal cost of capital is constant at 12 percent up to $100 million of capital. Beyond $100 million the marginal cost of capital rises as the firm begins to use more expensive new common stock. Of course, if GPP does not retain all of its earnings, the MCC will begin to rise before $100 million. For example, if GPP retained only $30 million, the MCC would begin to rise at $30 million retained earnings + $20 million debt = $50 million.

Next, suppose GPP's director of capital budgeting constructs an investment opportunity schedule and plots it on a graph. The investment opportunity curves for three different years — one for a good year (IOS_G), one for a normal year (IOS_N), and one for a bad year (IOS_B) — are shown in Figure 21-2. IOS_G shows that GPP can invest more money, and at higher rates of return, than it can when the investment opportunities are as given by IOS_N and IOS_B.

In Figure 21-3 the investment opportunity schedules are combined with the cost of capital schedule. The point where the IOS curve intersects the MCC curve defines the proper level of new investment. When investment opportunities are relatively bad (IOS_B), the optimal level of investment is $40 million; when opportunities are normal (IOS_N), $70 million should be invested; and when opportunities are relatively good (IOS_G), GPP should make new investments in the amount of $150 million.

Figure 21-3 **Interrelations among Cost of Capital, Investment Opportunities, and New Investment**

A firm's optimal level of new investment can be determined by combining the MCC and IOS curves. In this figure, for example, the IOS_N curve is crossed by the MCC curve at an investment level of $70 million. Any investment beyond $70 million, in a normal year, would generate returns lower than the 12 percent cost of capital and thus should not be undertaken.

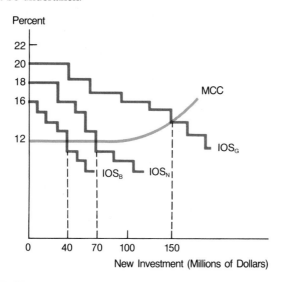

Consider the situation in which IOS_G is the appropriate schedule. GPP has $60 million in earnings and a 40 percent target debt ratio. Thus it can finance $100 million, consisting of $60 million of retained earnings plus $40 million of new debt, at a cost of 12 percent if it retains all of its earnings. If it pays out part of the earnings in dividends, it will have to begin using expensive new common stock earlier than need be, so the MCC curve will rise before it otherwise would. This suggests that under the conditions of IOS_G, GPP should retain all of its earnings. According to the residual theory, its payout ratio should be zero, and new common stock must be issued as well.

Under the conditions of IOS_N, however, GPP should invest only $70 million. How should this investment be financed? First, notice that if it retains the full amount of its earnings, $60 million, it will need to sell only $10 million of new debt. However, if GPP retains $60 million and sells only $10 million of new debt, it will move away from its target capital structure. To stay on target, GPP must finance 60 percent of the required $70 million by equity (retained earnings) and 40 percent by debt; this means retaining $42 million and selling $28 million of new debt. Since GPP retains only $42 million of its $60 million total earnings, it must distribute the residual $18 million to its stockholders.

Thus its optimal payout ratio is $18 million/$60 million = 30 percent, if IOS_N applies.

Under the conditions of IOS_B, GPP should invest only $40 million. Because it has $60 million in earnings, it could finance the entire $40 million out of retained earnings and still have $20 million available for dividends. Should this be done? Under our assumptions, this would not be a good decision, because this action would move GPP away from its optimal capital structure. To stay at the 40 percent target debt/assets ratio, GPP must retain $24 million of earnings and sell $16 million of debt. When the $24 million of retained earnings is subtracted from the $60 million total earnings, GPP is left with a residual of $36 million, the amount that should be paid out in dividends. Thus the payout ratio as prescribed by the residual theory is 60 percent.

DIVIDEND POLICY AND THE VALUE OF THE FIRM

From the previous example, it is clear that the firm's investment opportunity schedule and its optimal payout rate are interrelated. In this section, we take that concept a step further to show that the firm's dividend policy directly affects the value of the firm's stock and thus the value of the firm itself.

The basic constant growth stock price model, $P_0 = D_1/(k_s - g)$, first appeared in the financial literature in a slightly different form:

$$P_0 = E_1(1 - b)/(k_s - br).$$

P_0 and k_s retain the same definitions today as in the original model, whereas

E_1 = earnings expected at the end of Year 1.

b = the proportion of net income to be retained.

r = the rate of return on equity, ROE.

$(1 - b)$ = the dividend payout ratio; therefore, $E_1(1 - b) = D_1$.

br = the sustainable growth rate, g.

The logic behind the internally generated or sustainable growth is as follows. The funds available to finance growth come from the annual increase in retained earnings. These retained earnings are, of course, the proportion of net income that is not paid as dividends each period. These equity funds are to be invested, but at what rate? They will be invested to yield the firm's rate of return on equity. The firm will grow at a rate equal to the ROE times the retention rate; thus the rate of growth in both earnings and dividends, g, is equal to br.

Table 21-1 demonstrates the effect of dividend policy on stock prices under three situations: (1) the firm's return on equity, r, is greater than investors' required rate of return, k_s; (2) the firm's return on equity is less than the firm's required rate of return; and (3) the firm's return on equity equals the required

Table 21-1 **Dividend Policy and the Value of Common Stock**

$$P = \frac{E_1(1 - b)}{k_s - br}$$

$r > k_s$	$r < k_s$	$r = k_s$
$r = 15\%$	$r = 10\%$	$r = 12\%$
$k_s = 12\%$	$k_s = 12\%$	$k_s = 12\%$
$E_1 = \$8.00$	$E_1 = \$8.00$	$E_1 = \$8.00$

High Retention Dividend Policy

$b = 75\%$	$b = 75\%$	$b = 75\%$
$(1 - b) = 25\%$	$(1 - b) = 25\%$	$(1 - b) = 25\%$
$P = \dfrac{\$8(25\%)}{12\% - (75\%)(15\%)}$	$P = \dfrac{\$8(25\%)}{12\% - (75\%)(10\%)}$	$P = \dfrac{\$8(25\%)}{12\% - (75\%)(12\%)}$
$= \$2/(12\% - 11.25\%)$	$= \$2/(12\% - 7.5\%)$	$= \$2/(12\% - 9\%)$
$= \$266.67.$	$= \$44.44.$	$= \$66.67.$

High Dividend Payout Policy

$b = 25\%$	$b = 25\%$	$b = 25\%$
$(1 - b) = 75\%$	$(1 - b) = 75\%$	$(1 - b) = 75\%$
$P = \dfrac{\$8(75\%)}{12\% - (25\%)(15\%)}$	$P = \dfrac{\$8(75\%)}{12\% - (25\%)(10\%)}$	$P = \dfrac{\$8(75\%)}{12\% - (25\%)(12\%)}$
$= \$6/(12\% - 3.75\%)$	$= \$6/(12\% - 2.5\%)$	$= \$6/(12\% - 3\%)$
$= \$72.73.$	$= \$63.16.$	$= \$66.67.$

return on equity. Assuming that the firm is financed entirely with equity, what is the implication for the firm's dividend policy under each situation?

As shown on the left-hand side of Table 21-1, as long as $r > k_s$, the firm has projects available with positive NPVs. If the firm pays large dividends, it will be unable to take advantage of these investment opportunities. However, if the firm retains a large proportion of available earnings for the period, it will be able to invest these retained earnings in the profitable projects, which will increase the firm's future cash flow. Shareholders, recognizing that the firm has projects available that have positive NPVs, reward the firm for the correct dividend policy (high earnings retention) by purchasing the stock, thereby increasing its price. Similarly, a lower value of the firm's stock reflects the shareholders' realization that an incorrect dividend policy decision has been made. The relatively high payout means that the firm is forgoing investment in positive NPV projects and is therefore reducing the firm's future cash flow opportunities which reduces the value of its stock.

The opposite situation is portrayed in the center section of Table 21-1. Here the firm's required return is greater than its return on equity; $k_s > r$. In this situation only projects with negative NPVs are available for investment. If the firm retained earnings to invest in projects with negative NPVs, the value of the firm would be reduced. However, if management paid out a large percentage of the firm's earnings, investors could use the resulting cash flow to invest in other firms that did provide a return of k_s or higher. Therefore, the correct dividend policy would be a large payout, up to 100 percent.[1]

When the firm's required return and its return on equity are equal, the firm's dividend policy will not affect the value of the firm, as shown in the right-hand column of Table 21-1. As long as the firm earns exactly the required rate of return, the investor is no better off having dividends invested in other firms to yield k_s than having the funds invested in this firm, where they yield exactly the same k_s.

FACTORS THAT INFLUENCE DIVIDEND POLICY

The residual theory of dividends is only a starting point in establishing a dividend policy. Other factors that influence dividend policy may be grouped into four broad categories: (1) constraints on dividend payments, (2) investment opportunities, (3) availability and costs of alternative sources of capital, and (4) effects of dividend policy on the required rate of return, k_s. These categories and factors related to them are discussed in the following sections.

Constraints on Dividend Payments

constraints on dividend payments
Restrictions or limitations on the payment of dividends.

1. Bond indentures. Debt contracts generally restrict dividend payment to earnings generated after the loan was granted. Also, debt contracts often stipulate that no dividends can be paid unless the current ratio, the times-interest-earned ratio, and other safety ratios exceed stated minimums.

2. Impairment of capital rule. Dividend payments cannot exceed the balance sheet item "retained earnings." This legal restriction, known as *the impairment of capital rule,* is designed to protect creditors.

3. Availability of cash. Cash dividends can be paid only with cash. Thus a shortage of cash in the bank can restrict dividend payments. Unused borrowing capacity can offset this factor, however.

4. Penalty tax on improperly accumulated earnings. To prevent wealthy individuals from using corporations to avoid personal taxes, the tax code provides for a special surtax on improperly accumulated income. Thus,

---

[1]Unfortunately, the optimal payout ratio cannot be determined by this model. It indicates only that when $r > k_s$, more earnings should be retained; the model indicates that optimal retention in this situation is 100 percent. Similarly, the model implies that a larger proportion of net income should be paid as dividends when $k_s > r$; the optimal dividend policy, according to the model, would be 100 percent payout. Thus the model does not provide the optimal payout percentage, but it does indicate the direction dividend policy should take.

if the IRS can demonstrate that the dividend payout ratio is being deliberately held down to help stockholders avoid personal taxes, the firm may be subject to heavy penalties. To date, this factor has been applied only to closely held firms.

Investment Opportunities

1. Location of the IOS schedule. If the relevant IOS schedule in Figure 21-3 is far to the right, this will tend to produce a low payout, and, vice versa, if the IOS is far to the left, a large dividend payout is likely to result. The steeper the slope of the IOS, the more costly it is not to use the payout prescribed by the residual theory.

2. Possibility of accelerating or delaying projects. If the firm can accelerate or postpone projects, this will permit more flexibility in its dividend policy.

Alternative Sources of Capital

1. Cost of selling new stock. If a firm wishes to finance a given level of investment, it can obtain equity by retaining earnings or by selling new common stock. If flotation costs are high, k_e will be well above k_s, making it much better to finance through retention versus sale of new common stock (see Chapter 19). On the other hand, if flotation costs are low, dividend policy will be less important. Flotation costs differ among firms (for example, they are higher for small firms). Hence the importance of dividend policy and the optimal policy varies among firms.

2. Control. If management is concerned about maintaining control, it may be reluctant to sell new stock, and hence may retain more earnings than it otherwise would. This factor is especially important for small, closely held firms.

3. Capital structure flexibility. A firm can finance a given level of investment with either debt or equity. If the firm is willing to adjust its debt ratio, it can maintain a constant dollar dividend by using a variable debt ratio. The shape of the average cost of capital curve (left panel in Figure 21-1) determines the practical extent to which the debt ratio can be varied. If the average cost of capital curve is relatively flat over a wide range, dividend policy is less critical than it is if the curve has a distinct minimum.

Effects of Dividend Policy on k_s

1. Stockholders' desire for current versus future income. Some stockholders desire current income; retired individuals and university endowment funds are examples. Other stockholders have no need for current investment income and simply reinvest any dividends received, after first paying income taxes on the dividend income. If the firm retains and reinvests income rather than paying dividends, those stockholders who need

INDUSTRY PRACTICE

Dividend Plow Back Plans

Some companies pay out regular dividends. Others put all of their earnings back into the business. But about 1,000 U.S. corporations leave part of that decision to their shareholders. These are the companies that sponsor dividend-reinvestment plans, which allow shareholders to automatically plow back payouts into the purchase of more shares, sometimes at 3 to 5 percent below market price and usually without brokerage fees. Companies with reinvestment plans generally give shareholders the option to be credited with additional whole and fractional shares of stock instead of being sent dividend checks.

Reinvesting dividends is a form of dollar-cost averaging, an effective strategy of putting roughly equal amounts of money into a stock at regular intervals so that more shares are purchased when the price is low and fewer when the price is high. The acronym for dividend reinvestment plans — DRIPs — pretty well describes the Chinese water torture one would expect from a few shares of a $50 stock paying, for example, a $2 annual dividend. For an investor holding 100 shares of a company that boosts its dividend 10 percent every year, however, 100 shares could be effortlessly parlayed into 268 over ten years.

Aside from convenience, one of the most immediate benefits of dividend reinvestment plans is that shareholders are able to acquire extra stock without having to pay a brokerage commission, which often can make small purchases of stock uneconomical. "It's an easy way to save regularly," explains Marie Block, 68, of West Hartford, Connecticut, who reinvests all the dividends from her holdings of about 1,600 American Telephone and Telegraph shares. "It's like a payroll-savings plan."

DRIPs are not without their benefits to corporations as well. Reinvestment plans are an ideal way to encourage long-term investments and to boost shareholder commitment. Companies also find that stock plow-back plans can be an efficient way to raise capital by keeping the cash and issuing new shares. Ohio Edison Company has raised more than $460 million this way since it began its reinvestment plan more than a decade ago.

To spur reinvestment, a number of firms offer shareholders newly issued shares at cut-rate prices. "That's a way to make a small but quick gain with little risk," notes Louis Morrell, a vice president at Chemical Bank in New York. Chemical lets shareholders use dividends to buy shares at 5 percent below market price. Among others, Carter Hawley Hale Stores, Sperry Corporation, Timken Company, and Hospital Corporation of America also offer 5 percent discounts. Bankers Trust Company in New York offers 3 percent. The number of firms offering discounts has fallen off in recent years, partly because of the declining need for additional capital.

Reinvestment plans do have their drawbacks. One is the small number of extra shares that typically can be acquired with dividends alone. However, many firms allow investors to fatten their dividend reinvestment with additional cash. McDonald's Corporation allows a cash addition of $3,000 a quarter; Hospital Corporation of America allows up to $12,500 a quarter. A number of firms used to give discounts on these extra purchases. Even though discounting has become rare, shareholders still save on brokerage fees.

Dividend-reinvestment plans do not appeal to all shareholders. Investors who need dividend income to cover current expenses

Source: Leonard Wiener, "Making Money by Plowing Back Your Dividends," *U.S. News & World Report,* May 19, 1986, 72; and J. Howard Green, "Stocks That Reinvest Your Dividends," *Money,* September 1987, 147.

shouldn't participate, and the plans aren't suited for people who want to time purchases precisely. In addition, unless shareholders make specific arrangements to take receipt of the actual stock certificates, the plans make impromptu sales of shares difficult.

Investors also need to be aware of the tax consequences of stock-reinvestment plans. Cautions Bruce Barr, director of AT&T investor relations, "There are a number of substantial benefits to these plans, but taxes aren't one of them." Even though shareholders reinvest their dividends, they must pay taxes on them as if they had taken the cash. In addition, if shares are purchased at a discount, the amount of the discount is considered taxable income. Until 1985, investors in public utilities were allowed to defer tax on up to $1,500 a year in reinvested dividends, but that tax break has now expired.

Nevertheless, stockholders continue to flock to the reinvestment plans. About a third of AT&T's 3 million investors buy extra stock with their quarterly dividends of 30 cents a share. At Hospital Corporation of America, almost half of the 30,000 shareholders reinvest their 16½ cents-per-share quarterly payouts. All told, more than 600 companies listed on the New York and American stock exchanges, plus hundreds of firms traded over the counter, have reinvestment plans.

Although they have their drawbacks, dividend-reinvestment plans are an easy way for shareholders to compound growth in a stock. For companies they can have an extra payoff, too. Says Mary Healy, an official at McDonald's: "Long-term shareholders make excellent customers."

current income will be disadvantaged. Although they will presumably receive capital gains, they will be forced to sell off some of their shares to obtain cash. This will involve brokerage costs, which are relatively high unless large sums are involved. Some institutional investors (or trustees for individuals) may be precluded from selling stock and then "spending capital." In addition, stockholders who are saving rather than spending dividends will have to incur brokerage costs to reinvest their dividends. (However, as noted in a later section, many firms today have automatic dividend reinvestment plans that minimize the expense of reinvestment.)

Investors can, of course, switch companies if they own stock in a firm whose dividend policy differs from the policy they desire; this is an example of the **clientele effect.** However, there are costs associated with such changes (brokerage and capital gains taxes), and there may be a shortage of investors to replace those seeking to switch, in which case the stock price may fall and remain low.

clientele effect
The tendency of a firm to attract a certain type of investor according to its dividend policy.

2. Risk of dividends versus risk of capital gains. Gordon has argued that investors regard returns coming in the form of dividends as being less risky than capital gains returns. Others disagree. If an investor receives dividends, then turns around and reinvests them in the same firm or one of similar risk, there is little difference in risk between this action and that of the company retaining and reinvesting the earnings in the first place. This question has been subjected to statistical studies but without conclusive results.

3. Information content of dividends. It has been observed that an increase in the dividend (for example, the annual dividend per share is raised from $2 to $2.50) is often accompanied by an increase in the price of the stock, whereas an unexpected dividend cut generally leads to a stock price decline. This suggests to some observers that investors like dividends more than capital gains. However, others argue differently. They state that corporations are always reluctant to cut dividends, so firms do not raise dividends unless they anticipate higher, or at least stable, earnings in the future. Thus a dividend increase is a signal to investors that the firm's management forecasts good future earnings. Conversely, a dividend reduction signals that management is forecasting poor earnings in the future. Therefore, the price changes following a change in dividend policy may not reflect investors' preference for either dividends or earnings growth but in reality may be a reflection of the important information contained in the dividend announcement. As with many other controversies about dividend policy, empirical studies on the **information content of dividends** have been inconclusive. There is clearly some information content in dividend announcements, but it may or may not completely explain the stock price changes that follow increases or decreases in dividends.

> **information content of dividends**
>
> A theory that investors regard dividend changes as signals of management forecasts.

These points are considered by financial executives when they are establishing their firms' dividend policies, but the only real generalizations we can make are these:

1. The optimal dividend policy for a firm is influenced by many factors. Some factors suggest a higher payout than would be called for by the residual theory, whereas others suggest a lower optimal payout.

2. Much research has been done on dividend policy, but many points are still unresolved. Researchers are far from being able to specify a precise model for establishing corporate dividend policy.

Although no one has been able to construct a usable model for finding an optimal dividend policy, the residual theory does at least provide a good starting point, and there is a checklist of factors to consider before finalizing the dividend policy. Later in the chapter we return to the process of establishing a dividend policy, but first we must take up three other components of dividend policy — actual payment procedures, stock splits, and stock dividends.

DIVIDEND PAYMENT POLICIES

Corporations tend to use one of three major dividend payment policies: (1) *constant, or steadily increasing, dividends,* (2) *constant payout ratio,* or (3) *low regular dividends plus extras.* These alternatives are discussed in this section.

Figure 21-4 **Shoal Creek Engineering:
Dividends and Earnings Over Time**

Many firms use a stable dividend payment policy, maintaining a specific dividend
amount and raising it only if earnings increase on an apparently permanent basis. As
shown in this figure, Shoal Creek Engineering paid a dividend of $1.00 beginning in
1955 and maintained it over the period, along with several small dividend increases.
Note that a temporary drop in earnings below the dividend level in 1970 did not
affect the amount of dividend paid.

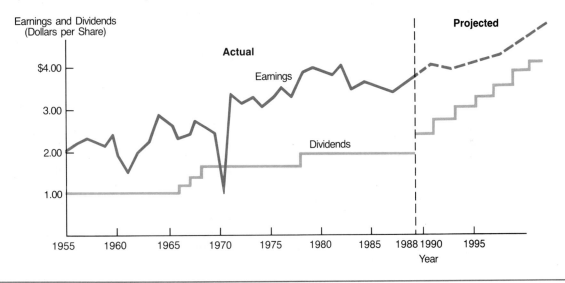

Constant, or Steadily Increasing, Dividend per Share

Some firms set a specific annual dividend per share and then maintain it, increasing the annual dividend only if it seems clear that future earnings will be
sufficient to allow the dividend to be maintained. A corollary of the policy is
this rule: *Avoid ever reducing the annual dividend.* The fact that most corporations do in fact follow, or attempt to follow, such a policy lends support to
the information content hypothesis described in the preceding section.

Figure 21-4, which illustrates a stable payment policy, presents data for
Shoal Creek Engineering from 1955 to 1988 with earnings and dividends projected to 1995. Initially, earnings were $2 and dividends were $1 a share, so
the payout ratio was 50 percent. Earnings rose for four years, while dividends
remained constant; thus the payout ratio fell during this period. During 1960
and 1961 earnings fell substantially; however, the dividend was maintained and
the payout rose above the 50 percent target. During the period between 1961
and 1965 earnings experienced a sustained rise. Dividends were held constant
while management sought to determine whether the earnings increase would
be permanent. By 1966, when it was apparent that the earnings gain would be
maintained, dividends were raised in three steps to reestablish the 50 percent

target payout. During 1970 a strike caused earnings to fall below the regular dividend. Expecting the earnings decline to be temporary, management maintained the dividend. Earnings fluctuated on a fairly high plateau from 1972 through 1977, during which time dividends remained constant. A new increase in earnings permitted management to raise the dividend in 1978 to reestablish the 50 percent payout ratio.

A variant of this policy is the "stable growth rate" policy. Here the firm sets a target growth rate for dividends (say, 6 percent per year) and strives to increase dividends by this amount each year. Obviously, earnings must be growing at a reasonably steady rate for this policy to be feasible. If Shoal Creek's earnings continue to grow as projected after 1988, the firm plans to adopt a constant growth rate dividend policy as illustrated in Figure 21-4.

There are several rationales for these policies. First, given the existence of the information content theory, a fluctuating payment policy might lead to fluctuating stock prices, which in turn could lead to a higher k_s. Second, because stockholders who use dividends for current consumption want to be able to count on receiving dividends regularly, irregular dividends might lower demand for the stock, causing a decline in its price. Third, even though the optimal payout (in the residual theory sense) might vary somewhat from year to year, delaying some investment projects, departing from the target capital structure during a particular year, or even selling common stock might all be preferable to cutting the dividend or reducing its growth rate. Finally, setting a steady dividend growth rate will confirm investors' estimates of the g factor and thus enhance the price of the stock; that is, investors will think of the stock as a growth stock.

Constant Payout Ratio

A very few firms follow a policy of paying out a constant percentage of earnings. Because earnings surely will fluctuate, following this policy necessarily means that the dollar amount of dividends will fluctuate. For reasons discussed in the preceding section, this policy is not likely to maximize a firm's stock price. However, before its bankruptcy Penn Central Railroad did follow the policy of paying out one half its earnings: "A dollar for the stockholders and a dollar for the company," as one director put it. Logic like this could drive any company to bankruptcy!

Low Regular Dividend plus Extras

extra dividend
A supplementary dividend paid in years when excess funds are available.

The low regular dividend plus a year-end extra is a compromise between the first two policies. It gives the firm flexibility, but it leaves investors somewhat uncertain about what their dividend will be. Still, if a firm's earnings and cash flows are quite volatile, using **extra dividends** may well be its best choice. The directors can set a relatively low regular dividend — low enough that it can be maintained even in low-profit years or in years when a considerable amount of reinvestment is needed — and then supplement it with an extra dividend in years when excess funds are available. General Motors, whose earnings fluctuate widely from year to year, has long followed this practice. However, after a period of time, the shareholders often expect extra dividends under this policy and consider them to be part of the firm's normal dividend, thus negating the concept of the extra dividend.

THE ACTUAL DIVIDEND PAYMENT

Dividends are normally paid quarterly. For example, IBM paid dividends of $4.40, $1.10 each quarter, during 1986. In common financial language, we say that IBM's regular quarterly dividend is $1.10 or that its regular annual dividend is $4.40. The actual dividend payment procedure is as follows:

1. Declaration date. The directors of IBM meet each quarter to declare a dividend. When they met on July 29, 1986, they issued a statement similar to the following: "On July 29, 1986, the directors of International Business Machines met and declared the regular quarterly dividend of $1.10 a share, payable to holders of record on August 13, payment to be made on September 10, 1986."

declaration date

Date on which a firm's directors issue a statement declaring a regular dividend.

2. Holder-of-record date. At the close of business on the **holder-of-record date,** August 13, the company closes its stock transfer books and makes up a list of the shareholders as of that date. If IBM is notified of the sale and transfer of some stock before 5 P.M. on August 13, the new owner receives the dividend. However, if notification is received on or after August 14, the old stockholder gets the dividend check.

holder-of-record date

The date on which registered security owners are entitled to receive the forthcoming cash or stock dividend.

3. Ex dividend date. Suppose Jean Buyer purchases 100 shares of IBM stock from John Seller on August 11. Will the company be notified of the transfer in time to list Buyer as the new owner and thus pay the dividend to her? To avoid conflict, the stock brokerage business has set up a convention of declaring that the right to the dividend remains with the stock until four business days prior to the holder-of-record date; on the fourth business day before the holder-of-record date, the right to the dividend no longer goes with the shares. The date when the right to the dividend leaves the stock is called the **ex dividend date.** In this case the ex dividend date is four business days before August 13, or August 7:

ex dividend date

The date on which the right to the current dividend no longer accompanies a stock; for a listed stock this date is four working days prior to the date of record.

	August 6
Ex dividend date:	August 7
	August 8
Weekend:	August 9 & 10
	August 11
	August 12
Holder-of-record date:	August 13

Therefore, if Buyer wishes to receive the dividend, she must buy the stock by August 6. If she buys it on August 7 or later, Seller will receive the dividend.

The dividend is $1.10 per share, so the ex dividend date is important. Barring fluctuations in the stock market, we would normally expect the price of a stock to drop by approximately the amount of the dividend on the ex dividend date. Thus, if IBM closed at $120.10 on August 6, it would probably open at about $119 on August 7.

4. Payment date. The company actually mailed the checks to the holders of record on September 10, 1986, the **payment date.**

payment date
Date on which a firm actually mails dividend checks.

DIVIDEND REINVESTMENT PLANS

dividend reinvestment plan (DRP)
A plan that enables a stockholder to automatically reinvest dividends received back into the stock of the paying corporation.

During the 1970s most of the larger companies instituted **dividend reinvestment plans (DRPs),** whereby stockholders can automatically reinvest dividends received in the stock of the paying corporation.[2] There are two types of DRPs: one involves only stock that is already outstanding, whereas the other involves newly issued stock. In either case the stockholder must pay income taxes on the amount of the dividends, even though stock rather than cash is received.

Under the "old-stock" type of plan, the stockholder elects either to continue receiving dividend checks or to have the dividends used to buy more stock in the corporation. If the stockholder elects reinvestment, a bank acting as trustee, takes the total funds available for reinvestment (minus a fee), purchases the corporation's stock on the open market, and allocates the shares purchased to the participating stockholders' accounts on a pro rata basis. The transactions costs of buying shares (brokerage costs) are low because of volume purchases, so these plans benefit small stockholders who do not need cash dividends for current consumption.

The "new-stock" type of DRP provides for dividends to be invested in newly issued stock; hence these plans raise new capital for the firm. AT&T, Florida Power & Light, Union Carbide, and many other companies have had such plans in effect, using them to raise substantial amounts of new equity capital. No fees are charged to stockholders, and many companies offer stock at a discount of 5 percent below the actual market price. The companies absorb these costs as a trade-off against flotation costs that would be incurred on stock sold through investment bankers rather than through the dividend reinvestment plans.[3]

---

[2]See R. H. Pettway and R. P. Malone, "Automatic Dividend Reinvestment Plans," *Financial Management,* Winter 1973, 11–18, for an excellent discussion of the topic.

[3]One interesting aspect of DRPs is that they are forcing corporations to reexamine their basic dividend policies. A high participation rate in a DRP suggests that stockholders might be better off if the firm simply reduced cash dividends, as this would save stockholders some personal income taxes. Quite a few firms are surveying their stockholders to learn more about their preferences and to find out how they would react to a change in dividend policy. A more rational approach to basic dividend policy decisions may emerge from this research.

STOCK REPURCHASE

Many firms are using **stock repurchase** plans as an alternative to paying dividends. The number of firms repurchasing their own stock has grown dramatically in the past few years. Before the 1980s, most repurchases amounted to only a few million dollars. By 1987, however, many large firms, including Atlantic Richfield, CBS, Coca Cola, Gulf Oil, IBM, Teledyne, and Texaco, had repurchased their own shares. The largest such transaction thus far was the repurchase by Phillips Petroleum of 81 million shares at a cost of more than $4.1 billion.

Several reasons exist for a firm to repurchase stock. First, the firm may wish to distribute cash to its shareholders in the form of a repurchase rather than a dividend. Prior to the 1986 tax act, capital gains were taxed at a lower rate than dividends, so wealthy individuals preferred selling stock to receiving dividends. Since dividends and capital gains are now taxed by the federal government at the same rate, it may seem that there is no advantage to the repurchase plan from the investor's point of view. However, profits earned on repurchases typically are not taxed until the stockholder sells the stock and receives a capital gain. Thus a repurchase allows the stockholder to decide when to sell (or not sell), thereby allowing her or him to make optimal use of tax planning. On the other hand, the investor must accept dividend payments and pay taxes whenever dividends are issued. For years Teledyne, a $3 billion conglomerate earning $4 million annually, appeared to be using repurchases as an alternative to dividends. Teledyne had not paid a dividend since its inception, and many analysts did not expect it to do so in the near future. However, in 1987 Teledyne declared and paid cash dividends of $4 per share.

A second reason that a firm utilizes repurchase is to change its capital structure. A firm may conclude that its capital structure is too heavily weighted with equity and may decide to sell debt, using the proceeds to buy back its stock. Consolidated Edison was confronted with a similar situation in 1985, when it repurchased $400 million of its common stock to affect changes in its capital structure. Had the firm changed its capital structure by financing all capital budgeting needs exclusively with debt, it would have taken years to reach the higher debt ratio. The repurchase program allowed Con Ed to reach its target capital structure instantaneously. Union Carbide and CBS followed similar plans in 1986.

A third reason that a firm uses a stock repurchase program is to fend off hostile takeovers. First, a firm with a high debt ratio is less attractive to an unwanted suitor. Second, by buying up excess shares, the firm reduces the ability of the suitor to purchase a controlling number of shares. For example, St. Joe Minerals held off a takeover bid by Seagram by borrowing heavily and using the funds to repurchase 7 million of its own shares at a cost of more than $400 million. Another type of takeover-related repurchase is represented by Disney's repurchase of its stock from Saul Steinberg and Mobil's repurchase from T. Boone Pickens. These "raiders" had acquired stock in Disney and Mo-

stock repurchase
A means by which a firm distributes income to stockholders by buying back shares of its own stock, thereby decreasing shares outstanding, increasing EPS, and increasing the price of the stock.

bil and had announced plans to take over the companies. Management bought them out, paying a premium price that is often called *greenmail.*

A fourth reason often cited for the repurchase of common stock is that it raises the value of the firm's stock. Stock that has been repurchased by the issuing firm is called *treasury stock.* If some of the outstanding stock is repurchased, fewer shares remain outstanding. Assuming that the repurchase does not adversely affect the firm's earnings, the earnings per share on the remaining shares will increase, resulting in a higher market price per share. As a result, capital gains will have been substituted for dividends.

Stock repurchases are commonly made in one of three ways: (1) A publicly owned firm can simply buy its own stock through a broker on the open market. (2) The firm can make a *tender offer,* under which it permits stockholders to send in (that is, "tender") their shares to the firm in exchange for a specified price per share, generally at a premium over the current market price. When a firm makes a tender offer, it generally indicates that it will buy up to a specified number of shares within a particular time period (usually about two weeks). If more shares are tendered than the firm wishes to purchase, purchases are made on a pro rata basis. (3) The firm can purchase a block of shares from one large shareholder on a negotiated basis.

In conclusion, the benefits of repurchase programs merit their continuance. Repurchase programs benefit investors by providing them with an opportunity to delay taxes on cash flows provided by the firm. Repurchases also can be especially valuable to the firm that wishes to make significant changes in its capital structure within a short period of time. However, repurchases on a regular, systematic basis may not be possible because of uncertainties about market price of the shares, how many shares would be tendered, and so forth.

On balance, companies probably should be doing more repurchasing and distributing fewer cash dividends than they are. Increases in the size and frequency of repurchases in recent years suggest that companies are increasingly reaching this same conclusion. The April 29, 1985, issue of *Fortune* contained an article on repurchases entitled, "Beating the Market by Buying Back Stock." It noted that in 1984 alone, more than 600 major firms had repurchased a significant amount of their own stock. The article concluded that ". . . buybacks have made a mint for shareholders who stuck with the companies carrying them out." However, the 1986 tax law revisions that limit the favorable treatment of capital gains reduce one of the major advantages of repurchases, and this could lead to a slowdown of repurchase activity.

STOCK DIVIDENDS AND STOCK SPLITS

Another aspect of dividend policy is the concept of stock dividends and stock splits. The rationale for stock dividends and splits can best be explained through an example; we will use Carter Chemical Company to illustrate.

As Carter Chemical continues to grow and retain earnings, its book value per share will also grow. More important, earnings per share and the market

Telephone & Data Systems Inc. declared a 3-for-2 stock split and increased its quarterly dividend on the post-split shares.

The telecommunications concern said the split is payable March 17 to stock of record March 3. It raised the quarterly to nine cents per post-split share, payable March 31 to stock of record March 17. The dividend is equivalent to 13.5 cents on pre-split shares. The company last paid a quarterly of 12 cents a share in December plus a special year-end of 5.5 cents.

The company, which has about 10.3 million common shares outstanding, said that beginning this year it will discontinue the special dividend and will incorporate it into its quarterly payouts.

Comerica Inc. announced a 3-for-2 stock split and increased its quarterly dividend 12.4%.

The banking company said it increased the dividend because of record earnings in 1987 and a strong financial outlook for 1988. On a pre-

split basis, the dividend was raised to 67.5 cents a share from 60 cents. On a post-split basis, the dividend is 45 cents a share and payable April 1 to holders of record March 15. The dividend will be paid on existing shares and shares created by the split.

The split will increase Comerica's shares outstanding to about 15.5 million.

LDBrinkman Corp., Kerrville, Texas, said holders at its annual meeting approved a 1-for-5 reverse split of the company's common stock, payable next Wednesday to stock of record last Monday. Before the split LDBrinkman had 10.6 million common shares outstanding. The company said holders also approved changing the corporate name to LDB Corp. and approved amending the company's articles of incorporation to limit the monetary liability of its directors under certain circumstances. LDBrinkman distributes carpeting and floor products, sells pizzas, and makes trailer homes and modular housing.

Stock splits, which increase the number of shares of a company's stock available for ownership, are often reported in the business press. These excerpts from *The Wall Street Journal* announce splits for three different companies and indicate how each split affects dividend payments as well as the value of the stock. Notice that stock splits need not be even, such as 2-for-1; two of the three companies announced 3-for-2 stock splits. LDBrinkman reports a reverse split whereby the company *reduced* the number of shares outstanding. Immediately after such a split the total number of shares have the same market value as before it, but each share is worth more. Splits of this nature are usually initiated by companies wanting to raise the price of their outstanding shares because they think the price is too low to attract investors.

Source: *The Wall Street Journal,* February 10, 1988, 39; February 12, 1988, 29; and February 24, 1988, 34.

price per share will rise. The firm began with only a few thousand shares outstanding. After some years of growth, each share had a very high EPS and DPS. When a "normal" P/E ratio was applied to the stock, the derived market price was so high that few people could afford to buy it. This limited demand for the stock, thus keeping the total market value of the firm below what it would have been if more shares, at a lower price, were outstanding. The solution for Carter's dilemma was resolved by splitting the stock.

Although there is little empirical evidence to support the contention, there is nevertheless a widespread belief in financial circles that an *optimal price range* exists for stocks. Here *optimal* means that, if the price is in this range, the price/earnings ratio will be maximized. Many observers, including Carter Chemical's management, believe that the best range for most stocks is from $20 to $80 per share. Accordingly, if at some future point the price of Carter's

stock split
An action to increase the
number of shares out-
standing; for example, in
a 3-for-1 split shares outstanding are tripled and
each stockholder re-
ceives 3 new shares for
each share formerly held.

stock dividend
A dividend paid in addi-
tional shares of stock
rather than cash.

stock rose to $80, management would probably declare a 2-for-1 **stock split,**
thus doubling the number of shares outstanding, halving the earnings and dividends per share, and lowering the price of the stock. Each stockholder would
have more shares, but each share would be worth less. If the post-split price
were $40, Carter's stockholders would be exactly as well off as they were be-
fore the split. If the price of the stock were to stabilize above $40, stockholders
would be better off. Stock splits can be of any size. For example, the stock
could be split 2-for-1, 3-for-1, 1.5-for-1, or in any other way.[4]

   Stock dividends are similar to stock splits in that they divide the "pie"
into smaller slices without affecting the fundamental position of the company
or each of its investors. On a 5 percent stock dividend, the holder of 100
shares would receive an additional 5 shares (without cost); on a 20 percent
stock dividend, the same holder would receive 20 new shares; and so on.
Because the total number of shares is increased, earnings, dividends, and the
price per share all decline.

   If a firm wants to reduce the price of its stock, should a stock split or a
stock dividend be used? Stock splits are generally used after a sharp price run-
up, when a large price reduction is sought. Stock dividends are frequently
used on an annual basis to keep the stock price more or less constrained. For
example, if a firm's earnings and dividends are growing at about 10 percent
per year, the price would tend to go up at about that same rate, and it would
soon be outside the desired trading range. A 10 percent annual stock dividend
would maintain the stock price within the optimal trading range.

   The economic effects of stock splits and stock dividends are virtually identical. Even so, the New York Stock Exchange has adopted a policy of calling a
distribution of stock under 25 percent a *dividend* and a distribution greater
than 25 percent a *split,* even if the issuing corporation calls its action something else.

   Accounts also treat stock splits and stock dividends somewhat differently.
Section 1 of Table 21-2 shows the equity portion of Carter Chemical Company's balance sheet before any action is taken on a stock dividend or split. In a
2-for-1 split, the shares outstanding are doubled and the par value is halved.
This treatment is shown in Section 2 of the table, where the only accounting
change to Carter's 1988 stockholders' equity pro forma statement is the adjustment to the par value of the stock. Had Carter decided to have a larger split,
say a 5-for-1 split, we would have only had to divide the par value by 5 to
reflect all necessary accounting changes. Since we can find the number of
shares outstanding by dividing the common stock account by the par value of
the stock, the new $0.20 par value and $50 million common stock account

---

[4]*Reverse splits,* which reduce the shares outstanding, can also be used; for example, a company
whose stock sells for $5 might employ a 1-for-5 reverse split, exchanging 1 new share for 5 old
shares and raising the value of the shares to about $25, which is within the optimal range.

Table 21-2 **Carter Chemical Company:**
Stockholders' Equity Accounts, Pro Forma
December 31, 1988

1. *Before a Stock Split or a Stock Dividend:*
Common stock (60 million shares authorized,
   50 million outstanding, $1 par) $ 50,000,000
Additional paid-in capital   100,000,000
Retained earnings   1,850,000,000
    Total common stockholders' equity $2,000,000,000

2. *After a 2-for-1 Stock Split:*
Common stock (120 million shares authorized,
   100 million outstanding, $0.50 par) $ 50,000,000
Additional paid-in capital   100,000,000
Retained earnings   1,850,000,000   Changes: Par value/2
    Total common stockholders' equity $2,000,000,000

3. *After a 20 Percent Stock Dividend:*
Common stock (60 million shares authorized,
   60 million outstanding, $1 par) $ 60,000,000   + $ 1 per share
Additional paid-in capital   890,000,000   + $79 per share
Retained earnings   1,050,000,000   − $80 per share
    Total common stockholders' equity $2,000,000,000   = $ 0 net change per share

would indicate that the number of shares had grown fivefold to 250 million shares.

Section 3 of Table 21-2 demonstrates the accounting changes that would occur in the equity section if Carter proceeded with a 20 percent stock dividend rather than the stock split. If Carter's common stock were selling at $80 per share, a 20 percent stock dividend would result in an $800 million transfer (or recapitalization) of funds from retained earnings to the common stock and paid-in-capital accounts. The transfer from retained earnings is calculated as follows:

$$\begin{pmatrix} \text{Dollars} \\ \text{transferred from} \\ \text{retained} \\ \text{earnings} \end{pmatrix} = \begin{pmatrix} \text{Number} \\ \text{of shares} \\ \text{outstanding} \end{pmatrix}\begin{pmatrix} \text{Percentage} \\ \text{of the} \\ \text{stock dividend} \end{pmatrix}\begin{pmatrix} \text{Market} \\ \text{price of} \\ \text{the stock} \end{pmatrix}$$

$$= (50 \text{ million})(0.2)(\$80)$$

$$= \$800,000,000.$$

The common stock account would increase by the stock's par value ($1) per share for each of the 10 million new shares issued. The remaining $79 per share (price minus par value) would be added to paid-in capital (or as its older but more descriptive account title was known, capital in excess of par).

Table 21-3 **Price Effects of Stock Dividends**

	Price at Selected Dates (in Percentages)		
	Six Months before Ex Dividend Date	**At Ex Dividend Date**	**Six Months after Ex Dividend Date**
Cash dividend increase	100	109	108
No cash dividend increase	100	99	88

Price Effects

Several empirical studies have examined the effects of stock splits and stock dividends on stock prices.[5] The findings of the Barker study, which are typical of those reported in the financial literature, are presented in Table 21-3. When a stock dividend was associated with a cash dividend increase, the value of the company's stock 6 months after the ex dividend date had risen by 8 percent. On the other hand, when a stock dividend was not accompanied by a cash dividend increase, the stock value had fallen by 12 percent, which approximated the percentage of the average stock dividend.

These data seem to suggest that stock dividends are seen for what they are — simply additional pieces of paper — and that they do not represent true income. When they are accompanied by higher earnings and cash dividends, investors bid up the value of the stocks. However, when stock dividends are not accompanied by increases in earnings and cash dividends, the dilution of earnings and dividends per share causes the prices of the stocks to drop by about the same percentage as the stock dividends. The fundamental determinants of price are the underlying earnings and dividends per share.

ESTABLISHING A DIVIDEND POLICY: SOME ILLUSTRATIONS

Many factors interact to determine a firm's optimal dividend policy. Because these interactions are too complex to permit the development of a rigorous model for use as a guide to dividend policy, firms are forced to consider their dividend policies in a relatively subjective manner. Some illustrations of how dividend policies are actually set follow.

---

[5]C. A. Barker, "Evaluation of Stock Dividends," *Harvard Business Review,* July–August 1958, 99–144. Barker's study has been replicated several times in recent years, and his results are still valid; they have withstood the test of time. Another excellent study, using an entirely different methodology yet reaching similar conclusions, is that of E. Fama, L. Fisher, M. C. Jensen, and R. Roll, "The Adjustment of Stock Prices to New Information," *International Economic Review,* February 1969, 1–21.

Shoal Creek Engineering

Shoal Creek Engineering analyzed its situation in terms of the residual theory, as shown in Figure 21-3. The residual theory suggested a dividend of $1.80 per share during 1988, or a 30 percent payout ratio. Shoal Creek's stock is widely held, and a number of tax-exempt institutions are important stockholders. A questionnaire to its stockholders revealed no strong preferences for dividends versus capital gains. Shoal Creek's long-range planning group projected a cost of capital and a set of investment opportunities during the next three to five years similar to those shown for this year.

Based on this information, Shoal Creek's treasurer recommended to the board of directors that it establish a dividend of $1.80 for 1988, payable 45 cents quarterly. The 1987 dividend was $1.70, so the $1.80 represented an increase of about 6 percent. The treasurer also reported to the board that, in the event of an unforeseen earnings downturn, the company could obtain additional debt to meet its capital expenditure requirements. The board accepted the treasurer's recommendation and in December 1987 declared a dividend of 45 cents per share, payable January 15, 1988. The board also announced its intention of maintaining this dividend for the balance of 1988.

Hytec Electronics

Hytec Electronics has a residual theory position that *resembles* IOS$_G$ in Figure 21-3. This suggests that no dividend should be paid. Hytec has, in fact, paid no dividend since its inception in 1978, even though it has been continuously profitable and earnings have recently been growing at a 25 percent rate. Informal conversations with the firm's major stockholders, all of whom are in high tax brackets, suggest that they neither expect nor want dividends; they would prefer to have the firm retain earnings, have good earnings growth, and provide capital gains, which are not taxed until the shares are sold. The stock now sells for $126 per share. Hytec's treasurer recommended a 3-for-1 split, no cash dividend, and a future policy of declaring an annual stock dividend geared to earnings for the year. The board of directors concurred.

Northwest Electric Company

Northwest Electric Company has an acute need for new equity capital. The company has a major expansion program underway and absolutely must come up with the money to meet construction payments. The debt ratio is high, and if the times-interest-earned ratio falls any lower, (1) the company's bonds will be downgraded and (2) it will be barred by bond indenture provisions from further debt issues. These facts suggest a cut in dividends from the $3.75 per share paid last year. However, the treasurer knows that many of the stockholders rely on dividends for current living expenses, so if dividends are cut, these stockholders may be forced to sell, thus driving down the price of the stock. This would be especially bad in view of the treasurer's forecast that there will be a need to sell new common stock during the coming year. (New outside

Initial Public Offering: It's Not Over Yet

If you were to ask entrepreneurs what they were trying to obtain from their businesses, they would undoubtedly answer something like, "A lot of money" or "financial independence." If you delved further into their goals, one of them might respond like this: "Well, in five years I hope to be able to take the company public or have it acquired by a bigger firm. Then my hard work will be over and I'll have it made!"

Taking a company public is one of the ways the entrepreneur "harvests" the company. Typically, the stock issued when a new firm is created is restricted stock; it cannot be sold in the public equity markets. Although the entrepreneur has a piece of paper showing his or her ownership of the company, the paper cannot easily be sold because it has no liquidity. Cash cannot be obtained for the ownership interest (at least not easily). Thus, one of the owner's dreams may be to take the company public, which means to have a public offering of the firm's stock. Then the entrepreneur could sell a portion of his or her ownership in the firm and begin enjoying the financial rewards of a successful business.

Why not go public in the beginning and enjoy liquidity from the outset? Some small businesses do, in fact, go public very early in their lives. They may go public through the "penny stock" market, a market in which stocks tend to sell at very low prices (often less than a dollar a share). When a firm has a public offering early in its life, however, it is normally to inject capital into the business, not to allow the owner-manager to derive cash from it. In fact, at a very early stage the business may have such a poor track record (if indeed it has any record at all) that it has nothing to sell. It is only after the firm has established a record and created some value that a public offering can successfully allow the entrepreneur to capitalize on that value.

In addition, even though the entrepreneur may firmly believe in an idea, convincing the public to have faith in it is a different story for several reasons. First, if no products have been sold or no market has been established for the products, the idea has no record of performance. Investors in the security markets would have to act on faith when buying the stock, and generally this means that the markets would value the stock far less than the entrepreneur. Second, if the idea is novel, the revelations the entrepreneur must make about the idea to have a successful offering invites competition. The public disclosures required for a public offering, then, can destroy the opportunity facing the small business.

Thus let's assume we are not talking about a public offering done very early in the life of a firm. Suppose instead that the entrepreneur has created the products, has developed a reputation for the company in its marketplace, and has achieved some financial success to point to. Now the firm is ready for a public offering. To reach this point, the entrepreneur has perhaps devoted many years of his or her life working untold hours, perhaps suffering a divorce or strained family relationships because of the time demands and pressures. The company is successful and it is time to reap the benefits. Or is it?

If the entrepreneur's desire is to haul off a wheelbarrow full of money to a tropic island retreat for a life of ease, there are some obstacles. Put yourself in the place of Hardy, an investor thinking of buying stock in Laurel's new public offering. One question Hardy would certainly want answered is, "Does Laurel really believe in this business?" If on the day of the public offering, Laurel is selling *ALL* of her stock and is getting out of the company, Hardy would be worried. It was Laurel who built this business. Is she bailing out? If so, who will give the firm the spirit and drive she gave it? The entrepreneur who built the business may be the single most valuable asset the business has.

As long as the entrepreneur continues to work for the firm, how serious is the problem of the entrepreneur bailing out? It can be quite serious. As an example, a venture capital firm in Dallas once provided capital to three different office supply businesses. One of them grew by leaps and bounds and was very profitable; the other two performed adequately but not well. The difference was a hard-charging, motivated entrepreneur in the first firm. Therefore the venture capitalist bought out the companies and merged them into one business to be run entirely by the successful entrepreneur. He was paid $2,000,000 in cash for his ownership interests. Almost immediately, his behavior changed. He came in late and left early, and he no longer worked on weekends. He quit at noon on Fridays to play golf. Eventually, he had to be replaced as CEO of the company.

What was the entrepreneur's problem? Very simply, he had worked hard to build some equity for himself and his family. The $2,000,000 was the payoff — he was ready to begin enjoying it and was no longer motivated to build a successful business. Many similar examples have taught investors that management motivation is fundamental to a firm's continued success. Any hint that management's motivation has declined or might decline is a negative signal to prospective investors.

Further, Hardy understands that Laurel knows more about this company's prospects than anyone else. If Laurel is bailing out entirely or to a large extent, what must she think about the company's *future?* Isn't her decision to sell her stock a signal to Hardy that its value is not likely to rise very much? An initial public offering may comprise newly-issued stock sold by the company to obtain cash for business purposes, or it may include stock sold by the entrepreneurs and other owners. Hardy will probably interpret stock sold by Laurel as a negative signal if she sells too much of her stake in the company. Therefore, Laurel's decision to get out will, in and of itself, reduce the price at which Laurel can get out.

A final caveat is that a company may do everything right and still not have a public offering that pleases the entrepreneurs. The reason is that one other variable has to be right — the timing of the issue in the market. Consider the case of CML Group, Inc., which was founded in 1969. By 1983, the company had annual revenues of $125,000,000 and was earning over $2.5 million net. The company was stable and solid, and management had taken its time to develop the company carefully before considering a public offering. Management and early investors expected to be able to sell about 2 million shares in an initial public offering — 1 million by the company for its internal needs and another 1 million by the investors to enable them to derive some liquidity from their investment. Even though prices were not yet firm, it was thought that the shares could be sold at a price-to-earnings ratio of around 25-to-1, bringing the offering in at around $19 per share and providing good returns to management and other investors.

During the three or four months that it took to prepare the issue, the roof caved in on the market for new issues. In one month's time, the prices of new issues fell precipitously, as did the number of issues brought to market. By the time the offering was ready for market, the decision had been made that no insiders would be able to sell their shares and only the company's stock would be sold. Even that would be sold at a price 30 percent below what was thought possible only a month earlier.

In another incident, a company that we will call XYZ was five years old at the time it was the target of an acquisition-minded company we'll call ACQ. Although XYZ was profitable, it was not big enough to have a public offering of the size or at a price the owners found desirable. ACQ made an offer for an exchange of stock, and XYZ agreed to the deal. One month later, at the end of January 1984, the stock market had fallen and ACQ's price had fallen by 50 percent. The deal was off; there was no merger. Again, the culprit wasn't XYZ's management; it was an unpredictable market that valued shares at one price one month and at half (or double) that amount the following month.

In building a company's value, the outcome is not entirely in the hands of the entrepreneurs and managers. Even in the best of circumstances, the capital markets can change rapidly and diminish a firm's value through no fault of management. Therefore, when considering a public offering, the entrepreneur must take timing carefully into account. Many opportunities have been missed by an entrepreneur who waited for the markets to rise, only to see them fall.

equity would be needed even if the company totally eliminated the dividend.) The treasurer is aware that many other utilities face similar problems. Some have cut their dividends, and their stock prices invariably have fallen by amounts ranging from 30 to 70 percent.

Northwest's earnings were forecast to increase from $5.00 to $5.26. The treasurer recommended that the dividend be raised from $3.75 to $4.05, with the dividend increase being announced a few weeks before the company floated a new stock issue. The hope was that this action would cause the price of the stock to increase, after which the company could sell a new issue of common stock at a better price.

Pacific Industries

Pacific Industries' 1987 dividend was $3.80 per share, up from $3.57 in 1986. Both dividend figures represented about 50 percent of earnings, and this payout was consistent with a residual theory analysis. The company's growth rate in EPS and DPS had been in the 5 to 10 percent range during the past few years, and management projected a continuation of this trend. The financial vice president foresaw a cash flow problem in 1988 — earnings were projected to increase in line with the historical average, but an especially large number of good investment opportunities (along with some unprofitable but required pollution control expenditures) were expected. A preliminary analysis using the residual theory suggested that the dividend in 1987 should be cut back sharply, if not eliminated.

The financial vice president quickly rejected this cutback and recommended instead a 6 percent *increase* in the dividend, to $4.03, noting that the company could easily borrow funds during the coming year to meet its capital requirements. Even though the debt ratio would rise somewhat above the target, the firm's average cost of capital curve is relatively flat, and cash flows from 1988 investments should permit a reduction in the debt ratio over the next few years. The vice president thought that it was more important to maintain the steady growth in dividends than to adhere strictly to the target debt ratio.

SUMMARY

Dividend policy involves the decision to pay out earnings or to retain them for reinvestment in the firm. Any change in dividend policy has both favorable and unfavorable effects on the price of the firm's stock. Higher dividends mean higher cash flows to investors, which is good, but lower future growth, which is bad. The optimal dividend policy balances these opposing forces and maximizes the price of the stock.

A number of factors bear on dividend policy, including legal constraints such as bond indenture provisions, the firm's investment opportunities, the availability and cost of funds from other sources (new stock and debt), stockholders' desire for current income, and the information content of dividend changes. Because of the large number of factors that affect dividend policy, and also because of the relative importance of these factors' changes over time and across companies, it is impossible to develop a precise, generalized model for use in establishing dividend policy. Firms can, however, consider the *residual theory model* in reaching a judgment about the most appropriate dividend policy.

Firms tend to use one of three payment policies: (1) a stable or continuously increasing dollar dividend per share; (2) a low regular dividend plus extras that depend on annual earnings; and (3) a constant payout ratio, which will cause the dollar dividend to fluctuate. Most firms follow the first policy, a few use the second, and almost none use the third. Also, many firms today are using dividend reinvestment plans to help stockholders reinvest dividends at minimal brokerage costs, and some firms use stock repurchase plans in lieu of increasing cash dividends.

Stock splits and stock dividends were also discussed. These actions may be beneficial if the firm's stock price is quite high, but otherwise they have little effect on the value of the firm.

RESOLUTION TO DECISION IN FINANCE

The Last Conglomerate

James L. Ketelsen believes that Tenneco's high dividend is a bet on his company's future and, in turn, is gambling that a few other of his strategically placed bets will pay off. First, he is gambling that oil and gas prices will rebound, an absolute must for a company with such a major stake in that field, and hardly a farfetched expectation. Second, he is counting on a turnaround at J.I. Case, the tractor and construction equipment company into which Ketelsen has been steadily plowing cash. And third, he is depending on continuing strength in Tenneco's nonenergy sectors, including shipbuilding, packaging, and automotive products, thus validating management's belief in diversification.

If all these bets pay off, record earnings could surface in as few as two to three years, with the option of corporate restructuring if things don't pan out. "I feel pretty good because we are doing a lot of things right for the long pull," Ketelsen declares. He believes that the $3.04 dividend is justified by Tenneco's cash flow. Although it was down from previous years, cash flow is still about $9 per share from continuing operations and should run higher in the near future. He believes that it is more than adequate to cover the dividend without starving Tenneco's other needs.

"If we looked ahead to 1990 and thought the cash flow wouldn't be high enough, then maintaining the dividend rate would be a different matter," Ketelsen says.

Sales of operations that were no longer deemed to fit Tenneco's desired mix of businesses have fattened company bank accounts and helped to trim the company's staggering debt somewhat, even though, as often happens in asset disposals, Tenneco has booked losses on some sales.

However, the jury is still out on the course that Ketelsen has charted for Tenneco. Many analysts contend that the company's stock is undervalued because the company has many divisions, such as automotive components and shipbuilding, that are solid moneymakers and basic stand-alone companies. They would, Ketelsen's critics say, be wonderful candidates for sale or spinoff. Indeed, many analysts think that if Tenneco would restructure by selling off several of its divisions, the market would salute Tenneco's shares with a sharp markup.

Vague takeover rumors have floated around from time to time. In 1987 Tenneco shares climbed several points after corporate raider T. Boone Pickens made a fairly innocuous comment to a *Houston Post* reporter that Tenneco stock was undervalued. Pickens also was quoted as saying that Tenneco management hadn't been aggressive enough in "transferring value from the company's assets to the stockholders."

Source: Harlan S. Byrne, "The Last Conglomerate," *Barrons,* April 27, 1987; Jo Ellen Davis, "Does Tenneco Have Too Much Riding on Tractors?" *Business Week,* December 1, 1986, 118–120; and Peter Nulty, "Plowing Different Fields," *Fortune,* August 3, 1987.

QUESTIONS

21-1 As an investor, would you rather invest in a firm that has a policy of maintaining **(a)** a constant payout ratio, **(b)** a constant dollar dividend per share, **(c)** a target dividend growth rate, or **(d)** a constant regular quarterly dividend plus a year-end extra when earnings are sufficiently high or corporate investment needs are sufficiently low? Explain your answer, stating how these policies would affect your k_s. Discuss also how your answer might change if you were a 21-year-old student, a 48-year-old professional in your peak earning years, or a retiree.

21-2 How would each of the following changes probably affect aggregate (that is, the average for all corporations) payout ratios? Explain your answers.
a. An increase in the personal income tax rate.
b. A liberalization in depreciation policies for federal income tax purposes; that is, faster tax write-offs.
c. A rise in interest rates.
d. An increase in corporate profits.
e. A decline in investment opportunities.

21-3 What are the pros and cons of having the directors formally announce what a firm's dividend policy will be in the future?

21-4 Most firms would like to have their stock selling at high P/E ratios and also have an extensive public ownership (many different shareholders). How may stock dividends or stock splits be compatible with these aims?

21-5 What is the difference between a stock dividend and a stock split? As a stockholder, would you prefer to see your company declare a 100 percent stock dividend or a 2-for-1 split? Assume that either action is feasible.

21-6 "The cost of retained earnings is less than the cost of new outside equity capital. Consequently, it is totally irrational for a firm to sell a new issue of stock and to pay dividends during the same year." Is this a true statement? Why or why not?

21-7 Would it ever be rational for a firm to borrow money in order to pay dividends? Explain.

SELF-TEST PROBLEM

ST-1 Campos Aircraft Corporation (CAC) has an all-equity capital structure that includes no preferred stock. It has 500,000 shares of $2 par value common stock outstanding.

When CAC's founder and chief engineer, Jennifer Campos, retired suddenly in late 1988, CAC was left suddenly and permanently with materially lower growth expectations and relatively few attractive new investment opportunities. Unfortunately, there was no way to replace the founder's contributions to the firm. Previously, CAC had found it necessary to plow back most of its earnings to finance growth, which had averaged 12 percent per year. Future growth of 5 percent appears to be realistic, but that would call for an increase in the dividend payout. Further, it now appears that new investment projects with at least the 14 percent rate of return required by CAC's shareholders (k_s = 14%) would amount to only $2,800,000 for 1989, in comparison to a projected $7 million of net income after taxes. If the existing 25 percent dividend payout were continued, retained earnings would be $5.25 million in 1989, but, as noted, investments that yield the 14 percent cost of capital amount to only $2.8 million.

The one encouraging thing is that the high earnings from existing assets are expected to continue, and net income of $7 million is still expected for 1989. Given the dramatically changed circumstances, CAC's management is reviewing the firm's dividend policy.
a. Assuming that the acceptable 1989 investment projects would be financed entirely by retained earnings during the year, calculate DPS in 1989, assuming that CAC uses the residual payment dividend policy.

b. What payout policy does this imply for 1989?

c. If the increased payout ratio is maintained for the foreseeable future, what should be the present market price of the common stock? How does this compare with the market price that should have prevailed under the assumptions existing just before the news about the retirement of CAC's founder? If the two values of P_0 are different, explain why.

d. What are the implications of continuing the 25 percent payout? Assume that if this payout is maintained, the average rate of return on retained earnings will be 8 percent and the new growth rate will be as follows:

$$g = (1.0 - \text{Payout rate})(\text{ROE})$$

$$= (1.0 - 0.25)(8.0\%)$$

$$= (0.75)(8.0\%)$$

$$= 6.0\%.$$

PROBLEMS

21-1   **Dividend payout.** Van Kirk Enterprises had net income for 1988 of $8 million.
a. What was the firm's payout ratio if it paid $5 million in dividends?
b. If the firm's payout was 25 percent, what was the dividend payment?
c. If the payout ratio was 40 percent, what was the retention ratio?
d. In 1987 the firm's payout ratio was 60 percent, and $4.2 million was paid in dividends. What was Van Kirk's net income in 1987?

21-2   **Sustainable growth.** With the following financial information for Babcock Supply, determine the growth rate, g, that the firm can support through internal resources:

Net margin $= 5\%$

Total asset turnover $= 2.0$

Equity financing $= 100\%$

Retention ratio $= 60\%$

21-3   **Sustainable growth.** Luthor Incorporated has reached a mature stage in its product life cycle, and although it remains profitable, it will have zero growth in earnings in the future. If Luthor's return on equity, ROE, is 12 percent and net income is $500,000, determine the firm's payout ratio.

21-4   **Sustainable growth.** Bolten Brothers has a rate of return on equity of 15 percent and a constant growth rate of 6 percent. What is Bolten Brothers' payout ratio?

21-5   **External equity financing.** Telecomp is expanding its productive capacity with a $12 million investment. The board of directors approved the expansion under the following conditions:
1. The firm would not exceed its current 40 percent debt/assets ratio.
2. The dividend payout ratio would remain at 30 percent.
If net earnings are expected to be $7.5 million this year, how much external equity must Telecomp seek during the year?

21-6 **Stock dividend.** Solectron has the following common stock equity accounts on its balance sheet:

Common stock ($2 par) $ 2,000,000
Paid-in capital   15,000,000
Retained earnings   40,000,000
    Total equity $57,000,000

The market price of the firm's stock is $40. Restate the equity accounts of Solectron to reflect a 20 percent stock dividend.

21-7 **Stock split.** New York Publishing Company has just announced a three-for-one stock split. Prior to the split, dividends were $5.50 per share. The firm plans to pay a dividend of $2.00 per share after the split. What is the percentage increase in the cash dividend that occurs after the split?

21-8 **Stock split.** After a five-for-one split, Como Enterprises paid a dividend of $3 per new share, which represents an 11 percent increase in last year's pre-split dividend. What was last year's dividend per share?

21-9 **Cash and stock dividends.** Findlay Metals declared a 10 percent stock dividend and a cash dividend of $0.50 per share. The cash dividend is paid on both the old shares and the shares received in the stock dividend. Construct a pro forma balance sheet showing the effect of these actions; use one new balance sheet that incorporates both actions. The stock sells for $40 per share. A condensed version of Findlay's end-of-year balance sheet (before dividends) is given below (in millions of dollars):

Cash	$ 50	Debt	$1,000
Other assets	1,950	Common stock	50
		(30 million shares authorized, 25 million outstanding, $2 par)	
		Paid-in capital	200
		Retained earnings	750
Total assets	$2,000	Total claims	$2,000

21-10 **Alternate dividend policies.** In 1987 Mississippi Equipment Company (MEC) paid dividends of $2.5 million. The firm's net income for 1987 was $10 million. For the past 5 years MEC's earnings and dividends have grown at a constant 7 percent rate. However, 1988 was an especially profitable year, with net income totaling $20 million. For 1989 MEC has $16 million of profitable investment opportunities planned. Even so, the surge in earnings enjoyed in 1988 cannot last, and the firm's profits are expected to return to the previous 7 percent stable growth rate. Calculate the 1988 dividends for MEC under each of the following dividend policies:
a. A stable and growing dividend payment.
b. Stable payout based on the 1987 payout ratio.
c. Passive residual dividend policy if the firm uses no debt to finance investment opportunities.
d. Passive residual dividend policy if the firm maintains a 40 percent debt/assets ratio.

21-11 **Payout policy.** The following financial information applies to Almaden Athletic Equipment:

$$\text{Net margin} = 6 \text{ percent}$$

$$\text{Total asset turnover} = 1.5 \text{ times}$$

$$\text{Debt/assets ratio} = 40 \text{ percent}$$

$$\text{Investors' required rate of return, } k_s = 17 \text{ percent}$$

$$\text{Earnings per share} = \$5.00$$

Almaden is trying to determine whether its payout ratio should be 20 percent or 80 percent.

a. What is the implied growth rate under each payout ratio?

b. What is the stock's value under each payout alternative?

c. Which payout ratio should the firm adopt?

21-12 **Dividend policy and capital structure.** Georgia Tobacco Company has for many years enjoyed a moderate but stable growth in sales and earnings. However, cigar consumption and consequently Georgia's sales have been falling recently, primarily because of an increasing awareness of the dangers of smoking to health. Anticipating further declines in tobacco sales in the future, Georgia's management hopes eventually to move almost entirely out of the tobacco business and into a newly developed, diversified product line in growth-oriented industries. The company is especially interested in the prospects for pollution-control devices, because its research department has already done much work on the problems of filtering smoke. Right now the company estimates that an investment of $24 million is necessary to purchase new facilities and to begin operations on these products, but the investment could be earning a return of about 18 percent within a short time. The only other available investment opportunity totals $9.6 million, is expected to return about 10.2 percent, and is indivisible; that is, it must be accepted in its entirety or else be rejected.

The company is expected to pay a $2.40 dividend on its 6 million outstanding shares, the same as its dividend last year. The directors may change the dividend, however, if there are good reasons for doing so. Total earnings for the year are expected to be $22.8 million; the common stock is currently selling for $45; the firm's target debt ratio (debt/assets ratio) is 45 percent; and its tax rate is 40 percent. The costs of various forms of financing are as follows:

New bonds, $k_d = 11\%$. This is a before-tax rate.

New common stock sold at $45 per share will net $41.

Required rate of return on retained earnings, $k_s = 14\%$.

a. Calculate Georgia's expected payout ratio, the break point where the MCC rises, and its marginal cost of capital above and below the point of exhaustion of retained earnings at the current payout. (*Hint:* k_s is given, and D_1/P_0 can be found. Then, knowing k_s and D_1/P_0, g can be determined.)

b. How large should Georgia's capital budget be for the year?

c. What is an appropriate dividend policy for Georgia? How should the capital budget be financed?

d. How might risk factors influence Georgia's cost of capital, capital structure, and dividend policy?

e. What assumptions, if any, do your answers to the preceding questions make about investors' preferences for dividends versus capital gains — that is, their preferences regarding the D_1/P_0 and g components of k_s?

(Do Part f only if you are using the computerized problem diskette.)

f. Assume that Georgia's management is considering changing the company's capital structure to include more debt, and thus it would like to analyze the effects of an increase in the debt ratio to 60 percent. However, the treasurer believes that such a move would cause lenders to increase the required rate of return on new bonds to 12 percent and that k_s would rise to 14.5 percent. How would this change affect the optimal capital budget? If k_s rose to 16 percent, would the low-return project be acceptable? Would the project selection be affected if the dividend were reduced to $1.50 from $2.40, still assuming $k_s = 16\%$?

ANSWER TO SELF-TEST PROBLEM

a.

Projected net income	$7,000,000
Less: Projected capital investments	2,800,000
Available residual	$4,200,000

Shares outstanding   500,000

$$DPS = \$4,200,000/500,000 \text{ shares} = \$8.40 = D_1.$$

b.
$$EPS = \$7,000,000/500,000 \text{ shares} = \$14.$$

$$\text{Payout ratio} = DPS/EPS = \$8.40/\$14 = 60\% \text{ or}$$

$$\text{Total dividends/NI} = \$4,200,000/7,000,000 = 60\%.$$

c.
$$P_0 = D_1/k_s - g = \$8.40/0.14 - 0.05 = \$8.40/0.09 = \$93.33.$$

Under the former circumstances, D_1 would have been equal to the 25 percent payout on the $14 EPS; therefore DPS = $3.50. With $k_s = 14\%$ and $g = 12\%$, we solve for P_0:

$$P_0 = D_1/k_s - g = \$3.50/0.14 - 0.12 = \$3.50/0.02 = \$175.$$

Although CAC has suffered a severe setback, its existing assets will continue to provide a good income stream. More of these earnings should now be passed on to the shareholders, as the slowed internal growth has reduced the need for funds. However, the net result is a whopping 47 percent decrease in the value of the shares.

d. If the dividend payout ratio were held at 25 percent even after internal investment opportunities had declined, the price of the stock would drop to $3.50/(0.14 − 0.06) = $43.75 rather than $93.33. Thus the increase in dividend payout is consistent with maximizing shareholder wealth.

Because of the downward sloping IOS curve (see Figure 21-3), the greater the firm's level of investment, the lower the average ROE. Thus, if CAC retains and invests more money, its average ROE will decline further. We can determine the average ROE under different conditions as follows:

Old Situation (with Founder Active and a 25 Percent Payout):

$$g = (1.0 - \text{Payout ratio})(\text{Average ROE})$$

$$= (1.0 - 0.25)(\text{Average ROE}).$$

$$\text{Average ROE} = 12\%/0.75 = 16\% > k_s = 14\%.$$

Note that the *average* ROE is 16 percent whereas the *marginal* ROE is presumably equal to 14 percent.

New Situation (with Founder Retired and a 60 Percent Payout):

$$g = 6\% = (1.0 - 0.6)(\text{ROE})$$

$$\text{ROE} = 6\%/0.4 = 15\% > k_s = 14\%.$$

This suggests that the new payout is appropriate and that the firm is taking on investments down to the point where marginal returns are equal to the cost of capital. Note, however, that if the 25 percent payout were maintained, the *average* ROE would be only 8.0 percent, which would imply a marginal ROE far below the 14 percent cost of capital.

Part VII

SELECTED TOPICS IN FINANCIAL MANAGEMENT

Throughout this text we have been developing the basic framework for making financial decisions. At this point we still have several important topics to discuss. We deferred these final topics so that they could be analyzed on an integrated basis using analytical tools developed in earlier chapters. Chapter 22 deals with mergers and acquisitions; Chapter 23 provides an analytical framework within which to evaluate leases; and Chapter 24 covers international finance.

Chapter 22

Mergers

One Tough Poker Match

Fred Hartley was a refinery maintenance worker with a cast-iron will and a flair for chemical engineering. He had $25 in his pocket when he joined Union Oil Company in 1942, but by the mid-1950s he was pushing the company into unproved technologies. A decade later, as president of what was to become Unocal, the nation's twelfth largest oil company, he expanded the company's operations to South Korea, Thailand, and the North Sea.

An equally flinty oil man, T. Boone Pickens used his stake of $1,300 to buy a 1955 Ford station wagon to hold his exploration gear and set out to find oil. He spent his days chasing rumors over the dusty back roads of Texas and Oklahoma and nights bent over maps studying geological strata. Ten years later his company, Mesa Petroleum, employed 650 people, and Pickens had become a real-life J. R. Ewing.

Pickens, the most powerful takeover artist in the oil field, has gone eyeball to eyeball with the biggest and strongest U.S. oil companies and forced them to blink. To his fans, he is a modern David, a champion of the little guy who takes on the Goliaths of Big Oil and more often than not gives them a costly "whupping." To his enemies, he is a dangerous upstart, a veritable rattlesnake in the woodpile bent on enriching himself and his cronies under the guise of pro-

moting the interests of shareholders.

At no time could Hartley be classified as T. Boone Pickens's fan. In 1985 Mesa Partners II, Pickens's group acquired 13.6 percent of Unocal's stock, becoming its biggest shareholder. Thus was launched a corporate poker match between two iron-willed opponents.

Pickens presented Unocal with an $8.1 billion two-step takeover plan, offering $54 a share for 64 million of Unocal's 173.7 million outstanding shares. The offer, coupled with shares Mesa already held, would have given Pickens' group slightly more than a 50 percent stake in the company. To justify his bid for Unocal, Pickens cited examples of mismanagement, among them the $600 million that Unocal spent on an oil shale plant that had produced no revenues in 30 years. If he gained control of Unocal, Pickens promised to end corporate waste and boost shareholder value.

Unocal's board of directors, in a special emergency meeting, voted unanimously to reject Mesa's bid, stating that it was "grossly inadequate" and promised to "promptly make recommendations to its shareholders."

As you read this chapter, think of what you would do if you were in Hartley's shoes. How would you balance your goals of maximizing shareholder value with trying to preserve a strategy of corporate management that you believed in? How might you fight off Mesa Partners II? How would you finance the battle?

See end of chapter for resolution.

Most corporate growth occurs through *internal expansion,* which takes place when the firm's existing divisions grow through normal capital budgeting activities. However, the most dramatic growth, and often the largest changes in firms' stock prices, are the result of **mergers.** Recently newspapers and business periodicals have reported a large number of business combinations, including those of Du Pont with Conoco, Texas Air with Eastern Airlines and Continental Airlines, Chrysler with American Motors, Burroughs with Sperry (to form Unisys), and many others. There are many important legal distinctions among the various means by which two or more economic units can combine. Our emphasis, however, is on the fundamental business and financial aspects of mergers and acquisitions.

merger
Any combination that forms one company from two or more previously existing companies.

THE ECONOMIC IMPLICATIONS OF MERGERS

The primary motivation for mergers is to increase the value of the combined enterprise. If Companies A and B merge to form Company C, and if C's value exceeds that of A and B taken separately, **synergy** is said to exist. Synergy has often been described as the "2 plus 2 equals 5 effect." Thus, when synergy exists, the new business entity is worth more than the simple sum of the merged firms. Such a merger is, of course, beneficial to both A's and B's stockholders. Synergistic effects can arise from four sources: (1) *operating economies* resulting from economies of scale in production or distribution; (2) *financial economies,* which can include a higher P/E ratio, a lower cost of debt, or greater debt capacity; (3) *differential management efficiency,* which implies that one firm's management is relatively inefficient, so the firm's profitability can be improved by merger; and (4) *increased market power* because of reduced competition. Operating and financial economies as well as mergers that increase managerial efficiency are socially desirable, but mergers that reduce competition are both undesirable and illegal.

synergy
The condition wherein the whole is greater than the sum of its parts; in a synergistic merger the postmerger value exceeds the sum of the separate companies' premerger values.

After the discussion of risk in Chapter 15, one may naturally assume that risk reduction would be an important economic implication in the combination of two firms. Indeed, managers often cite the stabilization of earnings and the resulting reduction of corporate risk as a prime motivation for mergers. Stabilization of the earnings stream through diversification should be beneficial to the firm's employees, customers, and suppliers, but is it beneficial to the firm's stockholders? After all, an investor can diversify more easily and cheaply than a firm. The shareholder can merge any combination of firms by purchasing shares of each stock. For example, if a merger of Delta and American Airlines would stabilize their earnings, an investor could purchase stock in each and efficiently create a merged firm at a much lower cost than would be possible if these firms merged in actuality.

When two firms begin merger negotiations, or when one firm begins thinking about acquiring another, one of the first considerations is antitrust: Is the Justice Department likely to try to block the merger, and would it be able to do so? If the answer to either part of this question is yes, chances are high that the merger will be aborted because of the legal expenses involved in fighting the Justice Department. However, how the Justice Department will view the merger is often uncertain; this was especially true during the Reagan era when mergers were constrained less than in some previous administrations. Occasionally firms believe that they will be allowed to merge and later find that they cannot. Southern-Pacific and Santa Fe Railroads spent millions in the belief that their merger would be allowed, but after three years of deliberation the Justice Department denied their merger.

TYPES OF MERGERS

Economists classify mergers into four groups: (1) horizontal, (2) vertical, (3) congeneric, and (4) conglomerate. A **horizontal merger** occurs when, for example, one automobile manufacturer acquires another, as Chrysler did with American Motors in 1987, or when one retail food chain merges with another. The merger of Nestle and Carnation was a horizontal merger because both firms manufacture food products. An example of a **vertical merger** is a steel producer's acquisition of an iron or coal mining firm, or a chemical producer's acquisition of a petroleum company that can supply it with a stream of raw materials. Thus Du Pont's acquisition of Conoco was a vertical merger. *Congeneric* means "allied in nature or action"; hence a **congeneric merger** involves related enterprises but not producers of the same product (horizontal) or firms in a producer-supplier relationship (vertical). Examples of congeneric mergers include American Express's takeover of Shearson Hammill, a stock brokerage firm, or Phillip Morris's acquisition of General Foods. A **conglomerate merger** occurs when unrelated enterprises combine; Mobil Oil's acquisition of Montgomery Ward illustrates a conglomerate merger.

Operating economies (and also anticompetitive effects) are partially dependent on the type of merger involved. Vertical and horizontal mergers provide the greatest operating benefits, but they are also the ones most likely to be attacked by the Justice Department. In any event, it is useful to think of these economic classifications when analyzing the feasibility of a prospective merger.

PROCEDURES FOR COMBINING FIRMS

In the majority of mergers, one firm (generally the larger of the two) simply decides to buy another company, negotiates a price for it, and acquires the target company. Occasionally the acquired firm will initiate the action, but it is much more common for a firm to seek acquisitions than to seek to be acquired. Following convention, we shall call a company that seeks to acquire another the **acquiring company** and the one that it seeks to acquire the **target company.**

Once an acquiring company has identified a possible target, it must establish a suitable price, or range of prices, that it is willing to pay. With this in

horizontal merger
The combination of two firms that produce the same type of goods or service.

vertical merger
A merger between a firm and one of its suppliers or customers.

congeneric merger
A merger of firms in the same general industry but in which no customer or supplier relationship exists.

conglomerate merger
A merger between companies in different industries.

acquiring company
A company that seeks to acquire another company.

target company
A company that another firm, generally a larger one, seeks to acquire through merger.

Announcements of *friendly mergers,* such as this advertisement in *The Wall Street Journal,* appear frequently in the business press. In this case, managements of both the acquiring company, Grolier, Inc., and the target company, Regensteiner Publishing Enterprises, Inc., approved the terms of the merger. Drexel Burnham Lambert Incorporated is the investment banking firm that handled the merger.

Regensteiner Publishing Enterprises, Inc.

has been acquired by

Grolier, Inc.

The undersigned initiated this transaction, assisted in the negotiations and acted as financial advisor to Regensteiner Publishing Enterprises, Inc.

Drexel Burnham Lambert
INCORPORATED

mind, the acquiring firm's managers must decide how to approach the target company's managers. If the acquiring firm has reason to believe that the target company's management will approve the merger, it will simply propose a merger and hope to work out suitable terms. The two management groups will then issue statements to their stockholders recommending that they approve the merger. Assuming that the stockholders do approve, the acquiring firm will buy the target company's shares from its stockholders, paying for them either with its own shares (in which case the target company's stockholders become stockholders of the acquiring company) or with cash. Situations in which the terms of the merger are approved by both management groups are called **friendly mergers.**

Under other circumstances the target company's management may resist the merger. Perhaps it believes that the price offered for the stock is too low,

friendly merger

A merger in which the terms are approved by the managements of both companies.

or perhaps the target firm's management simply wants to maintain its independence. In either case the target firm's management is said to be *hostile,* and the acquiring firm must make a direct appeal to the target firm's stockholders. In **hostile mergers,** or **takeovers,** the acquiring company generally makes a **tender offer,** in which it asks the stockholders of the firm it is seeking to control to submit, or "tender," their shares in exchange for a specified price. The price is generally stated as so many dollars per share of the stock to be acquired, although it can be stated in terms of shares of stock in the acquiring firm. The tender offer is a direct appeal to stockholders, so it need not be approved by the management of the target firm. Tender offers are not new, but the frequency of their use has increased greatly in recent years.

FINANCIAL ANALYSIS OF A PROPOSED MERGER

In theory, merger analysis is quite simple. The acquiring firm simply performs a capital budgeting analysis to determine whether the present value of the expected cash flows from the merger exceeds the price paid for the target company. The target company's stockholders should accept the proposal if the price offered exceeds the present value of the firm's expected future cash flows discounted at the cost of equity, assuming that it operates independently. Theory aside, however, some difficult decisions are involved. First, the acquiring company must estimate the incremental cash flow benefits, including any synergistic effects, that will be obtained from the acquisition and must determine what effect, if any, the merger will have on the required rate of return on equity. Then the acquiring company must decide how to pay for the merger — with cash, its own stock, or some other type or package of securities. Finally, having estimated the benefits of the merger, it is necessary for the acquiring and target firms' managers and stockholders to bargain over how to share these benefits.

Operating Mergers versus Financial Mergers

From the standpoint of financial analysis, there are two basic types of mergers:

1. Operating mergers, in which the operations of two companies are integrated with the expectation of obtaining synergistic effects. General Motors' purchases of Electronics Data Systems (EDS) and Hughes Aircraft were attempts at operating mergers.

2. Pure financial mergers, in which the merged companies will not be operated as a single unit and from which no operating economies are expected. Coca-Cola's acquisition of Columbia Pictures with $748 million in "surplus" cash is an example of a financial merger.

Of course, a merger may actually be a combination of these two types.

Estimating Future Operating Income

In a pure financial merger, the postmerger cash flows are simply the sum of the expected cash flows of the two companies as a result of the merger. If the two firms' operations are to be integrated in order to achieve better financial results, however, accurate predictions of future cash flows, which are absolutely essential to sound merger decisions, will be difficult to construct.

The basic rationale for any operating merger is synergy. Del Monte Corporation provides a good example of a series of well-thought-out, successful operating mergers. Del Monte merged and integrated numerous small canning companies into a very efficient, highly profitable organization. It used standardized production techniques to increase the efficiency of all its plants, a national brand name and national advertising to develop customer loyalty, a consolidated distribution system, and a centralized purchasing office that obtained substantial discounts from volume purchases. Because of these economies, Del Monte became perhaps the nation's most efficient and profitable canning company, and its merger activities helped make possible the size that produced these economies. Consumers also benefited because Del Monte's efficiency enabled the company to sell high-quality products at relatively low prices.

An example of poor pro forma analysis that resulted in a disastrous merger is the consolidation of the Pennsylvania and New York Central Railroads. The premerger analysis, which suggested large cost savings, was highly misleading. It failed to reveal the fact that certain key elements in the two rail systems were incompatible and hence could not be meshed together. Rather than gaining synergistic benefits, the combined system actually incurred additional overhead costs that helped lead to its bankruptcy.

In planning operating mergers, the development of accurate pro forma cash flow estimates is *the single most important aspect* of the merger analysis. In fact, many firms that are actively engaged in mergers have acquisition departments. These departments evaluate merger candidates, develop pro forma statements that forecast under varying assumptions the results of the mergers, and evaluate plans for making the projections materialize.

Terms of the Merger

The terms of a merger include two important elements: (1) Who will control the combined enterprise? (2) How much will the acquiring firm pay for the acquired company?

Postmerger Control. The employment/control situation is of vital importance. Consider a situation in which a small, owner-managed firm sells out to a larger concern. The owner-manager may be anxious to retain a high position and also may be concerned about keeping operating control of the organization after the merger. Thus these points are likely to be stressed during the merger negotiations. When a publicly owned firm, not controlled by its managers, is merged into another company, the acquired firm's management also worries about its postmerger position. If the acquiring firm agrees to keep the

INDUSTRY PRACTICE

Negotiations in a Fishbowl?

The Securities and Exchange Commission's campaign for fuller disclosure of merger talks is beginning to resemble a failed takeover attempt: lots of saber-rattling followed by little change.

In recent months, the agency has garnered big headlines and shocked Wall Street's legal community by filing charges against Allied Stores Corp. and other companies for allegedly violating disclosure rules. But the flurry of activity isn't helping the SEC create the "level playing field" it seeks for all investors. A slew of recent merger and restructuring announcements have been preceded by stock run-ups, indicating that market professionals continue to know far more about coming news than individual investors.

A major problem, many companies say, lies with the laws themselves. Executives, lawyers, and takeover specialists say there isn't any clear definition of when a company must publicize merger talks, leaving them confused about their obligations to investors. And they are sharply divided over the merits of early disclosure, with some companies even resisting it.

"It's stupid to think that you can run a negotiation that's good for shareholders if you're going to do it in a fishbowl," says Joseph Flom, a top takeover lawyer in New York who says he's seen several deals killed by premature publicity.

Counters Wayne Cross, a New York securities lawyer, "Early disclosure tends to equalize the inequity between market insiders and the moms and pops."

SEC officials concede that their rules, which require companies to publicize "material developments," are vague. But the agency is pushing

companies to err on the side of disclosure. "This is something we're very serious about," says Gary Lynch, the SEC's enforcement chief. "It's in everyone's interest to make disclosure as soon as possible."

But when is that? Consider:

On July 17, 1987, a Friday, Standard Brands Paints Co. received — but didn't disclose — a takeover bid from a New Zealand company. The bid, however, was announced by the suitor in New Zealand over the weekend. Standard executives didn't disclose the offer until the following Tuesday.

Dan Bane, Standard Brands' chief financial officer, says the Torrance, California-based company didn't immediately understand its disclosure obligations. "We really didn't know what to release, so we waited for more information on the offer," he says. In the meantime, however, the company's stock rose $2 a share Monday to $28.625 and an additional $2.375 Tuesday, prior to the Standard Brands announcement of the bid.

This sort of pre-announcement trading is widespread, and the run-up in stock prices is often substantial. According to an SEC study released in February 1987, average trading volume in a stock begins to increase about ten days before a takeover announcement. By three days before the announcement, it has tripled; two days before, it is five times normal. Volume surges to almost 20 times normal on the day of the announcement. On average, a company's stock price rises 38.8% before a takeover offer is announced.

Such a run-up doesn't necessarily mean an illegal leak of inside information — although that certainly prompts much activity, takeover professionals agree. The SEC study argues that most pre-announcement stock activity is fueled by Wall Street professionals using computers to track trading, educated guesses, and a variety of legal tips to make their assumptions. SEC officials, while acknowledging the continued presence of pre-announcement run-ups, believe their campaign has, if nothing else, increased awareness of disclosure issues among companies.

In June 1987, in its most highly publicized case, the SEC filed charges against Allied Stores and lawyer George Kern of the New York law firm of Sullivan & Cromwell for allegedly failing to promptly disclose merger talks and a prospective sale of six shopping centers to Edward J. DeBartolo Corp., a Youngstown, Ohio, developer of shopping malls.

While Allied Stores and Mr. Kern argued that the shopping center transaction was in the very early stages and that the proposed merger with DeBartolo was subject to financing, the SEC said that both moves were "material developments" and should have been disclosed.

The basis of the Allied Stores case was regulations for public filings that require companies subject to a tender offer to disclose merger talks or other "extraordinary" transactions. The SEC has made similar arguments in cases not involving tender offers; in one such brief, it pointed to the large sums paid by fallen arbitrager Ivan Boesky for inside information on preliminary merger talks to show the value market professionals place on it.

Opponents of early disclosure respond that the SEC overlooks the harm that can result from such publicity. In addition to simply killing such actions outright, disclosure may actually hurt less sophisticated investors, the opponents argue. Stock prices may be driven up — but may crash if the transaction falls through.

That argument, however, hasn't held water with some courts. "To attribute to investors a child-like simplicity, an inability to grasp the probabilistic significance of negotiations, implies that they should not be told about new plants, new products (or) new managers," the Seventh U.S. Circuit Court of Appeals recently said.

The SEC's opponents have at least one major court ruling in their favor. In a 1984 case that conflicts with current SEC policy, a federal appeals court ruled that Heublein Inc. didn't have to disclose merger talks with RJR Nabisco because the companies hadn't agreed on the transaction's price and structure.

To be on the safe side, many companies now believe that "no comment" is better than any comment at all. "To do anything else is too risky and cuts their flexibility later," says David Gunning, a lawyer with the Cleveland firm of Jones, Day, Reavis & Pogue whose clients include such rumored takeover targets as Gillette Co.

But the SEC has indicated in Allied Stores and other cases that when negotiations are judged "material," a "no comment" won't suffice.

An example of the quandary some companies find themselves in is Southland Corp. When the New York Stock Exchange in June 1987 inquired about trading that boosted Southland's stock $9.50 in a single week, the company said it didn't know what was behind the activity — even though, SEC documents revealed later, the company had been approached by the Belzberg brothers of Canada.

Southland repeated the assertion when rumors of the Belzbergs' interest grew so strong that Southland stock didn't open because of a trade imbalance. By then the company had created a committee of outside directors to evaluate a leveraged buyout or recapitalization plan. Southland, which eventually agreed to be acquired by its major shareholder, has defended its actions, saying that the Belzberg and other talks were preliminary and "inappropriate" to disclose.

old management, management may be willing to support the merger and recommend its acceptance to the stockholders. If the old management is to be removed, it probably will resist the merger.

The Price Paid. Another key element in a merger is the price to be paid for the acquired company — the cash or shares of stock to be given in exchange for the firm. If the merger is to be for cash, the analysis is similar to a regular capital budgeting analysis: the incremental cash flows are estimated; a discount rate is applied to find the present value of these cash flows; and, if the present value of the future incremental flows exceeds the price to be paid for the acquired firm, the merger is approved. If, because of operating economies or financial considerations, the acquired firm is worth more to the acquiring firm than its market value as a separate entity, the merger is feasible. Obviously, the acquiring firm tries to buy at as low a price as possible, whereas the acquired firm tries to sell out at the highest price possible. The final price is determined by negotiations, with the side that negotiates best capturing most of the incremental value. *The larger the synergistic benefits, the more room there is for bargaining and the higher the probability that the merger actually will be consummated.*

MERGER ANALYSIS

To illustrate how a merger may be analyzed, consider a proposed merger between Acquisition Technology and Target Industry, Inc. For Acquisition to determine the value of Target, two key items are needed: (1) a set of pro forma financial statements that develop Target's expected cash flows and (2) a discount rate, or cost of capital, to apply to these projected cash flows.

Pro Forma Income Statements

The merger team at Acquisition Technology, including the financial staff, accountants, engineers, and marketing specialists, has produced the projected income statements in Table 22-1. The data reflect all postmerger synergy that may be expected in the merger of Acquisition Technology and Target Industry.

The accuracy of the projected cash flows is critical to a successful evaluation of Target. Of course, the postmerger cash flows attributable to the firm to be acquired are extremely difficult to estimate. Because it is a friendly merger, Acquisition has sent part of the merger team, including dozens of financial analysts, accountants, engineers, and others, to Target's headquarters to go over its books, to estimate required maintenance expenses and future fixed asset investments, to set values on patents and research and development projects, and the like.

The data in Table 22-1 reflect the incremental changes in Acquisition's cash flows that will directly result from its merger with Target. Some of the net income generated through the merger will be retained by Acquisition to

Table 22-1 **Target Industry:**
Projected Postmerger Income Statement
(Millions of Dollars)

	1989	1990	1991	1992	1993
Net sales	$147	$176	$211	$244	$267
Cost of goods sold	112	132	155	178	192
Sales & administrative expenses	14	17	18	21	22
EBIT	$ 21	$ 27	$ 38	$ 45	$ 53
Interest	4	5	5	6	6
EBT	$ 17	$ 22	$ 33	$ 39	$ 47
Taxes	4	7	11	13	16
Net income	$ 13	$ 15	$ 22	$ 26	$ 31
Retention	7	12	14	15	16
Annual cash flow	$ 6	$ 3	$ 8	$ 11	$ 15
Terminal value					$275
Total cash flow	$ 6	$ 3	$ 8	$ 11	$290

finance its own asset growth, and some will be transferred to Target for investment in assets, for dividends, or for other purposes. The pro forma statement assumes that depreciation-generated funds will be used to replace worn-out and obsolete plant and equipment. The merger team projects that cash flows will grow at a constant rate of 10 percent after 1993. The value to Acquisition of all post-1993 cash flows as of December 31, 1993, is estimated by the constant growth model to be $275 million:

$$\text{Value in 1993} = CF_{1993}(1 + g)/(k_s - g)$$

$$= \$15(1.10)/(0.16 - 0.10)$$

$$= \$275 \text{ million.}$$

In the next section we discuss the determination of the appropriate discount rate. Target currently uses 30 percent debt in its capital structure, but if the merger occurs, Acquisition will increase Target's debt ratio to 50 percent.

Estimating the Discount Rate

Up to this point, our merger analysis has been quite similar to the analysis of capital budgeting projects, but an important difference exists between merger analysis and capital budgeting. It involves the choice of the discount rate used to determine the present value of the future cash flows. In capital budgeting the cash flows are discounted by the cost of capital; in merger analysis, however, the cost of equity is the appropriate discount rate.

Note that the net cash flows shown at the bottom of Table 22-1 are equity cash flows, so they should be discounted at the cost of equity rather than at the overall cost of capital. The cost of equity must reflect the risk of the cash flows shown in the table. Also, the cost of equity that is used should be Target's not Acquisition's or that of the consolidated postmerger firm. Target's market-determined premerger beta was 1.15, which reflects a debt ratio of 30 percent. Acquisition's investment bankers estimate that Target's beta will rise to 1.4 if its debt ratio is increased to 50 percent.

The Security Market Line can be used to determine Target's new cost of equity capital. If the risk-free rate is 9 percent and the market risk premium is 5 percent, Target's after-merger cost of equity, k_s, is estimated to be 16 percent:

$$k_s = R_F + b(k_s - R_F)$$

$$= 9\% + 1.4(5\%)$$

$$= 16\%.$$

Determining the Acquisition's Value

Target's value to Acquisition in 1988 can be determined by discounting at 16 percent the cash flows that are expected to accrue to Acquisition:

Year	Cash Flow	DF at 16%	Discounted Cash Flow
1989	$ 6,000,000	0.8621	$ 5,172,600
1990	$ 3,000,000	0.7432	2,229,600
1991	$ 8,000,000	0.6407	5,125,600
1992	$ 11,000,000	0.5523	6,075,300
1993	$290,000,000	0.4761	138,069,000
			$156,672,100

Therefore, if Acquisition could acquire Target for $156,672,100 or less, the merger would be acceptable from Acquisition's point of view.

ROLE OF THE INVESTMENT BANKER

The investment banking community not only helps with the sale of new securities but also is involved with mergers in a number of ways. First investment bankers help to arrange mergers. Also, because they are experts in arranging mergers, they have the expertise to help target companies *resist* mergers. Finally, investment bankers help acquiring firms to value target companies.

These merger-related activities have proved to be quite profitable to the investment banking community. For example, the investment bankers who arranged RCA's recent acquisition of C.I.T. Financial earned fees of $5.8 million. Du Pont's investment banker in the Conoco contest, First Boston, earned fees of more than $15 million, whereas Morgan Stanley, Conoco's investment banker, had an arrangement under which it would earn fees of about $15 million regardless of who won. No wonder investment banking houses are able to make top offers to finance graduates!

Arranging Mergers

The major investment banking firms have merger and acquisition groups that operate within their corporate finance departments. (Corporate finance departments offer advice rather than underwriting services for business firms or brokerage services for individuals.) Members of these groups strive to identify firms with excess cash that might want to buy other firms, companies that might be willing to be bought, and firms that might be attractive to others for a number of reasons. If a chemical company decided to expand into agribusiness, it might enlist the aid of an investment banker to help it locate and then negotiate with a target agribusiness operation. Similarly, dissident stockholders of firms with poor track records might work with investment bankers to oust management by helping to arrange a merger. Drexel Burnham Lambert, the investment banking house that developed junk bond financing, has offered financing packages to corporate raiders; such a package includes (1) designing the securities to be used in the tender offer and (2) getting people and firms to buy the target firm's stock now and then to tender it once the final offer is made.

MERGER DEFENSES

A target firm that does not want to be acquired usually enlists the help of an investment banking firm, along with a law firm that specializes in helping to block mergers. Defenses include such tactics as (1) changing the firm's by-laws so that only one-third of the directors are elected each year or so that a 75 percent approval rate, rather than a simple majority, is required to approve a merger; (2) trying to convince the target firm's stockholders that the price being offered is too low; (3) raising antitrust issues in the hope that the Justice Department will intervene; (4) repurchasing stock in the open market in an effort to push the price above that being offered by the potential acquirer; (5) finding a **white knight** that is more acceptable to the target firm's management to compete with the potential acquirer; and (6) "taking a poison pill."

Some examples of **poison pills** — which really do amount to virtually committing suicide to avoid a takeover — involve such tactics as borrowing on terms that require immediate repayment of all loans if the firm is acquired, selling off at bargain prices the assets that originally made the firm a desirable target, granting such lucrative **golden parachutes** to the firm's executives that the cash drain from these payments would render the merger infeasible, and planning defensive mergers that would leave the firm with assets of questionable value or with a huge amount of debt to service. Companies have even given their stockholders the right to buy the stock of an acquiring firm at half-price should the firm be acquired. The blatant use of poison pills is constrained by directors' awareness that such actions could trigger personal suits by stockholders against directors who voted for them. Perhaps in the near future there will be laws that limit management's use of these tactics; in the

white knight
A company that is more acceptable to a firm subject to a hostile takeover attempt than the potential acquirer.

poison pill
A self-destructive action that will seriously hurt a company if it is acquired by another.

golden parachutes
Large payments made to the managers of a firm as a poison pill defense against acquisition in a hostile merger.

meantime, investment bankers are busy thinking up new poison pill formulas, and others are just as actively trying to come up with antidotes.

VALUATION FUNCTION

If a friendly merger is being worked out between two firms' managements, it is important for them to be able to document that the agreed-upon price is a fair one; otherwise the stockholders of either company may sue to block the merger. Therefore, in many large mergers, each side will engage an investment banking firm to evaluate the target company and to help establish the fair price. For example, General Electric employed Morgan Stanley to determine a fair price for Utah International, as did Royal Dutch to help establish the price it paid for Shell Oil in 1985. Even if the merger is not friendly, investment bankers may still be asked to help establish a price. If a surprise tender offer is to be made, the acquiring firm will want to know the lowest price at which it might be able to acquire the stock, while the target firm may seek help in proving that the price being offered is too low.

DIVESTITURES

Although corporations do more buying than selling of productive facilities, a good deal of selling also occurs. There are four types of **divestitures:** (1) sale of an operating unit to another firm; (2) sale of the unit being divested to the managers; (3) setting up the business to be divested as a separate corporation and then giving (or "spinning off") its stock on a pro rata basis to the divesting firm's stockholders; and (4) outright liquidation of assets.

Sale to another firm generally involves the sale of an entire division or unit, usually for cash but sometimes for the acquiring firm's stock. ITT, for example, sold 27 separate companies with a value of $1.2 billion. In a *managerial buyout,* the managers or employees of the division purchase the division themselves, usually for cash plus notes; then, as owner-managers, they reorganize the division as a closely held firm. RCA recently sold Gibson Greeting Cards for $81 million to a group that included Gibson's managers and some financiers. In mid-1987, the pilots of American Airlines attempted to purchase the airline from its parent company, Allegis. In a *spin-off* the firm's existing stockholders are given new stock representing separate ownership rights in the company being divested. The new company establishes its own board of directors and officers and operates as a separate company. The stockholders end up owning shares of two firms instead of one, but no cash is transferred. IU International, a multimillion-dollar conglomerate, recently spun off three major subsidiaries—an ocean shipping company, a Canadian electric utility, and a gold mining company. After the spin-offs IU's stock price rose from $10 to $25 per share. Finally, in a *liquidation,* the assets of a division are sold off piecemeal rather than as a single entity. When Lawrence Tisch gained control

divestiture
The selling off of an asset or a division by its parent company; if the asset is given to the parent company's stockholders, the divestiture is called a *spin-off.*

of CBS, one of his first moves was to sell CBS Publishing to Harcourt Brace Jovanovich.

HOLDING COMPANIES

holding company
A corporation that owns sufficient common stocks of other firms to achieve working control over them.

parent company
A holding company that controls other firms by owning large blocks of their stock.

operating company
A subsidiary of a holding company; a separate legal entity.

Holding companies date from 1889, when New Jersey became the first state to pass a law permitting corporations to be formed for the sole purpose of owning the stocks of other companies. Strictly defined, any company that owns stock in another firm could be called a holding company. However, a holding company is generally considered to be a firm that holds large blocks of stock in other companies and exercises control over those firms. The holding company is often called the **parent company**, and the controlled companies are known as subsidiaries or **operating companies.** The parent can own 100 percent of a subsidiary's stock, but frequently control is exercised with less than this amount.

Many of the advantages and disadvantages of holding companies are identical to the advantages and disadvantages of large-scale operations already discussed in connection with mergers and consolidations. Whether a company is organized on a divisional basis or with the divisions kept as separate companies does not affect the basic reasons for conducting a large-scale, multiproduct, multiplant operation. However, the holding company form of large-scale operations has some advantages and disadvantages that differ from those of completely integrated divisionalized operations.

Advantages of Holding Companies

Control with Fractional Ownership. Through a holding company operation a firm may buy 5, 10, or 50 percent of the stock of another corporation. Such fractional ownership may be sufficient to give the acquiring company effective working control or substantial influence over the operations of the company in which it has acquired stock ownership. Working control is usually considered to entail more than 25 percent of the common stock, but it can be as low as 10 percent if the stock is widely distributed. One financier noted that the attitude of management is more important than the number of shares owned, adding that "if they think you can control the company, then you do." In addition, a very slim margin of control can be held through friendship with large stockholders outside the holding company group.

Isolation of Risks. Because the various operating companies in a holding company system are separate legal entities, the obligations of any one unit are separate from those of the other units. Catastrophic losses incurred by one unit of the holding company system are therefore not transmitted as claims on the assets of the other units.

Although this is the customary generalization on the nature of risk in a holding company system, it is not completely valid. First, the parent company may feel obligated to make good on the subsidiary's debts, even though it is not legally bound to do so, in order to keep its good name and thus retain customers. Examples of this include American Express's payment of more than $100 million in connection with a swindle that was the responsibility of one of its subsidiaries, and United California Bank's coverage of a multimillion-dollar fraud loss incurred by its Swiss affiliate. Second, a parent company may feel obligated to supply capital to an affiliate to protect its initial investment; General Public Utilities' continued support of its affiliate's Three Mile Island nuclear plant is an example. Third, when lending to one of the units of a holding company system, an astute loan officer may require a guarantee or a claim on the assets of the parent or of other elements in the holding company system. Finally, an accident such as the one at Union Carbide's Bhopal, India, plant may be deemed the responsibility of the parent company, voiding the limited liability rules that would otherwise apply. To some degree, therefore, the assets in the elements of a holding company are joined. Holding companies can at times prevent losses in one unit from bringing down other units in the system.

Legal Separation. Regulated companies such as certain financial institutions and utilities find it easier to operate as holding companies than as divisional corporations. Many banks, insurance companies, and other financial service corporations have found it convenient to be organized as holding companies. For example, Transamerica is a holding company that owns insurance companies, small loan companies, title companies, auto rental companies, and an airline. Similarly, Citicorp is a holding company that owns Citibank of New York, a leasing company, and a mortgage service company, among others.

Utilities also find the holding company format beneficial for operations. All of the Bell telephone companies are part of holding company systems. Southern Company, an electric utility that operates in and is regulated by several states, found it most practical to set up a holding company (Southern), which in turn owns a set of subsidiaries throughout several southern states (Georgia Power, Alabama Power, Mississippi Power, and Gulf Power). However, even utilities that operate within only a single state are finding it beneficial to operate as holding companies in order to separate those assets under the control of regulators from those not subject to utility commission regulation. Florida Power & Light recently reorganized and changed its corporate name to FPL Group, which owns a utility (Florida Power and Light) as well as subsidiaries engaged in insurance, real estate development, agriculture, and the like.

Disadvantages of Holding Companies

Partial Multiple Taxation. Provided that the holding company owns at least 80 percent of a subsidiary's voting stock, the Internal Revenue Service permits the filing of **consolidated returns,** in which case dividends received by the parent are not taxed. If less than 80 percent of the stock is owned, returns may not be consolidated. However 80 percent of the dividends received by the

consolidated return
An income tax return that combines the income statements of several affiliated firms.

SMALL BUSINESS

Merging as a Means to Exit a Closely Held Business

Imagine a small business that was started by a member of a family and that has achieved some success. Perhaps the entire family fortune is tied up in the firm. Such might be the case if a successful entrepreneur — say, Grandpa to whom we will refer throughout this section — started a business, brought the sons and daughters in as they reached adulthood, and continued to run the enterprise as it grew.

In such a situation, particularly if the firm is worth several million dollars or more, the family's entire financial well-being may be determined by the success of this one business. As long as Grandpa is healthy and continues to run the show, things are fine. Grandpa may, in fact, be reluctant to sell the business; it gives him something to pass on to his family and provides a place for the children and grandchildren to work.

Tightly-held family businesses like the one described here are fairly common in the United States. Yet there may be several reasons maintaining the business in its tightly held form may not be in the family's best interests.

First, there is the problem of succession. Because at some point Grandpa will retire or die, the issue of who will succeed him is important. Sometimes there is a clear choice for the successor, and everyone agrees with the choice. More often, however, even in families that are very close, the problem of succession can be an issue that splits the family apart. The problem is especially severe if Grandpa dies unexpectedly. At a time when emotions are already high, a key business decision needs to be made, and the choice is not a simple one. It is, therefore, very important for Grandpa and the other principals to take the time early on to set up a plan of succession. If the issue is irresolvable, plans should be made for the outright sale of the business in the event of Grandpa's death.

A second problem is that even though the business represents the family's primary asset of value, family members have no easy way to use that value when they need cash for various reasons: the business has no liquidity. Sometimes a plan will be made to buy a family member's stock at a predetermined rate, such as at its book value per share. This enables a family member to obtain cash, but the price paid probably bears little relation to the market value of the shares. Thus a family member gives up a valuable asset for the sake of liquidity, taking a potential loss in the process. An alternative, as discussed in the previous chapter, is to register the shares and take the company public so that family members can use their equity as they choose. A disadvantage to this approach is the potential loss of control as the number of shares held by the public increases.

A perhaps even more serious problem is that the family's entire wealth is tied up in a single business; the family holds an *undiversified portfolio*. As was explained in earlier chapters, diversification through investment in a variety of securities reduces a portfolio's risk. Thus the goals of maintaining control and reducing risk are in conflict in this situation. Again, a public offering would allow some family members to sell their stock and diversify their own personal portfolios. However, if Grandpa began a business that created wealth for the family, it may be desirable to take steps to ensure the security of that wealth, and diversification is a great aid to that process.

Both the diversification motives and family members' liquidity needs argue for changing the ownership structure of the business. There is another alternative — that of selling the entire business outright to another company or merging it into a larger firm. This alternative is often overlooked by tightly held businesses because it obviously means an immediate and complete loss of control in most cases. It deserves special consideration, however, because it can often be accomplished at far greater values than a public offering.

With the sale of the business, the family gives up control, yet that control is also exactly what makes the firm more valuable in a merger than in a public offering. Merger premiums for public companies often range up to as high as 50 to 70 percent over the market price. Therefore, a company worth, say, $10 million in the public market might instead be acquired for a price of $15 to $17 million.

What are the disadvantages of the merger? Obviously, the loss of control is one disadvantage. Also, family members might lose employment in the firm. If so, however, they will have additional wealth to sustain them while they seek another job.

The advantages of the acquisition by a bigger firm are in some respects the same as those gained in a public offering. Assuming that the acquisition is for stock in a public company, family members can sell off their holdings, gain instant liquidity, and use the proceeds to build a diversified portfolio that protects the wealth that Grandpa worked so hard to create.

A merger has advantages *over* a public offering as well. One is that if there is a public offering and family members want to sell off all of their stock in order to diversify their holdings, they will probably have to sell at a price below the quoted market price. When a large block comes to the market for sale, it usually has to be sold at a slightly reduced price. The price premium paid in an acquisition make it a better deal. Also, if family members hold the stock of the larger acquiring company, the larger firm's stock probably is more liquid, meaning that more of it can be sold at a price close to market.

Owners of the closely held family business must consider the cost-benefit trade-offs of continuing to be closely held, going public, and being acquired in a merger. Of the three alternatives, the acquisition alternative is likely to provide the most immediate wealth and security to the owners of the business.

holding company are excluded from taxation, so only 20 percent of the dividends are taxable. With a tax rate of 34 percent and only 20 percent of the dividends subject to taxation, the effective intercorporate tax rate on dividends is 34% × 20% = 6.8%. This partial double taxation somewhat offsets the benefits of holding company control with limited ownership, but whether or not a penalty of 6.8 percent of dividends received is sufficient to offset other possible advantages is a matter that must be decided in individual situations.

Ease of Enforced Dissolution. It is relatively easy for the U.S. Department of Justice to require dissolution of a holding company operation it finds unacceptable by disposal of stock ownership. For instance, Du Pont was required to dispose of its 23 percent stock interest in General Motors Corporation, acquired in the early 1920s. Because there was no fusion between the corporations, there were no difficulties, from an operating standpoint, in requiring the separation of the two companies. If complete amalgamation had taken place, however, it would have been much more difficult to break up the company after so many years, and the likelihood of forced divestiture would have been reduced.

Leverage in Holding Companies

The holding company vehicle has been used to obtain huge degrees of financial leverage. In the 1920s several tiers of holding companies were established in the electric utility and other industries. In those days an operating company might have $100 million of assets, financed by $50 million of debt and $50 million of equity. A first-tier holding company might own the stock of the operating firm as its only asset and be financed with $25 million of debt and $25 million of equity. A second-tier holding company, which owned the stock of a first-tier company as its only asset, might be financed with $12.5 million of debt and $12.5 million of equity. The system could be extended to many more levels, but even with only two holding companies, we can see that $100 million of operating assets are controlled at the top by $12.5 million of equity, and that these assets must provide enough cash income to support $87.5 million of debt. Such a holding company system is highly leveraged, even though the individual components have only 50 percent debt/assets ratios. Because of this *consolidated leverage,* even a small decline in profits at the operating company level could bring the whole system down like a house of cards. In fact, many analysts regard the existence of highly leveraged holding companies as a major contributor to the severity of the stock market crash of 1929 and the resulting depression of the 1930s.

SUMMARY

A merger involves the consolidation of two or more firms. Mergers can provide economic benefits through economies of scale or through more efficient management. However, they also have the potential for reducing competition, and for this reason they are carefully regulated by governmental agencies.

In most mergers one company (the *acquiring firm*) initiates action to take over another (the *target firm*). The acquiring company must analyze the situation and determine the target company's value. Often there will be *operating economies,* or *synergistic benefits,* which will raise the earnings of the combined enterprise more than the sum of the earnings of the two separate companies. In this circumstance the merger is potentially beneficial to both sets of stockholders, but the two firms' managers and stockholders must agree about how the net benefits will be shared. This all boils down to how much the acquiring company is willing to pay, either in cash or in shares of its own stock, for the target company.

In a merger one firm disappears. An alternative, however, is for one firm to buy all or a majority of the common stock of another and to run the acquired firm as an operating subsidiary. When this occurs, the acquiring firm is said to be a *holding company.* Holding company operations have both advantages and disadvantages. The major advantages are that (1) control can often be obtained for a smaller cash outlay, (2) risks may be separated, and (3) regulated companies can separate regulated from unregulated assets. The disadvantages include tax penalties and the fact that incomplete ownership, if it exists, can lead to control problems.

Divestitures, on the other hand, involve the selling of its productive facilities. An entire division or unit of one firm may be sold to another firm or to the current managers and/or employees of the divested unit. In a spin-off, shares of stock of the newly divested division are distributed to the shareholders of the existing firm. In the event of a liquidation, the sale of a division's assets are sold on an individual basis rather than as a complete entity.

 RESOLUTION TO DECISION IN FINANCE

One Tough Poker Match

During the spring of 1985, the newspapers chronicled the Hartley-Pickens poker game as the stakes began to mount. Unocal sued Mesa and Security Pacific, its principal bank, charging that Security made loans to Mesa Partners II knowing that it planned to use the money to buy Unocal shares. As several banks bowed out of Mesa's lending pool, Pickens alleged that Hartley had pressured them to withdraw financing.

Unocal also brought a lawsuit against Mesa Partners II, T. Boone Pickens, and seven others, contending that the group had purchased Unocal's stock in violation of federal laws. The purpose of the suit was to prevent Pickens and Mesa from voting any of the shares of Unocal stock. Unocal also reduced the quorum needed for its annual meeting in an effort to stymie plans by Pickens to delay the meeting past the closing date of Mesa's offer.

Mesa countered by suing Unocal and several of its directors, seeking a declaratory judgment that recent anti-takeover amendments to Unocal's bylaws were void and thereby unenforceable at Unocal's annual meeting. In a separate suit, Mesa also charged that Unocal violated the laws governing proxy solicitation in connection with the annual meeting.

As Unocal's stock price continued to rise in anticipation of Pickens' success in his bid for Unocal, Hartley launched a defense based on restructuring Unocal's balance sheet. In an effort

Source: John S. DeMott, "High Times for T. Boone Pickens," *Time,* March 4, 1985; Laurie P. Cohen and Daniel Hertzberg, "Mellon Bank Said Ready to Leave Mesa Lending Pool," *The Wall Street Journal,* April 1, 1985; Frederick Rose and James B. Stewart, "Unocal, in Bid to Thwart Pickens, Cuts Votes Needed to Hold Annual Meeting," *The Wall Street Journal,* April 3, 1985; Charles F. McCoy and Frederick Rose, "Unocal Rejects Pickens Takeover Offer as Group Sets $3.9 Billion of Financing," *The Wall Street Journal,* April 15, 1985; Thomas C. Hayes, "Unocal's Chairman Digs In," *New York Times,* April 16, 1985; Frederick Rose and Charles F. McCoy, "Unocal Sets Plan to Buy 49% of Its Stock in Effort to Thwart Takeover by Pickens," *The Wall Street Journal,* April 17, 1985; Fred R. Bleakley, "Spinoff Planned by Unocal: A New Effort to Halt Bid by Pickens," *New York Times,* April 20, 1985; "Unocal, in New Counter to Pickens, Seeks 29% of Its Shares for $72 Each in Notes," *The Wall Street Journal,* April 24, 1985; Laurie P. Cohen and Michael Cieply, "Unocal Is Ordered to Include Pickens in Buyback Offer," *The Wall Street Journal,* April 30, 1985; Frederick Rose, Laurie P. Cohen, and James B. Stewart, "Unocal, Mesa Group Reach Pact to End Takeover Battle for Firm," *The Wall Street Journal,* May 21, 1985; and Fred R. Bleakley, "Pickens to End Bid for Unocal," *New York Times,* May 21, 1985.

to thwart the takeover, he unveiled a conditional plan to buy as much as 49 percent of the company's stock with notes having a total face value of $6.28 billion. The $72-a-share offer would go into effect only if Mesa were successful in its $54-a-share bid for a majority of Unocal's outstanding shares, thereby loading the company with debt and making it a less attractive acquisition.

Pickens dismissed Unocal's offer as "a highly conditional poison pill" and filed lawsuits challenging the offer in the courts. When major institutional shareholders of Unocal stock reacted negatively to the company's buy-back offer, Unocal's executive committee voted to recommend that the company spin off a large portion of its assets into a limited partnership, much of which would be available for sale to the public. The purpose of such a spinoff would be to increase the value of Unocal's assets while making the company a much less attractive target for Mesa.

A week after it made its original offer to conditionally buy back some of its shares at $72, Unocal agreed to buy back 29 percent of its shares at that price unconditionally. In response, Pickens tendered some of the shares held by Mesa in an effort to profit from the $72-per-share offer. A Delaware chancery court ruled that Unocal's $3.6 billion buyback had to include shares tendered by Mesa. However, Mesa's victory was short lived. A few days later the partners were unsuccessful in their attempt to delay the company's annual meeting, and a slate of pro-management directors were elected for the forthcoming year. Then, the Delaware Supreme Court voted to support Unocal's exclusion of Mesa shares from its exchange offer. The group was then faced with the potential of a stock loss amounting to about $300 million once Unocal's share price fell to reflect the impact of the completed offer. As a result, Mesa had no choice but to head to the bargaining table.

One month later, Mesa Partners II headed by T. Boone Pickens reached a settlement with Hartley's Unocal under terms that handed Mr. Pickens his first major defeat in a takeover battle. Under the terms of the agreement, Unocal agreed to expand its announced $72-a-share buyback offer to include 7.7 million of the 23.7 million Unocal shares held by Mesa. In addition, Mesa agreed to sell its remaining Unocal shares under carefully controlled terms as part of an elaborate standstill agreement in which the group won't buy any additional Unocal stock for 25 years.

It was somewhat of a Pyrrhic victory for Fred L. Hartley, Unocal's feisty chairman. In addition to the $3.6 billion in debt the company was forced to take on under its exchange offer, Unocal was expected to add even more debt in order to eventually buy back all of Pickens' group's shares.

QUESTIONS

22-1 Four economic classifications of mergers are *horizontal, vertical, conglomerate,* and *congeneric.* What is the significance of these terms in merger analysis with regard to **(a)** the likelihood of Justice Department intervention and **(b)** possibilities for operating synergy?

22-2 Firm A wants to acquire Firm B. Firm B's management thinks the merger is a good idea. Might a tender offer be used?

22-3 What is the difference between an operating merger and a pure financial merger?

22-4 Two large, publicly owned firms are contemplating a merger. No operating synergy is expected, but returns on the two firms are not perfectly positively correlated, so σ_{EBIT} will be reduced for the combined corporation. One group of consultants argues that this risk reduction is sufficient grounds for the merger. Another group thinks that this type of risk reduction is irrelevant because stockholders can already hold the stock of both companies and thus gain the risk reduction benefits of merger. Whose position is correct?

SELF-TEST PROBLEM

ST-1 Perrin-Stewart, a large conglomerate that has grown in the past through mergers, is analyzing its latest takeover target, Cleburne Pharmaceuticals (CP). Perrin-Stewart's financial analysts have made a projection of CP's cash flows for the next four years. The analysts have assumed that depreciation expense is negligible for this firm. They predict that Cleburne's market value in 1992 will equal 10 times that year's after-tax earnings. Their 4-year projection of CP's postmerger year-end cash flows (in millions of dollars) is reproduced in the following table:

	1989	1990	1991	1992
Sales	$300	$345	$375	$405
Cost of goods sold	195	210	220	225
Sales & administrative expenses	30	40	45	50
EBIT	$ 75	$ 95	$110	$130
Interest	15	18	20	21
EBT	$ 60	$ 77	$ 90	$109
Taxes (34%)	20	26	31	37
Net income	$ 40	$ 51	$ 59	$ 72
Retained earnings	20	26	24	22
Cash available to owners	$ 20	$ 25	$ 35	$ 50
Terminal value				$720
Net cash flow	$ 20	$ 25	$ 35	$770

Cleburne currently has a capital structure of 17 percent debt, but if Perrin-Stewart's merger plans are successful, CP's debt ratio will rise to 55 percent of assets. CP's marginal tax rate will remain at 34 percent after the merger. However, its market-determined beta will rise because of the large increase in debt from a premerger beta of 1.3 to an estimated beta of 1.8. The risk-free rate is 7 percent and the market risk premium, $k_M - R_F$, is 5 percent.

The estimated cash flows that were presented in the table include the additional interest payments required by the increase in leverage and asset expansion. Retained earnings will be used in addition to the new debt to finance required asset expansion. Therefore, the preceding estimated net cash flows are the flows that are expected to accrue to Perrin-Stewart's shareholders.

a. What is the appropriate discount rate for valuing the proposed acquisition?

b. What is Cleburne Pharmaceuticals' value to Perrin-Stewart?

c. Cleburne Pharmaceuticals has 9 million shares outstanding, and its common stock currently sells for $39.75. What is the maximum price per share that Perrin-Stewart should offer for Cleburne's stock?

PROBLEMS

22-1   **Capital budgeting analysis.** Biotech wishes to acquire Garcia Industries for $3,000,000. Biotech expects the merger to provide incremental after-tax earnings of about $550,000 a year for 10 years. At the end of the 10-year period, the book and market value of Garcia Industries will be zero. Management has calculated the marginal cost of capital for this investment to be 14 percent. Conduct a capital budgeting analysis for Biotech to determine whether or not it should purchase Garcia Industries.

22-2   **Capital budgeting analysis.** Shannon Industries wishes to acquire Kennedy Corporation for $3,000,000. Shannon expects the merger to provide incremental after-tax earnings of about $550,000 a year for 10 years. At the end of the 10-year period, the book value of Kennedy will be $1 million, but its cash value will only be $400,000. Management has calculated the marginal cost of capital for this investment to be 12 percent. Conduct a capital budgeting analysis for Shannon to determine whether or not it should purchase Kennedy Corporation.

22-3   **Capital budgeting analysis.** The Lupin Corporation is contemplating the purchase of Sunno Corporation, a maker of tanning preparations and sun screens. Lupin has determined that Sunno's after-tax cash flows, which are $5 million today, will grow at 12 percent annually for the next three years. The growth will slow to a constant 5 percent after that time. If Lupin requires a 14 percent rate of return, what is the maximum price it should be willing to pay for Sunno?

22-4   **Merger analysis.** Universal Products has just purchased Little Corporation for $8 million. Universal's management has decided, however, that Little is "worth more dead than alive," because the expected synergistic advantages of the merger are not possible. Therefore, Universal will sell Little's assets, which have the following book and expected cash values:

Asset	Book Value	Cash Value
Cash	$ 500,000	$ 500,000
Accounts receivable	2,500,000	2,000,000
Inventory	5,000,000	3,000,000
Fixed assets	10,000,000	1,500,000
Total	$18,000,000	$7,000,000

Little has a $500,000 short-term bank loan outstanding with the First National Bank. Universal's marginal tax rate is 40 percent, and its required rate of return is 15 percent.

a. If all divestitures can be accomplished in a one-year period from the date of Little's purchase, what is Universal's rate of return from the divestiture? (*Hint:* Don't forget the tax write-offs that occur when assets are sold at less than book value.)

b. If Universal's growth is largely dependent on acquisitions, what effect might this divestiture have on future growth?

22-5   **Merger analysis.** Simatec, a large conglomerate, is evaluating the possible acquisition of Sunshine Manufacturing Corporation (SMC). Simatec's analysts project the following postmerger data for SMC (in thousands of dollars):

	1989	1990	1991	1992
Net sales	$200	$230	$250	$270
Selling and administrative expenses	20	25	30	32
Interest	10	12	13	14

Tax rate after merger: 40%
Cost of goods sold as a percent of sales: 65%
Beta after merger: 1.63
Risk-free rate: 8%
Market risk premium: 5%
Terminal growth rate of.cash flow available to Simatec: 10%

Note: Data do not add exactly because of rounding errors.

If the acquisition is made, it will occur on January 1, 1989. All cash flows shown in the income statements are assumed to occur at the end of the year. SMC currently has a market value capital structure of 40 percent debt, but Simatec would increase that to 50 percent if the acquisition were made. SMC, if independent, would pay taxes at a rate of 30 percent, but its income would be taxed at 40 percent if it were consolidated. SMC's current market-determined beta is 1.50, and its investment bankers think that its beta would rise to 1.63 if the debt ratio were increased to 50 percent. The cost of goods sold is expected to be 65 percent of sales, but it could vary somewhat. Depreciation-generated funds would be used to replace worn-out equipment, so they would not be available to Simatec's shareholders. The risk-free rate is 8 percent, and the market risk premium is 5 percent.

a. What is the appropriate discount rate for valuing the acquisition?

b. What is the terminal value? What is SMC's value to Simatec?

(Do Part c only if you are using the computerized problem diskette.)

c. 1. If sales in each year were $100 higher than the base case amounts, and if the cost of goods sold/sales ratio were 60 percent, what would SMC be worth to Simatec?

2. With sales and the cost of goods sold ratio at the Part c-1 levels, what would SMC's value be if its beta were 1.8, k_{RF} rose to 10 percent, and RP_M rose to 6 percent?

3. Leaving all values at the Part c-2 levels, what would be the value of the acquisition if the terminal growth rate rose to 18 percent or dropped to 3 percent?

22-6 **Merger analysis.** Cowtown Computer Corporation is considering a merger with Mega Memory, Inc. Mega is a publicly traded company, and its current beta is 1.40. Mega has been barely profitable, so it has paid an average tax rate of only 25 percent in taxes during the last several years. It also uses little debt, having a market-value debt ratio of just 15 percent.

If the acquisition is made, Cowtown plans to operate Mega as a separate, wholly owned subsidiary. Cowtown would pay taxes on a consolidated basis, and thus the tax rate would increase to 34 percent. In addition, Cowtown would increase the debt capitalization in the Mega subsidiary on a market-value basis to 45 percent of assets, which would increase beta to 1.50. Cowtown's acquisition department estimates that Mega, if acquired, would provide the following net cash flows to Cowtown's shareholders (in millions of dollars):

Year	Net Cash Flow
1989	$1.60
1990	1.92
1991	2.25
1992	2.50
1993 and beyond	Constant growth at 6%

These cash flows include all acquisition effects. Cowtown's cost of equity is 12 percent, its beta is 1.0, and its cost of debt is 9.5 percent. The risk-free rate is 8 percent.

a. What discount rate should be used to discount the estimated cash flows? (*Hint:* Use Cowtown's k_s to determine the market risk premium.)

b. What is Mega's dollar value to Cowtown?

c. Mega has 1.5 million common shares outstanding. What is the maximum price per share that Cowtown should offer for Mega? If the tender offer were accepted at this price, what would happen to Cowtown's stock price?

ANSWER TO SELF-TEST PROBLEM

a. The appropriate discount rate, k, is determined as follows:

$$k = R_F + \beta(k_M - R_F)$$

$$= 7\% + 1.8(5\%)$$

$$= 7\% + 9\%$$

$$= 16\%.$$

b. Cleburne Pharmaceuticals' value to Perrin-Stewart is determined by discounting the cash flows that will be available to Perrin-Stewart if it acquires CP. Therefore:

Year	Cash Flow	Discount Factors	Present Value (Millions of Dollars)
1989	$ 20	0.8621	$ 17.2
1990	25	0.7432	18.6
1991	35	0.6407	22.4
1992	770	0.5523	425.3
			$483.5

c. The maximum price that Perrin-Stewart should offer for Cleburne's stock on a per-share basis is:

$$\$483.5 \text{ million/9 million shares} = \$53.72.$$

Therefore, Perrin-Stewart should make its initial offer above the current market price of $39.75 but below its maximum offering price of $53.72.

Chapter 23

Leasing

Although firms generally own fixed assets and report them on their balance sheets, it is the *use* of buildings and equipment that is important, not their ownership per se. One way of obtaining the use of facilities and equipment is to buy them, but an alternative is to lease them. Prior to the 1950s leasing was generally associated with real estate — land and buildings. Today, however, it is possible to lease virtually any kind of fixed asset, and in 1987 about 25 percent of all new capital equipment acquired by businesses was financed through a lease arrangement.

Conceptually, as we show in this chapter, leasing is quite similar to borrowing, and it provides financial leverage. In effect, a lease is a type of debt.[1] Leasing takes several different forms, the three most important of which are (1) *sale-and-leaseback* arrangements, (2) *operating leases,* and (3) straight *financial or capital leases.*

SALE AND LEASEBACK

sale-and-leaseback
An operation whereby a firm sells land, buildings, or equipment to a purchaser and that simultaneously leases the property back for a specified period under specific terms.

lessee
The party leasing a property.

lessor
The owner of the leased property.

Under a **sale-and-leaseback** arrangement, a firm owning land, buildings, or equipment sells the property to another firm and simultaneously executes an agreement to lease the property back for a specified period under specific terms. The purchaser could be an insurance company, a commercial bank, a specialized leasing company, or an individual investor. A sale-and-leaseback arrangement is an alternative to a mortgage.

Note that the seller, or **lessee,** immediately receives the purchase price put up by the buyer, or **lessor.** At the same time the seller-lessee retains the use of the property. This parallel to borrowing is carried over to the lease payment schedule. Under a mortgage loan arrangement, the lending institution receives a series of equal payments just sufficient to amortize the loan and to provide the lender with a specified rate of return on investment. Under a sale-and-leaseback arrangement, the lease payments are set up in exactly the same manner; the payments are sufficient to return the full purchase price to the investor, plus a stated return on the investment.

OPERATING LEASES

operating lease
A lease under which the lessor maintains and services the asset; also called a *service lease.*

An **operating lease,** sometimes called a *service lease,* provides for both *financing* and *maintenance.* IBM is one of the pioneers of the operating lease contract. Computers and office copying machines, as well as automobiles and trucks, are the primary types of equipment involved in service leases. These leases ordinarily call for the lessor to maintain and service the leased equipment, and the maintenance cost is built into the lease payments.

---

[1]Some instructors will prefer to cover this chapter immediately after Chapter 17, which deals with long-term debt. If this is done, it will be necessary to discuss separately the after-tax cost of debt.

Another important characteristic of operating leases is the fact that they are frequently *not fully amortized*. In other words, the payments required under the lease contract are not sufficient to recover the full cost of the equipment. However, the lease contract is written for a considerably shorter period than the expected life of the leased equipment, and the lessor expects to recover all costs either from subsequent renewal payments, by leasing the equipment to others, or through sale of the leased equipment.

A final feature of operating leases is that they often contain a *cancellation clause* giving the lessee the right to cancel the lease and return the equipment before the expiration of the basic lease agreement. This is an important consideration, for it means that the equipment can be returned if it is rendered obsolete by technological developments or is simply no longer needed by the lessee.

FINANCIAL LEASES

A **financial lease,** sometimes called a *capital lease,* is different from an operating lease in three respects: (1) it does *not* provide for maintenance, (2) it is *not* cancelable, and (3) it *is* fully amortized (that is, the lessor receives rental payments equal to the full price of the leased equipment plus a return on investment). The typical arrangement involves the following steps:

Step 1 The firm that will use the equipment (the lessee) selects the specific items it requires and negotiates the price and delivery terms with the manufacturer.

Step 2 The user firm then negotiates terms with the leasing company and, once the terms are set, arranges to have the lessor buy the equipment from the manufacturer or the distributor. When the equipment is purchased, the user firm simultaneously executes the lease agreement. The terms of the lease call for full amortization of the lessor's investment, plus a rate of return on the unamortized balance close to the percentage rate the lessee would have to pay on a secured term loan. For example, if the lessee would have to pay 12 percent for a term loan, a rate of about 12 percent would be built into the lease contract. The lessee is generally given an option to renew the lease at a reduced rental on expiration of the basic lease. However, the basic lease usually cannot be canceled unless the lessor is completely paid off. Also, the lessee generally pays the property taxes and insurance on the leased property. Because the lessor receives a return *after,* or *net of,* these payments, this type of lease is often called a "net, net" lease.

Financial leases are almost the same as sale-and-leaseback arrangements, the major difference being that the leased equipment is new and the lessor buys it from a manufacturer or a distributor instead of from the user-lessee. A sale and leaseback then, may be thought of as a special type of financial lease. Both sale-and-leaseback arrangements and financial leases are analyzed in the same manner.

financial lease
A lease that does not provide for maintenance service, is not cancelable, and covers the entire expected life of the equipment; also called a *capital lease.*

INDUSTRY PRACTICE

Microcomputers: To Buy, Or . . . To Lease?

Small businesses have entered the computer age. All kinds of businesses — from auto parts stores to physicians' offices — are using microcomputers for data processing, accounting, preparing invoices, and word processing. For more and more small businesses, the question is no longer should we buy a computer but what sort of computer should we buy? Often, the most important question is how should we pay for it? Indeed, choosing a computer and software package may be the easiest part of acquiring one.

Small businesses are confronted with an often baffling array of lease and purchase options made more complex by the Tax Reform Act of 1986, which changed the incentives for purchasers of computers. To make matters even more complicated, smaller companies are particularly vulnerable to the consequences of poor decisions regarding choosing and paying for computer systems.

It is no wonder that leasing has become such an attractive option to so many businesses. For one thing, equipment leasing passes the risk of fast-changing technology on to someone else (the lessor). It also conserves cash, hedges against inflation, involves less documentation and paperwork than a purchase, and requires no depreciation schedule.

Besides the non-tax reasons for leasing, there are two tax-related incentives. First, companies that can't use all of their depreciation deductions may be able to lower their leasing costs by leasing from someone who can use the depreciation credits — and is willing to charge a lower lease rate for the privilege. Also, compa-

Source: "Tax Incentives Make Leasing Look Better," John Pierson, *The Office,* July 1987, 56, and "Micros in Small Business: Lease Vs. Buy Decision," James Deliale, Ph.D., Larry Giunipero, Ph.D., and William Hillison, Ph.D., *Journal of Systems Management* May 12, 1987, 12–17.

nies that acquire their equipment during the last quarter of the tax year may be able to boost the number of their depreciation deductions by leasing.

The second tax incentive boils down to three letters: AMT, otherwise known as the Alternative Minimum Tax. This provision of the Tax Reform Act of 1986 is a radically new tax provision designed to make sure that all companies pay at least some tax. The new AMT is separate from the regular corporate tax and increases the amount of liability for many companies. If a company plans to acquire computer equipment, leasing can be part of its strategy for reducing AMT's impact. Lease and rental payments can be recorded as an ordinary expense item instead of as a liability. Lease rentals do not require an AMT adjustment and will not push book income higher than tax income.

Here's a simplified example of how the AMT system works and how it can make equipment leasing attractive.

Say a company has a net revenue of $350,000 and acquires a $1 million piece of equipment. If the company has an AMT adjustment of $75,000, which is the amount by which its first-year accelerated depreciation exceeds its straight-line book depreciation, the AMT will be $4,800 more than the regular tax. In fact, AMT has boosted the company's effective tax rate from 34% to 39%.

A company acquiring either computers or general, industrial machinery would pay about 3% less in equipment costs if it leased, rather than bought, the equipment, according to Barry L. Dennis, a senior manager for tax economics at Price Waterhouse.

But the decision is often not just a simple one of whether to lease or to buy. There are a variety of lease forms from which to choose. They can be classified into two basic types: "capital" and "operating." A capital lease is treated in almost the same way as a purchase and must be capitalized (shown as an asset and a corresponding liability) on the balance sheet of the lessee. The asset is systematically depreciated over time and the depreciation reflected as an expense on the income statement. The Financial Accounting Standards Board establishes four major criteria for capital leases. If any one of the criteria is met, the lease is considered a capital lease: (1) The lease transfers ownership of the property to the lessee by the end of the lease term; (2) the lease contains an option for the lessee to purchase the equipment at significantly less than current market value; (3) the lease term is equal to 75% or more of the estimated economic life of the leased property; or (4) the present value of the minimum lease payments is equal to 90% or more of the equipment cost (less any tax credit) when retained by the lessor.

A lease that does not fall into one or more of these categories would be considered an operating lease. Typically, the term of an operating lease is for a period considerably less than the asset's useful life. Operating leases are essentially a form of rental agreement. The monthly payments are treated as expenses and reflected as deductions from revenue on the income statement. The operating lease is not reflected on the balance sheet.

Operating leases have very specific advantages. A short-term operating lease can be used as a trial period during which the new system can be tested in the actual operating environment prior to making a long-term commitment for the system. If the system is not a success, the small business owner suffers only a short-term loss over the lease period and is not confronted with the problem of how to get rid of a system that really isn't filling the company's needs.

Operating leases also leave capital available for other, more profitable purposes. Instead of requiring a large, lump-sum outlay, the lessee is required to make a series of smaller payments. This can be critical for a small business since profits result from the use of the equipment, not its ownership.

Another benefit of leasing is that many of the responsibilities of ownership are sidestepped by the lessee. For example, the lessor is usually responsible for maintenance and often leases provide for replacement equipment for the lessee while equipment is being serviced, cutting down on downtime and its associated costs.

But leasing is not without its drawbacks and the choice is by no means always clear. In general, leasing is more expensive than purchase both in terms of direct dollar outlays and present value terms. This is true because the lessor must charge a premium for accepting the risk of obsolescence of the equipment, overhead costs, and profit. The lessee may also restrict equipment use in order to regulate wear-and-tear on mechanical and electrical components. The lessor may also restrict use of off-brand expansion boards and peripherals, forcing the lessee to pay a premium for name brands.

INTERNAL REVENUE SERVICE REQUIREMENTS FOR A LEASE

The full amount of the annual lease payment is a deductible expense for income tax purposes *provided the Internal Revenue Service agrees that a particular contract is a genuine lease and not simply an installment loan called a lease.* It is therefore important for a lease contract to be written in a form acceptable to the Internal Revenue Service. The IRS will emphasize the follow-

Table 23-1 **Balance Sheet Effects of Leasing**

Before Asset Increase			After Asset Increase						
Firms P and L			**Firm P, Which Borrows and Purchases**			**Firm L, Which Leases**			
Total assets		Debt	$ 50	Total assets		Debt	$150	Total assets		Debt	$ 50

Firms P and L: Total assets $100; Debt $50; Equity $50; $100.
Firm P, Which Borrows and Purchases: Total assets $200; Debt $150; Equity $50; $200.
Firm L, Which Leases: Total assets $100; Debt $50; Equity $50; $100.

ing factors when deciding whether or not a given contract is a bona fide lease transaction for tax purposes:

1. Length of the lease period. A lease that calls for payments approximating the cost of the asset over a relatively short period may be considered a sale by the IRS.

2. Renewal options. After the initial lease period, the original lessee may be given an opportunity to match an outside offer to lease the equipment but may not be given preferential consideration over other potential lessees.

3. Purchase options. After the initial lease period, the original lessee should be given equal parity with an outside offer to purchase the property.

Therefore, a rapid payment period followed by a noncompetitive renewal or purchase option is a clear sign to the IRS that the so-called lease is indeed a purchase for tax purposes. The IRS is concerned that without restrictions, a company could set up a "lease" transaction calling for very rapid payments, which would be tax deductible. The effect would be to depreciate the equipment over a much shorter period than its ACRS-class life. For example, if a $3 million airplane with a 10-year life were leased for 3 years, then purchased under a purchase option for $1 or renewed for $1 a year, this would have the same cash flow effect as depreciating the airplane in 3 years rather than over 10 years.

EFFECTS OF LEASING ON A FIRM'S BALANCE SHEET

off-balance-sheet financing

Financing wherein for many years neither the leased assets nor the liabilities under the lease contract appeared on the lessee's balance sheet; problem corrected by FASB #13.

Even though lease payments are shown as operating expenses on the income statement, under certain conditions neither the leased assets nor the resulting liabilities created by these lease contracts appear on a firm's balance sheet. For this reason, leasing is sometimes referred to as **off-balance-sheet financing.** This point is illustrated in Table 23-1 by the balance sheets of two hypothetical firms, P (for Purchase) and L (for Lease). Initially the balance sheets of both firms are identical, and both firms have debt ratios of 50 percent. Next, each firm decides to acquire assets costing $100. Firm P borrows $100 to make the purchase, so both an asset and a liability go on its balance sheet, and its debt ratio is increased to 75 percent. Firm L leases the equipment. The lease may call for fixed charges as high as or even higher than the loan, and the obligations assumed under the lease may be equally or more dangerous from the standpoint of financial analysis, but the firm's debt ratio will remain at 50 percent.

To correct this problem, the Financial Accounting Standards Board issued FASB #13, which requires that, for an unqualified audit report, firms entering into financial (or capital) leases must restate their balance sheets to report the leased asset under fixed assets and the present value of the future lease payments as a debt.[2] This process is called **capitalizing the lease,** and its net effect is to cause Firms P and L to have similar balance sheets, both of which will, in essence, resemble the one shown in the table for Firm P.

The logic behind FASB #13 is as follows. If a firm signs a lease contract, its obligation to make lease payments is just as binding as payments under a loan agreement; the failure to make lease payments can bankrupt a firm just as fast as the failure to make principal and interest payments on a loan. Therefore, for all intents and purposes, a financial lease is identical to a loan. This being the case, a firm's signing of a lease agreement has the effect of raising its debt ratio and thus changing its current capital structure. If the firm had previously established a target capital structure, additional equity financing would be required to return the capital structure to its optimal point whether debt or lease financing was implemented.

If disclosure of the lease in the Table 23-1 example was not made, Firm L's investors could be deceived into thinking that its financial position is stronger than it really is. Even if the lease was disclosed in a footnote, investors might not fully recognize the impact of leases and might perceive Firms P and L as being in the same financial position. If this were the case, leasing could alter the capital structure decision in a really significant manner; a firm could increase its true leverage through a lease arrangement with a smaller effect on its cost of conventional debt (k_d) and on its cost of equity (k_s). Consequently its average cost of capital, k_a, would increase less than that for Firm P, which borrowed directly. Thus investors would be willing to pay a higher price for Firm L because they would view it as being in a stronger financial position than Firm P. These benefits would accrue to existing investors at the expense of new investors, who were deceived because the balance sheet did not reflect the firm's true liability situation. This is why FASB #13 was issued.

A lease is classified as a capital lease, and hence is capitalized and shown directly on the balance sheet, if one or more of the following conditions exist:

1. Under the terms of the lease, ownership of the property is effectively transferred from the lessor to the lessee.

2. The lessee can purchase the property at less than its true market value when the lease expires.

capitalizing the lease
Incorporating the lease provisions into the balance sheet by reporting the leased asset under fixed assets and reporting the present value of future lease payments as debt; required by FASB #13.

---

[2]FASB #13, "Accounting for Leases" (November 1976). This document spells out in detail the conditions under which the lease must be capitalized and the procedures for doing so.

3. The lease runs for a period equal to or greater than 75 percent of the asset's life. Thus, if an asset has a 10-year life and the lease is written for 8 years, the lease must be capitalized.

4. The present value of the lease payments is equal to or greater than 90 percent of the initial value of the asset, minus any tax credit taken by the lessor.[3]

These rules, together with strong footnote disclosure rules for operating leases, certainly should be sufficient to insure that no one will be fooled by lease financing and thus that leases will be regarded as debt and will have the same effects as debt on k_d and k_s. Therefore, leasing is not likely to permit a firm to use more financial leverage than could be obtained with conventional debt.

EVALUATING LEASE PROPOSALS

In the typical case, the events leading to a lease arrangement follow the sequence described in this section. There is a great deal of uncertainty about the theoretically correct way to evaluate lease versus purchase decisions, and some complex decision models have been developed to aid in the analysis. However, the simple **lease evaluation** analysis given here is accurate enough for every case we have encountered.

lease evaluation
The analysis of the firm's cash flows under lease or purchase alternatives to determine the lower present value of costs.

1. The firm decides to acquire a particular building or piece of equipment; this decision is based on regular capital budgeting procedures. The decision to acquire the machine is not at issue in the typical lease analysis — this decision was made previously as part of the capital budgeting process. In a lease analysis the firm's management is concerned simply with whether to obtain the use of the asset by lease or by purchase via a loan. However, if the effective cost of the lease is substantially lower than the cost of debt (and this could occur for a number of reasons, including the situation in which the lessor is able to use depreciation tax shelters but the lessee is not) the cost of capital used in capital budgeting will have to be recalculated, and, perhaps, projects formerly deemed unacceptable may become acceptable.

2. Once the firm has decided to acquire the asset, the next question is how to finance its acquisition. Because well-run businesses do not have excess cash lying around, new assets must be financed in some manner.

3. Funds to purchase the asset could be obtained by borrowing, by retaining earnings, or by selling stock, or the asset could be leased.

As indicated at the beginning of this chapter, a financial lease is comparable to a loan in the sense that the firm is required to make a specified series

---

[3]The discount rate used to calculate the present value of the lease payments must be the lower of (1) the rate used by the lessor to establish the lease payments or (2) the rate of interest the lessee would have to pay for new debt with a maturity equal to that of the lease.

of payments and that failure to meet these payments can result in bankruptcy. Thus, it is most appropriate to compare lease financing with debt financing. The lease versus borrow-and-purchase analysis is illustrated with data on the Carter Chemical Company. The following conditions are assumed:

1. Carter plans to acquire equipment costing $2 million delivered and installed.

2. Carter can borrow the required $2 million through a 10 percent loan to be amortized over 5 years. The loan will call for payments of $527,593.12 per year, calculated as follows:

$$\text{Payment} = \frac{\$2,000,000}{\text{DFa } (10\%, 5 \text{ years})} = \frac{\$2,000,000}{3.7908} = \$527,593.12.$$

3. The equipment definitely will be used for 5 years, at which time its estimated after-tax salvage value will be $143,000. If the operation is profitable, Carter will continue to use the equipment.

4. Carter can lease the equipment for 5 years at a rental charge of $560,000 per year, but the lessor will own it at the expiration of the lease. (The lease payment schedule is established by the potential lessor, and Carter can accept it, reject it, or negotiate.) If Carter plans to continue using the equipment, a purchase arrangement will have to be negotiated with the lessor. We assume that Carter will be able to buy the equipment at its estimated salvage value, $143,000.

5. The lease contract calls for the lessor to maintain the equipment.[4] If Carter borrows and purchases, it will have to bear the cost of maintenance, which will be performed by the equipment manufacturer at a contracted cost of $100,000 per year.

6. The equipment falls in the ACRS 5-year-class life, and for this analysis we assume that Carter's effective tax rate is 40 percent.

Table 23-2 shows the steps involved in the analysis. Columns 2 through 10 are devoted to the costs of borrowing and purchasing. Within this set, Columns 2 through 5 give the loan amortization schedule; Column 6 shows the maintenance expense; and Column 7 gives depreciation charges. Tax-deductible expenses — interest, maintenance, and depreciation — are summed and presented in Column 8, whereas Column 9 shows the taxes saved because Carter has these deductions. Column 10 summarizes the preceding columns and gives the annual net cash outflows Carter will incur if it borrows and purchases the equipment.

---

[4]We have distinguished between operating leases, which usually provide maintenance, and financial leases, which usually do not. Most issues are negotiable, however, and in this case we have a financial lease in which the lessor has agreed to provide maintenance. In all other respects this lease is similar to the financial leases discussed earlier in the chapter.

Table 23-2 **Carter Chemical Company:**
Lease versus Purchase Analysis
(Thousands of Dollars)

Applicable to Net Cost of Owning

	Loan Amortization Schedule					
Year (1)	**Total Payment (2)**	**Interest (3)**	**Amortization Payment (4)**	**Remaining Balance (5)**	**Maintenance Cost (6)**	**Depreciation (7)**
1	$ 527.6	$200.0	$ 327.6	$1,672.4	100	$ 400
2	527.6	167.2	360.4	1,312.0	100	640
3	527.6	131.2	396.4	915.6	100	400
4	527.6	91.6	436.0	479.6	100	280
5	527.6	48.0	479.6	0	100	280
5[a]	—	—	—	—	—	
	$2,638.0	$638.0	$2,000.0			$2,000

[a]Two lines are shown for Year 5 in order to account for the salvage value, $143,000.
[b]Assume the appropriate ACRS percentages are: Year 1, 20%; Year 2, 32%; Year 3, 20%; Years 4 and 5, 14%.

Notes:
1. The net advantage to leasing could be calculated by subtracting Column 11 from Column 10, then discounting these differences. This procedure is more efficient, hence preferable in actual practice, but the procedure used here is better for explanatory purposes.
2. Leases often involve payments at the *beginning* of the period rather than at the end. Also, a down payment may be required under either the lease or the loan. In either event, it would be necessary to set up a "0" year to show payments made at time zero.
3. Students may wish to review the construction of loan amortization tables in Chapter 13.

The lease payments are to be $560,000 per year; this rate, which includes maintenance, was established by the prospective lessor and offered to Carter. If Carter accepts the lease, the full $560,000 will be a deductible expense, so the after-tax cost of the lease will be calculated as follows:

$$After\text{-}tax\ cost = Lease\ payment - Tax\ savings$$

$$= Lease\ payment - (Tax\ rate)(Lease\ payment)$$

$$= Lease\ payment\ (1 - Tax\ rate)$$

$$= \$560,000(1 - 0.4)$$

$$= \$336,000.$$

This amount is shown in Column 11, Years 1 through 5.

Notice that the last entry in Column 11, the $143,000 shown under Year 5, represents the $143,000 expected Year 5 purchase price. We include this

			Applicable to Lease		Comparative Costs	
Tax-Deductible Expense = 3 + 6 + 7 (8)	Tax Savings = (0.4)(8) (9)	Cash Outflow If Owned = 2 + 6 − 9 (10)	Lease Cost after Tax = (1 − 0.4) (Lease Cost) (11)	DFs for 6% (12)	Present Value of the Cost of Owning = 10 × 12 (13)	Present Value of the Cost of Leasing = 11 × 12 (14)
$700.0	$280.0	$347.6	$336.0	0.9434	$ 327.9	$ 317.0
907.2	362.9	264.7	336.0	0.8900	235.6	299.0
631.2	252.5	375.1	336.0	0.8396	314.9	282.1
471.6	188.6	439.0	336.0	0.7921	347.7	266.1
428.0	171.2	456.4	336.0	0.7473	341.1	251.1
			143.0	0.7473	—	106.9
					$1,567.2	$1,522.2

Net advantage to leasing = $1,567.2 − $1,522.2 = $45

amount as a cost of leasing on the assumption that Carter will want to continue the operation and thus will be forced to purchase the equipment from the lessor. If we assumed that the operation would not be continued, we would put the $143,000 into Column 10 as an inflow; that is, it would have a minus sign.

The next step is to compare the net cost of owning with the net cost of leasing. However, the annual cash flows of leasing and borrowing must first be put on a common basis. This requires converting them to present values, which brings up the question of the proper rate at which to discount the costs. In Chapter 15 we saw that the riskier the cash flow, the higher the discount rate used to find present values. This principle, observed in our discussion of capital budgeting, applies to lease analysis as well. Just how risky are the cash flows under consideration here? Most of them are relatively certain, at least compared to the types of cash flow estimates that were developed in capital budgeting. For example, the loan payment schedule is set by contract, as is the lease payment schedule. The depreciation expenses are also established and not subject to change, and the $100,000 annual maintenance cost is fixed by contract as well. The tax savings are somewhat uncertain, but they will be as projected so long as Carter's effective tax rate remains at 40 percent. The residual value is the least certain of the cash flows, but even here Carter's management is fairly certain that it will want to acquire the property, and hence will incur the $143,000 outlay in Year 5.

Because the cash flows under the lease and the borrow-and-purchase alternatives are both relatively certain, they should be discounted at a relatively low rate. Most analysts recommend that the company's cost of debt be used, and this rate seems reasonable in this instance. In this instance, since all the cash flows are on an after-tax basis, *the after-tax cost of debt, which is 6 percent, should be used.* Accordingly, we multiply the cash outflows in Columns 10 and 11 by the 6 percent DFs given in Column 12. The resulting present values are shown in Columns 13 and 14; when these columns are summed, we have the net present values of the costs of owning and leasing. The financing method that produces the smaller present value of cost is the one that should be selected. The example shown in Table 23-2 indicates that leasing has the advantage over buying: the present value of the cost of leasing is $45,000 less than that of buying. In this instance it is to Carter's advantage to lease.

Lease Evaluation by the Lessor

A lease must be economically viable for both the lessee and the lessor. So far we have considered a lease only from the lessee's viewpoint, but, of course, any prospective lease must also be evaluated by the lessor, who may be a specialized leasing company, a bank or bank affiliate, a manufacturer like IBM that uses leasing as a sales tool, or even an individual or a group of individuals. The lessor needs to know the potential profitability of the lease, and this information is also useful to the prospective lessee. Since lease terms are often negotiated, it is helpful to have an idea of how far negotiations can go before the lease is unprofitable for either party.

The lessor's analysis involves (1) determining the net cash outlay, which is usually the invoice price of the leased property minus any lease payments made in advance; (2) determining the periodic cash inflows, which consist of the lease payments minus both income taxes and the lessor's maintenance expense (if maintenance has been negotiated into the lease agreement); (3) estimating the *residual value* of the property at the end of the lease period; and (4) determining whether the rate of return on the lease exceeds the lessor's opportunity cost, or equivalently, whether the NPV of the proposed lease exceeds zero.

To illustrate the lessor's analysis, we will assume the same facts from the lease evaluation made in the previous section by Carter Chemical. Carter Chemical wishes to lease the equipment from General Leasing Corporation, one of the nation's largest general leasing firms. General Leasing can purchase the equipment desired by Carter Chemical for $2 million. The leasing firm's combined state and federal tax rate is 40 percent. If the lease is not consummated, General Leasing will invest the funds in a project that yields 5 percent after taxes. The property's estimated after-tax residual value at the end of the lease period is $143,000.

The lease analysis from General Leasing's standpoint is developed in Table 23-3. Here we see that the net present value of the lease is $10,000. Thus the

Table 23-3 **General Leasing's Lease Analysis (Thousands of Dollars)**

Year (1)	Lease Payment (2)	Maintenance Expense (3)	Depreciation (4)	Taxes (2 − 3 − 4)(t) (5)	Cash Flow (2 − 3 − 5) (6)	DF at 5.0% (7)	PV of After-Tax Cash Flow (8)
1	$560	$100	$400	$24	$436	0.9524	$ 415
2	560	100	640	(72)	532	0.9070	483
3	560	100	400	24	436	0.8638	377
4	560	100	280	72	388	0.8227	319
5	560	100	280	72	388	0.7835	304
5		After-tax residual value			143	0.7835	112
					PV of the lease investment		$2,010
					Less: Cost		$2,000
					NPV of the lease investment		$ 10

firm is better off leasing the equipment to Carter Chemical than investing in the alternative project. Because the lease is also advantageous to Carter Chemical, the transaction should be completed.

FACTORS THAT AFFECT LEASING DECISIONS

Although the basic method of analysis set forth in Table 23-2 is sufficient to handle most situations, certain factors warrant additional comment.

Estimated Residual Value

It is important to note that the lessor owns the property at the expiration of a lease. The value of the property at that time is called its **residual value.** Superficially, it appears that when residual values are expected to be large, owning has an advantage over leasing. This apparent advantage of owning is subject to substantial qualification, however. If residual values are large, as they may be under inflation for certain types of equipment and also if real estate is involved, competition among leasing companies and other financial sources will force leasing rates down to the point where potential residual values are fully recognized in the lease contract rates. Thus the existence of large residual values on equipment is not likely to result in materially lower costs of owning.

residual value
The market value of an asset at the end of its lease term.

Increased Credit Availability

Leasing is sometimes said to provide an advantage for firms seeking the maximum degree of financial leverage. First, it is frequently stated that firms can obtain more money for longer terms under a lease arrangement than under a secured loan agreement for the purchase of a specific piece of equipment. Second, because some leases do not appear on the balance sheet, lease financing has been said to give the firm the appearance of being stronger in a *super-*

ficial credit analysis and thus to permit the firm to use more leverage than it could use if it did not lease.

There is probably some truth to these claims for smaller firms. Now that large firms are required to capitalize major leases and report them on their balance sheets, however, this point is of questionable validity for these firms.

SUMMARY

This chapter has analyzed the three major types of leases: (1) *operating leases,* (2) *sale-and-leaseback plans,* and (3) *financial leases for new assets.* Operating, or service, leases provide for the financing of an asset as well as for its maintenance, whereas both sale-and-leaseback plans and regular financial leases provide only financing and are alternatives to debt financing.

Financial leases (and sale-and-leaseback plans) are evaluated by a cash flow analysis. First it is assumed that an asset will be acquired and that the acquisition will be financed either by debt or by a lease. Next, the annual net cash outflows associated with each financing plan are determined. Finally, the two sets of outflows are discounted at the company's after-tax cost of debt, and the alternative with the lower present value of costs is chosen.

Leasing sometimes represents off-balance-sheet financing, which can permit firms to obtain more financial leverage if they employ leasing than if they use straight debt. This was formerly cited as a major reason for leasing. Today, however, taxes are the primary reason for the growth of financial leasing. Leasing permits the tax savings to be transferred from the user of an asset to the supplier of capital, and if these parties are in different tax brackets, both can benefit from the lease arrangement.

 ## RESOLUTION TO DECISION IN FINANCE

Sandy's Gamble

By tradition, airplane manufacturers have always insisted on selling their products either directly to the airlines or to leasing companies that then lease to the carriers for 15 years or longer. But Sandy McDonnell decided to break that tradition with short-term, fly-before-buy

Source: Adapted from "Sandy's Gamble," *Forbes,* December 20, 1982, 79–85; and "A Leasing Plan to Keep Jet Production Rolling," *Business Week,* October 11, 1982, 34–35.

leasing deals that he hoped to convert to sales when the economy improved.

McDonnell's first customer, in October 1982, was American Airlines, which took a 5-year lease on 20 DC-9-80s, with the option of a 13-year extension. The plan called for American to make lease payments of about $180,000 per plane per month — roughly what the interest would have been on the original price. To sweeten the deal, the airline would run virtually no risk: it would have no cash tied up in down payments, and on 30 days' notice, it could return the planes for a penalty of less than $2 million per plane. McDonnell worked out similar deals with TWA and Alitalia shortly thereafter.

Leasing was a daring route for Sandy McDonnell to take. He had to raise around $450 million to fund production and finance ownership on the American and TWA deals. McDonnell Douglas itself put up about 75 percent of the money, while its suppliers, such as engine maker Pratt & Whitney, put up the rest. The net effect of the leasing deals would depress McDonnell Douglas's earnings for at least 3 years. From Sandy McDonnell's point of view, that was a necessary price to pay for all the benefits the company would receive.

Most important was the fact that the leasing deals filled the production lines and averted the plant shutdown that everyone had dreaded. In the process they attracted new interest in the company's products, squelched rumors that McDonnell Douglas might abandon the commercial airplane market, and instilled confidence that the DC-9-80 would not become obsolete for at least 5 years. The leases also created goodwill because they enabled airlines to acquire the efficient planes they needed but couldn't afford to buy or lease conventionally.

Of course, the biggest risk to McDonnell Douglas is that the planes might be returned. But the company is sure that once the airlines fly the planes, they'll like them and keep them. Even if American does return its planes after 5 years, it will have paid between 25 percent and 40 percent of their cost and McDonnell Douglas will have depreciated them to less than market value. "We're strong enough financially to get them all back," says a company official.

Although the leases may penalize McDonnell Douglas's short-term profits, they may ensure the viability of the company that Sandy McDonnell's uncle founded more than 45 years ago. It's still too soon to predict the final outcome of Sandy's gamble, but you have to give him and his board credit for courage, innovation, and farsightedness.

QUESTIONS

23-1 Distinguish between operating and financial leases. Would a firm be more likely to finance a fleet of trucks or a manufacturing plant with an operating lease?

23-2 The 1986 Tax Act lowered tax rates for individuals and corporations and eliminated the Investment Tax Credit. How might these changes affect the economic viability of leasing in the future?

23-3 Discuss a sale-and-leaseback arrangement.

23-4 One alleged advantage of leasing voiced in the past was that it kept liabilities off the balance sheet, thus making it possible for a firm to obtain more leverage than it otherwise could have. This raised the question of whether or not both the lease obligation and the asset involved should be capitalized and shown on the balance sheet. Discuss the pros and cons of capitalizing leases and the related assets.

23-5 Suppose that there were no IRS restrictions on what constituted a valid lease. Why should some restrictions be imposed? Explain in a manner that a legislator might understand.

23-6 What are the advantages and disadvantages of leveraged leases from the standpoint of **(a)** the lessee, **(b)** the equity investor in the lease, and **(c)** the supplier of the debt capital?

23-7 Suppose Congress enacted new tax law changes that would (1) permit equipment to be depreciated over a shorter period, (2) lower corporate tax rates, and (3) reinstate and increase the investment tax credit. How would each of these potential changes affect the relative volume of leasing (versus conventional debt) in the U.S. economy?

SELF-TEST PROBLEM

ST-1 It is January 2, 1990, and the Bay City Construction Company has decided to acquire a new earthmover immediately. One alternative is to lease the earthmover from the manufacturer on a 4-year contract, with payments of $25,000 per year to be made at the *beginning* of each year. The lease would include maintenance. Alternatively, Bay City could purchase the earthmover outright for $100,000, financing it with a loan from a bank for the net purchase price and amortizing the loan over a 4-year period at an interest rate of 10 percent per year. Under the borrow-to-purchase arrangement, Bay City would have to maintain the earthmover at a cost of $2,500 per year, payable at year-end. The earthmover falls into the ACRS 3-year class, and it has an after-tax salvage value of $16,500 after 4 years, at which time Bay City plans to replace it regardless of whether it leases or buys. Bay City's marginal tax rate is 34 percent.
  a. What is Bay City's present value (PV) cost of leasing?
  b. What is Bay City's PV cost of owning? Should the earthmover be leased or purchased?
  c. The appropriate discount rate for use in Bay City's analysis is the firm's after-tax cost of debt. Why?
  d. The salvage value is the least certain cash flow in the analysis. How might Bay City incorporate the higher riskiness of this cash flow into the analysis?

PROBLEMS

23-1 **Establishing lease payments.** Sav-U-Lease specializes in leasing trucks and equipment to construction firms in the metropolitan Miami area. Wells-Crocker Construction wishes to lease $1.5 million in equipment from Sav-U-Lease for a 5-year period. What is the annual lease payment Wells-Crocker would pay if the lease is based on a 12 percent lease rate? The lease payments are to be made at the end of each year. (Note that the 12 percent rate is simply the rate used to establish the lease payments; it is not Sav-U-Lease's rate of return.)

23-2 **Establishing lease payments.** Refer to Problem 23-1. What would the annual lease payments be if Sav-U-Lease required lease payments to be made at the beginning of the year rather than at the end of the year? Note that 5 payments will be made, with the first due immediately.

23-3 **Balance sheet effects.** Two trucking firms, Fast Freight and Robertson Transfer, began operations with identical balance sheets. A year later, both required additional trucks and trailers that cost $1 million. Fast Freight obtained a 5-year, $1 million loan at a 12 percent interest rate from its bank. Robertson, on the other hand, decided to lease the trucks from Alabama Leasing for 5 years; a 12 percent return was built into the lease. The balance sheet for each company, before the asset increases, was as follows:

		Debt	$1,000,000
		Equity	2,000,000
Total assets	$3,000,000	Total claims	$3,000,000

    a. Show the balance sheet of each firm after the asset increase, and calculate each firm's new debt ratio.

    b. Show how Robertson's balance sheet would look immediately after the financing if it had capitalized the lease.

    c. Would the rate of return on assets and equity be affected by the choice of financing. How?

23-4   **Lessor's analysis.** Golden State Leasing Company has been approached by Dallas Paper to arrange lease financing for $25 million in equipment. The lease would cover a 10-year period. The leased assets are expected to have little or no residual value at the end of the lease period. If Dallas Paper proposes a lease payment of $5.5 million at the end of each of the next 10 years, what rate of return would Golden State earn? Assume that Golden State depreciates assets on a straight-line basis and has a combined state and federal marginal tax rate of 40 percent.

23-5   **Lessor's analysis.** Refer to Problem 23-4. If the leased assets are 5-year class property for tax purposes and ACRS is used to depreciate these assets (rather than straight line), what is the effect on the NPV and IRR of the lease for Golden State? No computations are necessary.

23-6   **Lessor's analysis.** Hemphill Leasing is negotiating a lease contract with Cochran Research Corporation. Cochran claims it can lease equipment worth $3 million from Rival Leasing for an annual payment of $1.3 million payable at the end of each year. In light of their long-standing business relationship, Cochran asks Hemphill if it will match Rival's lease terms.

    If Hemphill enters into the lease agreement, it would depreciate the equipment on a straight-line basis. This equipment will be valueless at the end of the 3-year lease period. If Hemphill requires a 12 percent rate of return and has a 40 percent marginal tax rate, should it meet Rival's proposed lease terms?

23-7   **Lease versus buy.** Condor Air Service, a small commuter airline, is negotiating a lease of a small airplane with Capital Leasing. The airplane can be purchased by Capital from Airway Engineering for $5 million. Capital's lease terms call for 5 annual end-of-year payments of $1.2 million each. As an alternative to leasing, the firm can borrow from a regional bank and buy the airplane. The $5 million would be borrowed on an amortized term loan at a 12 percent interest rate for 5 years. Airplanes of this type fall into the ACRS 5-year class and have an expected after-tax residual value of $500,000. Maintenance costs would be included in the lease. If the airplane is purchased, a maintenance contract can be obtained that calls for $50,000 payments made at the beginning of each year. Condor will sell the fully depreciated airplane at the end of 5 years, or if the airplane is leased, it will not renew the lease. Condor's marginal tax rate is 20 percent. Should Condor lease the airplane from Capital Leasing? Assume the ACRS percentages in effect during the lease period are: Year 1, 20%; Year 2, 30%; Year 3, 20%; Years 4 and 5, 15%.

23-8   **Lease versus buy.** West Virginia Coal Company must install $1 million of new machinery in its Kanawha Valley mine. It can obtain a bank loan for 100 percent of the required amount. Alternatively, a Charleston investment banking firm which represents a group of investors believes that it can arrange for a lease financing plan. Assume that these facts apply:

1. The equipment falls in the ACRS 5-year class.

2. Estimated maintenance expenses are $50,000 per year.

3. West Virginia Coal's tax rate is 20 percent.

4. If the money is borrowed, the bank loan will be at a rate of 14 percent, amortized in 5 equal installments at the end of each year.

5. The tentative lease terms call for payments of $240,000 per year for 5 years.

6. Under the proposed lease terms, the lessee must pay for insurance, property taxes, and maintenance.

7. West Virginia Coal must use the equipment if it is to continue in business, so it will almost certainly want to acquire the property at the end of the lease. If it does, under the lease terms it can purchase the machinery at its fair market value at that time. The best estimate of this market value is the $200,000 salvage value, but it could be much higher or lower under certain circumstances.

To assist management in making the proper lease-versus-buy decision, you are asked to answer the following questions:

a. Assuming that the lease can be arranged, should West Virginia Coal lease or borrow and buy the equipment? Explain. (*Hints:* PV cost of owning = $848,402 versus $823,683 for leasing; use these as check figures. Also, we used a discount rate of 11.2%. PVIFA$_{11.2\%,3}$ = 2.4352 and PVIF$_{11.2\%,3}$ = 0.7273. Loan payment = $291,284.)

b. Consider the $200,000 estimated salvage value. Is it appropriate to discount it at the same rate as the other cash flows? What about the other cash flows — are they all equally risky? (*Hint:* Riskier cash flows are normally discounted at higher rates, but when the cash flows are *costs* rather than *inflows,* the normal procedure must be reversed.)

(Do Parts c and d only if you are using the computerized problem diskette.)

c. Determine the lease payment at which West Virginia Coal would be indifferent to buying or leasing — that is, the lease payment that equates the NPV of leasing to that of buying. (*Hint:* Use trial-and-error.)

d. Using the $240,000 lease payment, what would be the effect if West Virginia Coal's tax rate rose to 34 percent? What generalization does this suggest?

ANSWER TO SELF-TEST PROBLEM

a. *Cost of leasing:*

	Beginning of Year			
	1990	**1991**	**1992**	**1993**
After-tax lease payment[a]	$16,500	$ 16,500	$ 16,500	$ 16,500
DFs (6.6%)[b]	×1.000	×0.9381	×0.8800	×0.8255
PV of leasing	$16,500	$ 15,479	$ 14,520	$ 13,621

Total PV cost of leasing = $60,120

[a]After-tax lease payment = $25,000(1 − t) = $25,000(1 − 0.34) = $16,500.
[b]This is the after-tax cost of debt: 10%(1 − t) = 10%(1 − 34%) = 6.6%.

b. *Cost of owning:*

$$\text{Purchase price} = \$100,000$$

$$\text{Annual loan payment} = \$100,000/(DFa_{10\%,4n})$$

$$= \$100,000/3.1699$$

$$= \$31,547.$$

Amortization schedule:

Year	Payment	Interest	Principal	End-of-Year Balance	Interest Tax Savings[c]
1990	$31,547	$10,000	$21,547	$78,453	$3,400
1991	31,547	7,845	23,702	54,751	2,667
1992	31,547	5,475	26,072	28,679	1,862
1993	31,547	2,868	28,679	0	975

[c]Interest tax savings = Interest(t).

Depreciation schedule:

$$\text{Depreciable asset value} = \$100,000.$$

Year	ACRS Factor[d]	Depreciation Expense	Depreciation Tax Savings[e]
1990	0.33	$33,000	$11,220
1991	0.45	45,000	15,300
1992	0.22	22,000	7,480

[d]Assume that these are the appropriate ACRS percentages for the lease period.
[e]Depreciation tax savings = Depreciation expense(t).

Cash outflows:

	End of Year			
	1990	**1991**	**1992**	**1993**
Lease payment	$31,547	$31,547	$31,547	$31,547
Interest tax savings	(3,400)	(2,667)	(1,862)	(975)
Depreciation tax savings	(11,220)	(15,300)	(7,480)	-0-
After-tax maintenance[f]	1,650	1,650	1,650	1,650
Salvage value (AT)				(16,500)
Total cash outflows	$18,577	$15,230	$23,855	$15,722
DFs (at 6.6%)	0.9381	0.8800	0.8255	0.7744
PV of outflows	$17,427	$13,402	$19,692	$12,175
Total PV cost of owning	$62,696			

[f]After-tax maintenance expense = $2,500(1 − t) = $2,500(66%) = $1,650.

Because the present value of the cost of leasing is less than the present value cost of borrowing and buying the earthmover, the equipment should be leased ($62,696 − $60,120 = $2,576 net advantage to leasing).

c. The discount rate is based on the cost of debt because most cash flows are fixed by contract and, consequently, are relatively certain. Thus the lease cash flows have about the same risk as the firm's debt. Also, leasing is considered to be a substitute for debt. An after-tax rate is used because the cash flows are stated net of taxes.

d. Bay City could increase the discount rate on the salvage value cash flow. This would increase the PV cost of owning, possibly by enough to give the advantage to leasing.

Chapter 24

International Financial Management

Lessons from Ireland

Industrial development has become an increasingly competitive and risky business. Nearly every state in the United States has some kind of program, which includes everything from just plain informal talks to tax breaks and employee training grants. In Europe, with unemployment in the Common Market countries averaging around 11 percent, the Scots, French, Dutch, Spanish, and Austrians are all ferociously fighting for new Japanese or U.S. plants.

Ireland's Industrial Development Authority (IDA), one of the first into the fray, is still regarded as the wisest and best-staffed of the agencies trolling the world for investment. Today some 800 multinational companies have operations in Ireland, accounting for 40 percent of the country's manufacturing employment, well over half of manufactured exports. An enviable record.

The IDA hasn't become the most savvy development agency in the world without its share of stumbles. Consider Ireland's experience with Hyster Co., the Portland, Oregon,

forklift maker. When Hyster's 200 Irish workers showed up for work at the Blanchardstown factory west of Dublin on June 10, 1987, they got a rude welcome. Hyster abruptly announced it was closing the five-year-old plant. Blanchardstown was making warehouse automation systems, and Hyster explained that sales were too slow to keep going.

The workers were so irate that they occupied the plant for several days, but they weren't the only ones who were angry. After all, back in 1982 the Industrial Development Authority had been so taken with Hyster's rosy business projections (450 jobs by 1987, the company had estimated) that it put up some $16 million, an exceedingly generous 60 percent of the operation's cost. That excluded the $8.2 million IDA had used to build the Blanchardstown plant. Even though the IDA got the plant back when Hyster folded its Irish operations, the rest of the money turned into a gift from the IDA.

As you read this chapter, think of ways that the IDA could have averted the Hyster disaster. How might it decide how much money to sink into a venture? What lessons do you think the IDA learned from its experience with Hyster?

See end of chapter for resolution.

multinational corporation

A firm that operates in two or more countries.

The term **multinational corporation** is used to describe a firm that operates in two or more nations. Such a simple characterization obscures some essential attributes of the modern corporation, however. In the period since World War II, a new and fundamentally different format for international commercial activity has developed, and it has greatly increased the degree of worldwide economic and political interdependence. The distinguishing characteristic between the new form of commercial transaction and earlier forms is that rather than merely buying resources from foreign concerns, firms now make direct investments in fully integrated operations, with worldwide entities controlling all phases of the production process — from extraction of raw materials, through the manufacturing process, to distribution to consumers throughout the world. Today, multinational corporate networks control a large and growing share of the world's technological, marketing, and productive resources.

The rapid expansion of foreign investment by U.S. companies has been in large part because of lower overseas labor costs, which result in generally higher rates of return on foreign investments, especially in developing nations, as compared with equivalent-risk domestic projects. General Electric maintains production and assembly plants in Mexico, South Korea, and Singapore; many high-tech firms including IBM have computer hardware manufacturing and servicing subsidiaries in many parts of Europe and the Far East; and Caterpillar produces tractors and farm equipment in the Middle East, Europe, the Far East, and Africa. U.S. executives frequently travel and live abroad, and U.S. multinational corporations have come to exert significant economic and political influence in many parts of the world.

Companies move into multinational operations for a number of reasons. First, many of the present U.S. multinational firms commenced their international operations because raw materials were located abroad; this is true of oil, mining, and some food processing companies. Other firms expanded overseas to obtain an outlet for their finished products. Frequently, these firms first set up sales offices and then developed manufacturing plants when it became clear that the market would support such plants. Still other firms have moved their manufacturing facilities overseas to take advantage of low production costs in cheap labor areas; the electronics and textile industries are good examples. Finally, banks, accounting firms, and other service corporations have expanded overseas both to better serve their primary customers and to take advantage of new investment opportunities that are expected to be profitable.

The past decade has also seen an increasing amount of investment in the United States by foreign corporations. This "reverse" investment, which is of growing concern to U.S. government officials, has actually been occurring at a higher rate in the past few years than has U.S. investment abroad. The level of foreign investment in the United States has been concentrated in manufacturing operations, trading companies, and the petroleum industry. The fastest

---

This chapter was coauthored by Professor Roy L. Crum of the University of Florida.

growth has been by Japanese firms, such as Toyota in California and Honda in Tennessee, in the trade and manufacturing sectors.

These trends are important because of their implications for eroding the traditional doctrine of independence and self-reliance that has always been a hallmark of U.S. policy. Just as American corporations with extensive overseas operations are said to use their enormous economic power to exert substantial economic and political influence over host governments in many parts of the world, it is feared that foreign corporations are gaining similar sway over U.S. policy. These developments suggest an increasing degree of mutual influence and interdependence among business enterprises and nations, from which the United States is not immune.

MULTINATIONAL VERSUS DOMESTIC FINANCIAL MANAGEMENT

In theory, the concepts and procedures discussed in various parts of the text are valid for both domestic and multinational operations. However, several problems uniquely associated with the international environment increase the complexity of the manager's task in a multinational corporation, and often they force the manager to alter the way alternative courses of action are evaluated and compared. Five complicating factors distinguish financial management as practiced by firms operating entirely in a single country from those that operate in several different countries:

1. Different Denominations. Cash flows in various parts of a multinational corporate system will be denominated in different currencies. Hence, an analysis of exchange rates and the effects of changing currency values must be included in all financial analyses.

2. Economic and Legal Ramifications. Each country in which the firm operates has its own unique political and economic institutions. Institutional differences among countries can cause significant problems when the corporation tries to coordinate and control the worldwide operations of its subsidiaries. For example, differences in tax laws among countries can cause a given economic transaction to have strikingly dissimilar after-tax consequences, depending on where the transaction occurred. Similarly, differences in legal systems of host nations, such as the Common Law of Great Britain versus the French Civil Law, complicate many matters, from the simple recording of a business transaction to the role played by the judiciary in resolving conflicts. Such differences can restrict multinational corporations' flexibility to deploy resources as they wish and can even preclude procedures in one part of the company that are required in another part. These differences also make it difficult for executives trained under one system to control operations effectively in another.

3. Cultural Differences. Even within geographic regions that have long been considered relatively homogeneous, different countries have unique cultural heritages that shape values and influence the role of business in the society. Multinational corporations find that such matters as definition of the appropriate goals of the firm, attitudes toward risk-taking, dealings with employees, the ability to curtail unprofitable operations, and so on, can vary dramatically from one country to the next.

4. Role of Governments. Most traditional models in finance assume the existence of a competitive marketplace, in which the terms of competition are determined through the actions of participants. The government, through its power to establish basic ground rules, is only slightly involved in this process. Thus the market provides both the primary barometer of success and an indicator of the actions that must be taken to remain competitive. This view of the process is reasonably correct for the United States and a few other major Western industrialized nations, but it does not accurately describe the situation in the majority of countries. Frequently, the terms under which companies compete, the actions that must be taken or avoided, and the terms of trade on various transactions are determined not in the marketplace, but by direct negotiation between the host government and the multinational corporation. This is essentially a political process, and it must be treated as such. Thus traditional financial models have to be recast to include political and other noneconomic facets of the decision.

5. Political Risk. The distinguishing characteristic of a nation state that differentiates it from multinational corporation is that the nation state exercises sovereignty over the people and property in its territory. Hence, a nation state is free to place constraints on the transfer of corporate resources and even to expropriate without compensation the assets of the firm. This is a political risk, and it tends to be largely a given rather than a variable that can be changed by negotiation. Political risk varies from country to country, and it must be addressed explicitly in financial analyses.

These five factors complicate financial management within the multinational firm, and they increase the risk faced by the firms involved. However, higher prospects for profit often make it well worthwhile for firms to accept these risks and to learn how to minimize or at least live with them.

EXCHANGE RATES AND THE INTERNATIONAL MONETARY SYSTEM

exchange rate
The number of units of a given currency that can be purchased for one unit of another currency.

An **exchange rate** specifies the number of units of a given currency that can be purchased for one unit of another currency. Exchange rates for the leading trading partners of the United States appear in the financial sections of newspapers each day. Selected rates from the September 3, 1987, issue of *The Wall Street Journal* are given in Table 24-1. The value shown in Column 1 of Table 24-1 is the number of U.S. dollars required to purchase one unit of foreign currency; this is called a *direct quotation*. Thus the direct U.S. dollar quotation for the West German mark is $0.5583, as one German mark can be bought for

Table 24-1 **Illustrative Exchange Rates, September 3, 1987**

	Direct Quotation U.S. Dollars Required to Buy One Unit of Foreign Currency (1)	**Indirect Quotation Number of Units of Foreign Currency per U.S. Dollar (2)**
British pound	$1.6570	0.6035
Canadian dollar	0.7608	1.3144
Dutch guilder	0.4953	2.0191
French franc	0.1667	6.0000
Greek drachma	0.0073	137.00
Indian rupee	0.0769	13.000
Italian lira	0.00077	1,298.00
Japanese yen	0.00709	141.05
Mexican peso	0.00067	1,488.0
Norwegian krone	0.1520	6.5800
Saudi Arabian riyal	0.2666	3.7510
Singapore dollar	0.4766	2.0980
South African rand	0.4935	2.0263
Spanish peseta	0.0083	120.35
Swedish krona	0.1682	5.9453
Swiss franc	0.6754	1.4805
West German mark	0.5583	1.7913

Note: Column 2 equals 1.0 divided by Column 1.
Source: *The Wall Street Journal,* September 4, 1987.

55.83 cents. The exchange rates given in Column 2 represent the number of units of foreign currency that can be purchased for one U.S. dollar; these are *indirect quotations*. The indirect quotation for the mark is DM1.7913. (The "DM" stands for "deutsche mark"; it is equivalent to the symbol "$".) Normal practice in the United States is to use indirect quotations (Column 2) for all currencies other than British pounds, for which direct quotations are given. Thus we speak of the pound as "selling at $1.66" but of the mark as "being at 1.79."

It is also a universal convention on the world's foreign currency exchanges to state all exchange rates except British pounds on a "dollar basis" — that is, the foreign currency price of one U.S. dollar as reported in Column 2 of Table 24-1. Thus, in all currency trading centers, whether in New York, Frankfurt, London, Tokyo, or anywhere else, the exchange rate for the German mark on September 3, 1987, would be displayed as DM1.7913. This convention eliminates confusion when comparing quotations from one trading center with those from another.

Let us use the rates in Table 24-1 to show how one figures exchange rates. Suppose an American tourist on holiday flies from New York to London, then to Paris, then on to Munich, and finally back to New York. When she arrives at

London's Heathrow Airport, she goes to the bank to check the foreign exchange listing. The rate she observes for U.S. dollars is $1.6570; this means that 1 pound will cost her $1.6570. Assume that she exchanges $2,000 for $2,000/$1.6570 = £1,207.00 and enjoys a week's vacation in London, spending £707.00 while there.

At the end of the week she travels to Dover to catch the Hovercraft to Calais on the coast of France and realizes that she needs to exchange her 500 remaining British pounds for French francs. However, what she sees on the board is the direct quotation between pounds and dollars ($1.6570) and the indirect quotation between francs and dollars (FF6.000). The exchange rate between pounds and francs is called a *cross rate,* and it is computed as follows:

$$\text{Cross rate} = \frac{\text{Dollars}}{\text{Pound}} \times \frac{\text{Francs}}{\text{Dollar}} = \frac{\text{Francs}}{\text{Pound}}$$

$$= 1.657 \text{ dollars per pound} \times 6.000 \text{ francs per dollar}$$

$$= 9.942 \text{ francs per pound}.$$

Therefore, for every British pound she would receive 9.942 French francs. Thus she would receive $9.9420 \times 500 = 4,971$ francs.

When she finishes touring in France and arrives in Germany, the American tourist again needs to determine a cross exchange rate, this time between French francs and West German marks. The dollar-basis quotes she sees are FF6.000 per dollar and DM1.7913 per dollar. To find the cross rate, she must divide the two dollar-basis rates:

$$\text{Cross rate, francs to marks} = \frac{\text{DM1.7913/\$}}{\text{FF6.000/\$}} = \text{DM0.2986}.$$

Thus, if she had FF3,000 remaining, she could exchange them for $0.2986 \times 3,000 = \text{DM895.8}$ or 895.8 marks.

Finally, when her vacation ends and she returns to New York, the quotation she sees is DM1.7913, which tells her that she can buy 1.7913 marks for a dollar. She now holds marks (50 of them) and not dollars, however, she wants to know how many U.S. dollars she will receive for her marks. First, she must find the reciprocal of the quoted indirect rate:

$$\frac{1}{\text{DM1.7913}} = \$0.5583.$$

Then she will end up with

$$0.5583 \times 50 = \$27.92.$$

In this example, we have made two very strong and probably incorrect assumptions. First, we assumed that our traveler had to calculate the appropriate cross rates. For retail transactions, it is customary to display the cross rates directly instead of a series of dollar rates. Second we assumed that exchange rates remain constant over time. Actually, exchange rates vary every day, often dramatically. For instance, in 1984 the pound was selling for about $1.50, but in the spring of 1985 it was down to $1.10, a 27 percent decline. Thus it took fewer dollars to purchase a given number of pounds in 1985 than in 1984, and this strengthening of the dollar (or cheapening of the pound) would have been of sufficient magnitude to introduce serious errors into financial decisions if it had not been anticipated. For example, if a U.S. firm had invested $1 million in Britain in 1984, its pound investment would have been $1,000,000/ 1.5 = £666,667. If its pound investment appreciated by a healthy 15 percent, the pound value of the investment would be 1.15(£666,667) = £766,667. However, those pounds would now be worth only $1.10(766,667) = $843,333, down from the original $1,000,000. Although the U.S. firm's British investment was superficially profitable, the exchange rate differential turned its 15 percent profit into a substantial loss.

We see, then, that exchange rate fluctuations can have a considerable effect on the profitability of foreign investments. To understand what causes exchange rates to change over time, and thus to be able to predict exchange rates, it is necessary to look at the factors that affect currencies and the world monetary system.

Recent History of the World Monetary System

From the end of World War II until August 1971, the world was on a **fixed exchange rate system** administered by the International Monetary Fund (IMF). Under this system the U.S. dollar was linked to gold ($35 per ounce), and other currencies were then tied to the dollar. Exchange rates between other currencies and the dollar were controlled within narrow limits. For example, in 1964 the British pound was fixed at 2.80 dollars for 1 pound, with a 1 percent permissible fluctuation about this rate:

fixed exchange rate system
The world monetary system in existence prior to 1971 under which the value of the U.S. dollar was tied to gold and the values of the other currencies were pegged to the U.S. dollar.

	Value of the Pound **(Exchange Rate in Dollars per Pound)**
Upper limit (+ 1%)	2.828
Official rate	2.800
Lower limit (− 1%)	2.772

Fluctuations in exchange rates tend to occur because of changes in the supply of and demand for dollars, pounds, and other currencies. These supply and demand changes have two primary sources. First, changes in the demand for currencies depend on changes in imports and exports of goods and services. For example, U.S. importers must buy British pounds to pay for British goods, whereas British importers must buy U.S. dollars to pay for U.S. goods. If U.S. imports from Britain were to exceed U.S. exports to Britain, there would be a greater demand for pounds than for dollars; this would drive up the price

deficit trade balance

A country's trade balance resulting from an excess of its imports over its exports.

of the pound relative to that of the dollar. In terms of Table 24-1, the dollar cost of pounds might rise from $1.657 to $2.0000. The U.S. dollar would be said to be *depreciating,* whereas the pound would be *appreciating.* In this example the root cause of the change would be the U.S. **deficit trade balance** with Britain. Of course, if U.S. exports to Britain were greater than U.S. imports from Britain, Britain would have a deficit trade balance with the United States.[1] (Still, under the old fixed rate system, the change in relative currency values was subject to the artificial 1 percent limit.)

Changes in the demand for a currency, and hence exchange rate fluctuations, also depend on capital movements. For example, suppose interest rates in Britain were higher than those in the United States. To take advantage of the high British interest rates, U.S. banks, corporations, and even sophisticated individuals would buy pounds with dollars and then use those pounds to purchase high-yielding British securities. These purchases would tend to drive up the price of pounds.[2]

Before 1972 these fluctuations were kept within the narrow 1 percent limit by regular intervention of the British government in the market. When the value of the pound was falling, the Bank of England would step in and buy pounds, offering gold or foreign currencies in exchange. These government purchases would push up the pound rate. Conversely, when the pound rate was too high, the Bank of England would sell pounds. The central banks of other countries operated similarly. Of course, a central bank's ability to control its exchange rate was limited by its supply of gold and foreign currencies.

devaluation

The process of officially reducing the value of a country's currency relative to other currencies.

With the approval of the IMF, a country could **devalue** its currency — which means officially to lower its value relative to other currencies — if it experienced persistent difficulty over a long period in preventing its exchange rate from falling below the lower limit, and if its central bank was running out of the gold and other currencies that could be used to buy its own currency

---

[1]If the dollar value of the pound moved up from $1.657 to $2.00, this increase in the value of the pound would mean that British goods would now be more expensive in the U.S. market. For example, a box of candy costing 1 pound in England would rise in price in the United States from $1.657 to $2.00. Conversely, U.S. goods would be cheaper in England. For example, the British could now buy goods worth $2.00 for 1 pound, whereas before the exchange rate change, 1 pound would buy merchandise worth only $1.657. These price changes would, of course, tend to *reduce* British exports and *increase* imports, and this, in turn, would lower the exchange rate, because people in the United States and other nations would be buying fewer pounds to pay for English goods. However, in the old days the 1 percent limit severely constrained the market's ability to reach an equilibrium between trade balances and exchange rates.

[2]Such capital inflows would also tend to drive down British interest rates. If rates were high in the first place because of efforts by the British monetary authorities to curb inflation, the international currency flows would have helped to thwart that effort. This is one of the reasons why domestic and international economics are so closely linked.

A good example of this occurred during the summer of 1981. In an effort to curb inflation, the Federal Reserve Board helped push U.S. interest rates to record levels. This, in turn, caused an outflow of capital from European nations to the United States. The Europeans were suffering from a severe recession and wanted to keep interest rates down in order to stimulate investment, but the U.S. policy made this difficult because of the ease of international capital flows.

and thus prop up its price. For just these reasons the British pound was devalued from $2.80 per pound to $2.50 per pound in 1967. This lowered the price of British goods in the United States and elsewhere and raised the prices of foreign goods in Britain, thus stopping the deficit British trade balance that had been putting pressure on the pound in the first place. Conversely, a nation with an export surplus and a strong currency might **revalue** its currency upward, as West Germany did twice in the 1960s.

Today's Floating Exchange Rate System

Devaluations and revaluations occurred only rarely before 1971. They were usually accompanied by severe international financial repercussions, partly because nations tended to postpone these needed measures until economic pressures had built up to explosive proportions. For this and other reasons the old international monetary system came to a dramatic end in the early 1970s, when the U.S. dollar, the foundation upon which all other currencies were anchored, was cut loose from the gold standard and, in effect, allowed to "float."

Under a system of **floating exchange rates,** currency prices are allowed to seek their own levels without much governmental intervention. The present world monetary system is known as a **managed floating system:** major world currency rates move (float) with market forces, largely unrestricted by any internationally agreed-upon limits. However, the central bank of each country does intervene in the foreign exchange market, buying and selling its currency to smooth out exchange rate fluctuations to some extent. There have also been agreements by groups of countries to keep the relative values of their currencies within a predetermined range. Such an agreement by the "group of seven" at the Seoul Economic Summit in October 1985 caused the U.S. dollar to fall substantially against most major currencies. This action was endorsed as appropriate at the Washington Economic Summit in September 1987. The "group of seven" was also responsible for helping to stabilize the falling dollar in early 1988. Each central bank also tries to keep its average exchange rate at a level deemed desirable by its government's economic policy. This is important, because exchange rates have a profound effect on the levels of imports and exports, which in turn influence the level of domestic employment. For example, if a country was having a problem with unemployment, its central bank might encourage a *decline* in the value of its currency. This would cause its goods to be cheaper in world markets and thus stimulate exports, production, and domestic employment. Conversely, the central bank of a country that is operating at full capacity and experiencing inflation might try to raise the value of its currency to reduce exports and increase imports. Under the current floating rate system, however, such intervention can affect the situation only temporarily; market forces will prevail in the long run.

Figure 24-1 shows how German marks, Japanese yen, and British pounds moved in comparison to the dollar from 1962 to 1987. Until 1971, when the fixed rate system was terminated, rates were quite stable. The pound's fluctua-

revaluation
The process of officially increasing the value of a country's currency relative to other currencies.

floating exchange rates
Exchange rates not fixed by government policy but allowed to float up or down in accordance with supply and demand.

managed floating system
A system in which major currency rates move with market forces, unrestricted by any internationally agreed-upon limits.

Figure 24-1 **Changes in the Values of Marks, Yen, and Pounds Relative to the Value of the Dollar, 1960–1987**

Prior to 1971, world currencies were narrowly controlled and changes in relative values were minimal. Since 1971, currencies have been allowed to float, resulting in marked fluctuations in values. As the figure shows, until 1985, the pound, relative to the dollar, had generally drifted down, whereas the yen had risen. The mark rose against the dollar until 1979, but it fell in value till 1985. The dollar fell precipitiously against all of these currencies starting in early 1985.

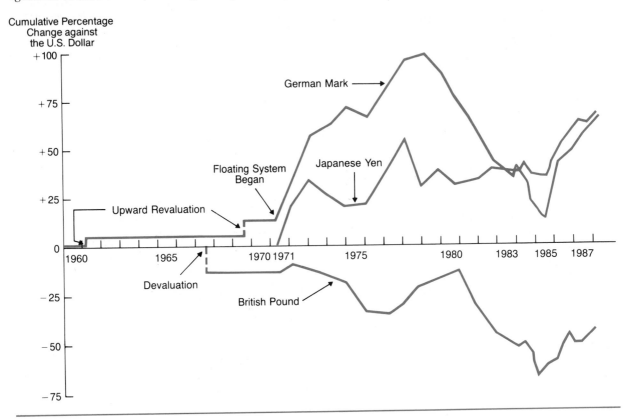

tions against the dollar were too small to even show up on the graph prior to 1967, when a devaluation occurred. The mark was revaluated in 1969. The yen was stable until 1971, when the dollar was allowed to float. After 1971, economic forces became the major factor in setting relative currency values, and Figure 24-1 illustrates the volatility that has occurred since then. (Note that Figure 24-1 plots cumulative changes in relative value.) From the late 1970s until 1985, the German mark fell in value rapidly against the dollar while the Japanese yen remained relatively stable during the period. The value of the British pound, on the other hand, generally drifted down from 1980 to 1985.

Since early 1985 the dollar's value has fallen precipitously against all of these currencies.

The volatility of exchange rates that is inherent under a floating system increases the uncertainty of the cash flows for a multinational corporation. Because these cash flows are generated in many parts of the world, they are denominated in numerous currency units. But since exchange rates change, the dollar-equivalent value of the consolidated cash flows is uncertain. This is known as *exchange rate risk,* and it is a major factor differentiating the multinational corporation from a purely domestic one. However, there are numerous ways for a multinational corporation to manage and limit its exchange rate risk, several of which are discussed below.

Trading in Foreign Exchange

Importers, exporters, and tourists, as well as governments, buy and sell currencies in the foreign exchange market. For example, when a U.S. trader imports automobiles from West Germany, payment will probably be made in German marks. The importer buys marks (through its bank) in the foreign exchange market, much as one buys common stocks on the New York Stock Exchange or pork bellies on the Chicago Mercantile Exchange. However, whereas stock and commodity exchanges have organized trading floors, the foreign exchange market consists of a network of brokers and banks based in New York, London, Tokyo, and other financial centers. Most buy and sell orders are conducted by cablegram and telephone.[3]

Spot Rates and Forward Rates

The exchange rates shown earlier in Table 24-1 are known as **spot rates,** which means the rate paid for delivery of the currency "on the spot" or, in reality, two days after the day of the trade. For most of the world's major currencies, it is also possible to buy (or sell) currency for delivery at some agreed-upon future date, usually 30, 90, or 180 days from the day the transaction is negotiated. This rate is known as the **forward exchange rate.** For example, if a U.S. firm must make payment to a Swiss firm in 90 days, the U.S. firm's treasurer can buy Swiss francs today for delivery in 90 days, paying the 90-day forward rate. Forward rates are exactly analogous to futures prices on commodity exchanges, where contracts are drawn up for wheat or corn to be delivered at agreed-upon prices at some future date. The contract is signed today, and the dollar cost of the Swiss francs is then known with certainty. Purchase of a forward contract is one technique for eliminating the volatility of future cash flows caused by fluctuations in exchange rates.

Forward rates for 30-, 90-, and 180-day delivery, along with the spot rates for September 3, 1987, are given in Table 24-2. If one can obtain *more* of the

spot rate
The effective exchange rate for a foreign currency for delivery on (approximately) the current day.

forward exchange rate
An agreed-upon price at which two currencies are to be exchanged at some future date.

---

[3]For a more detailed explanation of exchange rate determination and operations of the foreign exchange market, see Steven Bell and Bryan Kettell, *Foreign Exchange Handbook* (Westport, Conn.: Quorum Books, 1983).

Table 24-2 **Selected Spot and Forward
Exchange Rates, September 3, 1987
(Number of Units of Foreign Currency per U.S. Dollar)**

	Spot Rate	Forward Rates			Spot Rate at a Premium or Discount
		30 Days	90 Days	180 Days	
British pound	0.6035	0.6048	0.6075	0.6106	Discount
French franc	6.0000	6.0027	6.0105	6.0300	Discount
Japanese yen	141.05	140.65	139.86	138.64	Premium
Swiss franc	1.4805	1.4757	1.4666	1.4526	Premium
West German mark	1.7913	1.7863	1.7762	1.7611	Premium

Note: These are representative quotes as provided by a sample of New York banks. Forward rates for other currencies and for other lengths of time can often be negotiated.

Source: *The Wall Street Journal,* September 4, 1987.

discount on forward rate

The situation when the spot rate is less than the forward rate and the quotation is based on the number of units of foreign currency per U.S. dollar.

premium on forward rate

The situation when the spot rate is greater than the forward rate and the quotation is based on the number of units of foreign currency per U.S. dollar.

hedging exchange rate exposure

The process whereby a firm protects itself against losses due to future exchange rate fluctuations.

foreign currency for a dollar in the forward than in the spot market, the forward currency is less valuable than the spot currency, and the forward currency is said to be selling at a **discount.** Thus, because 1 dollar could buy 0.6035 British pounds in the spot market but 0.6106 pounds in the 180-day forward market, forward pounds sell at a discount as compared with spot pounds. Conversely, if a dollar will buy *fewer* units of a currency in the forward than in the spot market, the forward currency is worth more dollars than the spot currency, and the forward currency is said to be selling at a **premium.** Thus we see in Table 24-2 that on September 3, 1987, the pound and the French franc were selling at a discount but the forward yen, Swiss franc, and mark were selling at a premium.

Hedging in the Exchange Markets

Individuals and corporations buy or sell forward currencies as a means of **hedging exchange rate exposure.** For example, suppose that on September 3, 1987, a U.S. jeweler buys watches from a Swiss manufacturer for 1 million Swiss francs. Payment is to be made in Swiss francs 90 days after the goods are shipped, or on December 1, so the Swiss firm is extending trade credit for 90 days. The Swiss franc has been strong recently, and the U.S. company is apprehensive that the dollar will weaken because of large trade deficits. If the Swiss franc appreciates rapidly, more dollars will be required to buy the million francs, and the profits on the watches will be lost. Still, the U.S. firm does not want to forgo 90 days of free trade credit by paying cash. It can take the trade credit and protect itself by purchasing 1 million Swiss francs for delivery in 90 days. The 90-day rate is SF1.4666, so the dollar cost is SF1,000,000/ SF1.4666 = $681,849. When payment comes due on December 1, 1987, regardless of the spot rate on that day, the U.S. firm can obtain the needed Swiss francs at the agreed-upon price of $681,849. The U.S. firm is said to have *covered* its trade payables with a *forward market hedge.*

Inflation, Interest Rates, and Exchange Rates

Relative inflation rates, or the rates of inflation in foreign countries compared to that at home, have many implications for multinational financial decisions. Obviously, relative inflation rates will greatly influence production costs at home and those abroad. Equally important, they have a dominant influence on relative interest rates as well as exchange rates. Both relative interest rates and exchange rates influence the methods chosen by multinational corporations for financing their foreign investments, and both of these factors have a notable effect on the profitability of foreign investments.

The currencies of countries with higher inflation rates than that of the United States tend over time to depreciate against the dollar. Some countries for which this is the case are France, Italy, Mexico, and all the South American nations. On the other hand, the currencies of countries such as West Germany, Switzerland, and Japan, which have had less inflation than the United States, have appreciated relative to the dollar. *In fact, a foreign currency will, on average, depreciate (appreciate) at a percentage rate approximately equal to the amount by which its inflation rate exceeds (is less than) our own.*

Relative inflation rates are also reflected in interest rates. The interest rate in any country is largely determined by its inflation rate; this point was made in Chapter 5. Therefore, countries currently experiencing higher rates of inflation than the United States also tend to have higher interest rates, whereas the reverse is true for countries with lower inflation rates.

It is tempting for the treasurer of a multinational corporation to borrow in countries with the lowest interest rates. However, this is not always the best strategy. Suppose for example, that interest rates in West Germany are lower than those in the United States because of Germany's lower inflation rate. A U.S. multinational firm could save interest by borrowing in Germany, but the German exchange rate can be expected to appreciate in the future, causing annual interest and principal payments on this debt to cost an increasing number of dollars over time. Thus the lower interest rate could be more than offset by losses from currency appreciation. Similarly, one should not expect multinational corporations to avoid borrowing in a country like Brazil, where interest rates are very high, because future depreciation of the Brazilian cruzeiro might well make such borrowing relatively inexpensive.

PROCEDURES FOR ANALYZING POTENTIAL FOREIGN INVESTMENTS

Although the same basic principles of investment analysis apply to both foreign and domestic operations, there are some key differences. First, cash flow analysis is much more complex for overseas investments. Most multinational firms set up a separate subsidiary in each foreign country in which they operate. The relevant cash flows are the dividends and royalties repatriated by each subsidiary to the parent company. These cash flows must be converted to the currency of the parent company and thus are subject to future exchange rate

INDUSTRY PRACTICE

The Selling of America

The Japanese are about to descend on Pearl Harbor again, but this time they have come not to bomb but to build. Construction is underway for a billion-dollar vacationland including lagoons, golf courses, and luxury hotels that they hope will rival Waikiki. The resort at Pearl Harbor epitomizes the onslaught of foreign investment in the U.S. In addition to real estate, offshore investors are buying up stocks, bonds, Treasury securities, assembly plants, factories, fish, forests, and entire companies, both large and small.

Suddenly, it seems, the United States has become a country for sale, a huge shopping mart in which foreigners are energetically filling up their carts. As a result, foreign ownership in the United States, including everything from real estate to securities, rose to a remarkable $1.33 trillion in 1986, up 25 percent from the previous year. By contrast, in a complete reversal of the situation only a decade ago, U.S. holdings abroad now total only $1.07 trillion. The foreign buying boom has spurred fabulous hikes in real estate values, ignited corporate takeovers, and helped drive Wall Street's bull market.

The selling of America is, to a large extent, a by-product of the nation's gargantuan trade deficit. The U.S. has stuffed the world's pockets with the dollars it pays for foreign products. The biggest beneficiary of America's import binge has been Japan. Despite its obsession with U.S. bagels, burgers, and diapers, Japan invariably comes out tens of billions of dollars ahead in trade.

The U.S. not only welcomes foreign money but courts it. Mayors and governors bump into each other in Europe and Asia at trade shows

staged to woo foreign investment. Flat Rock, Michigan, seduced Mazda Motor into building an assembly plant there by waiving property taxes for 14 years. The state of Oklahoma has hired the London investment bank of Morgan Grenfell to help it lure capital from abroad.

Response to the foreign buying spree has not been uniformly positive, however. Critics ask: How does foreign investment affect America's industrial strength and ability to compete? Just how much overseas investment is good for the country, and how much of America should foreigners be allowed to buy? What other kinds of control might follow? Warns Lawrence Brainard, chief international economist for Manhattan's Bankers Trust: "By the end of this century, the U.S. may have the most modern manufacturing sector in the world, but it won't own it."

But proponents of foreign investment see clear benefits in the trend. Just as foreign investment by Coca-Cola, Ford, and other multinationals has benefited the rest of the world, capital coming the other way enriches the United States, they maintain. Says Lord Lever, a British businessman who served in the cabinets of prime ministers Harold Wilson and James Callaghan, "Europe got 20 times more out of American investment after the war than the multinationals did. Every country gains by productive investment."

Jobs are the most unequivocal benefit of capital immigration. Foreign companies directly employ some three million Americans, or about 3 percent of the work force, and create jobs for countless more in shops where those workers spend their paychecks. Proponents of foreign investment argue that the U.S. is hardly being colonized. Foreigners own just 1 percent of U.S. real estate and farmland and claim less than 5 percent of corporate earnings. Even though foreign companies do get to repatriate their prof-

Source: Stephen Koepp, "For Sale: America," *Time*, September 14, 1987, 52–62; Jaclyn Fierman, "The Selling Off of America," *Fortune,* December 22, 1986, 48–56.

its, the wages they pay and the value added in their manufacturing plants bolster America's gross national product.

Tax reform makes the United States more attractive than ever. The new maximum corporate tax rate—34 percent in 1988—is the lowest in the industrial world. Foreigners also see the U.S. as a technology hothouse and are supplying almost one-quarter of America's venture capital to ensure themselves a stake in new discoveries.

Japan, the world's largest creditor country, where consumers save 17 percent of their earnings (versus 4 percent in the U.S.) has the mightiest bankroll of all to engage in buying America. Bereft of enough investment opportunities at home to absorb their astonishing pile of savings, the Japanese are hungrily looking abroad for places to park the excess cash. As a result, the Japanese have taken America's skylines by storm. They have invested more than $7 billion in office towers and other buildings. American real estate agents love the trend: by some estimates, the Japanese have single-handedly boosted the selling prices of prime Manhattan real estate by 10 to 15 percent, to roughly $500 per square foot. Those prices are still a bargain compared with costs in Tokyo, where office towers sell for an astronomical $20,000 or more per square foot, on those rare occasions when anything comes up for sale.

The Japanese are buying more than buildings and businesses. They have been busy fattening their portfolio investments as well. Their appetite for corporate debt has been voracious.

While investors in many different nations have been riding the recent U.S. bull market, the biggest takers by far are the Japanese. The Security Dealers Association of Japan estimates that Japan's purchases of Treasury securities have been averaging more than $8 billion a month since the Japanese government recently eased restrictions on offshore investments by institutions.

One corporate arena in which Japan's huge bankroll is prompting intense jitters is the U.S. financial-services industry. Tokyo's largest banks and investment firms, which already eclipse American companies like Citicorp (assets: $196 billion) and Merrill Lynch ($53 billion), openly aim to grab a large share of the U.S. financial marketplace. They have established a major beachhead in California, where four of the top ten banks are now Japanese owned. On Wall Street, Japan's Sumitomo Bank shelled out $500 million for a 12.5 percent share of profits in the Goldman, Sachs investment-banking firm, whereas Nippon Life Insurance paid $538 million for a 13 percent slice of Shearson Lehman Brothers.

Xenophobia aside, most experts agree that the current crush of foreign buyers offers more opportunities than threats. The size of the $4.5 trillion U.S. economy, they point out, is its best defense against being swamped by an invasion of foreign investors. Says Theodore Moran, a professor of international business diplomacy at Georgetown University, "We are not going to have our economy taken over by foreigners unless it continues to decline for 50 or 60 years."

changes. In other words, General Motors' German subsidiary may make a profit of 100 million marks in 1987 and again in 1988, but the value of these profits to GM will depend on the dollar/mark exchange rate. How many *dollars* is 100 million marks worth?

Dividends and royalties are normally taxed by both foreign and domestic governments. Furthermore, a foreign government may restrict the amount of the cash flows that may be **repatriated** to the parent company. For example,

repatriation of earnings
The process of sending cash flows from a foreign subsidiary to its parent company.

some governments place a ceiling, stated as a percentage of the company's net worth, on the amount of cash dividends that may be paid by a subsidiary to its parent company. Such restrictions are normally intended to force multinational firms to reinvest earnings in the foreign country, although restrictions are sometimes imposed to prevent large currency outflows, which might destabilize exchange rates.

Whatever the host country's motivation, the result is that the parent corporation cannot use cash flows blocked in the foreign country to pay current dividends to its shareholders, nor does it have the flexibility to reinvest cash flows elsewhere in the world, where expected returns may be higher. Hence, from the perspective of the parent organization, the cash flows relevant for the analysis of an international investment are the financial cash flows that the subsidiary can legally send back to the parent. The present value of these cash flows is found by applying an appropriate discount rate; this present value is then compared to the parent's investment in the project to determine the project's NPV.

In addition to the complexities of the cash flow analysis, *the cost of capital may be different for a foreign project than for an equivalent domestic project because foreign projects may be more or less risky*. A higher risk could arise from two primary sources — (1) exchange risk and (2) sovereign risk — while a lower risk might result from international diversification.

exchange risk
The risk that the basic cash flows of a foreign project will be worth less in the parent company's home currency.

Exchange risk refers to the fact that exchange rates fluctuate. This increases the inherent uncertainty about the home currency value of cash flows sent back to the parent. In other words, foreign projects have an added risk element that relates to what the basic cash flows will be worth in the parent company's home currency. As we have seen, although it is sometimes possible to hedge against exchange rate fluctuations, it may not be possible to hedge completely, and, in addition, the costs of hedging must be subtracted from the project's cash flows.

sovereign risk
The risk of an unanticipated restriction or reduction in the cash flows of a foreign subsidiary caused by a foreign power. The ultimate sovereign risk is expropriation of assets without compensation to the parent company.

Sovereign risk refers to any action (or the probability of an action) by a host government in exercising its political power, which reduces the value of a company's investment. It includes at one extreme the expropriation without compensation of the subsidiary's assets. Sovereign risk also includes less drastic actions that reduce the value of the parent firm's investment in the foreign subsidiary such as higher taxes, tighter repatriation or currency controls, and restrictions on prices or markets, among others. The risk of expropriation of U.S. assets abroad is small in traditionally friendly and stable countries such as Britain or Switzerland. However, in many parts of the developing world of Latin America, Africa, and the Far East, the risk may be substantial. Examples of expropriations include those of ITT and Anaconda in Chile, Gulf Oil in Bolivia, Occidental Petroleum in Libia, International Petroleum in Peru, and the assets of many companies in Iran and Cuba. In recent years, however, there have been very few examples of governments expropriating the assets of foreign firms.

INTERNATIONAL CAPITAL MARKETS

Direct foreign investment by U.S. multinational corporations is one way for U.S. citizens to invest in world markets. Another way is to purchase stocks, bonds, or various money market instruments issued in foreign countries. U.S. citizens actually do invest substantial amounts in the stocks and bonds of large corporations headquartered in Europe and to a lesser extent in the Far East and South America. They also buy securities issued by foreign governments. Such investments in foreign capital markets are known as *portfolio investments,* and they are distinguished from *direct investments* in physical assets by U.S. corporations.

Eurodollars

A **Eurodollar** is a U.S. dollar deposited in a time account such as a Certificate of Deposit (CD) in a bank outside the United States. Note however that demand deposits abroad are not considered to be Eurodollars. The bank in which the deposit is made may be a host country institution, such as Barclay's Bank in London, the foreign branch of a U.S. bank, such as Citibank's Paris branch, or even a foreign branch of a third-country bank, such as Barclay's Munich branch. Most Eurodollar deposits are for $500,000 or more, and they have maturities ranging from call money (or overnight funds) up to 5 years. Approximately 85 percent of all Eurodollars are held as withdrawable, interest-bearing deposits; the remaining 15 percent take the form of negotiable certificates of deposit (CDs).

Eurodollar
A U.S. dollar in a time deposit in a foreign bank — generally, but not necessarily, a European bank.

Eurodollar Interest Rates

Eurodollars are always held in interest-bearing accounts. The interest rate paid on these deposits depends (1) on the bank's lending rate, as the interest a bank earns on loans determines its willingness and ability to pay interest on deposits, and (2) on rates of return available on U.S. money market instruments. If rates in the United States are above Eurodollar deposit rates, these funds will be sent back and invested in the United States, whereas if Eurodollar deposit rates are significantly above U.S. rates, more dollars will be sent out of the United States.

International Bond Markets

The Eurodollar market is essentially a short-term market; most loans and deposits are for less than one year. However, there are also two important types of international bond markets: foreign bonds and Eurobonds. **Foreign bonds** are bonds sold by a foreign borrower but denominated in the currency of the country in which the issue is sold. For instance, Bell Canada may need U.S. dollars to finance the operations of its subsidiaries in the United States. If it decides to raise the needed capital in the domestic U.S. bond market, the bond

foreign bond
A bond sold by a foreign borrower but denominated in the currency of the country in which it is sold.

will be underwritten by a syndicate of U.S. investment bankers, denominated in U.S. dollars, and sold to U.S. investors in accordance with SEC and applicable state regulations. Except for the foreign origin of the borrower (Canada), this bond will be indistinguishable from those issued by equivalent U.S. corporations. Since Bell Canada is a foreign corporation, however, the bond will be called a foreign bond.

Eurobond
A bond sold in a country other than the one in whose currency the bond is denominated.

The term **Eurobonds** is used to designate any bond sold in some country *other than* the one in whose currency the bond is denominated. Examples include a British firm's issue of pound bonds sold in France, a Ford Motor Company issue denominated in dollars and sold in West Germany, or a German firm's sale of mark-denominated bonds in Switzerland. The institutional arrangements by which Eurobonds are marketed are different than those for most other bond issues, with the most important distinction being a far lower level of required disclosure than is usually found for bonds issued in domestic markets, particularly in the United States. Governments tend to not apply regulations on securities denominated in foreign currencies that are as strict as they would be on home-currency securities because of the nature of the bond's probable purchasers. This often leads to lower total transaction costs for Eurobonds.

More than half of all Eurobonds are denominated in dollars; bonds in German marks and Dutch guilders account for most of the rest. Although centered in Europe, Eurobonds are truly international. Their underwriting syndicates include investment bankers from all parts of the world, and the bonds are sold to investors not only in Europe but also in such faraway places as Bahrain and Singapore. Thus multinational corporations, together with international financial institutions and national governments, play an important role in mobilizing capital in all parts of the world to finance production and economic growth. For better or for worse, this has resulted in great interdependence among world economies.

SUMMARY

As the world economy becomes more integrated, the role of multinational firms is increasing, and new companies are joining the ranks of the multinationals every day. Although the same basic principles of financial management apply to multinational corporations as to domestic ones, the financial manager of a multinational firm faces a much more complex task. The primary problem, from a financial standpoint, is that cash flows must cross national boundaries. These flows may be constrained in various ways, and, equally important, their value in dollars may rise or fall depending on exchange rate fluctuations. This means that the multinational manager must be constantly aware of the many complex interactions among national economies and the effects of these interactions on multinational operations.

Efficient markets for foreign currencies and securities tie together the various national money and capital markets, and the forward and spot currency markets can be used to smooth out the effects of exchange rate fluctuations over time. Because of the central role the U.S. dollar plays in international commerce, large markets have developed for U.S. dollar deposits (Eurodollars) and dollar-denominated bonds (Eurobonds) in the world. These markets represent important sources of capital for multinational corporations.

The ability to redeploy worldwide resources quickly in response to environmental signals gives multinational corporations a distinct advantage over domestic firms. Many complex issues must be taken into consideration in order to make good decisions, thus making multinational financial management both important and challenging. The risks of international operations are high, but so are the potential rewards. In a world economy that grows more interdependent each year, the multinational manager can look forward to an ever-expanding role in corporate decision making.

 RESOLUTION TO DECISION IN FINANCE

Lessons from Ireland

The government of Ireland lost over $16 million dollars when the Hyster Co. shut down its operations in Ireland. The money, which the country could ill-afford to lose, went down the drain because the IDA had gotten so starry-eyed over the project that it never required Hyster Ireland's parent to guarantee repayment in case the plant failed.

The Irish were seduced and ignored this fact: Hyster, even as early as 1982, was already a pro at playing state industrial agencies, in Europe as well as in the U.S., against one another. Hyster was particularly adept at getting the agencies to pay most of the costs as it wandered into risky new markets. Great for Hyster. Lousy for Ireland. And instructive for other countries and states trying to attract long-term jobs to bolster their economies.

Fortunately for Ireland, the IDA has learned a thing or two in its 30 years of hustling the corporations of the world for new business:

Source: Adapted by permission from Kathleen K. Wiegner, "Lessons from Ireland," *Forbes,* September 7, 1987, 37–39. © Forbes Inc., 1987.

Never try to underprice the Third World. Always remember that the object of a development agency is to work itself out of a job. And finally (Hyster Co. notwithstanding), never give away the store.

Although the IDA's fiasco with Hyster is an instance when the agency failed to follow its own rules, in the numerous cases when it has followed these edicts, it has been remarkably successful. Maynard, Mass.-based Digital Equipment Corporation (DEC) is a case in point. Digital had begun selling computers to the Common Market and opened a simple test and assembly operation in Galway 15 years ago. Pleased with the quality of local work, DEC soon was manufacturing components there as well. That led, in 1979, to a second plant in Clonmel, to design and build network connections and power supplies, further tying DEC to local vendors of components, who had to be brought in at the design stage.

Mentec, a $12 million (revenues) software and hardware company, would not exist today if not for DEC. Situated in a small, one-story building in an industrial park on the outskirts of

Dublin, Mentec was started in 1977 by Michael Peirce, an engineer with a doctorate from Trinity College. Mentec was formed under the aegis of the IDA's Enterprise Development Program, which assists companies that want to be vendors for multinationals based in Ireland, through loan guarantees and a good deal of hand-holding.

Peirce and his 75 employees build computer-integrated manufacturing software systems for DEC products such as its VAX and single-board computers. From that base Mentec has even designed its own single-board computer, which can be slipped into a DEC machine. Today Peirce lists among his customers Michelin, Unilever, Guinness, and General Electric Co. of the U.K. Which is the way development should be done, says Peirce. Pick your most promising opportunities and nurture them gently.

QUESTIONS

24-1 Under the fixed exchange rate system, what was the currency against which all other currency values were defined?

24-2 Exchange rates fluctuate under both the fixed exchange rate and floating exchange rate systems. What, then, is the difference between the two systems?

24-3 If the French franc depreciates against the U.S. dollar, can a dollar buy more or fewer French francs as a result?

24-4 If the United States imports more goods from abroad than it exports, foreigners will tend to have a surplus of U.S. dollars. What will this do to the value of the dollar with respect to foreign currencies? What is the corresponding effect on foreign investments in the United States?

24-5 Why do U.S. corporations build manufacturing plants abroad when they could build them at home?

24-6 Most firms require higher rates of return on foreign projects than on identical projects located at home. Why?

24-7 What is a Eurodollar? If a French citizen deposits $10,000 in Chase Manhattan Bank in New York, have Eurodollars been created? What if the deposit is made in Barclay's Bank in London? Chase Manhattan's Paris branch?

PROBLEMS

24-1 **Exchange rate.** If British pounds sell for $1.66 (U.S.) per pound, what should dollars sell for in pounds per dollar?

24-2 **Currency appreciation.** Suppose that 1 French franc could be purchased in the foreign exchange market for 20 U.S. cents today. If the franc appreciated 10 percent tomorrow against the dollar, how many francs would a dollar buy tomorrow?

24-3 **Cross exchange rates.** Recently the exchange rate between U.S. dollars and the French franc was fr. 8 = $1, and the exchange rate between the dollar and British pound was £1 = $1.50. What was the exchange rate between francs and pounds?

24-4 **Cross exchange rates.** Look up the same three currencies as in Problem 24-3 in the foreign exchange section of a current issue of *The Wall Street Journal.* What is the current exchange rate between francs and pounds?

24-5 **Exchange rates.** Table 24-1 lists foreign exchange rates for September 3, 1987. On that day how many dollars would be required to purchase 1,000 units of each of the following: Indian rupees, Italian lira, Japanese yen, Mexican pesos, and Saudi Arabian riyals?

24-6 **Exchange rates.** Look up the same five currencies as in Problem 24-5 in the foreign exchange section of a current issue of *The Wall Street Journal.*
   a. What is the current exchange rate for changing dollars into 1,000 units of rupees, lira, yen, pesos, and riyals?
   b. What is the percentage gain or loss between the September 3, 1987, exchange rate and the current exchange rate for each of the currencies in Part a?

24-7 **Results of exchange rate changes.** Early in September 1983, it took 245 Japanese yen to equal $1. Four years later, in September 1987, that exchange rate had fallen to 141 yen to $1. Assume the price of a Japanese manufactured automobile was $8,000 in September 1983 and that its price changes were in direct relation to exchange rates.
   a. Has the price in dollars of the automobile increased or decreased during the 4 year period because of changes in the exchange rate?
   b. What would the dollar price of the automobile be today, again assuming that the car's price changes only with exchange rates?

24-8 **Hedging.** La Belle France Imports has agreed to purchase 15,000 cases of French wine for 16 million francs at today's spot rate. The firm's financial manager, Frank O'File, has noted the following current spot and forward rates:

	U.S. Dollar/Franc	Franc/U.S. Dollar
Spot	0.1667	6.0000
30-day forward	0.1653	6.0500
60-day forward	0.1634	6.1200
90-day forward	0.1600	6.2500

On the same day Mr. O'File agrees to purchase 15,000 more cases of wine in 3 months at the same price of 16 million francs.
   a. What is the price of the wine, in U.S. dollars, if it is purchased at today's spot rate?
   b. What is the cost, in dollars, of the second 15,000 cases if payment is made in 90 days and the spot rate at that time equals today's 90-day forward rate?
   c. If Mr. O'File is concerned about the dollar losing value relative to the franc in the next 90 days, what can he do to reduce his exposure to exchange risk?
   d. If he does not hedge his exposure to exchange risk, and the exchange rate for the French franc is 5.75 to $1 in 90 days, how much will he have to pay for the wine (in dollars)?

24-9 **Foreign investment analysis.** After all foreign and U.S. taxes, a U.S. corporation expects to receive 3 pounds of dividends per share from a British subsidiary this year. The exchange rate at the end of the year is expected to be $1.50 per pound, and the pound is expected to depreciate 5 percent against the dollar each year for an indefinite period. The dividend (in pounds) is expected to grow at 10 percent a year indefinitely. The parent U.S. corporation owns 10 million shares of the subsidiary. What is the present value of its equity ownership of the subsidiary? Assume a cost of equity capital of 14 percent for the subsidiary.

24-10   **Translation gains and losses.** You are vice president of International InfoTec, headquartered in Detroit, Michigan. All shareholders of the firm live in the United States. Earlier this month you obtained a loan of 10 million Canadian dollars from a bank in Toronto to finance the construction of a new plant in Montreal. At the time the loan was received, the exchange rate was 85 U.S. cents to the Canadian dollar. By the end of the month it has unexpectedly dropped to 80 cents. Has your company made a gain or loss as a result, and by how much?

APPENDIXES

Appendix A **Future Value of $1 at the End of n Periods: IF $= (1 + k)^n$**

Period	1%	2%	3%	4%	5%	6%	7%	8%	9%	10%
1	1.0100	1.0200	1.0300	1.0400	1.0500	1.0600	1.0700	1.0800	1.0900	1.1000
2	1.0201	1.0404	1.0609	1.0816	1.1025	1.1236	1.1449	1.1664	1.1881	1.2100
3	1.0303	1.0612	1.0927	1.1249	1.1576	1.1910	1.2250	1.2597	1.2950	1.3310
4	1.0406	1.0824	1.1255	1.1699	1.2155	1.2625	1.3108	1.3605	1.4116	1.4641
5	1.0510	1.1041	1.1593	1.2167	1.2763	1.3382	1.4026	1.4693	1.5386	1.6105
6	1.0615	1.1262	1.1941	1.2653	1.3401	1.4185	1.5007	1.5869	1.6771	1.7716
7	1.0721	1.1487	1.2299	1.3159	1.4071	1.5036	1.6058	1.7138	1.8280	1.9487
8	1.0829	1.1717	1.2668	1.3686	1.4775	1.5938	1.7182	1.8509	1.9926	2.1436
9	1.0937	1.1951	1.3048	1.4233	1.5513	1.6895	1.8385	1.9990	2.1719	2.3579
10	1.1046	1.2190	1.3439	1.4802	1.6289	1.7908	1.9672	2.1589	2.3674	2.5937
11	1.1157	1.2434	1.3842	1.5395	1.7103	1.8983	2.1049	2.3316	2.5804	2.8531
12	1.1268	1.2682	1.4258	1.6010	1.7959	2.0122	2.2522	2.5182	2.8127	3.1384
13	1.1381	1.2936	1.4685	1.6651	1.8856	2.1329	2.4098	2.7196	3.0658	3.4523
14	1.1495	1.3195	1.5126	1.7317	1.9799	2.2609	2.5785	2.9372	3.3417	3.7975
15	1.1610	1.3459	1.5580	1.8009	2.0789	2.3966	2.7590	3.1722	3.6425	4.1772
16	1.1726	1.3728	1.6047	1.8730	2.1829	2.5404	2.9522	3.4259	3.9703	4.5950
17	1.1843	1.4002	1.6528	1.9479	2.2920	2.6928	3.1588	3.7000	4.3276	5.0545
18	1.1961	1.4282	1.7024	2.0258	2.4066	2.8543	3.3799	3.9960	4.7171	5.5599
19	1.2081	1.4568	1.7535	2.1068	2.5270	3.0256	3.6165	4.3157	5.1417	6.1159
20	1.2202	1.4859	1.8061	2.1911	2.6533	3.2071	3.8697	4.6610	5.6044	6.7275
21	1.2324	1.5157	1.8603	2.2788	2.7860	3.3996	4.1406	5.0338	6.1088	7.4002
22	1.2447	1.5460	1.9161	2.3699	2.9253	3.6035	4.4304	5.4365	6.6586	8.1403
23	1.2572	1.5769	1.9736	2.4647	3.0715	3.8197	4.7405	5.8715	7.2579	8.9543
24	1.2697	1.6084	2.0328	2.5633	3.2251	4.0489	5.0724	6.3412	7.9111	9.8497
25	1.2824	1.6406	2.0938	2.6658	3.3864	4.2919	5.4274	6.8485	8.6231	10.834
26	1.2953	1.6734	2.1566	2.7725	3.5557	4.5494	5.8074	7.3964	9.3992	11.918
27	1.3082	1.7069	2.2213	2.8834	3.7335	4.8223	6.2139	7.9881	10.245	13.110
28	1.3213	1.7410	2.2879	2.9987	3.9201	5.1117	6.6488	8.6271	11.167	14.421
29	1.3345	1.7758	2.3566	3.1187	4.1161	5.4184	7.1143	9.3173	12.172	15.863
30	1.3478	1.8114	2.4273	3.2434	4.3219	5.7435	7.6123	10.062	13.267	17.449
40	1.4889	2.2080	3.2620	4.8010	7.0400	10.285	14.974	21.724	31.409	45.259
50	1.6446	2.6916	4.3839	7.1067	11.467	18.420	29.457	46.901	74.357	117.39
60	1.8167	3.2810	5.8916	10.519	18.679	32.987	57.946	101.25	176.03	304.48

Period	12%	14%	15%	16%	18%	20%	24%	28%	32%	36%
1	1.1200	1.1400	1.1500	1.1600	1.1800	1.2000	1.2400	1.2800	1.3200	1.3600
2	1.2544	1.2996	1.3225	1.3456	1.3924	1.4400	1.5376	1.6384	1.7424	1.8496
3	1.4049	1.4815	1.5209	1.5609	1.6430	1.7280	1.9066	2.0972	2.3000	2.5155
4	1.5735	1.6890	1.7490	1.8106	1.9388	2.0736	2.3642	2.6844	3.0360	3.4210
5	1.7623	1.9254	2.0114	2.1003	2.2878	2.4883	2.9316	3.4360	4.0075	4.6526
6	1.9738	2.1950	2.3131	2.4364	2.6996	2.9860	3.6352	4.3980	5.2899	6.3275
7	2.2107	2.5023	2.6600	2.8262	3.1855	3.5832	4.5077	5.6295	6.9826	8.6054
8	2.4760	2.8526	3.0590	3.2784	3.7589	4.2998	5.5895	7.2058	9.2170	11.703
9	2.7731	3.2519	3.5179	3.8030	4.4355	5.1598	6.9310	9.2234	12.166	15.916
10	3.1058	3.7072	4.0456	4.4114	5.2338	6.1917	8.5944	11.805	16.059	21.646
11	3.4785	4.2262	4.6524	5.1173	6.1759	7.4301	10.657	15.111	21.198	29.439
12	3.8960	4.8179	5.3502	5.9360	7.2876	8.9161	13.214	19.342	27.982	40.037
13	4.3635	5.4924	6.1528	6.8858	8.5994	10.699	16.386	24.758	36.937	54.451
14	4.8871	6.2613	7.0757	7.9875	10.147	12.839	20.319	31.691	48.756	74.053
15	5.4736	7.1379	8.1371	9.2655	11.973	15.407	25.195	40.564	64.358	100.71
16	6.1304	8.1372	9.3576	10.748	14.129	18.488	31.242	51.923	84.953	136.96
17	6.8660	9.2765	10.761	12.467	16.672	22.186	38.740	66.461	112.13	186.27
18	7.6900	10.575	12.375	14.462	19.673	26.623	48.038	85.070	148.02	253.33
19	8.6128	12.055	14.231	16.776	23.214	31.948	59.567	108.89	195.39	344.53
20	9.6463	13.743	16.366	19.460	27.393	38.337	73.864	139.37	257.91	468.57
21	10.803	15.667	18.821	22.574	32.323	46.005	91.591	178.40	340.44	637.26
22	12.100	17.861	21.644	26.186	38.142	55.206	113.57	228.35	449.39	866.67
23	13.552	20.361	24.891	30.376	45.007	66.247	140.83	292.30	593.19	1178.6
24	15.178	23.212	28.625	35.236	53.108	79.496	174.63	374.14	783.02	1602.9
25	17.000	26.461	32.918	40.874	62.668	95.396	216.54	478.90	1033.5	2180.0
26	19.040	30.166	37.856	47.414	73.948	114.47	268.51	612.99	1364.3	2964.9
27	21.324	34.389	43.535	55.000	87.259	137.37	332.95	784.63	1800.9	4032.2
28	23.883	39.204	50.065	63.800	102.96	164.84	412.86	1004.3	2377.2	5483.8
29	26.749	44.693	57.575	74.008	121.50	197.81	511.95	1285.5	3137.9	7458.0
30	29.959	50.950	66.211	85.849	143.37	237.37	634.81	1645.5	4142.0	10143.
40	93.050	188.88	267.86	378.72	750.37	1469.7	5455.9	19426.	66520.	*
50	289.00	700.23	1083.6	1670.7	3927.3	9100.4	46890.	*	*	*
60	897.59	2595.9	4383.9	7370.1	20555.	56347.	*	*	*	*

*IF > 99,999.

Appendix B **Present Value of $1: DF $= 1/(1 + k)^n$**

Period	1%	2%	3%	4%	5%	6%	7%	8%	9%	10%
1	.9901	.9804	.9709	.9615	.9524	.9434	.9346	.9259	.9174	.9091
2	.9803	.9612	.9426	.9246	.9070	.8900	.8734	.8573	.8417	.8264
3	.9706	.9423	.9151	.8890	.8638	.8396	.8163	.7938	.7722	.7513
4	.9610	.9238	.8885	.8548	.8227	.7921	.7629	.7350	.7084	.6830
5	.9515	.9057	.8626	.8219	.7835	.7473	.7130	.6806	.6499	.6209
6	.9420	.8880	.8375	.7903	.7462	.7050	.6663	.6302	.5963	.5645
7	.9327	.8706	.8131	.7599	.7107	.6651	.6227	.5835	.5470	.5132
8	.9235	.8535	.7894	.7307	.6768	.6274	.5820	.5403	.5019	.4665
9	.9143	.8368	.7664	.7026	.6446	.5919	.5439	.5002	.4604	.4241
10	.9053	.8203	.7441	.6756	.6139	.5584	.5083	.4632	.4224	.3855
11	.8963	.8043	.7224	.6496	.5847	.5268	.4751	.4289	.3875	.3505
12	.8874	.7885	.7014	.6246	.5568	.4970	.4440	.3971	.3555	.3186
13	.8787	.7730	.6810	.6006	.5303	.4688	.4150	.3677	.3262	.2897
14	.8700	.7579	.6611	.5775	.5051	.4423	.3878	.3405	.2992	.2633
15	.8613	.7430	.6419	.5553	.4810	.4173	.3624	.3152	.2745	.2394
16	.8528	.7284	.6232	.5339	.4581	.3936	.3387	.2919	.2519	.2176
17	.8444	.7142	.6050	.5134	.4363	.3714	.3166	.2703	.2311	.1978
18	.8360	.7002	.5874	.4936	.4155	.3503	.2959	.2502	.2120	.1799
19	.8277	.6864	.5703	.4746	.3957	.3305	.2765	.2317	.1945	.1635
20	.8195	.6730	.5537	.4564	.3769	.3118	.2584	.2145	.1784	.1486
21	.8114	.6598	.5375	.4388	.3589	.2942	.2415	.1987	.1637	.1351
22	.8034	.6468	.5219	.4220	.3418	.2775	.2257	.1839	.1502	.1228
23	.7954	.6342	.5067	.4057	.3256	.2618	.2109	.1703	.1378	.1117
24	.7876	.6217	.4919	.3901	.3101	.2470	.1971	.1577	.1264	.1015
25	.7798	.6095	.4776	.3751	.2953	.2330	.1842	.1460	.1160	.0923
26	.7720	.5976	.4637	.3607	.2812	.2198	.1722	.1352	.1064	.0839
27	.7644	.5859	.4502	.3468	.2678	.2074	.1609	.1252	.0976	.0763
28	.7568	.5744	.4371	.3335	.2551	.1956	.1504	.1159	.0895	.0693
29	.7493	.5631	.4243	.3207	.2429	.1846	.1406	.1073	.0822	.0630
30	.7419	.5521	.4120	.3083	.2314	.1741	.1314	.0994	.0754	.0573
35	.7059	.5000	.3554	.2534	.1813	.1301	.0937	.0676	.0490	.0356
40	.6717	.4529	.3066	.2083	.1420	.0972	.0668	.0460	.0318	.0221
45	.6391	.4102	.2644	.1712	.1113	.0727	.0476	.0313	.0207	.0137
50	.6080	.3715	.2281	.1407	.0872	.0543	.0339	.0213	.0134	.0085
55	.5785	.3365	.1968	.1157	.0683	.0406	.0242	.0145	.0087	.0053

Period	12%	14%	15%	16%	18%	20%	24%	28%	32%	36%
1	.8929	.8772	.8696	.8621	.8475	.8333	.8065	.7813	.7576	.7353
2	.7972	.7695	.7561	.7432	.7182	.6944	.6504	.6104	.5739	.5407
3	.7118	.6750	.6575	.6407	.6086	.5787	.5245	.4768	.4348	.3975
4	.6355	.5921	.5718	.5523	.5158	.4823	.4230	.3725	.3294	.2923
5	.5674	.5194	.4972	.4761	.4371	.4019	.3411	.2910	.2495	.2149
6	.5066	.4556	.4323	.4104	.3704	.3349	.2751	.2274	.1890	.1580
7	.4523	.3996	.3759	.3538	.3139	.2791	.2218	.1776	.1432	.1162
8	.4039	.3506	.3269	.3050	.2660	.2326	.1789	.1388	.1085	.0854
9	.3606	.3075	.2843	.2630	.2255	.1938	.1443	.1084	.0822	.0628
10	.3220	.2697	.2472	.2267	.1911	.1615	.1164	.0847	.0623	.0462
11	.2875	.2366	.2149	.1954	.1619	.1346	.0938	.0662	.0472	.0340
12	.2567	.2076	.1869	.1685	.1372	.1122	.0757	.0517	.0357	.0250
13	.2292	.1821	.1625	.1452	.1163	.0935	.0610	.0404	.0271	.0184
14	.2046	.1597	.1413	.1252	.0985	.0779	.0492	.0316	.0205	.0135
15	.1827	.1401	.1229	.1079	.0835	.0649	.0397	.0247	.0155	.0099
16	.1631	.1229	.1069	.0930	.0708	.0541	.0320	.0193	.0118	.0073
17	.1456	.1078	.0929	.0802	.0600	.0451	.0258	.0150	.0089	.0054
18	.1300	.0946	.0808	.0691	.0508	.0376	.0208	.0118	.0068	.0039
19	.1161	.0829	.0703	.0596	.0431	.0313	.0168	.0092	.0051	.0029
20	.1037	.0728	.0611	.0514	.0365	.0261	.0135	.0072	.0039	.0021
21	.0926	.0638	.0531	.0443	.0309	.0217	.0109	.0056	.0029	.0016
22	.0826	.0560	.0462	.0382	.0262	.0181	.0088	.0044	.0022	.0012
23	.0738	.0491	.0402	.0329	.0222	.0151	.0071	.0034	.0017	.0008
24	.0659	.0431	.0349	.0284	.0188	.0126	.0057	.0027	.0013	.0006
25	.0588	.0378	.0304	.0245	.0160	.0105	.0046	.0021	.0010	.0005
26	.0525	.0331	.0264	.0211	.0135	.0087	.0037	.0016	.0007	.0003
27	.0469	.0291	.0230	.0182	.0115	.0073	.0030	.0013	.0006	.0002
28	.0419	.0255	.0200	.0157	.0097	.0061	.0024	.0010	.0004	.0002
29	.0374	.0224	.0174	.0135	.0082	.0051	.0020	.0008	.0003	.0001
30	.0334	.0196	.0151	.0116	.0070	.0042	.0016	.0006	.0002	.0001
35	.0189	.0102	.0075	.0055	.0030	.0017	.0005	.0002	.0001	*
40	.0107	.0053	.0037	.0026	.0013	.0007	.0002	.0001	*	*
45	.0061	.0027	.0019	.0013	.0006	.0003	.0001	*	*	*
50	.0035	.0014	.0009	.0006	.0003	.0001	*	*	*	*
55	.0020	.0007	.0005	.0003	.0001	*	*	*	*	*

*The factor is zero to four decimal places.

Appendix C **Sum of an Annuity of $1 per Period for n Periods:**

$$IFa = \sum_{t=1}^{n} (1 + k)^{n-t} = \frac{(1 + k)^n - 1}{k}$$

Number of Periods	1%	2%	3%	4%	5%	6%	7%	8%	9%	10%
1	1.0000	1.0000	1.0000	1.0000	1.0000	1.0000	1.0000	1.0000	1.0000	1.0000
2	2.0100	2.0200	2.0300	2.0400	2.0500	2.0600	2.0700	2.0800	2.0900	2.1000
3	3.0301	3.0604	3.0909	3.1216	3.1525	3.1836	3.2149	3.2464	3.2781	3.3100
4	4.0604	4.1216	4.1836	4.2465	4.3101	4.3746	4.4399	4.5061	4.5731	4.6410
5	5.1010	5.2040	5.3091	5.4163	5.5256	5.6371	5.7507	5.8666	5.9847	6.1051
6	6.1520	6.3081	6.4684	6.6330	6.8019	6.9753	7.1533	7.3359	7.5233	7.7156
7	7.2135	7.4343	7.6625	7.8983	8.1420	8.3938	8.6540	8.9228	9.2004	9.4872
8	8.2857	8.5830	8.8923	9.2142	9.5491	9.8975	10.259	10.636	11.028	11.435
9	9.3685	9.7546	10.159	10.582	11.026	11.491	11.978	12.487	13.021	13.579
10	10.462	10.949	11.463	12.006	12.577	13.180	13.816	14.486	15.192	15.937
11	11.566	12.168	12.807	13.486	14.206	14.971	15.783	16.645	17.560	18.531
12	12.682	13.412	14.192	15.025	15.917	16.869	17.888	18.977	20.140	21.384
13	13.809	14.680	15.617	16.626	17.713	18.882	20.140	21.495	22.953	24.522
14	14.947	15.973	17.086	18.291	19.598	21.015	22.550	24.214	26.019	27.975
15	16.096	17.293	18.598	20.023	21.578	23.276	25.129	27.152	29.360	31.772
16	17.257	18.639	20.156	21.824	23.657	25.672	27.888	30.324	33.003	35.949
17	18.430	20.012	21.761	23.697	25.840	28.212	30.840	33.750	36.973	40.544
18	19.614	21.412	23.414	25.645	28.132	30.905	33.999	37.450	41.301	45.599
19	20.810	22.840	25.116	27.671	30.539	33.760	37.379	41.446	46.018	51.159
20	22.019	24.297	26.870	29.778	33.066	36.785	40.995	45.762	51.160	57.275
21	23.239	25.783	28.676	31.969	35.719	39.992	44.865	50.422	56.764	64.002
22	24.471	27.299	30.536	34.248	38.505	43.392	49.005	55.456	62.873	71.402
23	25.716	28.845	32.452	36.617	41.430	46.995	53.436	60.893	69.531	79.543
24	26.973	30.421	34.426	39.082	44.502	50.815	58.176	66.764	76.789	88.497
25	28.243	32.030	36.459	41.645	47.727	54.864	63.249	73.105	84.700	98.347
26	29.525	33.670	38.553	44.311	51.113	59.156	68.676	79.954	93.323	109.18
27	30.820	35.344	40.709	47.084	54.669	63.705	74.483	87.350	102.72	121.09
28	32.129	37.051	42.930	49.967	58.402	68.528	80.697	95.338	112.96	134.20
29	33.450	38.792	45.218	52.966	62.322	73.639	87.346	103.96	124.13	148.63
30	34.784	40.568	47.575	56.084	66.438	79.058	94.460	113.28	136.30	164.49
40	48.886	60.402	75.401	95.025	120.79	154.76	199.63	259.05	337.88	442.59
50	64.463	84.579	112.79	152.66	209.34	290.33	406.52	573.76	815.08	1163.9
60	81.669	114.05	163.05	237.99	353.58	533.12	813.52	1253.2	1944.7	3034.8

Number of Periods	12%	14%	15%	16%	18%	20%	24%	28%	32%	36%
1	1.0000	1.0000	1.0000	1.0000	1.0000	1.0000	1.0000	1.0000	1.0000	1.0000
2	2.1200	2.1400	2.1500	2.1600	2.1800	2.2000	2.2400	2.2800	2.3200	2.3600
3	3.3744	3.4396	3.4725	3.5056	3.5724	3.6400	3.7776	3.9184	4.0624	4.2096
4	4.7793	4.9211	4.9934	5.0665	5.2154	5.3680	5.6842	6.0156	6.3624	6.7251
5	6.3528	6.6101	6.7424	6.8771	7.1542	7.4416	8.0484	8.6999	9.3983	10.146
6	8.1152	8.5355	8.7537	8.9775	9.4420	9.9299	10.980	12.135	13.405	14.798
7	10.089	10.730	11.066	11.413	12.141	12.915	14.615	16.533	18.695	21.126
8	12.299	13.232	13.726	14.240	15.327	16.499	19.122	22.163	25.678	29.731
9	14.775	16.085	16.785	17.518	19.085	20.798	24.712	29.369	34.895	41.435
10	17.548	19.337	20.303	21.321	23.521	25.958	31.643	38.592	47.061	57.351
11	20.654	23.044	24.349	25.732	28.755	32.150	40.237	50.398	63.121	78.998
12	24.133	27.270	29.001	30.850	34.931	39.580	50.894	65.510	84.320	108.43
13	28.029	32.088	34.351	36.786	42.218	48.496	64.109	84.852	112.30	148.47
14	32.392	37.581	40.504	43.672	50.818	59.195	80.496	109.61	149.23	202.92
15	37.279	43.842	47.580	51.659	60.965	72.035	100.81	141.30	197.99	276.97
16	42.753	50.980	55.717	60.925	72.939	87.442	126.01	181.86	262.35	377.69
17	48.883	59.117	65.075	71.673	87.068	105.93	157.25	233.79	347.30	514.66
18	55.749	68.394	75.836	84.140	103.74	128.11	195.99	300.25	459.44	700.93
19	63.439	78.969	88.211	98.603	123.41	154.74	244.03	385.32	607.47	954.27
20	72.052	91.024	102.44	115.37	146.62	186.68	303.60	494.21	802.86	1298.8
21	81.698	104.76	118.81	134.84	174.02	225.02	377.46	633.59	1060.7	1767.3
22	92.502	120.43	137.63	157.41	206.34	271.03	469.05	811.99	1401.2	2404.6
23	104.60	138.29	159.27	183.60	244.48	326.23	582.62	1040.3	1850.6	3271.3
24	118.15	158.65	184.16	213.97	289.49	392.48	723.46	1332.6	2443.8	4449.9
25	133.33	181.87	212.79	249.21	342.60	471.98	898.09	1706.8	3226.8	6052.9
26	150.33	208.33	245.71	290.08	405.27	567.37	1114.6	2185.7	4260.4	8233.0
27	169.37	238.49	283.56	337.50	479.22	681.85	1383.1	2798.7	5624.7	11197.9
28	190.69	272.88	327.10	392.50	566.48	819.22	1716.0	3583.3	7425.6	15230.2
29	214.58	312.09	377.16	456.30	669.44	984.06	2128.9	4587.6	9802.9	20714.1
30	241.33	356.78	434.74	530.31	790.94	1181.8	2640.9	5873.2	12940.	28172.2
40	767.09	1342.0	1779.0	2360.7	4163.2	7343.8	22728.	69377.	*	*
50	2400.0	4994.5	7217.7	10435.	21813.	45497.	*	*	*	*
60	7471.6	18535.	29219.	46057.	*	*	*	*	*	*

*IFa > 99,999.

Appendix D **Present Value of an Annuity of $1 per Period for n Periods:**

$$DFa = \sum_{t=1}^{n} \frac{1}{(1 + k)^t} = \frac{1 - \dfrac{1}{(1 + k)^n}}{k}$$

Number of Periods	1%	2%	3%	4%	5%	6%	7%	8%	9%
1	0.9901	0.9804	0.9709	0.9615	0.9524	0.9434	0.9346	0.9259	0.9174
2	1.9704	1.9416	1.9135	1.8861	1.8594	1.8334	1.8080	1.7833	1.7591
3	2.9410	2.8839	2.8286	2.7751	2.7232	2.6730	2.6243	2.5771	2.5313
4	3.9020	3.8077	3.7171	3.6299	3.5460	3.4651	3.3872	3.3121	3.2397
5	4.8534	4.7135	4.5797	4.4518	4.3295	4.2124	4.1002	3.9927	3.8897
6	5.7955	5.6014	5.4172	5.2421	5.0757	4.9173	4.7665	4.6229	4.4859
7	6.7282	6.4720	6.2303	6.0021	5.7864	5.5824	5.3893	5.2064	5.0330
8	7.6517	7.3255	7.0197	6.7327	6.4632	6.2098	5.9713	5.7466	5.5348
9	8.5660	8.1622	7.7861	7.4353	7.1078	6.8017	6.5152	6.2469	5.9952
10	9.4713	8.9826	8.5302	8.1109	7.7217	7.3601	7.0236	6.7101	6.4177
11	10.3676	9.7868	9.2526	8.7605	8.3064	7.8869	7.4987	7.1390	6.8052
12	11.2551	10.5753	9.9540	9.3851	8.8633	8.3838	7.9427	7.5361	7.1607
13	12.1337	11.3484	10.6350	9.9856	9.3936	8.8527	8.3577	7.9038	7.4869
14	13.0037	12.1062	11.2961	10.5631	9.8986	9.2950	8.7455	8.2442	7.7862
15	13.8651	12.8493	11.9379	11.1184	10.3797	9.7122	9.1079	8.5595	8.0607
16	14.7179	13.5777	12.5611	11.6523	10.8378	10.1059	9.4466	8.8514	8.3126
17	15.5623	14.2919	13.1661	12.1657	11.2741	10.4773	9.7632	9.1216	8.5436
18	16.3983	14.9920	13.7535	12.6593	11.6896	10.8276	10.0591	9.3719	8.7556
19	17.2260	15.6785	14.3238	13.1339	12.0853	11.1581	10.3356	9.6036	8.9501
20	18.0456	16.3514	14.8775	13.5903	12.4622	11.4699	10.5940	9.8181	9.1285
21	18.8570	17.0112	15.4150	14.0292	12.8212	11.7641	10.8355	10.0168	9.2922
22	19.6604	17.6580	15.9369	14.4511	13.1630	12.0416	11.0612	10.2007	9.4424
23	20.4558	18.2922	16.4436	14.8568	13.4886	12.3034	11.2722	10.3711	9.5802
24	21.2434	18.9139	16.9355	15.2470	13.7986	12.5504	11.4693	10.5288	9.7066
25	22.0232	19.5235	17.4131	15.6221	14.0939	12.7834	11.6536	10.6748	9.8226
26	22.7952	20.1210	17.8768	15.9828	14.3752	13.0032	11.8258	10.8100	9.9290
27	23.5596	20.7069	18.3270	16.3296	14.6430	13.2105	11.9867	10.9352	10.0266
28	24.3164	21.2813	18.7641	16.6631	14.8981	13.4062	12.1371	11.0511	10.1161
29	25.0658	21.8444	19.1885	16.9837	15.1411	13.5907	12.2777	11.1584	10.1983
30	25.8077	22.3965	19.6004	17.2920	15.3725	13.7648	12.4090	11.2578	10.2737
35	29.4086	24.9986	21.4872	18.6646	16.3742	14.4982	12.9477	11.6546	10.5668
40	32.8347	27.3555	23.1148	19.7928	17.1591	15.0463	13.3317	11.9246	10.7574
45	36.0945	29.4902	24.5187	20.7200	17.7741	15.4558	13.6055	12.1084	10.8812
50	39.1961	31.4236	25.7298	21.4822	18.2559	15.7619	13.8007	12.2335	10.9617
55	42.1472	33.1748	26.7744	22.1086	18.6335	15.9905	13.9399	12.3186	11.0140

Number of Periods	10%	12%	14%	15%	16%	18%	20%	24%	28%	32%
1	0.9091	0.8929	0.8772	0.8696	0.8621	0.8475	0.8333	0.8065	0.7813	0.7576
2	1.7355	1.6901	1.6467	1.6257	1.6052	1.5656	1.5278	1.4568	1.3916	1.3315
3	2.4869	2.4018	2.3216	2.2832	2.2459	2.1743	2.1065	1.9813	1.8684	1.7663
4	3.1699	3.0373	2.9137	2.8550	2.7982	2.6901	2.5887	2.4043	2.2410	2.0957
5	3.7908	3.6048	3.4331	3.3522	3.2743	3.1272	2.9906	2.7454	2.5320	2.3452
6	4.3553	4.1114	3.8887	3.7845	3.6847	3.4976	3.3255	3.0205	2.7594	2.5342
7	4.8684	4.5638	4.2883	4.1604	4.0386	3.8115	3.6046	3.2423	2.9370	2.6775
8	5.3349	4.9676	4.6389	4.4873	4.3436	4.0776	3.8372	3.4212	3.0758	2.7860
9	5.7590	5.3282	4.9464	4.7716	4.6065	4.3030	4.0310	3.5655	3.1842	2.8681
10	6.1446	5.6502	5.2161	5.0188	4.8332	4.4941	4.1925	3.6819	3.2689	2.9304
11	6.4951	5.9377	5.4527	5.2337	5.0286	4.6560	4.3271	3.7757	3.3351	2.9776
12	6.8137	6.1944	5.6603	5.4206	5.1971	4.7932	4.4392	3.8514	3.3868	3.0133
13	7.1034	6.4235	5.8424	5.5831	5.3423	4.9095	4.5327	3.9124	3.4272	3.0404
14	7.3667	6.6282	6.0021	5.7245	5.4675	5.0081	4.6106	3.9616	3.4587	3.0609
15	7.6061	6.8109	6.1422	5.8474	5.5755	5.0916	4.6755	4.0013	3.4834	3.0764
16	7.8237	6.9740	6.2651	5.9542	5.6685	5.1624	4.7296	4.0333	3.5026	3.0882
17	8.0216	7.1196	6.3729	6.0472	5.7487	5.2223	4.7746	4.0591	3.5177	3.0971
18	8.2014	7.2497	6.4674	6.1280	5.8178	5.2732	4.8122	4.0799	3.5294	3.1039
19	8.3649	7.3658	6.5504	6.1982	5.8775	5.3162	4.8435	4.0967	3.5386	3.1090
20	8.5136	7.4694	6.6231	6.2593	5.9288	5.3527	4.8696	4.1103	3.5458	3.1129
21	8.6487	7.5620	6.6870	6.3125	5.9731	5.3837	4.8913	4.1212	3.5514	3.1158
22	8.7715	7.6446	6.7429	6.3587	6.0113	5.4099	4.9094	4.1300	3.5558	3.1180
23	8.8832	7.7184	6.7921	6.3988	6.0442	5.4321	4.9245	4.1371	3.5592	3.1197
24	8.9847	7.7843	6.8351	6.4338	6.0726	5.4510	4.9371	4.1428	3.5619	3.1210
25	9.0770	7.8431	6.8729	6.4642	6.0971	5.4669	4.9476	4.1474	3.5640	3.1220
26	9.1609	7.8957	6.9061	6.4906	6.1182	5.4804	4.9563	4.1511	3.5656	3.1227
27	9.2372	7.9426	6.9352	6.5135	6.1364	5.4919	4.9636	4.1542	3.5669	3.1233
28	9.3066	7.9844	6.9607	6.5335	6.1520	5.5016	4.9697	4.1566	3.5679	3.1237
29	9.3696	8.0218	6.9830	6.5509	6.1656	5.5098	4.9747	4.1585	3.5687	3.1240
30	9.4269	8.0552	7.0027	6.5660	6.1772	5.5168	4.9789	4.1601	3.5693	3.1242
35	9.6442	8.1755	7.0700	6.6166	6.2153	5.5386	4.9915	4.1644	3.5708	3.1248
40	9.7791	8.2438	7.1050	6.6418	6.2335	5.5482	4.9966	4.1659	3.5712	3.1250
45	9.8628	8.2825	7.1232	6.6543	6.2421	5.5523	4.9986	4.1664	3.5714	3.1250
50	9.9148	8.3045	7.1327	6.6605	6.2463	5.5541	4.9995	4.1666	3.5714	3.1250
55	9.9471	8.3170	7.1376	6.6636	6.2482	5.5549	4.9998	4.1666	3.5714	3.1250

Appendix E

Answers to Selected End-of-Chapter Problems

In this appendix we present some intermediate steps and final answers to selected end-of-chapter problems. Please note that your answer may differ slightly from ours due to rounding errors. Also, although we hope not, some of the problems may have more than one correct solution, depending on the assumptions made in working the problem. Finally, many of the problems involve some verbal discussion as well as numerical calculations; that verbal material is not presented here.

2-1   **a.** $61,250
        b. 30.625%
        c. 39%

2-2 $76,850

2-3   **a.** $61,250
        b. $7,800
        c. $1,560

2-5   **a.** $22,599
        b. 33%; 27.5%
        d. 18.2%

2-6   **a.** $53,000; $77,000; $41,000; $12,000; $17,000

2-7   **a.** $33,000; $45,000; $22,000
        b. $5,250; $6,000; $29,270
        c. $62,750; $79,000; $110,730

2-8   **a. 1.** $5,415; $8,415; $11,415
        a. 2. $6,240; $11,840; $17,650

4-1   **b.** $50,000,000

4-2   **b.** $64,000,000

5-1   **a.** $k_1 = 12.3\%$; $k_5 = 11.3\%$; $k_{20} = 11.45\%$

5-4 $I_2 = 12\%$

6-2 $1,750

6-3   **a.** $45,500

6-4   **a.** $200,000
      b. $250,000
      c. $333,333.33

6-6   Total equity = $83,500,000

6-7   **a.** $6.42
      b. $4.17
      c. Total equity = $97,000,000

6-8 $1,312,500

6-9   **b.** + $1,400,000
      f. − $100,000

6-10 **a.** $800,000,000
      b. $2.80

6-12 Total sources = $234 million

7-1   14.9%

7-2   24%

7-3   60%

7-4   2.448%

7-5   40 days

7-6   3; 120 days

7-7   **a.** 43 days
      b. 47.78 days

7-8 $700,000; quick ratio = 1.19

7-9 $1,875,000

7-10 $2,000,000, ACP = 30 days

7-11 Fixed assets = $450,000; Total assets = $1,350,000; Current liabilities = $450,000;
      Total debt = $540,000

7-12 **a.** Current ratio 1.98; ACP = 75 days; Total asset turnover = 1.7; Debt ratio = 61.9%

7-15 **a.** 16%
      b. ROE = 20.97%

7-16 **a.** Quick ratio = 0.8%; ACP = 37 days; ROE = 13.1%; Debt ratio 54.8%

8-1   **a.** Total assets = $10.8 million

8-1   **b.** $5,370,000

8-2   **a.** Total debt = $960,000
      b. $75,000

8-3   **a.** $370,000
      b. $81,000; $289,000
      c. 58.18%
      d. current ratio = 1.66
      e. ROA = 5.45%

8-4   **a.** $182,500
          b. $81,000; $101,500
          c. 52.1%
          d. current ratio = 2.06
          e. 6.24%

8-5   4.2%

8-6 $960,000

8-7 $1,440,000 excess funds

8-8   **a.** $16,325,000
          c. current ratio = 1.87, ROE = 14.72%
          d. 1. $6,175,000 excess funds
          d. 3. current ratio = 3.4, ROE = 11.37%

8-9   **b.** $1,080,000

8-10 **b.** 25% sales increase
          c. $5,400,000
          d. 10.6% ROE

8-11 **b.** $103,500
          d. 6.25%

8-12 **a.** AFN = $578,000

9-1   **a.** $900,000
          b. $610,000

9-2   **a.** 80 days
          b. $285,000
          c. 5 times

9-3   **a.** 30 days
          b. $270,000
          c. $45,000
          d. 28 days; $336,000

9-4   **a.** 10.1%; 11.52%
          b. 9.12%; 7.68%

9-5   **a.** current ratio 1.6; NWC $3,750,000; ROE 13.33%
          b. current ratio 2.4; NWC $8,750,000; ROE 11.2%

9-7   **a.** Inventory turnover 6.67
          b. Inventory turnover period 54 days
          c. ACP 70 days
          d. cash cycle 89 days
          e. ROA 8.04%

9-8   **a.** $200,000
          b. $250,000
          c. 55 days
          d. ROA 9.47%

9-9   **a.** ROE for: aggressive 11.75%; moderate 10.8%; conservative 9.16%

10-1 **b. 1.** $3,000,000
          b. 2. − $13,000,000

10-2   **a.** $2,100,000
         b. $189,000
         c. $15,750

10-3   June $66,975; July $101,925; August $123,675

10-4   August $248,800,000; September $223,000,000; October $132,800,000

10-5   **b.** $164,400

10-6   **a.** July surplus cash = $85,250; October loans = $26,500

11-1   ACP = 75 days

11-2   **a.** ACP = 29.25 days
         b. A/R = $40,625
         c. ACP = 21 days; A/R = $29,166.67

11-3   **a.** ACP before = 28 days; after = 22 days
         b. before $700,000; after $550,000

11-4   **a.** ACP before = 25 days; after = 20 days
         b. Discount costs are $10,000 before, $23,400 after change
         c. $4,861 before, $5,056 after change
         d. Bad debt loss is $20,000 before, $26,000 after change
         e. $42,243

11-5 NI_3 = $46,811; NI_4 = $15,467; NI_5 = $8,538

11-7   **a.** NI_0 = $496,500; NI_N = $509,156

11-8   **a.** 500 pounds
         b. 10 orders
         c. 250 pounds

11-10   **a.** 4,243 bags
          b. 5,243 bags
          c. 3,121.5 bags
          d. 12.7 days

11-11   **a.** 100,000 square yards
          b. $120,000
          c. $44,000
          d. 48,462 square yards

11-12   **a.** 20,400 units
          b. 38.2 orders
          c. 30,000 units

12-1   **a.** 18.18%
         b. 24.24%
         c. 36.73%
         d. 29.39%
         e. 7.27%
         f. 22.27%
         g. 111.34%

12-3   **a.** $166.667
         c. $500,000; 36.73%

12-4 **a.** 10%
      b. 11.1%
      c. 20%

12-5 **a.** 16.5%
      b. 16.25%
      c. 15.38%
      d. 18%

12-6 **a.** 12.9%
      b. $97,059

12-7 15.625%

12-8 **a.** 27.84%
      b. 17.5%

12-9 14.44%

12-10 13.4%

12-11 **a.** (1) 55.67% (2) 18.55% (3) 24.09%

12-12 **b.** 14.58%
      c. 14.25%
      d. 14.06%
      e. 14.00%

12-13 **a.** Bank 11.11%; trade 14.69%

12-14 **a.** $150,000

12-15 **a.** 60 days
      b. 14.69%

12-16 **a. 1.** Trade 18.18%
      a. 2. Bank 12.68%

13-1 **a.** $1,080.00
      b. $1,166.40
      c. $925.90
      d. $857.30

13-2 **a.** $1,790.83
      b. $3,105.80
      c. $558.40
      d. $1,000.07

13-3 **a.** 12 years
      b. 6 years
      c. 5 years
      d. 1 year

13-4 **a.** $15,937.00
      b. $11,051.20
      c. $5,000.00

13-5 **a.** $17,531.00
      b. $11,603.80
      c. $5,000.00

13-6 **a.** $6,144.60
         b. $8,659.00
         c. $5,000.00

13-7 **a.** $6,759.00
         b. $9,092.00
         c. $5,000.00

13-8 **a.** PV_A = $10,795.70
             PV_B = $11,948.50
         b. $15,000

13-9 $21,580.00

13-10 **a.** 15%

13-11 **a.** $17,252.10
         b. $18,459.90

13-12 **a.** 10%
         b. 10%
         c. 12%
         d. 9%

13-13 20%

13-14 15%

13-15 8%

13-16 9%

13-17 **a.** $39,745.20
         b. $30,924.82; $0.00

13-18 $620.90

13-19 **a.** $65,736.71
         b. $59,760.72

13-20 **a.** Year 1 $5.5 million; Year 5 $8,052,500

13-21 $2,000; $1,000.

13-22 **a.** $8,042.14

13A-1 **a.** $314.71
         b. $318.78
         c. $320.92
         d. $225.38

13A-2 **a.** $125.48
         b. $124.64
         c. $177.48

13A-3 **a.** $1,980.00
         b. $2,512.22

13A-4 10.38% vs. 11%

14-1 **a.** 2.79 years
         b. $166,761
         c. 32%

14-2 **a.** 3.7908 years
     b. $266,371.30
     c. 10.0%

14-3 **a.** 2.99 years
     b. $205,376.63
     c. 20.0%

14-4 **a.** 3.13 years
     b. Zero
     c. 14%

14-5 **a.** 3.17 years
     b. − $2,661.60

14-6 **a.** $3,612.70
     b. 14%

	NPV	IRR
14-7 Truck	$ 416.66	16.0%
Pulley	2,927.82	20.0%

	NPV	IRR
14-8 Elec.	$6,744.98	≈ 20%
Gas	5,483.09	≈ 20%

	X	Y
14-9 **a.**	2.17 years	2.86 years
b.	$5,301.00	$4,378.60
c.	18%	15%

	Year 1	Year 2	Year 3
14-10 **a.**	$220,000	$238,000	$256,000
b.	$ 59,584		

14-11 **a.** $286,410
      b. $54,037

	Year 1	Year 2	Year 3	Year 4	Year 5
14-12 Cash flow	$26,000	$31,000	$26,000	$23,600	$23,600

NPV = − $5,176

15-1 **a.** 15%
     b. 12.845%

15-2 **a.** 15%
     b. 27.73%

15-3 **a.** $38,442
     b. 20%

15-4 Alpha $92,872; Omega $76,952

15-5 **a.** 18%
     b. − $50,590

15-6   **a.** 9.5%
      b. 11%
      c. 14%

15-7   **a.** 17%

k_m	k_s

      b. 1. 16%   19%
          2. 12%   15%
      c. 1. $k_s = 20.2\%$
          2. $k_s = 13.8\%$

15-8 NPV_A $3,001.87; NPV_B $5,731.58

15-9   **a.** $10,000
      d. 1. $11,800
          2. 11.8%

15-10   **a.** k = 9% + 1.2 (14% − 9%)
      b. 15%
      c. 19%

15-11   **a.** Project A $9,000; Project B $10,200
      b. Project A $13,382.10; Project B $15,498.36

16-1   **a.** $45,600
      b. $14,378.88
      c. 15.8%

16-2 $54,224

16-4   **a.** 16%
      b. $0.00
      c. 16%

16-5   **a.** 15%
      b. ≈18%
      c. $18,176

16-6   **a.** Project E 12%; Project F 15%
      c. At 12% Project E = $7,356.64; at 15% Project F = − $2,786.20

16-7   **a.** $920,000
      b. Year 1: Depreciation $64,000; Year 5: Depreciation $35,200
      c. Cash flow: Year 1 = $184,000; Year 5 = $155,200
      d. After tax $60,000

16-10   **b.** NPV = $61,255

16-11   **a.** 16.5%
      b. Recap NPV = $8,682; Tire NPV = − $14,440

17-1   **a.** $57.14

17-2   **a.** 10%
      b. 13.26%
      c. 14%

17-3 $1,113.03

17-4   **a. 1.** $1,134.20
            2. $1,000.00
            3. $ 887.00
            b. 1. $1,018.50
            2. $1,000.00
            3. $ 982.14

17-5   **a.** (1) 10.0%; (2) 6.0%

17-6   **a.** $908.68

17-7   **a.** $514,178.47
            b. $311,638.13
            c. $554,815.80
            d. $353,969.77

	Year 1	Year 2	Year 3
17-9 **a.**	$303,537.75	$303,537.75	$603,539.65

b. $725,504

17-10   **a.** YTM = 9%; YTC = 7.75%

18-1 $60.00

18-2 $66.25

18-3 $78.90

18-4 $50.00

18-5   **a.** 10%
            b. 15%

18-6   **a.** 5%
            b. $58.34

18-7 $83.33

18-8   **a.** D_1 = $4.28; D_2 $4.5798; D_3 $4.9002
            b. $10.41
            c. $43.09
            d. $53.50
            e. $53.50

18-9   **a.** 8%
            b. 10%
            c. 18%

18-10   **a. 1.** $9.50
            2. $13.33
            3. $26.75
            4. $44.00
            5. $228.00
            b. 1. Undefined
            2. − $48.00

18-11 $28.72

18-12   **a.** $16.37

18-13 $24.41

18-14   **a.** $36.36
   b. $34.48
   c. $47.62
   d. $65.16

18-15   **a.** No, new price = $31.34
   b. Beta = 0.5

18-16   **a.**

	1983	1988
EPS	$8,160	$12,000
DPS	$4,200	$ 6,000
Book per Share		$90,000

   d.

	1983	1988
EPS	$2.04	$ 3.00
DPS	$1.05	$ 1.50
Book per Share		$22.50

   g.

	ROE
Gemex	15.00%
Dimson	13.64%
Atherton	13.33%

   h.

	Debt Ratio
Gemex	43%
Dimson	37%
Atherton	55%

   i.

	P/E
Gemex	8.00
Dimson	8.67

   k.

Gemex	15.2%
Dimson	12.54%

18-17   **a.** P_0 = $36.46

19-1   **a.** 14%
   b. 9.24%
   c. 8.4%
   d. 5.6%

19-2   8.1%

19-3   **a.** 923.95
   b. 10%

19-4   13.04%

19-5   **a.** 14%
   b. 14%

19-6   **a.** 12.2%
   b. 12%

19-7   17.7%

19-8   **a.** 9%
         b. $1.9075
         c. 16.988%

19-9   **a.** 15.4%
         b. 11.8%
         c. 13.0%

19-10   **a.** 14%
         b. 13.5%
         d. 14.0%

19-11   **a.** 16%
         b. 8%
         c. 16.78%

19-12   **a.** 15%
         b. 6.75%
         c. 16.75%

19-13   **a.** 29%; 15%; 14–16%

19-14   **a.** $6,000,000
         b. $14,000,000
         c. $23,333,333.33
         d. $37,500,000; $62,500,000

19-15 $478,300

19-16   13.782%

19-17   **a.** $k_d = 7.2\%$; $k_s = 16\%$
         b. 11.6%
         c. $7,800,000
         d. 17%

19-18   **a.** $30,000,000
         b. $18,000,000
         c. $6,000,000; $12,000,000
         d. $k_s = 15\%$; $k_e = 16.06\%$
         e. $10,000,000
         f. **1.** 11.64%
              2. 12.28%

19-19   **a.** 3
         c. 11.4%; 12.4%; 12.9%; 13.4%
         d. 16%; 14%

20-1   100%

20-2   **a.** 50,000 units
         b. $1,500,000
         c. DOL 6
         d. − $50,000

20-3   **a.** 70,000 units
         b. $2,100,000

c. DOL 8

d. − $100,000

20-4 **a.** $6,000,000

b. DOL 6

c. $9,600,000

e. $2,400,000

20-5 **a.**

Sales	Option 1	Option 2
$ 40,000	− 1.00	− 0.20
$120,000	3.00	∞
$240,000	1.50	2.00

20-6 $90

20-7 **a.** DOL = 2.15

b. DFL = 2.45

c. DTL = 5.28

20-8 **a.** DOL = 3

b. DFL = 2

c. DTL = 6

20-9 **a.** DOL = 11

b. DFL = − 5

c. DTL = − 55

20-10 $165,000

20-11 **a.** $2.85

20-12 **a.**

	DOL	
Sales	LOL	HOL
$1.2 million	3	∞
$1.6 million	2	4

b.

	DFL			
	LOL		HOL	
Sales	No Debt	$900,000 Debt	No Debt	$900,000 Debt
$1.2 million	1.00	10.00	1.00	0.00
$1.6 million	1.00	1.82	1.00	1.82

c.

	DTL	
Sales	LOL	HOL
$1.2 million	30.00	− 6.67
$1.6 million	3.64	7.27

20-14 **a.** Equity

b.

Financing	Stock Price
Equity	$67.20
Debt issue	$46.50
Preferred issue	$48.00

21-1   **a.** 62.5%
      b. $2,000,000
      c. 60%
      d. $7,000,000

21-2   6%

21-3   100%

21-4   60%

21-5 $1,950,000

21-6   Total equity = $57,000,000

21-7   9.09%

21-8 $13.5135

21-10   **a.** $2,675,000
      b. $5,000,000
      c. $4,000,000
      d. $10,400,000

21-11   **a.**

@ 20%	@ 80%
12%	3%

      b.

@ 20%	@ 80%
$22.40	$29.43

      c. 80% payout

21-12   **a.** Payout = 63.16%; Break point = $15.27 million; 10.67%; 10.96%
      b. $24 million

22-1   − $131,145

22-2 $313,690

22-3 $69,799,000

22-5   **a.** 16.2%
      b. Terminal value $520,000

22-6   **a.** 14%
      b. $25,493,000
      c. $17.00

23-1 $416,112

23-2 $371,535

23-4   11.3%

23-6   IRR = 8.76%

23-8   **c.** PMT = $248,402

24-1   0.6024 pounds per dollar

24-2   4.545 francs per dollar

24-3   .12 francs per pound

24-5

Dollars per 1,000 Units of			
Rupees	**Lira**	**Pesos**	**Riyals**
$76.90	$0.77	$0.67	$266.60

24-7   **b.** $13,900.71

24-8   **a.** $2,666,666.67
           b. $2,560,000
           d. $2,782,608.70

24-9 $50.00

24-10 $500,000

Appendix F

Selected Equations

Chapter 5

$$k = k^* + IP + DP + LP + MP.$$

Chapter 6

$$EPS = \frac{\text{Net income after tax}}{\text{Shares outstanding}}.$$

$$DPS = \frac{\text{Dividends paid to common shareholders}}{\text{Shares outstanding}}.$$

Chapter 7

$$\frac{\text{Current}}{\text{ratio}} = \frac{\text{Current assets}}{\text{Current liabilities}}.$$

$$\frac{\text{Quick}}{\text{ratio}} = \frac{\text{Current assets} - \text{Inventory}}{\text{Current liabilities}}.$$

$$\frac{\text{Fixed assets}}{\substack{\text{utilization} \\ \text{(or turnover)}}} = \frac{\text{Sales}}{\text{Net fixed assets}}.$$

$$\frac{\text{Inventory utilization}}{\text{(or turnover)}} = \frac{\text{Sales}}{\text{Inventory}}.$$

$$ACP = \frac{\text{Receivables}}{\text{Sales per day}} = \frac{\text{A/R}}{\text{Sales/360}}.$$

$$\frac{\text{Total assets utilization}}{\text{(or turnover)}} = \frac{\text{Sales}}{\text{Total assets}}.$$

$$\frac{\text{Profit}}{\text{margin}} = \frac{\text{Net profit after taxes}}{\text{Sales}}.$$

$$\frac{\text{Debt}}{\text{ratio}} = \frac{\text{Total debt}}{\text{Total assets}}.$$

$$ROA = \frac{\text{Net profit after taxes}}{\text{Total assets}}.$$

$$TIE = \frac{\text{EBIT}}{\text{I}}.$$

$$ROE = \frac{\text{Net profit after taxes}}{\text{Common equity}}.$$

$$P/E \text{ ratio} = \frac{\text{Price per share}}{\text{Earnings per share}}.$$

$$M/B \text{ ratio} = \frac{\text{Price per share}}{\text{Book value per share}}.$$

$$ROE = ROA \times \frac{\text{Assets}}{\text{Common equity}}.$$

$$ROA = \frac{\text{Profit}}{\text{margin}} \times \frac{\text{Total assets}}{\text{utilization}}.$$

$$BEP = \frac{\text{EBIT}}{\text{Total assets}}.$$

Chapter 8

$$AFN = A/S(\Delta S) - L/S(\Delta S) - MS_1(1 - d).$$

Chapter 11

$$EOQ = \sqrt{\frac{2FS}{CP}}.$$

Chapter 12

$$\frac{\text{Percentage}}{\text{cost}} = \frac{\text{Discount percent}}{100 - \text{Discount percent}} \times \frac{360}{\text{Days credit is outstanding} - \text{Discount period}}.$$

$$\frac{\text{Effective rate of interest}}{\text{on simple interest loan}} = \frac{\text{Interest}}{\text{Amount borrowed}}.$$

$$\frac{\text{Effective rate of interest}}{\text{on discounted loan}} = \frac{\text{Interest}}{\text{Amount borrowed} - \text{Interest}}.$$

$$= \frac{\text{Interest rate (\%)}}{1.0 - \text{Interest rate (fraction)}}.$$

$$\frac{\text{Approximate effective rate of interest on installment loan}}{} = \frac{\text{Annual interest}}{\text{Loan amount} \div 2}.$$

$$\frac{\text{Effective rate of interest on compensating balance loan}}{} = \frac{\text{Interest rate (\%)}}{1.0 - \text{Compensating balance fraction}}.$$

$$\frac{\text{Discount loan with compensating balance}}{} = \frac{\text{Interest rate (\%)}}{1.0 - \text{Stated interest rate (fraction)} - \text{Compensating balance (fraction)}}.$$

Chapter 13

$$FV = PV(IF). \qquad IF = (1 + k)^n.$$

$$PV = FV(DF). \qquad DF = [1/(1 + k)^n] = (1/IF).$$

$$FVa = Pmt(IFa). \qquad IFa = \frac{(1 + k)^n - 1}{k}.$$

$$PVa = Pmt(DFa). \qquad DFa = \frac{1 - \dfrac{1}{(1 + k)^n}}{k}.$$

Appendix 13A

$$FV_n = PV\left(1 + \frac{k_{Nom}}{m}\right)^{mn}$$

$$\text{Effective annual rate} = \left(1 + \frac{k_{Nom}}{m}\right)^m - 1.0.$$

Chapter 14

$$NPV = \sum_{t=1}^{n} \frac{CF_t}{(1 + k)^t} - C \qquad IRR = \sum_{t=1}^{n} \frac{CF_t}{(1 + r)^t} - C = 0.$$

$$= \sum_{t=1}^{n} CF_t(DF) - C. \qquad \sum_{t=1}^{n} CF_t(DF) - C = 0.$$

Chapter 15

$$k = R_F + b(k_M - R_F).$$

$$\hat{k} = \sum_{i=1}^{n} P_i k_i.$$

$$\sigma = \sqrt{\sum_{t=1}^{n} (k_i - \hat{k})^2 P_i}.$$

$$\sigma^2 = \sum_{i=1}^{n} (k_i - \hat{k})^2 P_i.$$

Chapter 16

$$1 + k_n = (1 + k_r)(1 + i).$$

$$NPV = \sum_{t=1}^{n} \frac{CF_t}{(1 + k_n)^t} - C.$$

$$NPV = \sum_{t=1}^{n} \frac{RCF_t}{(1 + k_r)^t} - C.$$

Chapter 17

$$V = \sum_{t=1}^{n} I\left(\frac{1}{1 + k_d}\right)^t + M\left(\frac{1}{1 + k_d}\right)^n$$

$$= I(DFa) + M(DF).$$

$$\text{Approximate YTM} = \frac{I + (M - V)/n}{(M + V)/2}.$$

$$P_p = \frac{D}{k_p}.$$

$$FCC = \frac{EBIT + \text{Lease payments}}{I + \text{Lease payments} + \dfrac{\text{Sinking fund payments}}{1 - t}}.$$

$$P_p = \frac{D_p}{k_p}.$$

Chapter 18

$$D_t = D_0(1 + g)^t.$$

$$P_0 = \frac{D_1}{k_s - g}.$$

Appendix 18A

$$V_w = (P_0 - P_s)(N).$$

Chapter 19

$$\text{After-tax } k_d = k_d (1 - t). \qquad k_e = \frac{D_1}{P_0(1 - F)} + g. \qquad k_s = \frac{D_1}{P_0} + g.$$

$$k_p = D_p/P_p. \qquad k_a = w_d(k_d)(1 - t) + w_s(k_s \text{ or } k_e) + w_p(k_p).$$

$$\text{Break point} = \frac{\$ \text{ of low-cost capital}}{\begin{array}{c} \% \text{ of this type of capital} \\ \text{in capital structure} \end{array}}.$$

$$k_p = \frac{D_p}{P_p}.$$

Chapter 20

$$DTL = \frac{Q(P - V)}{Q(P - V) - F - I}.$$

$$DTL = (DOL)(DFL).$$

$$EPS_1 = EPS_0[1 + (DTL)(\%\Delta S)].$$

$$\text{Breakeven } Q = \frac{F}{P - V}.$$

$$DFL = \frac{EBIT}{EBIT - I}.$$

$$EPS = \frac{(EBIT - I)(1 - t)}{\text{Shares outstanding}}.$$

$$DOL = \frac{Q(P - V)}{Q(P - V) - F}.$$

Chapter 21

$$g = br.$$

Glossary

ABC system A system used to categorize inventory items to ensure that the most critical inventory items are reviewed most often.

Accelerated Cost Recovery System (ACRS) A depreciation system that permits businesses to write off the cost of an asset over a period much shorter than its operating life.

accounting profit A firm's net income as calculated on its income statement.

account receivable A balance due from a customer.

accruals Continually recurring short-term liabilities, such as accrued wages, accrued taxes, and accrued interest.

acquiring company A company that seeks to acquire another company.

additional funds needed Funds that must be acquired by a firm through borrowing or by selling new stock.

add-on interest Interest calculated and added to funds received to determine the face amount of an installment loan.

after-tax cost of debt, $k_d(1 - t)$ The relevant cost to the firm for new debt financing, since interest is deductible from taxable income.

aggressive working capital policy A policy in which holdings of cash, securities, inventories, and receivables are minimized.

aging schedule A report showing how long accounts receivable have been outstanding; it gives the percentage of receivables past due by different lengths of time.

amortization schedule A schedule that shows precisely how a loan will be repaid; it gives the payment required on each specified date as well as a breakdown of each payment, showing how much of it constitutes interest and how much constitutes repayment of principal.

amortize To liquidate on an installment basis.

amortized loan A loan in which the principal amount is repaid in installments during the life of the loan.

annual report A report, issued annually by corporations to their stockholders, containing basic financial statements and management's opinion of operations and future prospects.

annuity A series of equal payments or receipts for a specified number of periods.

annuity due A series of payments of a fixed amount for a specified number of periods, with the payments occurring at the beginning of the period.

arrearage An unpaid dividend on preferred stock.

asked price The price at which a broker or dealer in securities will sell shares of stock out of inventory.

asset management ratios Set of several ratios, including inventory utilization, average collection period, and total assets utilization, that are designed to measure how effectively the firm's assets are being managed.

assets All things to which the firm holds legal claim.

average collection period (ACP) The ratio computed by dividing average credit sales per day into accounts receivable; indicates the average length of time the firm must wait after making a credit sale before receiving payment.

average tax rate The tax rate determined by dividing taxes paid by taxable income.

balance sheet A statement of the firm's financial status at a specific point in time.

bankruptcy A legal procedure for formally liquidating a business, carried out under the courts of law.

basic earning power ratio The ratio of operating profits to assets. This ratio indicates the power of the firm's assets to generate operating income.

best efforts An agreement for the sale of an issue of securities in which the investment banker handling the transaction gives no guarantee that the securities will be sold.

beta coefficient, b A measurement of the extent to which the returns of a given stock move with the stock market.

beta risk See *market risk*.

bid price The price a broker or dealer in securities will pay for a stock.

blanket inventory lien A claim on all of the borrower's inventories as security for a loan.

Blue Sky Laws State laws that prevent the sale of securities that have little or no asset backing.

Board of Governors of the Federal Reserve System Seven-member decision-making authority of the Fed.

bond A long-term debt instrument.

bond ratings Ratings assigned to bonds based on the probability of their firms' default. Those bonds with the smallest default probability are rated AAA and carry the lowest interest rates.

bracket creep An upward change in tax bracket that occurs when progressive tax rates combine with inflation to cause a greater portion of each taxpayer's real income to be paid as taxes.

break, or jump, in the MCC schedule A change in the weighted average cost of capital that occurs when there is a change in the component cost of capital.

break point The dollar value of new capital raised that corresponds to a jump in the MCC schedule.

breakeven point The level of operations at which total costs equal total revenues and therefore profits equal zero.

business risk The risk associated with future operating income; the risk that would exist even if the firm's operations were all equity financed.

bylaws A set of rules governing the management of a company.

call premium The amount in excess of par value that a company must pay when it calls a security.

call provision A provision in a bond contract that gives the issuer the right to redeem the bonds under specified terms prior to the normal maturity date.

capital account The account that represents a bank's total assets minus its liabilities.

Capital Asset Pricing Model (CAPM) A model based on the proposition that any stock's required rate of return is equal to the riskless rate of return plus the stock's risk premium.

capital budgeting The process of planning and analyzing expenditures on assets whose returns extend beyond one year.

capital components The items on the right-hand side of the balance sheet; various types of long-term debt, preferred stock, and common equity.

capital gain The profit from the sale of a capital asset for more than its purchase price.

capital gains yield The capital gain during any one year divided by the beginning price.

capital intensity ratio The amount of assets required per dollar of sales (A/S).

capital loss The loss from the sale of a capital asset for less than its purchase price.

capital market The financial market for long-term debt (one year or longer maturity) and equity securities.

capitalizing the lease Incorporating the lease provisions into the balance sheet by reporting the leased asset under fixed assets and reporting the present value of future lease payments as debt, as required under the conditions spelled out in FASB #13.

carrying costs The costs associated with carrying inventories, including storage, capital, and depreciation costs; generally increase in proportion to the average amount of inventory held.

cash The total of bank demand deposits plus currency.

cash account The account that represents a bank's vault cash, float, and funds required to be kept on deposit with the Federal Reserve.

cash budget A schedule showing cash flows (receipts, disbursements, and net cash) for a firm over a specified period.

cash conversion cycle The length of time between the purchase of raw materials and the collection of accounts receivable generated in the sale of the final product.

cash discount A reduction in price given for early payment.

cash flow The actual net cash, as opposed to accounting net income, that flows into or out of the firm during a specified period; equal to net income after taxes plus noncash expenses, including depreciation.

certificate of deposit (CD) A receipt for funds deposited for a specified time and interest rate.

change in net working capital The increased current assets resulting from a new project minus the increased spontaneous liabilities.

charter A formal legal document that describes the scope and nature of a corporation and defines the rights and duties of its stockholders and managers.

check clearing The process of converting a check, after it is written and mailed, into cash in the payee's account. Firms try to speed up the clearing process for checks received and to slow down the process for checks disbursed.

classified stock Common stock that is given special designations, such as Class A, Class B, and so forth, to meet special needs of the company.

clientele effect The tendency of a firm to attract a certain type of investor according to its dividend policy.

coefficient of variation Standardized measure of the risk per unit of return, calculated as the standard deviation divided by the expected return.

collateral Assets that are used to secure a loan.

collection policy Procedures that a firm follows to collect accounts receivable.

commercial paper Unsecured, short-term promissory notes of large, financially strong firms, usually issued in denominations of $100,000 or more and having an interest rate somewhat below the prime rate.

company-specific risk That part of a security's risk associated with random events. Such risk can be eliminated by proper diversification.

comparative ratio analysis The analysis based on comparison of a firm's ratios with those of other firms in the same industry.

compounding The arithmetic process of determining the final value of a payment or series of payments when compound interest is applied.

computerized inventory control system Inventory control through the use of computers to indicate order points and to adjust inventory balances.

congeneric merger A merger of firms in the same general industry but for which no customer or supplier relationship exists.

conglomerate merger A merger between companies in different industries.

conservative working capital policy A policy in which relatively large amounts of cash, marketable securities, and inventories are carried and in which sales are stimulated by a liberal credit policy, resulting in a high level of receivables.

consol A perpetual bond, such as that issued by the British government to consolidate past debts; in general, any perpetual bond.

consolidated return An income tax return that combines the income statements of several affiliated firms.

constraints on dividend payments Restrictions or limitations on the payment of dividends.

conversion price, P_c The effective price paid for common stock when the stock is obtained by converting either convertible preferred stocks or convertible bonds.

conversion ratio, R The number of shares of common stock that may be obtained by converting a convertible bond or share of convertible preferred stock.

convertible bond A security that is convertible into shares of common stock.

convertible securities Bonds or preferred stocks that are exchangeable at the option of the holder for common stock of the issuing firm.

corporate risk See *total risk.*

corporation A legal entity created by a state, separate and distinct from its owners and managers, having unlimited life, easy transferability of ownership, and limited liability.

cost of capital The discount rate that should be used in the capital budgeting process.

cost of external equity, k_e The cost of retained earnings adjusted for flotation costs.

cost of preferred stock, k_p The preferred dividend, D_p, divided by the net issuing price, P_n.

cost of retained earnings, k_s The rate of return stockholders require on the firm's common stock based on alternative investment opportunities available to stockholders if no earnings were retained.

costly trade credit Credit taken in excess of the free trade credit period, thereby forfeiting the discount offered.

coupon rate The stated or nominal rate of interest on a bond.

coverage The measure of a firm's ability to meet interest and principal payments; times interest earned (TIE) is the most common coverage ratio.

credit period The length of time for which credit is granted.

credit policy A set of decisions that determine a firm's credit period, credit standards, collection procedures, and discounts offered.

credit standards Standards that stipulate the minimum financial strength of acceptable credit customers.

cumulative dividends A protective feature on preferred stock that requires all past preferred dividends to be paid before any common dividends.

current ratio The ratio computed by dividing current assets by current liabilities.

current yield The annual interest payment of a bond divided by its market price.

debenture A long-term debt instrument that is not secured by a mortgage on specific property.

debt ratio The ratio of total debt to total assets.

declaration date The date on which a firm's directors issue a statement declaring a regular dividend.

default risk The risk that a borrower will not pay the interest or principal on a loan.

default risk premium (DP) The difference between the interest rate on a Treasury bond and that on a corporate bond.

deficit trade balance A country's trade balance resulting from an excess of its imports over its exports.

degree of financial leverage The percentage change in earnings available to common shareholders that is associated with a given percentage change in earnings before interest and taxes.

degree of operating leverage (DOL) The ratio of the percentage change in operating income to the percentage change in sales.

demand deposits Transaction deposits at commercial banks that are available on demand, usually through a check.

Depository Institutions Deregulation and Monetary Control Act of 1980 Act that eliminated many of the distinctions between commercial banks and other depository institutions.

depreciable basis The portion of an asset's value that can be depreciated for tax purposes.

depreciation An annual noncash charge against income that reflects a rough estimate of the dollar cost of equipment used in the production process.

devaluation The process of officially reducing the value of a country's currency relative to other currencies.

discount bond A bond that sells below its par value, which occurs when the coupon rate is lower than the going rate of interest.

discount factor (DF) The factor used to determine the present value of a lump sum in n periods in the future discounted at k percent per period.

discount on forward rate The situation when the spot rate is less than the forward rate.

discount rate The interest rate used in the discounting process. Also, the interest rate charged by the Fed for loans of reserves to depository institutions.

discounted cash flow (DCF) techniques Methods of ranking investment proposals that employ time value of money concepts, two of which are the net present value method and the internal rate of return method.

discounted interest Interest calculated on the face amount of a loan but deducted in advance.

discounting The process of finding the present value of a series of future cash flows. Discounting is the reverse of compounding.

divestiture The selling off of an asset or a division by its parent company. If the asset is given to the parent company's stockholders, the divestiture is called a *spin-off*.

dividend payout ratio The percentage of earnings paid out in dividends.

dividend policy Determination of the percentage of current earnings to be paid out as dividends to stockholders.

dividend reinvestment plan (DRP) A plan that enables a stockholder to automatically reinvest dividends received back into the stock of the paying corporation.

dividend yield A stock's current dividend divided by the current price of a share of stock.

Du Pont System A system of analysis designed to show the relationships among return on investment, asset turnover, and profit margin.

earnings per share (EPS) The net income of the firm divided by the number of shares of common stock outstanding.

economic ordering quantity (EOQ) The optimal (least-cost) quantity of inventory that should be ordered.

effective annual rate The annual rate of interest actually being earned as opposed to the stated rate; also called the *annual percentage rate (APR)*.

efficient capital market Market in which securities are fairly priced in the sense that the price reflects all publicly available information on each security.

EOQ model Formula for determining the order quantity that minimizes the total inventory cost: $EOQ = \sqrt{2FS/CP}$.

equity Money supplied by the firm's owners.

Eurobond A bond sold in a country other than the one in whose currency the bond is denominated.

Eurodollar A U.S. dollar on deposit in a foreign bank — generally, but not necessarily, a European bank.

Eurodollar bank time deposits Interest-bearing time deposits, denominated in U.S. dollars, placed in banks outside the United States.

ex dividend date The date on which the right to the current dividend no longer accompanies the stock. For a listed stock this date is four working days prior to the date of record.

excess capacity Capacity that exists when an asset is not being fully utilized.

exchange rate The number of units of a given currency that can be purchased for one unit of another currency.

exchange risk The risk that the basic cash flows of a foreign project will be worth less in the parent company's home currency.

expansion project A project that is intended to increase sales.

expectations theory The theory that the shape of the yield curve depends on investors' expectations about future inflation rates.

expected rate of return, k The rate of return expected to be realized from an investment; the mean value of the probability distribution of possible returns.

extra dividend A supplementary dividend paid in years when excess funds are available.

factoring Sale of accounts receivable to a financial institution.

federal funds market The market in which depository institutions lend reserve funds among themselves for short periods of time.

Federal Open Market Committee (FOMC) Committee of the Federal Reserve System that has responsibility for open-market operations.

Federal Reserve System The central banking system in the United States; the chief regulator of the banking system.

finance Evaluation and acquisition of productive assets, procurement of funds, and disbursement of profits.

financial intermediaries Specialized financial firms that facilitate the transfer of funds from savers to those who need capital.

financial lease A lease that does not provide for maintenance service, is not cancelable, and covers the entire expected life of the equipment; also called a *capital lease*.

financial leverage The extent to which fixed-income securities (debt and preferred stock) are used in a firm's capital structure.

financial management The acquisition and utilization of funds to maximize the efficiency and value of an enterprise.

financial risk The portion of total corporate risk over and above the basic business risk that results from using debt.

financial service corporations Institutions whose services include a wide variety of financial operations; usually includes banks, S&Ls, investment banking, insurance, pension plans, and mutual funds.

five Cs of credit Factors used to evaluate credit risk: character, capacity, capital, collateral, and conditions.

fixed assets utilization The ratio of sales to fixed assets; also known as *fixed assets turnover*.

fixed exchange rate system The world monetary system in existence prior to 1971 under which the value of the U.S. dollar was tied to gold and the values of the other currencies were pegged to the U.S. dollar.

float The amount of funds tied up in checks that have been written but are still in process and have not yet cleared.

floating exchange rates Exchange rates not fixed by government policy but allowed to float up or down in accordance with supply and demand.

floating rate bond A bond whose interest rate fluctuates with shifts in the general level of interest rates.

flotation costs The costs of issuing a new stock or bond issue.

foreign bond A bond sold by a foreign borrower but denominated in the currency of the country in which it is sold.

formula, or exercise, value The theoretical value of a warrant if it were exercised today; the actual value is determined in the marketplace.

forward exchange rate An agreed-upon price at which two currencies are to be exchanged at some future date.

founders' shares Classified stock that has sole voting rights and restricted dividends; it is owned by the firm's founders.

free trade credit Credit received during the discount period.

friendly merger A merger in which the terms are approved by the managements of both companies.

full underwriting Agreement for the sale of an issue of securities in which the investment banker guarantees the sale of the securities, thus agreeing to bear any risks involved in the transaction.

funded debt Long-term debt.

future value (FV) The amount to which a payment or series of payments will grow by a given future date when compounded at a given interest rate.

going public The act of selling stock to the public for the first time by a closely held corporation's principal stockholders.

golden parachute Large payments made to the managers of a firm as a poison pill defense against acquisition in a hostile merger.

half-year convention A feature of ACRS in which all assets are assumed to be put into service at mid-year and thus allowed a half-year's depreciation.

hedging exchange rate exposure The process whereby a firm protects itself against loss due to future exchange rate fluctuations.

holder-of-record date The date on which registered security owners are entitled to receive the forthcoming cash or stock dividend.

holding company A corporation that owns sufficient common stocks of other firms to achieve working control over them.

horizontal merger The combination of two firms that produce the same type of goods or service.

hostile merger (takeover) A merger in which the target firm's management resists acquisition.

improper accumulation Retention of earnings by a business for the purpose of enabling stockholders to avoid personal income taxes.

income bond A bond that pays interest to bondholders only if the interest is earned.

income statement A statement summarizing the firm's revenues and expenses over an accounting period.

incremental cash flow The net cash flow attributable to an investment project.

indenture A formal contract between the issuer of a bond and the bondholders.

independent project A project whose cash flows are unaffected by the decision to accept or reject some other project.

inflation An increase in the volume of money and credit relative to the available supply of goods, resulting in a rise in the general level of prices.

inflation risk premium (IP) A premium for anticipated or expected inflation that investors add to the pure rate of return to protect their purchasing power.

information content of dividends The theory that investors regard dividend changes as signals of management forecasts.

insiders Officers, directors, major stockholders, and others who may have access to information not available to the public about the company's operations.

interest rate The price paid by borrowers to lenders for the use of funds.

interest rate risk The risk of capital losses to which investors are exposed because of changing interest rates.

internal rate of return (IRR) The rate of return on an asset investment, calculated by finding the discount rate that equates the present value of future cash flows to the cost of the investment.

inventory management The balancing of a set of costs that increase with larger inventory holdings with a set of costs that decrease with larger order size.

inventory utilization The ratio of sales to inventories; also known as *inventory turnover*.

inverted ("abnormal") yield curve A downward-sloping yield curve.

investment banking house A financial firm that underwrites and distributes new investment securities and that helps businesses obtain financing.

investment opportunity schedule (IOS) A listing, or graph, of the firm's investment opportunities ranked in order of the projects' rates of return.

investment outlay Funds expended for fixed assets of a specified project plus working capital funds expended as a result of the project's adoption.

investment tax credit (ITC) A specified percentage of the cost of new assets that business firms can at times deduct as a credit against their income taxes.

junk bond A high-risk, high-yield bond used to finance mergers, leveraged buyouts, and troubled companies.

lease evaluation The analysis of the firm's cash flows under lease or purchase alternatives to determine the lower present value of costs.

lessee The party leasing a property.

lessor The owner of a property to be leased.

liabilities All the legal claims held against the firm by nonowners.

limited partnership An unincorporated business owned both by general partners having unlimited liability and by other partners having liability limited to their investment in the firm.

line of credit An arrangement whereby a financial institution commits itself to lend funds up to a designated maximum amount during a specified period.

liquid asset An asset that can be readily converted to spendable cash.

liquidity The ability to sell an asset at a reasonable price on short notice.

liquidity or marketability risk The risk that securities cannot be sold at a reasonable price on short notice.

liquidity preference theory The theory that lenders prefer to make short-term loans rather than long-term loans, and hence they will lend short-term funds at lower rates than long-term funds.

liquidity ratio The relationship of a firm's cash and other current assets to its current obligations.

liquidity risk premium (LP) A premium added to the equilibrium interest rate on a security that cannot be converted to cash on short notice.

lockbox plan A procedure used to speed up collections and to reduce float through the use of post office boxes in payers' local areas.

"lumpy" assets Those assets that cannot be acquired in small increments but must be purchased in large, discrete amounts.

managed floating system A system in which major currency rates move with market forces, unrestricted by internationally agreed-upon limits.

margin requirement The minimum percentage of equity that must be used to purchase a security.

marginal cost of capital (MCC) The cost of obtaining another dollar of new capital; the weighted average cost of capital at a particular dollar value of new capital. The MCC increases as more and more capital is raised.

marginal cost of capital (MCC) schedule A graph or table that relates the firm's weighted average cost of capital to the amount of new capital raised.

marginal tax rate The tax applicable to the last unit of income.

market/book ratio The ratio of a stock's market price to its book value.

market or beta risk That part of a security's risk that cannot be eliminated by diversification. It is measured by the beta coefficient.

market segmentation theory The theory that each borrower and lender has a preferred maturity and that the slope of the yield curve depends on the supply of and demand for funds in the long-term market relative to the short-term market.

market value ratios The ratios that relate a firm's stock price to its earnings and book value per share.

marketable securities Securities that can be sold on short notice for close to their quoted market prices.

maturity risk premium (MP) A premium for the risk to which investors are exposed because of the length of a security's maturity.

measuring risk Determining the amount of risk on the assumption that the tighter the probability distribution of expected future returns, the smaller the risk of a given investment.

merger Any combination that forms one company from two or more previously existing companies.

money market The financial market in which funds are borrowed or loaned for less than one year.

money market fund A mutual fund that invests in short-term, low-risk securities and that allows investors to write checks against their accounts.

mortgage bond A pledge of designated property (real assets) as security for a bond.

multinational corporation A firm that operates in two or more countries.

mutual fund A corporation that invests the pooled funds of savers, thus obtaining economies of scale in investing and reducing risk by diversification.

near-cash reserves Reserves that are quickly and easily converted to cash.

net present value (NPV) A method of ranking investment proposals. The NPV is equal to the present value of future returns, discounted at the marginal cost of capital, minus the present value of the cost of the investment.

net present value profile A curve showing the relationship between a project's NPV and the discount rate used to calculate it.

net working capital The difference between total current assets and total current liabilities.

net worth The capital and surplus of the firm; common stock, paid-in capital, and retained earnings.

New York Stock Exchange; American Stock Exchange The two major U.S. security exchanges.

nominal (stated) interest rate The contracted, or stated, interest rate.

normal profits/rates of return Those profits close to the average of all firms within an industry.

"normal" yield curve An upward-sloping yield curve.

NOW (Negotiable Order of Withdrawal) account A form of savings account that allows withdrawal by check.

off-balance-sheet financing Financing wherein for many years neither the leased assets nor the liabilities under the lease contract appeared on the lessee's balance sheet. The Financial Accounting Standards Board issued FASB #13 to correct this problem.

open-market operations The purchase and sale of U.S. Government securities by the Federal Reserve System.

operating cash flows Those cash flows that arise from normal operations; the difference between sales revenues and cash expenses plus taxes paid.

operating company A subsidiary of a holding company; a separate legal entity.

operating income Earnings before interest and taxes (EBIT).

operating lease A lease under which the lessor maintains and services the asset; also called a *service lease*.

operating leverage The extent to which fixed costs are used in a firm's operations.

operating merger A merger in which the operations of two companies are integrated with the expectation of achieving synergistic benefits.

opportunity cost The rate of return on the best alternative investment available — the highest return that will *not* be earned if the funds are invested in a particular project.

optimal dividend policy The dividend policy that strikes a balance between current dividends and future growth and thereby maximizes the firm's stock price.

option A contract giving the holder the right to buy or sell an asset at some predetermined price within a specified period of time.

order point Point at which stock on hand must be replenished.

ordering costs The costs of placing and receiving orders; these costs are fixed for each order regardless of the size of the order.

organized security exchanges Formal organizations that have tangible, physical locations and that conduct auction markets in designated ("listed") securities.

overdraft systems Systems wherein depositors may write checks in excess of their balances, with banks automatically extending loans to cover the shortages.

over-the-counter market A large collection of brokers and dealers, connected electronically by telephones and computers, that provides for trading in unlisted securities.

paid-in capital The funds received in excess of par value when the firm sells stock for the first time (that is, in the primary market).

par value The nominal or face value of a stock or bond.

parent company A holding company that controls other firms by owning large blocks of their stock.

partnership An unincorporated business owned by two or more persons.

payback (or payback period) The length of time required for cash flows to return the cost of an investment.

payment date Date on which a firm actually mails dividend checks.

percentage of sales method A method of forecasting financial requirements by expressing various balance sheet items as a percentage of sales and then multiplying these percentages by expected future sales to construct pro forma balance sheets.

permanent current assets The minimum level of current assets that are required when business activity is set at seasonal or cyclical lows.

perpetuity A stream of equal payments expected to last forever.

pledging of accounts receivable Borrowing when the loan is secured by accounts receivable.

poison pill A self-destructive action that will seriously hurt a company if it is acquired by another.

post-audit A comparison of the actual and expected results for a given capital project.

precautionary balances Cash balances held in reserve for random, unforeseen fluctuations in inflows and outflows.

preemptive right A provision contained in the corporate charter and bylaws that gives holders of common stock the right to purchase on a pro rata basis new issues of common stock (or securities convertible into common stock).

preferred stock A long-term equity security paying a fixed dividend.

premium The amount that a bond sells for above its par value, which occurs when the coupon rate is above the going rate of interest.

premium on forward rate The situation when the spot rate is greater than the forward rate.

present value (PV) The value today of a future payment or series of payments, discounted at the appropriate discount rate.

price/book ratio See *market/book ratio*.

price/earnings (P/E) ratio The ratio of price to earnings; shows how much investors are willing to pay per dollar of profits.

primary markets The markets in which newly issued securities are bought and sold for the first time.

prime rate A published rate of interest that commercial banks charge very large, strong corporations.

pro forma statement A financial statement that shows how an actual statement will look if certain specified assumptions are realized; used to forecast financial requirements.

probability distribution A listing of all possible outcomes or events, with the probability (the chance of the event's occurrence) assigned to each outcome.

production opportunity The return available within an economy from investment in productive (cash-generating) investments.

profit margin on sales Profit per dollar of sales, computed by dividing net income after taxes by sales.

profit maximization The maximization of the firm's net income; does not consider risk or timing of earnings and thus is not an appropriate standard for financial decisions.

profitability ratios The ratios that show the combined effects of liquidity, asset management, and debt management on operating results.

progressive tax A tax that requires a higher percentage payment on higher incomes. The personal income tax in the United States, which goes from a rate of zero percent on its lowest increments of income to 28 percent on the highest increments, is progressive.

promissory note A document specifying terms and conditions of a loan, such as the amount, percentage interest rate, and repayment schedule.

proprietorship A business owned by one individual.

prospectus A document issued for the purpose of describing a new security issue and the issuing company.

proxy A document giving one person the authority to act for another. Typically, it is the authority to vote shares of common stock.

proxy fight An attempt by a person, group, or company to gain control of a company by getting the stockholder to vote a new management into office.

purchasing power risk The risk that inflation will reduce the purchasing power of a given sum of money.

pure financial merger A merger in which the merged companies will not be operated as a single unit and from which no operating economies are expected.

pure rate of interest, k* The real, risk-free rate of interest. It is that rate of return that would cause investors to postpone current consumption if no risks existed in the financial environment.

quick (acid test) ratio The ratio computed by deducting inventories from current assets and dividing the remainder by current liabilities.

rate of return, k The rate of interest offered by or required of an investment.

ratio analysis Analysis of the relationships among financial statement accounts.

red-line method An inventory control procedure in which a red line drawn around the inside of an inventory-stocked bin indicates the order point level.

registration statement A statement of facts filed with the SEC about a company planning to issue securities.

regular annuity A series of payments of a fixed amount for a specified number of periods with the payments occurring at the end of the period.

reinvestment rate assumption The assumption that cash flows from a project can be reinvested (1) at the cost of capital, if using the NPV method, or (2) at the internal rate of return, if using the IRR method.

reinvestment rate risk Risk that a decline in interest rates will lead to lower income when short-term bonds mature and funds are reinvested.

repatriation of earnings Restriction on the amount of cash flows that may be directed from a foreign subsidiary to its parent company.

replacement decision The decision to replace an existing asset that is still productive with a new one; an example of mutually exclusive projects.

required rate of return The minimum rate of return on common stock that stockholders consider acceptable.

required reserves The minimum reserves that a bank must hold as vault cash or reserve deposits with the Federal Reserve.

residual theory of dividends The theory that dividends should equal the excess of earnings over retained earnings necessary to finance the optimal capital budget.

residual value The value of an asset at the end of its lease term.

restrictive covenant A provision in a bond indenture or term loan agreement that requires the bond issuer to meet certain stated conditions.

retention rate The percentage of earnings retained after payment of dividends.

return on common equity (ROE) The ratio of net profit after taxes to common equity; measures the rate of return on stockholders' investment.

return on total assets (ROA) The ratio of net income after taxes to total assets.

revaluation The process of officially increasing the value of a country's currency relative to other currencies.

revolving credit agreement A formal line of credit extended to a firm by a bank or other financial institution.

risk The probability that actual future returns will be below expected returns.

risk-adjusted discount rate The discount rate that applies to a particular risky (uncertain) stream of cash flows; the riskless rate plus a risk premium appropriate to the level of risk attached to a particular project's income stream.

risk aversion A dislike for risk. Risk-averse investors have higher required rates of return for higher-risk investments.

risk premium (RP) The difference between the required rate of return on a particular risky asset and the rate of return on a riskless asset with the same expected life.

safety stocks Additional inventories carried to guard against changes in sales rates or production/shipping delays.

sale and leaseback An operation whereby a firm sells land, buildings, or equipment to a purchaser who simultaneously leases the property back to the firm for a specified period under specific terms.

sales (demand) forecast Forecast of unit and dollar sales for some future period. Generally, sales forecasts are based on recent trends in sales plus forecasts of the economic prospects for the nation, region, industry, and so forth.

salvage value The market price of a capital asset at the end of a specified period. In a capital budgeting decision, it is also the current market price of an asset being considered for replacement.

seasonal dating Procedure that creates an invoice date during the purchaser's selling season, regardless of when the merchandise was shipped, to induce customers to buy early.

secondary markets The markets in which stocks are traded after they have been issued by corporations.

secondary reserves Excess reserves invested by banks in marketable securities.

secured loan A loan backed by collateral.

Securities and Exchange Commission (SEC) The U.S. Government agency that regulates the issuance and trading of stocks and bonds.

security agreement A standardized document that includes a description of the specific assets pledged for the purpose of securing a loan.

Security Market Line (SML) The line that shows the relationship between risk and rate of return for individual securities.

selling group A group of stock brokerage firms formed for the purpose of distributing a new issue of securities.

simple interest Interest calculated on funds received and paid on maturity of a loan.

sinking fund A required annual payment designed to retire a bond or a preferred stock issue.

social responsibility The concept that businesses should be responsible to some degree for the welfare of society at large.

sovereign risk The risk of expropriation of a foreign subsidiary's assets by the host country and of unanticipated restrictions on cash flows to the parent company.

speculative balances Cash balances that are held to enable a firm to take advantage of any bargain purchases that might arise.

spontaneously generated funds Funds that arise automatically from routine business transactions, such as accrued wages or trade credit.

spot rate The effective exchange rate for a foreign currency for delivery on (approximately) the current day.

spread The difference between the price a security dealer offers to pay for securities (the "bid" price) and the price at which the dealer offers to sell them (the "asked" price).

standard deviation, σ A statistical measurement of the variability of a set of observations.

statement of changes in financial position A statement reporting the firm's sources of financing and the uses of those funds during an accounting period.

statement of retained earnings A statement reporting the portion of earnings not paid out in dividends. The figure that appears on the balance sheet is the sum of retained earnings for each year of the company's history.

stock dividend A dividend paid in additional shares of stock rather than cash.

stock repurchase A means by which the firm distributes income to stockholders by buying back shares of its own stock, thereby decreasing shares outstanding, increasing EPS, and increasing the price of the stock.

stock split An action taken to increase the number of shares outstanding; for example, in a 3-for-1 split, shares outstanding are tripled and each shareholder receives 3 new shares for each share formerly held.

stockholder wealth maximization The appropriate goal for management decisions; considers the risk and timing associated with increasing earnings per share in order to maximize the firm's stock price.

stockholders' equity (net worth) The capital supplied by stockholders—capital stock, paid-in capital, and retained earnings. *Common equity,* or *stockholders' equity,* is that part of the total net worth belonging to the common stockholders.

"stretching" accounts payable The practice of deliberately paying accounts payable late.

subordinated debenture A bond having a claim on assets in the event of liquidation only after the senior debt has been paid off.

supernormal (nonconstant) growth The part of the life cycle of a firm in which its growth is much faster than that of the economy as a whole.

synchronized cash flows Cash flows that permit inflows to coincide with the timing of outflows, thereby holding transactions balances to a minimum.

synergy The condition wherein the whole is greater than the sum of its parts. In a synergistic merger, the postmerger value exceeds the sum of the separate companies' premerger values.

takeover The acquisition of one firm by another over the opposition of the acquired firm's management.

target capital structure The optimal capital structure; the capital structure that will minimize the firm's cost of capital and thereby maximize the price of its stock.

target cash balance The minimum cash balance that a firm must maintain to conduct business.

target company A company that another firm, generally a larger one, seeks to acquire through merger.

tax loss carry-back and carry-forward Corporate losses that can be carried back or carried forward to offset taxable income in a given year.

taxable income Gross income minus allowable deductions as set forth in the Tax Code.

temporary current assets Current assets that fluctuate with seasonal or cyclical variations in a firm's business.

tender offer The offer of one firm to buy the stock of another by going directly to the stockholders, frequently over the opposition of the target company's management.

term loan A loan, generally obtained from a bank or insurance company, with a maturity greater than one year.

term structure of interest rates The relationship between yields and maturities of securities.

time preferences for consumption The preferences of consumers for current consumption as opposed to saving for future consumption.

times interest earned (TIE) The ratio of earnings before interest and taxes to interest charges; measures the ability of the firm to meet its annual interest payments.

total assets utilization The ratio that measures the turnover of all of a firm's assets, computed by dividing sales by total assets.

total, or corporate, risk Risk not considering the effects of diversification; in capital budgeting, it relates to the probability that a project will incur losses that will destabilize profits.

total leverage effect The combination of operating leverage and financial leverage that results in a magnified effect of a small change in sales on the firm's earnings per share.

trade credit Interfirm debt arising through credit sales and recorded as an account receivable by the seller and as an account payable by the buyer.

transaction balances Cash balances associated with payments and collections; those balances necessary to conduct day-to-day business.

trend analysis The analysis of a firm's financial ratios over time to determine the improvement or deterioration of a financial situation.

trust receipt An instrument acknowledging that the borrower holds certain goods in trust for the lender.

trustee The representative of bondholders who acts in their interest and facilitates communication between them and the bond issuer.

two-bin method An inventory control procedure in which the order point is reached when one of two inventory-stocked bins is empty.

underwriting syndicate A syndicate of investment firms formed to spread the risk associated with the purchase and distribution of a new issue of securities.

uneven payment stream A series of payments in which the amount varies from one period to the next.

Uniform Commercial Code A system of standards that simplifies the procedure for establishing loan security.

venture capital Risk capital supplied to small companies by wealthy individuals, partnerships, or corporations, usually in return for an equity position in the firm.

vertical merger A merger between a firm and one of its suppliers or customers.

warehouse financing An arrangement under which the lending institution employs a third party to exercise control over the borrower's inventory and to act as the lender's agent.

warrant A long-term option to buy a stated number of shares of common stock at a specified price.

weighted average cost of capital, WACC = k_a A weighted average, or composite, of the after-tax component costs of debt, preferred stock, and common equity.

white knight A company that is more acceptable to a firm subject to a hostile takeover attempt than the potential acquirer.

window dressing Techniques used by a firm to make a financial statement look better to credit analysts.

working capital A firm's investment in short-term assets — cash, marketable securities, inventory, and accounts receivable.

working capital management The administration, within policy guidelines, of current assets and current liabilities.

working capital policy Basic policy decisions regarding target levels for each category of current assets and for the financing of these assets.

yield curve A graph showing the relationship between the yields and maturities of a group of equal-risk securities. Often Treasury securities are used because their risk varies only with their term to maturity.

yield to maturity (YTM) The rate of return earned on a bond if it is held to maturity.

zero coupon bond A bond that pays no annual interest but sells at a discount below par and therefore provides compensation to investors in the form of capital appreciation.

Index

Note: Boldface terms in the index refer to key terms in the text and the boldface number refers to the page on which the key term is defined. (DIF) refers to Decision in Finance and Resolution to Decision in Finance; (SB) to Small Business sections; and (IP) to Industry Practice.